D1608387

COMPLICATIONS OF
GLAUCOMA SURGERY

COMPLICATIONS OF
GLAUCOMA SURGERY

Robert M. Feldman, M.D.

Nicholas P. Bell, M.D.

MANAGING EDITOR
Kimberly A. Mankiewicz, Ph.D.

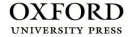
OXFORD
UNIVERSITY PRESS

OXFORD

UNIVERSITY PRESS

Oxford University Press is a department of the University of Oxford.
It furthers the University's objective of excellence in research, scholarship,
and education by publishing worldwide.

Oxford   New York

Auckland   Cape Town   Dar es Salaam   Hong Kong   Karachi
Kuala Lumpur   Madrid   Melbourne   Mexico City   Nairobi
New Delhi   Shanghai   Taipei   Toronto

With offices in

Argentina   Austria   Brazil   Chile   Czech Republic   France   Greece
Guatemala   Hungary   Italy   Japan   Poland   Portugal   Singapore
South Korea   Switzerland   Thailand   Turkey   Ukraine   Vietnam

Oxford is a registered trademark of Oxford University Press in the UK
and certain other countries.

Published in the United States of America by
Oxford University Press
198 Madison Avenue, New York, NY 10016

© Oxford University Press 2013

All rights reserved. No part of this publication may be reproduced, stored in a retrieval system, or
transmitted, in any form or by any means, without the prior permission in writing of Oxford University Press,
or as expressly permitted by law, by license, or under terms agreed with the appropriate reproduction rights
organization. Inquiries concerning reproduction outside the scope of the above should be sent to the Rights
Department, Oxford University Press, at the address above.

You must not circulate this work in any other form
and you must impose this same condition on any acquirer.

Library of Congress Cataloging-in-Publication Data

Complications of glaucoma surgery / [edited by] Robert M. Feldman, Nicholas P. Bell ; managing editor,
Kimberly A. Mankiewicz.
p. ; cm.
Includes bibliographical references.
ISBN 978-0-19-538236-5 (alk. paper)
I. Feldman, Robert M.   II. Bell, Nicholas P.
[DNLM: 1. Glaucoma—surgery.   2. Filtering Surgery—adverse effects.   3. Intraoperative
Complications—prevention & control.   4. Postoperative Complications—prevention & control. WW 290]
LC Classification not assigned
617.7'41059—dc23
2012020763

3 5 7 9 8 6 4 2
Printed in China
on acid-free paper

This book is dedicated to my professional mentors in glaucoma, Dr. George Spaeth, Dr. Robert Weinreb, and Dr. Ron Gross, who have shared their experiences with me and encouraged my interest in dealing with these difficult problems, and also to my family, who always has stood with me to become who I am today, and especially my wife, Ashley, who too often has shared her date night with this book and other professional projects.

—Robert M. Feldman

This book is for the patients, colleagues, and trainees who may benefit from the nuggets of wisdom found on these pages. I am grateful for the support of my wife, Kathy, and children, Zachary, Michael, and Elisabeth, who are often asked to share time with my "glaucoma family."

—Nicholas P. Bell

FOREWORD

"DON'T DO SURGERY." That is the answer to the question as to how to completely avoid surgical complications. For those of us who do surgery, it is incumbent on us to manage the predictable problems as well as maximize outcomes. What separates the good surgeon from the exceptional surgeon is not only the execution of the original procedure but also how he/she handles any complications. It is often the postoperative care that determines the success of the operation. In glaucoma, and all disciplines of ophthalmology for that matter, the stakes are high—how the complication is resolved may well have substantial impact on the visual outcome. Sight is not just our ability to look at things, but it is our emotional connection to the world around us. Thus our job as surgeons is certainly not trivial—our actions greatly affect a patient's quality of life.

While dozens of books are available on how to technically perform all kinds of glaucoma procedures, assemblies of information describing thoroughly how to handle the inevitable (and hopefully infrequent) complications are lacking. This book provides a unique comprehensive compendium for handling complications of glaucoma surgery, from common ones (such as hypotony) to those that fortunately happen rarely (i.e. endophthalmitis). The chapters cover a wide range of glaucoma surgical procedures including guarded filtration (trabeculectomy) and tube shunt surgeries, with additional chapters on angle and nonpenetrating surgery complications. The authors of these chapters represent the leading surgeons in the field of glaucoma, with extensive experience. As there are often many opinions how to best address a complication, alternative viewpoints are presented with commentaries, often from several different perspectives, that are part of each chapter, and reflect the multiplicities of approaches when addressing these difficult situations.

I have known both Robert Feldman and Nicholas Bell for many years. Although I am sure neither of them has actually experienced any of the complications discussed, we are all grateful that they undertook this noble effort for the benefit of the rest of us. They are both excellent surgeons with a great wealth of experience in dealing with wide and varied complications as members of a referral, academic glaucoma practice. They took on the task of identifying and recruiting very talented surgeons in the glaucoma world so we could all benefit from their expertise and varied points of view and actually accomplished the assignment, making them the perfect editors for this book.

This book is an essential manual for any glaucoma surgeon, from those that are just entering the field to those that have been practicing for many years. Although we may lose substantial sleep worrying about our patients after glaucoma surgery, this book gives us a good chance to sleep better. It is a vital component of any glaucoma library providing needed insight to optimize our surgical outcomes, a result that is of great benefit to both ourselves and our patients.

Ronald L. Gross, MD
Professor of Ophthalmology
Clifton R. McMichael
Chair of Ophthalmology
Baylor College of Medicine
May 2012
Houston, TX

PREFACE

GLAUCOMA SURGERY is difficult and fraught with complications. However, good outcomes are still likely if those complications encountered are managed properly. This book is intended for those surgeons wishing to improve their skill and ability to manage difficult problems that will come up during the care of glaucoma patients.

Some complications are common and mild, while others are rare and/or vision threatening. This text is intended to allow the reader to identify and manage complications as they encounter them in their surgical travels. The authors of each chapter have also been asked to provide surgical and clinical pearls not only for managing difficulties but in preventing them as well. There are key references placed in chapters where there is literature to support concepts. However, in many places the opinions of the authors are from experience and are not backed by any literature, as there is no-peer reviewed literature on many subjects covered. Additionally, because each surgeon has their own individual approach to addressing a particular situation, there is commentary at the end of each chapter to provide another opinion or strategy for dealing with a particular surgical scenario.

Section 1 addresses outflow mechanisms after glaucoma surgery, and Section 2 discusses wound healing processes and modulators. These chapters provide an overview on these topics in the context of treating complications of glaucoma surgery. Sections 3–7 discuss complications in filtering surgery (trabeculectomy and Ex-PRESS™ Glaucoma Filtration Device [Alcon Laboratories, Inc., Fort Worth, Texas]), tube shunt implantation, angle procedures (trabeculotomy, canaloplasty, and Trabectome® [NeoMedix, Inc, Tustin, California]), and nonpenetrating surgery (deep sclerectomy and viscocanalostomy). Some complications overlap and occur with several procedures, while others are specific to the procedure. Cross-referencing is provided throughout this book to direct the reader to as many helpful sections as possible.

Our hope is that this book will help both new and experienced glaucoma surgeons deal with complications and provide successful results for their patients.

Robert M. Feldman, MD
Nicholas P. Bell, MD

ACKNOWLEDGMENTS

THIS BOOK was the result of exceptional ability, experience, and many hours of hard work by a truly amazing group of people. We would like to thank firstly all of the authors and contributors for their chapters and commentary. This book would not have been what it is without all of your expertise and experience with these complications. Thank you for sharing your knowledge.

We would like to thank Dr. Richard Ruiz and the Ruiz Department of Ophthalmology and Visual Science for all of their support of this project. In particular, we would like to acknowledge Dr. David Lee and Dr. Rania Tabet for their help in formulating the initial outline and getting this project going.

A thank you also to Anabel Sherkat for her amazing ability to keep track of everything and everyone. This project would not have gotten off the ground without her.

A big thank you to Anne Dellinger, Catherine Barnes, and Catharine Carlin at Oxford University Press for their assistance, support, and patience in completing this project. Their guidance was truly invaluable.

Last but not least a big thanks to Dr. Kimberly Mankiewicz for her contributions not only as an author but also for organizing, editing, and managing this project to completion. Without her help, this book would never have reached reality.

Funding Support: The authors would like to acknowledge extensive grant support from Research to Prevent Blindness. The editors would also like to acknowledge support from Research to Prevent Blindness and the Hermann Eye Fund.

CONTENTS

CONTRIBUTORS

Ahmed Al-Ghoul, MD, FRCSC
Clinical Lecturer
Department of Surgery
Faculty of Medicine
University of Calgary
Calgary, Alberta, Canada

Charlotte Akor, MD
Pediatric Ophthalmologist

Annie K. Baik, MD
Assistant Health Sciences Clinical Professor
Department of Ophthalmology
University of California, Davis Eye Center
Sacramento, CA

Michael R. Banitt, MD, MHA
Assistant Professor of Clinical Ophthalmology
Bascom Palmer Eye Institute
Department of Ophthalmology
Miller School of Medicine
University of Miami
Miami, FL

Shai M. Bar-Sela, MD
Faculty of Medicine, Ophthalmology
Tel Aviv University
Tel Aviv, Israel

Nicholas P. Bell, MD
A.G. McNeese, Jr. Professor of
    Ophthalmology
Clinical Associate Professor
Ruiz Department of Ophthalmology
    and Visual Science
The University of Texas Medical School
    at Houston
Director of Glaucoma Service
Robert Cizik Eye Clinic
Chief of Ophthalmology Service
Lyndon B. Johnson General Hospital
Houston, TX

John P. Berdahl, MD
Vance Thompson Vision
Sanford Clinic
Sioux Falls, SD

James D. Brandt, MD
Professor and Director of Glaucoma Service
Department of Ophthalmology and Vision
    Science
University of California, Davis Eye Center
Sacramento, CA

Donald L. Budenz, MD, MPH
Professor and Chair
Department of Ophthalmology
University of North Carolina at Chapel Hill
Chapel Hill, NC

Peter T. Chang, MD
Assistant Professor of Ophthalmology
Director, Glaucoma Fellowship
Department of Ophthalmology
Cullen Eye Institute
Baylor College of Medicine
Houston, TX

Philip P. Chen, MD
Professor of Ophthalmology
Department of Ophthalmology
University of Washington
Chief of Ophthalmology
University of Washington Eye Institute
Seattle, WA

Teresa C. Chen, MD
Associate Professor of Ophthalmology
Harvard Medical School
Chief Quality Officer for Ophthalmology
Massachusetts Eye and Ear Infirmary
Glaucoma Service
Boston, MA

Gabriel T. Chong, MD
Raleigh Ophthalmology
Raleigh, NC

John S. Cohen, MD
Director Emeritus, Glaucoma Service
Cincinnati Eye Institute
Volunteer Clinical Professor
Department of Ophthalmology
University of Cincinnati College of Medicine
Cincinnati, OH

Anastasios P. Costarides, MD, PhD
Associate Professor of Ophthalmology
Pamela Humphrey Firman Professor of
    Ophthalmology
Emory Eye Center
Emory University School of Medicine
Atlanta, GA

Alan S. Crandall, MD
Professor and Senior Vice Chair
Director, Glaucoma and Cataract
Department of Ophthalmology and Visual
    Sciences
John A. Moran Eye Center
The University of Utah
Salt Lake City, UT

E. Randy Craven, MD
Associate Clinical Professor
Rocky Vista University
Director, Glaucoma Consultants of
    Colorado Research
Specialty Eye Care
Parker, CO

Andrew C. Crichton, MD, FRCSC
Specialist Ophthalmologist
Clinical Professor
Department of Surgery
Faculty of Medicine
University of Calgary
Calgary, Alberta, Canada

Marc R. Criden, MD
Assistant Professor of Ophthalmology
Neuro-Ophthalmology, Oculoplastics,
    and Orbital Diseases
Havener Eye Institute
Department of Ophthalmology
The Ohio State University
Columbus, OH

Garvin H. Davis, MD, MPH
Clinical Assistant Professor
Ruiz Department of Ophthalmology and
    Visual Science
The University of Texas Medical School
    at Houston
Robert Cizik Eye Clinic
Houston, TX

Francisco E. Fantes, MD†
Professor of Clinical Ophthalmology
Bascom Palmer Eye Institute
Department of Ophthalmology
Miller School of Medicine
University of Miami
Miami, FL

Robert D. Fechtner, MD
Professor of Ophthalmology
Director, Glaucoma Division
Institute of Ophthalmology and Visual
    Science
New Jersey Medical School
University of Medicine and Dentistry
    of New Jersey
Newark, NJ

Robert M. Feldman, MD
Richard S. Ruiz, MD Distinguished
    University Chair
Professor and Chairman
Ruiz Department of Ophthalmology and
    Visual Science
The University of Texas Medical School
    at Houston
Robert Cizik Eye Clinic
Houston, TX

Ronald L. Fellman, MD
Clinical Associate Professor Emeritus
Department of Ophthalmology
University of Texas Southwestern
    Medical Center
Dallas, TX
President
Glaucoma Associates of Texas
Dallas, TX

Edney R. Moura Filho, MD
Glaucoma and Cornea Specialist Director and
    Chief of the Glaucoma Service Hospital
    Pacini Brasília, Brazil

Brian A. Francis, MD, MS
Ralph and Angelyn Riffenburgh Professor of
    Glaucoma
Associate Professor
Department of Ophthalmology
Doheny Eye Institute
Keck School of Medicine
University of Southern California
Los Angeles, CA

**Jeffrey Freedman, MBBCh, PhD,
FRCSE, FCS(SA)**
Professor of Clinical Ophthalmology
Department of Ophthalmology
SUNY Downstate Medical Center, College
    of Medicine
Brooklyn, NY

Sharon F. Freedman, MD
Chief, Pediatric Ophthalmology and
    Strabismus Division
Professor of Ophthalmology
Professor of Glaucoma
Duke University Eye Center
Durham, NC

Steven J. Gedde, MD
Professor of Ophthalmology
Bascom Palmer Eye Institute
Department of Ophthalmology
Miller School of Medicine
University of Miami
Miami, FL

Megan M. Geloneck, MD
Resident Physician
Ruiz Department of Ophthalmology
    and Visual Science
The University of Texas Medical School at
    Houston
Houston, TX

David G. Godfrey, MD
Glaucoma Associates of Texas
Glaucoma Specialist
Clinical Associate Professor
University of Texas Southwestern Medical School
Dallas, TX

Parag A. Gokhale, MD
Eye Physician and Surgeon, Glaucoma
    and Cataract
Virginia Mason Medical Center
Seattle, WA

Jason A. Goldsmith, MD, MS
Assistant Clinical Professor
Department of Ophthalmology and Visual
    Sciences

John A. Moran Eye Center
The University of Utah
Chief of Ophthalmology
Department of Veterans Affairs Medical Center
Salt Lake City, UT

Ronald L. Gross, MD
Professor of Ophthalmology
Clifton R. McMichael Chair in
	Ophthalmology
Department of Ophthalmology
Cullen Eye Institute
Baylor College of Medicine
Houston, TX

Paul J. Harasymowycz, MD, MSc, FRCSC
Director and Chief of Glaucoma
Montreal Glaucoma Institute
University of Montreal
Montreal, Quebec, Canada

Malik Y. Kahook, MD
Professor of Ophthalmology
Director of Clinical and Translational
	Research
Chief, Glaucoma Service
University of Colorado Eye Center
Aurora, CO

L. Jay Katz, MD, FACS
Professor of Ophthalmology
Department of Ophthalmology
Jefferson Medical College
Thomas Jefferson University
Director, Glaucoma Service
Wills Eye Institute
Philadelphia, PA

Judianne Kellaway, MD
Steve A. Lasher III Professor in
	Ophthalmology
Clinical Associate Professor
Director, Residency Program
Ruiz Department of Ophthalmology and
	Visual Science
The University of Texas Medical School at
	Houston
Robert Cizik Eye Clinic
Houston, TX

Mahmoud A. Khaimi, MD
Clinical Associate Professor of
	Ophthalmology
Dean McGee Eye Institute
The University of Oklahoma College of
	Medicine
Oklahoma City, OK

Parul Khator, MD
Glaucoma Specialist
Georgia Eye Partners
Atlanta, GA

Albert S. Khouri, MD
Assistant Professor of Ophthalmology
Associate Director, Glaucoma Division
Institute of Ophthalmology and Visual
	Science
New Jersey Medical School
University of Medicine and Dentistry
	of New Jersey
Newark, NJ

Won I. Kim, MD
Assistant Professor of Surgery
Uniformed Services University of the Health
	Sciences
Department of Ophthalmology
Walter Reed National Military Medical Center
Bethesda, MD

Scott D. Lawrence, MD
Assistant Professor
Department of Ophthalmology
The University of North Carolina
	at Chapel Hill
Chapel Hill, NC

David A. Lee, MD, MS, MBA, FACS
Clinical Professor
Ruiz Department of Ophthalmology and
	Visual Science
The University of Texas Medical School
	at Houston
Robert Cizik Eye Clinic
Houston, TX

Richard A. Lewis, MD
Consultant in Glaucoma
Grutzmacher, Lewis, and Sierra Surgical
	Eye Specialists
Sacramento, CA

Shan C. Lin, MD
Professor of Clinical Ophthalmology
Co-Director, Glaucoma Service
Department of Ophthalmology
University of California, San Francisco
San Francisco, CA

John T. Lind, MD
Assistant Professor of Ophthalmology
Saint Louis University Eye Institute
Saint Louis, MO

Jeff Maltzman, MD, FACS
Partner
Fishkind, Bakewell, and Maltzman Eye Care
    and Surgery Center
Tucson, AZ
Clinical Instructor
Midwestern University School of Medicine
Glendale, AZ

Nick Mamalis, MD
Professor
Director, Ophthalmic Pathology
Director, Intermountain Ocular Research
    Center
Department of Ophthalmology and Visual
    Sciences
John A. Moran Eye Center
The University of Utah
Salt Lake City, UT

Kimberly A. Mankiewicz, PhD
Technical Writer III
Ruiz Department of Ophthalmology
    and Visual Science
The University of Texas Medical School
    at Houston
Houston, TX

Cynthia Mattox, MD, FACS
Vice Chair and Associate Professor
Department of Ophthalmology
Tufts University School of Medicine
Director, Glaucoma and Cataract Service
New England Eye Center
Boston, MA

Malcolm L. Mazow, MD, FACS
Houston Eye Associates
Houston, TX

Matthew G. McMenemy, MD
Lone Star Eye Care, P.A.
Sugar Land, TX

Richard P. Mills, MD, MPH
Glaucoma Consultants Northwest
Seattle, WA

Jonathan S. Myers, MD
Associate Attending Surgeon
Glaucoma Service
Wills Eye Institute
Philadelphia, PA

Kundandeep S. Nagi, MD
Assistant Professor
Department of Ophthalmology
The University of Texas Health Science Center
    at San Antonio
San Antonio, TX

Peter A. Netland, MD, PhD
DuPont Guerry III Professor and Chairman
Department of Ophthalmology
University of Virginia School of Medicine
Charlottesville, VA

Robert J. Noecker, MD, MBA
Ophthalmic Consultants of Connecticut
Fairfield, CT

Osman Oram, MD
Associate Professor of Ophthalmology
Chief, Department of Ophthalmology
VKF American Hospital,

Istanbul, Turkey
Eye Care Line Executive
Michael E. DeBakey VAMC

Silvia D. Orengo-Nania, MD
Professor of Ophthalmology
Department of Ophthalmology
Cullen Eye Institute
Baylor College of Medicine
Houston, TX

Richard K. Parrish, II, MD
Professor of Ophthalmology
Bascom Palmer Eye Institute
Department of Ophthalmology
Associate Dean of Graduate Medical
    Education
Miller School of Medicine
University of Miami
Miami, FL

Louis R. Pasquale, MD
Associate Professor of Ophthalmology
Department of Ophthalmology
Harvard Medical School
Director, Glaucoma Service
Director, Telemedicine
Massachusetts Eye and Ear Infirmary
Boston, MA

Omar Piovanetti, MD
Glaucoma Specialist
Centro Oftalmológico Metropolitano
San Juan, PR

Amir A. Pirouzian, MD, FACS
Instructor, Cornea
Department of Ophthalmology
Gavin Herbert Eye Institute
University of California, Irvine
Irvine, CA

Tony Realini, MD, MPH
Associate Professor of Ophthalmology
Department of Ophthalmology
West Virginia University Eye Institute
Morgantown, WV

Adam C. Reynolds MD
Intermountain Eye and Laser Centers.
Boise, ID
Jorge L. Rivera-Vélez , MD
Glaucoma Specialist
Centrode Oftalmología, Glaucomay
  Retina del Oeste.
Mayagüez, PR

Thomas W. Samuelson, MD
Consultant, Glaucoma and Anterior Segment
  Surgery
Minnesota Eye Consultants, P.A.
Attending Surgeon
Phillips Eye Institute
Adjunct Associate Professor
Department of Ophthalmology
University of Minnesota
Minneapolis, MN

Steven R. Sarkisian, Jr., MD
Clinical Associate Professor of Ophthalmology
Glaucoma Fellowship Director
Dean McGee Eye Institute
The University of Oklahoma College of
  Medicine
Oklahoma City, OK

Jeffrey S. Schultz, MD
Associate Professor and Director of Glaucoma
  Service
Department of Ophthalmology and Visual
  Sciences
Montefiore Medical Center, Albert Einstein
  College of Medicine
Bronx, NY

Leonard K. Seibold, MD
Assistant Professor
Glaucoma and Cataract
University of Colorado Eye Center
Department of Ophthalmology
University of Colorado Denver School
  of Medicine
Aurora, CO

Mark B. Sherwood, MD
Professor of Ophthalmology
Director, Center for Vision Research
Department of Ophthalmology
University of Florida College of Medicine
Gainesville, FL

Anurag Shrivastava, MD
Assistant Professor of Ophthalmology
Attending Surgeon - Glaucoma Service
Montefiore Medical Center
Albert Einstein College of Medicine

Bronx, NY

Paul A. Sidoti, MD, FACS
Professor of Ophthalmology
New York Medical College
The New York Eye and Ear Infirmary
New York, NY

Steven T. Simmons, MD
Associate Clinical Professor
Department of Ophthalmology
Albany Medical College
Albany, NY
Glaucoma Consultants of the Capital
  Region
Slingerlands, NY

Kuldev Singh MD MPH
Professor of Ophthalmology
Director, Glaucoma Service
Stanford University
Stanford, CA

Arthur J. Sit, SM, MD
Associate Professor
Department of Ophthalmology
Mayo Clinic
Rochester, MN

Alfred M. Solish, MD
Southern California Glaucoma
Los Angeles, CA

Detlev Spiegel, MD
Professor
Department of Ophthalmology
University of Regensburg
Regensburg, Germany
Glaucoma Specialist
Augenzentrum Muenchen Sued
Munich, Germany

Clark L. Springs, MD
Assistant Professor of Ophthalmology
Cornea, Cataract, and Refractive Surgery
Eugene and Marilyn Glick Eye Institute
Department of Ophthalmology
Indiana University School of Medicine
Indianapolis, IN

Robert L. Stamper, MD
Professor of Clinical Ophthalmology
Director, Glaucoma Service
Department of Ophthalmology
University of California, San Francisco
San Francisco, CA

Misha F. Syed, MD
Assistant Professor, Glaucoma
Director, Residency Program
Department of Ophthalmology and Visual
    Sciences
The University of Texas Medical Branch at
    Galveston
Galveston, TX
Angelo P. Tanna, MD

Associate Professor of Ophthalmology
Vice Chairman
Director, Glaucoma Service
Department of Ophthalmology
Northwestern University
Feinberg School of Medicine
Chicago, IL

James C. Tsai, MD, MBA
Robert R. Young Professor and Chairman
Department of Ophthalmology and Visual
    Science
Yale University School of Medicine
Chief of Ophthalmology, Yale-New
    Haven Hospital
New Haven, CT

Héctor J. Villarrubia, MD
Associate Professor
Universidad Central del Caribe School
    of Medicine
Caribbean Glaucoma Consultants
Bayamon, PR

Steven D. Vold, MD
Glaucoma and Cataract Surgery Consultant
Vold Vision, PLLC
Fayetteville, AR

Martin Wand, MD
Clinical Professor of Ophthalmology
University of Connecticut School of Medicine
Consulting Ophthalmologists, PC
Farmington, CT

Nan Wang, MD, PhD
Walter and Ruth Sterling Professor in
    Ophthalmology
Clinical Associate Professor
Ruiz Department of Ophthalmology and
    Visual Science
The University of Texas Medical School
    at Houston
Director, Cornea and Anterior Segment
    Service
Robert Cizik Eye Clinic
Houston, TX

Robert N. Weinreb, MD
Chair and Distinguished Professor of
Ophthalmology
Morris Gleich, MD Chair of Glaucoma
Director, Shiley Eye Center
Director, Hamilton Glaucoma Center
University of California, San Diego
La Jolla, CA

Jess T. Whitson, MD
Professor of Ophthalmology
Department of Ophthalmology
University of Texas Southwestern Medical
    Center Dallas, TX

Peter T. Wollan, MD
Glaucoma Specialist
Eye Physicians of Austin
Austin, TX

Huijuan Wu, MD, PhD
Associate Professor of Ophthalmology
Department of Ophthalmology
Peking University
People's Hospital
Key Laboratory of Vision Loss and
    Restoration
Ministry of Education
Beijing, China

Darrell WuDunn, MD, PhD
Professor of Ophthalmology
Eugene and Marilyn Glick Eye Institute
Department of Ophthalmology
Indiana University School of Medicine
Indianapolis, IN

PART ONE

AQUEOUS OUTFLOW MECHANISM AFTER GLAUCOMA SURGERY

A. TRABECULECTOMY AND TUBE SHUNTS

1

TRABECULECTOMY AND TUBE SHUNTS

DARRELL WUDUNN

TRABECULECTOMY AND TUBE SHUNTS

Trabeculectomy surgery is the most common operative procedure for managing glaucoma. Although the techniques have evolved over the decades, the basic procedure remains the same since filtering surgery was first performed a century ago: a scleral fistula enables aqueous fluid to drain into the subconjunctival space and create a bleb. Despite the long history of trabeculectomy surgery, the mechanisms of how aqueous fluid ultimately exits the eye after trabeculectomy are still not well characterized.

Aqueous tube shunts are becoming more popular among glaucoma surgeons as an alternative to trabeculectomy in eyes with previously failed blebs or in eyes at high risk for bleb failure.[1,2] Although the mechanism of

aqueous outflow following tube shunt implantation may be similar to the mechanism after trabeculectomy, key differences exist that may be important for future developments in glaucoma surgery.

Multiple potential routes of aqueous drainage exist for both trabeculectomy and tube shunt implants. Thus, aqueous drainage can be thought of as a complex system of pathways arranged in series and in parallel. In general, fluid flowing through any system will be directed according to the resistance along each potential pathway. After glaucoma surgery, the arrangement and resistance through these pathways will depend on the wound healing response (see Chapter 3), and thus the mechanism of aqueous drainage will alter as the wound healing response evolves. However, it is likely that one or 2 main routes of drainage will dominate as the tissue reaction stabilizes.

AQUEOUS OUTFLOW AFTER TRABECULECTOMY

When Cairns first described the trabeculectomy procedure, he argued that aqueous humor would flow out through the cut ends of Schlemm's canal without subconjunctival drainage.[3] However, as the procedure is currently performed, a filtering bleb is almost always created, and a block of trabecular meshwork is not consistently excised. Thus, modern trabeculectomy is a filtering procedure in which aqueous passes through the sclera into the subconjunctival space overlying the scleral flap. The existence of a filtering bleb does not eliminate the possibility of aqueous outflow through Schlemm's canal into the aqueous veins. Indeed, tracer studies suggest that some aqueous enters the aqueous veins.[4–6] However, histological studies indicate that after successful trabeculectomy, extracellular material accumulates in the trabecular meshwork and the diameter of Schlemm's canal decreases, suggesting that flow is reduced through the trabecular outflow pathway.[7,8]

The bulk of aqueous fluid reaches the subconjunctival space overlying the scleral flap. Aqueous may reach the subconjunctival space either through the gaps around the scleral flap or directly through the scleral flap tissue (transscleral). The transscleral route has been supported by histological and tracer studies, which show that aqueous fluid passes through the sclera.[9,10]

Recent developments in anterior segment imaging have revealed distinct routes of aqueous flow into the subconjunctival space. Anterior segment optical coherence tomography (ASOCT) demonstrates the outline of the scleral flap and a discernible route beneath the flap connecting the sclerostomy and the subconjunctival/suprascleral fluid collections.[11–14] However, it should be noted that the detection of a route beneath the scleral flap and suprascleral fluid does not indicate whether the aqueous drainage is adequate since outflow may still be impaired within the overlying bleb substance.

Aqueous fluid may also drain through newly developed vessels within the sclera. Histologic examination of eyes after trabeculectomy identified transscleral channels in the area of the incision that consist of cell-rich connective tissue with many endothelium-lined capillaries.[10] These new vessels may help carry collected aqueous as the fluid percolates transsclerally.

As the bulk of aqueous fluid reaches the subconjunctival space and creates a distinct bleb, the aqueous must exit the bleb by percolating through the conjunctiva into the tear film and/or by absorption into surrounding vessels. The exit mechanism likely depends on the bleb architecture, which is often reflected by the appearance of the bleb. A thin-walled, avascular bleb is more likely to have transconjunctival flow of aqueous than a thick-walled, vascularized bleb. For some blebs, painting the bleb with a fluorescein strip will reveal multiple pinpoint leaks of fluid or a "starry sky" appearance, signifying flow across the bleb wall. The presence of microcysts on the bleb surface is a likely indicator of robust transconjunctival flow. Indeed, impression cytology of blebs suggests that these microcysts represent modified goblet cells that contain aqueous rather than mucin and are responsible for aqueous flow across the bleb wall.[15] Other studies suggest that microcysts are epithelial cysts responsible for transconjunctival flow.[16] Thus, aqueous fluid may seep across the bleb wall through microbreaks in the bleb epithelial layer or transcellularly through these modified goblet cells or epithelial cysts.

It is not surprising that successful trabeculectomy surgery significantly increases outflow facility, since this is essentially the goal of filtration surgery.[17] What may not be well appreciated is that increased outflow facility associated with trabeculectomy should dampen short-term and diurnal variability of intraocular pressure.[18] Diurnal fluctuation in intraocular pressure is considerably less in eyes after successful trabeculectomy compared to eyes undergoing medical therapy.[19]

AQUEOUS OUTFLOW AFTER TUBE SHUNT SURGERY

Although aqueous may drain through the sclerostomy around the tube during the early postoperative period, implantation of a tube shunt will direct aqueous drainage through the tube into the reservoir created by the extra-ocular portion (plate) of the device. Like trabeculectomy, tube shunt implantation results in a conjunctival/Tenon's bleb. However, blebs associated with tube shunts are generally much thicker and more vascular than trabeculectomy blebs. It is likely, therefore, that aqueous exits the bleb from a tube shunt in a different manner.

Whereas aqueous flow through or around a trabeculectomy flap may encounter some resistance before it reaches the subconjunctival space, flow is unimpeded through a tube shunt (~300 micron internal diameter) lacking a valve or flow restrictor.[20] Even a small bore tube, such as an EX-PRESS™ Glaucoma Filtration Device (Alcon Laboratories, Inc., Fort Worth, Texas) with a 50 micron inside diameter (Chapter 29), does not provide appreciable resistance at physiological aqueous flow rates (~2 microliters/minute).[20] To avoid hypotony in nonvalved tube implants, a capsule must form around the plate and provide some resistance to aqueous flow. Without a capsule, aqueous can flow unimpeded throughout the subconjunctival potential space. Thus in the early postoperative period before a capsule develops, the surgeon must mitigate the flow of aqueous through the tube. A high viscosity viscoelastic device can also be used to slow the flow of fluid through the tube.[21] An absorbable or releasable suture (ligature) can be tied around the tube to occlude the lumen until a capsule forms. Slits or fenestrations in the tube proximal to the ligature can be created to enable some aqueous fluid to flow into the subconjunctival space[22] (see Chapter 35). The rate of flow through the slit or fenestration is dependent in part on the width and length of the slit. A capsule will eventually form around the tube and render the slit or fenestration ineffective (typically about 3 weeks postoperatively); however, by then a sufficient capsule has also formed around the plate, and the ligature can be released. Tube shunts with a valve, such as the Ahmed™ Glaucoma Valve (New World Medical, Inc., Rancho Cucamonga, California), do provide some resistance to flow, although the resistance is variable.[20]

It is important to be aware that even with a properly ligated or valved tube fluid can seep around the tube within the scleral tunnel during the initial day or 2 after surgery and cause hypotony (see Chapters 34 and 39).

After fluid reaches the reservoir over the plate, it percolates through the capsule into the surrounding orbital tissues by simple passive diffusion.[23] Thus, the rate at which aqueous fluid drains from the reservoir is dependent on the thickness of the surrounding capsule that forms around the plate and on the surface area of the plate (which determines the surface area of the capsule).[24] Tracer agents such as horseradish peroxidase and latex particles have been shown to move through the capsule wall in between collagen bundles and into the surrounding tissues.[23] Aqueous is then cleared away from ocular tissues via the venous system.

Unlike trabeculectomy blebs, fluid does not appear to flow through the bleb wall into the tear film at a significant rate but may instead enter the orbit. Tube shunt blebs typically resemble encapsulated trabeculectomy blebs and lack the conjunctival microcysts often seen on well-functioning mitomycin-C trabeculectomy blebs. Attempts to enhance trans-capsule flow from tube shunt blebs have generally been unsuccessful. Several studies using mitomycin-C have not shown improved intraocular pressure control when the antifibrotic agent was applied to the area of the plate.[25-27]

CONCLUSION

An understanding of the mechanisms of aqueous outflow through trabeculectomy filtering blebs and tube shunt devices is a prerequisite for the surgeon performing glaucoma surgery to effectively anticipate early or late postoperative complications. Now that what to expect has been discussed, Sections III and IV will address what can go wrong and how to manage or avoid complications of trabeculectomy and tube shunt surgery, respectively.

REFERENCES

1. Chen PP, Yamamoto T, Sawada A, Parrish RK, 2nd, Kitazawa Y. Use of antifibrosis agents and

glaucoma drainage devices in the American and Japanese Glaucoma Societies. *J Glaucoma*. Jun 1997;6(3):192–196.

2. Joshi AB, Parrish RK, 2nd, Feuer WF. 2002 survey of the American Glaucoma Society: practice preferences for glaucoma surgery and antifibrotic use. *J Glaucoma*. Apr 2005; 14(2):172–174.

3. Cairns JE. Trabeculectomy. Preliminary report of a new method. *Am J Ophthalmol*. Oct 1968;66(4):673–679.

4. Benedikt O. [Demonstration of aqueous outflow patterns of normal and glaucomatous human eyes through the injection of fluorescein solution in the anterior chamber (author's transl)]. *Albrecht von Graefes Archiv fur klinische und experimentelle Ophthalmologie. Albrecht von Graefe's archive for clinical and experimental ophthalmology*. Apr 1 1976;199(1):45–67.

5. Benedikt O. [The effect of filtering operations (author's transl)]. *Klinische Monatsblatter fur Augenheilkunde*. Jan 1977;170(1):10–19.

6. Teng CC, Chi HH, Katzin HM. Histology and mechanism of filtering operations. *Am J Ophthalmol*. Jan 1959;47(1 Part 1):16–33.

7. Johnson DH, Matsumoto Y. Schlemm's canal becomes smaller after successful filtration surgery. *Arch Ophthalmol*. Sept 2000;118(9): 1251–1256.

8. Lutjen-Drecoll E, Barany EH. Functional and electron microscopic changes in the trabecular meshwork remaining after trabeculectomy in cynomolgus monkeys. *Invest Ophthalmol*. Jul 1974;13(7):511–524.

9. Shields MB, Bradbury MJ, Shelburne JD, Bell SW. The permeability of the outer layers of limbus and anterior sclera. *Invest Ophthalmol Vis Sci*. Sept 1977;16(9):866–869.

10. van der Zypen E, Fankhauser F, Kwasniewska S. The mechanism of aqueous outflow following trabeculectomy. A light and electron microscopic study. *Int Ophthalmol*. May 1989;13(3): 219–228.

11. Leung CK, Yick DW, Kwong YY, et al. Analysis of bleb morphology after trabeculectomy with Visante anterior segment optical coherence tomography. *Br J Ophthalmol*. Mar 2007;91(3): 340–344.

12. Miura M, Kawana K, Iwasaki T, et al. Three-dimensional anterior segment optical coherence tomography of filtering blebs after trabeculectomy. *J Glaucoma*. Apr-May 2008; 17(3): 193–196.

13. Singh M, Chew PT, Friedman DS, et al. Imaging of trabeculectomy blebs using anterior segment optical coherence tomography. *Ophthalmology*. Jan 2007;114(1):47–53.

14. Zhang Y, Wu Q, Zhang M, Song BW, Du XH, Lu B. Evaluating subconjunctival bleb function after trabeculectomy using slit-lamp optical coherence tomography and ultrasound biomicroscopy. *Chin Med J (Engl)*. Jul 20 2008;121(14):1274–1279.

15. Amar N, Labbe A, Hamard P, Dupas B, Baudouin C. Filtering blebs and aqueous pathway an immunocytological and in vivo confocal microscopy study. *Ophthalmology*. Jul 2008;115(7):1154–1161.

16. Messmer EM, Zapp DM, Mackert MJ, Thiel M, Kampik A. In vivo confocal microscopy of filtering blebs after trabeculectomy. *Arch Ophthalmol*. Aug 2006;124(8):1095–1103.

17. Rossier A, Uffer S, Mermoud A. Aqueous dynamics in experimental ab externo trabeculectomy. *Ophthalmic Res*. Jul-Aug 2000; 32(4):165–171.

18. Brubaker RF. Targeting outflow facility in glaucoma management. *Surv Ophthalmol*. Apr 2003;48 (suppl 1):S17–S20.

19. Medeiros FA, Pinheiro A, Moura FC, Leal BC, Susanna R, Jr. Intraocular pressure fluctuations in medical versus surgically treated glaucomatous patients. *J Ocul Pharmacol Ther*. Dec 2002;18(6):489–498.

20. Prata JA, Jr., Mermoud A, LaBree L, Minckler DS. In vitro and in vivo flow characteristics of glaucoma drainage implants. *Ophthalmology*. Jun 1995;102(6):894–904.

21. Goulet RJ, 3rd, Phan AD, Cantor LB, WuDunn D. Efficacy of the Ahmed™ S2 glaucoma valve compared with the Baerveldt® 250-mm² glaucoma implant. *Ophthalmology*. Jul 2008;115(7): 1141–1147.

22. Trible JR, Brown DB. Occlusive ligature and standardized fenestration of a Baerveldt® tube with and without antimetabolites for early postoperative intraocular pressure control. *Ophthalmology*. Dec 1998;105(12): 2243–2250.

23. Minckler DS, Shammas A, Wilcox M, Ogden TE. Experimental studies of aqueous filtration using the Molteno® implant. *Trans Am Ophthalmol Soc*. 1987;85:368–392.

24. Prata JA, Jr., Santos RCR, LaBree L, Minckler DS. Surface area of glaucoma implants and perfusion flow rates in rabbit eyes. *J Glaucoma*. Aug 1995;4(4):274–280.

25. Cantor L, Burgoyne J, Sanders S, Bhavnani V, Hoop J, Brizendine E. The effect of mitomycin C on Molteno® implant surgery: a 1-year

randomized, masked, prospective study. *J Glaucoma.* Aug 1998;7(4):240–246.

26. Costa VP, Azuara-Blanco A, Netland PA, Lesk MR, Arcieri ES. Efficacy and safety of adjunctive mitomycin C during Ahmed™ Glaucoma Valve implantation: a prospective randomized clinical trial. *Ophthalmology.* Jun 2004;111(6):1071–1076.

27. Susanna R, Jr. Partial Tenon's capsule resection with adjunctive mitomycin C in Ahmed™ glaucoma valve implant surgery. *Br J Ophthalmol.* Aug 2003;87(8):994–998.

B. ANGLE AND NONPENETRATING SURGERY

2

ANGLE AND NONPENETRATING GLAUCOMA SURGERY

HUIJUAN WU AND TERESA C. CHEN

ANGLE AND NONPENETRATING GLAUCOMA SURGERY

Normal aqueous outflow

The outflow of aqueous via the anterior chamber angle is a constant process. The aqueous is formed by the ciliary processes and then passes through the pupil from the posterior chamber to the anterior chamber (Figure 2.1). About 83%–96% of the aqueous finally exits the eye into the anterior chamber angle via the trabecular meshwork—Schlemm's canal—venous system (i.e., the conventional or canalicular outflow pathway).[1,2] The other 5%–15% of aqueous outflow occurs via uveoscleral outflow (i.e., the unconventional or extracanalicular outflow pathway), with aqueous passing through the ciliary muscle and iris, then entering into the supraciliary and suprachoroidal spaces, and then finally exiting

the eye through the sclera or along the penetrating nerves and vessels.[1,3,4]

Glaucoma is usually associated with aqueous outflow problems through a variety of mechanisms. For the developmental glaucomas, the improper development of the outflow structures is the main reason for high eye pressures.[5] In the primary and secondary open-angle glaucomas, the theories to explain the diminished outflow facility are numerous. Possible etiologies are as follows: deposition of foreign material (such as pigment, red blood cells, glycosaminoglycans, extracellular lysosomes, plaque-like material, and proteins) into the trabecular meshwork (TM) and the wall of Schlemm's canal (SC),[6–10] loss of trabecular endothelial cells,[9,11] structural changes of the inner wall of SC,[9,12] and abnormal phagocytic activity of trabecular endothelial cells.[9,13] In angle closure glaucoma, the peripheral iris closes the entrance to the TM by the anterior

• 13

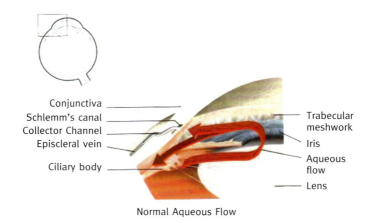

Normal Aqueous Flow

Conjunctiva
Schlemm's canal
Collector Channel
Episcleral vein
Ciliary body
Trabecular meshwork
Iris
Aqueous flow
Lens

FIGURE 2.1 **Normal aqueous outflow pathways.** Trabecular or conventional outflow pathway and uveoscleral or unconventional outflow pathway. Reproduced, with permission, from Cioffi GA, Basic and Clinical Science Course, Section 10, American Academy of Ophthalmology, 2010–2011.

pulling mechanism or the posterior pushing mechanism,[14,15] resulting in the direct blockage of conventional outflow.

The goal of angle and nonpenetrating procedures is to restore aqueous outflow, thereby lowering intraocular pressure (IOP). Angle surgery restores outflow by re-opening the natural channels for aqueous outflow, and nonpenetrating glaucoma surgery creates an artificial external filtration site and partly restores the normal physiologic pathways.

ANGLE GLAUCOMA SURGERY

Goniotomy

In 1936, Otto Barkan was the first to describe a surgical procedure that creates an internal incision into trabecular tissue under direct magnified view of the anterior chamber angle.[14-16] Indications for this surgery, known as goniotomy, include the primary developmental glaucomas,[17-21] secondary pediatric glaucomas,[22-24] and aniridic glaucoma prevention.[25,26] The success rate of goniotomy ranges from 72% to 94%.[19-21,27-31] Outcome rates are particularly good for primary developmental glaucoma[19-21,27-29,31] and chronic childhood uveitic glaucoma.[22] Goniotomy is not as successful in cases of aniridia with progressive angle closure by residual iris tissue; success rates of 20% or less have been

reported.[25,26,32] Success rates are also poor in patients with anterior segment dysgenesis with iridocorneal attachments; Wallace et al noted no surgical successes in 5 patients with this disorder.[24]

Under binocular magnified view through a direct gonioscopy lens, a goniotomy incision is made at the anterior one-third of the angle or the mid-trabecular meshwork using a goniotomy knife[24,33,34] or a needle (23- or 25-gauge) (Figure 2.2).[35]

The main indication for goniotomy is congenital glaucoma. When this surgery was originally described by Barkan, he believed the incision made a cleft through a membrane covering the angle in patients with congenital glaucoma.[16] However, an actual Barkan's membrane has not been proven histologically.[36,37] In pathogenesis theories, primary congenital glaucoma appears to result from a developmental arrest of the TM, which is derived from the neural crest cells, and this leads to aqueous outflow obstruction by one or more mechanisms.[31,38] One theory proposes that the goniotomy breaks the abnormal insertion of the ciliary muscle's longitudinal fibers onto the posterior portion of the TM, thereby decreasing the compaction of trabecular sheets in order to relieve outflow obstruction.[36,39,40] Another widely accepted theory of primary congenital glaucoma suggests that there are primary developmental defects not only at

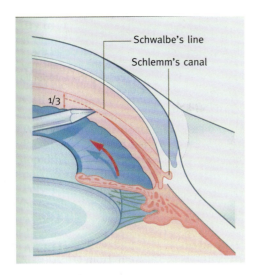

Schwalbe's line

Schlemm's canal

1/3

FIGURE 2.2 A successful goniotomy incision made through trabecular meshwork permits egress of aqueous humor into Schlemm's canal. (From Chen et al 2008[34], with permission of Elsevier)

various levels of the TM[36,41–44] but also in SC.[44,45] The poor surgical results of goniotomy in newborn glaucoma[46] imply that either an abnormality or absence of SC exists in some cases of congenital glaucoma that present at birth, even though a proper goniotomy incision has been made. The main reason why IOP may be lowered by successful goniotomy surgery is the re-establishment of the physiologic drainage pathway. This is accomplished by incising through TM tissue in order to re-establish entry of anterior chamber aqueous into the SC (Figure 2.2).[16] Since goniotomy surgery only bypasses abnormalities in the TM, a successful goniotomy operation is dependent on a relatively normal SC and on normal outflow pathways distal to SC.

Goniotomy has also been reported to be a safe and effective surgery for pediatric uveitic glaucoma with success rates of 71% and 75% at last follow-up, which was at 10.3±6.4 years and 32.4 months (range 6–84), respectively.[22,23] This secondary glaucoma is associated with chronic childhood uveitis and is thought to be due to progressive inflammatory damage to aqueous outflow pathways and closure of the anterior chamber

angle by peripheral anterior synechiae (PAS).[22] In open-angle cases of uveitic glaucoma, the likely pathologic site of inflammatory damage is the TM. Postgoniotomy gonioscopy reveals a circumferential slit of variable depth and vertical widening of the TM.[23] The mechanism of goniotomy surgery has been proven by both histology[48] and *in vivo* imaging.[47,48] After goniotomy surgery, histology has clearly shown the new artificial channel between the anterior chamber and SC through the incised TM.[49] With ultrasound biomicroscopy (UBM), the morphologic sign of a goniotomy incision is a triangular cleft within the chamber angle.[47,48] The success rate may decrease if the surgical technique is suboptimal (e.g., the incision goes into the sclera or involves the ciliary body, which may cause bleeding and fibrous proliferation).[49]

To summarize, goniotomy success rates are largely dependent on the type of glaucoma and the successful formation of an incisional opening into SC. Re-establishing normal outflow from the anterior chamber into SC is the core mechanism for lowering IOP with goniotomy surgery. This surgery appears to work best if SC and distal drainage pathways are relatively normal and if the primary site of obstruction is at the TM.

Trabeculotomy

The technique of external trabeculotomy or trabeculotomy *ab externo* was independently described in 1960 by both Hermann Burian[50,51] and Redmond Smith,[52–54] although the instruments each used were different. The technique was then modified by Harms[55,56] and McPherson,[57] and a double-armed probe was introduced (Figure 2.3). The surgery increased in popularity in the 1970s in Europe[55,56] and is considered an alternative to goniotomy surgery for congenital and childhood glaucomas,[58] especially in cases with cloudy corneas that would hinder a clear gonioscopic view of the angle. The success rates for this surgery are reported to be 70%–90%.[56,57,59] Trabeculotomy alone[60] or combined with cataract extraction[61,62] has success rates of 73.5%[60] and 92%,[62] respectively, for select patients with open-angle pseudoexfoliation glaucoma.

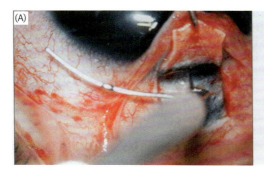
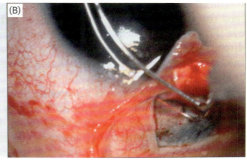

FIGURE 2.3 **Images of trabeculotomy surgery.** (A) Harms trabeculotome fully inserted into Schlemm's canal. (B) Harms trabeculotome after rotation into the anterior chamber, completing one-half of a standard trabeculotomy procedure. (From Chen et al 2008[59], with permission of Elsevier)

Trabeculotomy achieves a similar anatomic change in the angle as goniotomy, in that aqueous outflow is re-established from the anterior chamber into SC; however, the surgery is approached from outside the eye instead of from inside the eye. For trabeculotomy surgery, a partial-thickness scleral flap is created followed by a radial incision that enters SC.[58,63] At this point, 3 possible instruments can be used to enter SC: a metal trabeculotome[50,51,55,56,58,63] or a suture or catheter trabeculotome.[52–54,63] Once the trabeculotome is threaded into SC, the trabeculotome is used to break through the inner wall of SC and the TM, thereby entering the anterior chamber (Figure 2.3).

Therefore, trabeculotomy surgery allows aqueous entry into SC and the collector channels.[59] These morphologic changes after external trabeculotomy were demonstrated by UBM (Figure 2.4).[48] When suggesting possible mechanisms for this surgery, Grehn theorized that trabeculotomy triggers an "additional ripening" of the TM and the angle structures.[63] Many physiologic studies have also demonstrated that the facility of outflow may increase after trabeculotomy.[64–67] In one study, the authors noted that unroofing SC by using a nylon thread may increase intraoperative outflow facility by 4 times when actual outflow facility was measured during trabeculotomy surgeries in human glaucoma eyes.[64] In contrast, histopathological studies of eyes with unsuccessful trabeculotomy surgery showed the formation of fibrous scar tissue in the anterior chamber angle, which indicates that reclosure of the surgically created channel from the anterior chamber into SC results in failure.[68]

In summary, trabeculotomy restores normal outflow by 1) removing the resistance attributed to the TM and the inner wall of SC and 2) opening entry into SC. This procedure may also increase outflow facility. Both these structural and functional changes may contribute to final IOP reduction.

Trabeculodialysis

Trabeculodialysis was first described by Dellaporta[69] about 50 years ago but has not achieved widespread acceptance. Like goniotomy and external trabeculotomy, the development of this technique was based upon the theory that the main cause of increased IOP is obstruction at the level of the TM, the endothelium of SC, and the inner wall of SC.[69–73]

Inflammatory glaucoma responds modestly well to trabeculodialysis[74–78] with success rates around 60%.[76,78]

Trabeculodialysis involves detaching the corneoscleral TM from its natural bed and thereby allowing free communication of aqueous from the anterior chamber into SC (Figure 2.5). An angulated spatula or a similarly angulated instrument is often used for this procedure.[69,79,80] These anatomic changes have been confirmed by histology studies.[69,79,80]

Although the main mechanism for pressure reduction is direct communication between the anterior chamber and SC (Figure 2.6),[74] other sites of aqueous egress, such as the limited cyclodialysis cleft that often accompanies this surgery, may also be contributory.[80]

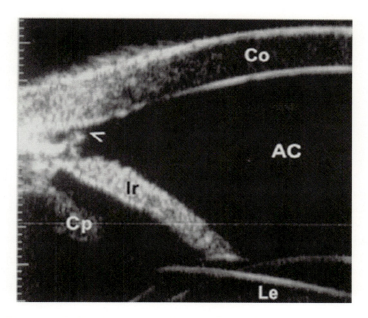

FIGURE 2.4 **Ultrasound biomicroscopy 3 months after trabeculotomy surgery**. The trabeculotomy incision is seen, leaving the trabecular meshwork and bridging iris strands ruptured (white arrow). AC – anterior chamber, Ir – iris, Co – cornea, Cp – ciliary process, Le – lens. (From Dietlein et al 2000[48], with permission of Elsevier.)

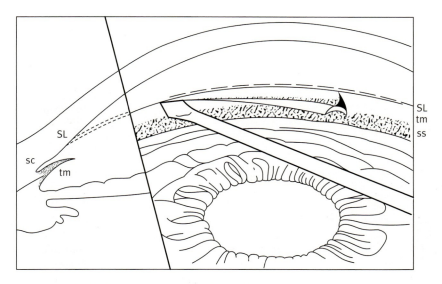

FIGURE 2.5 Trabeculodialysis involves detaching the corneoscleral trabecular meshwork (TM) from its natural bed. SL – Schwalbe's line, sc – Schlemm's canal, tm – trabecular meshwork, ss – scleral spur. This figure was published in Stamper RL, Marc FL, Michael VD, eds. Becker-Shaffer's Diagnosis and Therapy of the Glaucomas, page 673, Figure 39–14, Copyright Elsevier (2001).

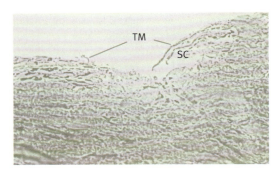

FIGURE 2.6 **Phase contrast photomicrograph illustrating trabeculodialysis surgery.** Specimen was obtained from trabeculectomy surgery done one month later. The trabecular meshwork (TM) has been disrupted and shows no signs of healing. Schlemm's canal (SC) has direct connection to the anterior chamber (paraphenylenediamine, ×275). (From Herschler et al. *Arch Ophthalmol.* Apr 1980;98(4):684–7[78]. Copyright © (1980) American Medical Association. All rights reserved)

Goniosynechiolysis

Although goniosynechiolysis was first described by Shaffer in 1957,[81] it was not often used due to difficulty maintaining the anterior chamber depth intraoperatively, which could potentially compromise the cornea, angle, and lens.[82] The procedure became more widely accepted after 1984 when Campbell and Vela introduced the modern technique of using sodium hyaluronate and an irrigating cyclodialysis spatula to maintain intraoperative anterior chamber depth.[81] Goniosynechiolysis is indicated when there are PAS causing primary or secondary angle closure glaucoma. Success rates range from 87% to 93%.[81–84]

The initial step of the operation is to release aqueous from the anterior and posterior chambers and then to deepen the anterior chamber with viscoelastic to a depth of 6–8 corneal thicknesses.[81,85] Under direct gonioscopic visualization, goniosynechiolysis can be performed with an irrigating cyclodialysis spatula,[81] a needle, or a goniotomy knife.[85] This instrument then disinserts the iris and PAS from the TM face using repetitive posterior depression movements (Figure 2.7).[81,85,86]

The mechanism of IOP reduction with goniosynechiolysis can be deduced from analysis and summary of the proper indications and successful outcomes of this surgery. The ideal result of this surgery is to facilitate conventional outflow by peeling back any iris tissue that had been blocking entry of aqueous into the TM face. However, reestablishing a normal open-angle configuration with

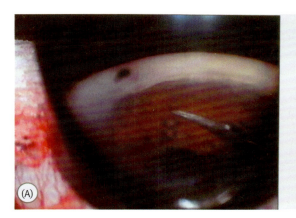
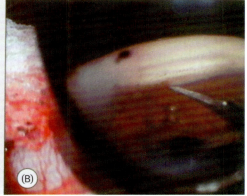

FIGURE 2.7 **Images of the anterior chamber angle in synechial angle closure glaucoma.** (A) Corneal opacity and edema reduced the quality of the view of the angle structures. (B) The angle that is free of synechiae is shown to the right of the spatula. (From Takanashi et al[147], with permission of Lippincott Williams & Wilkins)

goniosynechiolysis, as shown postoperatively by gonioscopy[81–84,87] and UBM,[88] is not sufficient to successfully lower IOP. In addition to physically removing iris or PAS covering the TM, having an adequate degree of functional TM is also very important. A study measuring tonographic C values after successful goniosynechiolysis suggests that goniosynechiolysis improves outflow facility via the TM.[83] Both laboratory evidence[70] and clinical experience show that better TM function preservation, as well as better surgical outcomes, is achieved in the eyes with PAS that were present for fewer than 6 months to one year.[77,82,85,86] Goniosynechiolysis is most effective in cases of synechial angle closure without chronic inflammation, endothelialization, or neovascularization.[82–85,88,89] Normal or near normal function of the TM is also a necessary condition for adequate pressure reduction. Furthermore, additional procedures such as phacoemulsification and/or laser peripheral iridoplasty may enhance surgical success by decreasing anterior chamber angle crowding and minimizing PAS recurrence.[90–92]

In summary, the main mechanism of successful goniosynechiolysis is relieving any mechanical blockage of the TM face by PAS in the presence of a functioning TM.

Ab interno trabeculectomy (Trabectome®)

Trabectome® (Neomedix, Inc., Tustin, California) surgery, invented by George Baerveldt and Roy Chuck, is most similar to goniotomy surgery.[93] The first clinical series using the Trabectome® was reported by Minckler et al in 2005.[94] The main indication for this surgery is adult open-angle glaucoma.[94–96]

In this procedure, a Trabectome® handpiece is used instead of a goniotomy knife (Figure 2.8). The footplate of the Trabectome handpiece is inserted *ab interno* and placed into SC while employing electrosurgical ablation of the TM, simultaneous infusion of saline, and aspiration of debris.[94] This new technique attempts to enhance conventional outflow via SC by improving aqueous access to collector channels, most numerous nasally.[96] Although Barkan's goniotomy surgery achieves a similar anatomic result,[16] the use of goniotomy surgery for adult open-angle glaucoma is limited in part by postoperative reapproximation and closing of the cut ends of the TM from

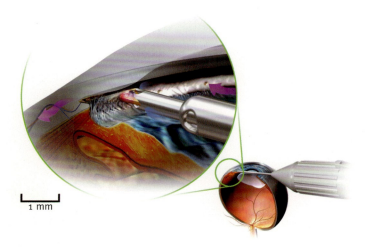

1 mm

FIGURE 2.8 The Trabectome® handpiece is inserted into Schlemm's canal and applies microelectrocautery ablation to the trabecular tissue in its pathway. (With permission of NeoMedix™ Corporation, Tustin, California)

fibrosis.[97] This closure does not occur as easily in pediatric patients because of the relatively more elastic surrounding tissues, which tend to gape and pull apart the edges of the goniotomy incision.[94,98] Excision or ablation of the TM with the microelectrocautery tip may facilitate retraction of the incision edges by heat effect.[97] After this microelectrocautery and ablation, less tissue remains at the surgical cleft compared to goniotomy or trabeculotomy surgery, and this may minimize scar formation at the incision.[94] In theory, these advantages may improve the success rate of Trabectome® surgery compared to regular goniotomy surgery in the treatment of adult open-angle glaucoma.

Histology of human autopsy eyes treated with the Trabectome® displays disruption of the TM and SC inner wall without damage to the surrounding structures.[97] Transmission electron microscopy demonstrates an intact SC outer wall, collector channels, and an intact cell after Trabectome® surgery (Figure 2.9).[99] Effective IOP lowering with Trabectome® surgery in adult open-angle glaucoma[94–96,99–101] supports these anatomic changes. However, further studies are needed to evaluate other potential mechanisms that may enhance outflow.[96]

In summary, by unroofing SC with ablation of its inner wall and adjacent TM,[94] Trabectome® surgery appears effective for improving aqueous outflow and reducing IOP. For more information on Trabectome®, see Chapter 50.

NONPENETRATING GLAUCOMA SURGERY

The concept of nonpenetrating glaucoma surgery (NPGS) was first introduced by Kraznov in the early 1960s as sinusotomy[102,103]; however, this technique was never popularized because of the surgical difficulties in removing a lamellar band of sclera and opening SC over 120 degrees from 10-o'clock to 2-o'clock without a microscope.[104] Another similar procedure called "ab externo trabeculectomy" was reported by Zimmerman et al in 1984,[105,106] and the main difference between it and sinusotomy are that Zimmerman's procedure involves a superficial scleral flap and the removal of a block of SC and juxtacanalicular TM.[104–106] At this point, deep sclerectomy (DS) and viscocanalostomy (Chapter 52) are the 2 most common modifications of NPGS for the treatment of open-angle glaucoma.[107]

Deep sclerectomy (DS)

Deep sclerectomy (DS) was first reported by Fyodorov and Koslov in the late 1980s and early 1990s.[108,109] This technique may be combined with ab externo trabeculectomy,[104,110]

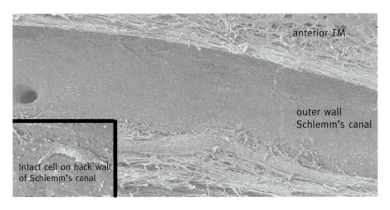

FIGURE 2.9 **Transmission electron microscopy of a human autopsy eye after Trabectome®** **surgery.** An intact outer wall of Schlemm's canal is seen with a collector channel on the left and an intact cell on the lower left. (From Nguyen 2008[99], with permission of Lippincott Williams & Wilkins.

device implantation,[109,111–115] or Nd:YAG gonio-puncture.[110] Various implantable devices may be employed to maintain an open scleral lake in the space left by removing the deep scleral flap.

The goal of DS is to remove a deep scleral flap along with some superficial corneal stroma anterior to the TM underneath a partial-thick-ness superficial scleral flap and expose a small area of intact Descemet's membrane (Figure 2.10A).[104,110] This may be combined with *ab externo* trabeculectomy, where the aqueous out-flow is enhanced by stripping the inner lining of SC (Figure 2.10B). Another variation of DS entails the additional implantation of different devices in the scleral bed or lake of the surgical site (Figure 2.10C). Such devices may include the collagen Aquaflow™ implant (Aquaflow™ Collagen Glaucoma Drainage Device, STAAR® Surgical Company, Monrovia, California),[111–116] a reticulated hyaluronic implant (SK GEL®, Corneal Laboratories, Paris, France),[117,118] the T-Flux® NV implant (Carl Zeiss Meditec SAS, La Rochelle, France),[119–121] or an autologous scleral implant.[122,123] Since DS does not achieve as low eye pressures as traditional trabeculec-tomy surgery,[124] Nd:YAG laser goniopuncture can be performed after the surgery if the IOP does not reach target levels.[110,124,125] By open-ing a direct communication to the anterior chamber, this laser effectively converts the DS to a penetrating trabeculectomy procedure.

The mechanism of this technique is appre-ciably complex since there are several associ-ated surgical adjunctive procedures.

First, there is the initial outflow mechanism from the anterior chamber to the scleral lake. In DS, initial aqueous outflow occurs through the anterior TM and Descemet's membrane in order to reach the scleral lake.[106,110,113] This hypothesis has been proven in an *in vitro* por-cine and human eye study, where outflow facility was significantly increased after DS.[126] In this study, DS was performed in 12 porcine enucleated eyes and 9 human enucleated eyes. Horse ferritin solution was then injected into the anterior chamber and was seen percolating through the newly created DS site. The histol-ogy slides dyed with ferritin showed that the aqueous outflow mainly occurred at the ante-rior TM.[126] Another *in vitro* study evaluated outflow rates through Descemet's membrane

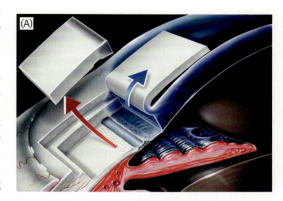

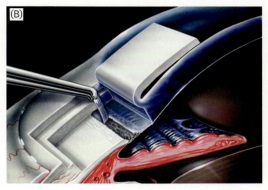

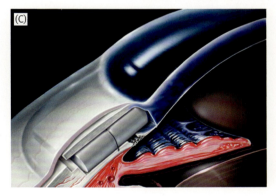

FIGURE 2.10 **Schematic of deep sclerectomy (DS) surgery.** (A) DS involves creating a superficial and then deeper flap of scleral tissue. The deeper scleral block is excised. This allows the aqueous fluid to begin to exit the eye at an increased but controlled rate. (B) The aqueous outflow is enhanced by stripping or removing the inner lining of Schlemm's canal. (C) The superficial flap is loosely closed with or without the collagen implant or other device to allow for the aqueous fluid to flow from underneath the flap to the bleb. (With permission of STAAR® Surgical Company, Monrovia, California)

at different levels of IOP in enucleated rabbit eyes.[127] This study showed high outflow resistance through Descemet's membrane at low pressures of around 20 mm Hg.[127] This indicates that the increase in aqueous outflow facility after DS is probably also due to surgical changes at the level of the inner wall of SC and the adjacent trabecular tissue.[110] In contrast, *ab externo* trabeculectomy largely facilitates drainage through the posterior TM.[104] Therefore, if *ab externo* trabeculectomy[128] is performed with DS (Figure 2.10 A, B), outflow could be facilitated in theory at the level of both the anterior TM and posterior TM.

Once the aqueous is at the level of the scleral lake, it may exit the eye through 3 potential pathways: the subconjunctival filtering bleb, transscleral outflow, or uveoscleral outflow.

1) Subconjunctival filtering bleb outflow: A filtering bleb often develops after NPGS,[112] although these blebs tend to be more shallow and diffuse than those seen after trabeculectomy.[110,129] UBM examination has demonstrated filtering bleb formation (Figure 2.11A, asterisks) in most eyes after DS with device implantation in the scleral bed or lake, and this implies that persistent filtration is one of the long-term mechanisms of aqueous resorption.[117,130,131] Studies have shown that aqueous in the filtering bleb usually filters through the conjunctiva, mixes with the tear film, or is absorbed by vascular or perivascular conjunctival tissue.[132–136]

2) Transscleral (or intrascleral bleb) outflow: this mechanism was proposed by Kozlov when describing DS with collagen implant.[109] Formation of an intrascleral "bleb" relies on the presence of a space-occupying device or implant (i.e., collagen implant, reticulated hyaluronic implant, etc.) in the scleral lake during the period of maximal healing response.[129] As the eye heals after DS, these devices, such as the collagen implant, slowly resorb within 6–9 months,[117,130] leaving behind an intrascleral aqueous lake.[115] UBM clearly showed that an intrascleral cavity was observed in 47%[117] of the cases implanted with reticulated hyaluronic acid implant and 92.8%[131] of the cases with collagen implant implantation 1 year after DS (Figure 2.11A, "ds" = decompression

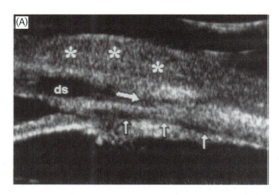

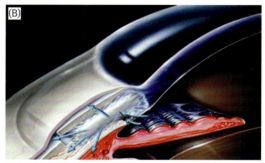

FIGURE 2.11 (A) Ultrasound biomicroscopy of an eye 12 months after deep sclerectomy surgery (DS) with reticulated hyaluronic acid implant (RHAI). New outflow pathways are shown and are as follows: a filtering bleb (asterisks), the decompression space (ds) or scleral lake, and a thin supraciliary hypoechoic area (small vertical arrows). There is also an area of scleral hyporeflectivity next to the decompression space (large arrow). (From Marchini et al 2001[117], with permission of Elsevier) (B) Schematic of an eye after deep sclerectomy surgery. The arrows illustrate the new aqueous outflow mechanisms. (With permission of STAAR® Surgical Company, Monrovia, California)

space or scleral lake). The T-Flux® NV implant is a nonabsorbable T-shaped hydrophilic acrylic device that creates a permanent intrascleral space maintained by the 2 arms at the top of the "T," which are inserted into SC. In theory, this device may promote intrascleral and physiologic aqueous drainage after DS.[121]

Aqueous in the intrascleral bleb or lake might also be resorbed by new aqueous drainage vessels, as showed by Delarive et al in an animal study.[137] In this study, DS was performed on rabbit eyes, and light microscopy revealed the appearance of new aqueous drainage vessels in the sclera adjacent to the dissection site of the DS.

3) Uveoscleral outflow: UBM has demonstrated a persistent supraciliary or suprachoroidal hypoechoic area in 45.2%–60% of DS cases with device implantation (Figure 2.11A, small vertical arrows), which suggests that some aqueous may drain through the uveoscleral pathway after DS.[117,121,130,131]

Despite the aforementioned outflow pathways, sometimes insufficient filtration occurs at the level of the trabeculo-Descemet's membrane (TDM) after DS. In these cases, Nd:YAG goniopuncture of the TDM can be performed.[110,125,138,139] This laser procedure is a safe and successful method to lower IOP after DS surgery,[139] and one or 2 laser applications through the TDM are usually sufficient to effectively convert this non-penetrating surgery to a penetrating operation.[140]

A final potential mechanism of IOP reduction after DS is chronic localized ciliary body detachment, which would result in decreased aqueous production.[129]

The complicated mechanism of aqueous drainage after DS has been studied by many researchers. In summary, aqueous drainage after DS initially occurs from the anterior chamber and then through anterior TM and Descemet's membrane to the scleral lake. After reaching the scleral lake, the aqueous may drain via 3 potential pathways: 1) through the classic subconjunctival filtering bleb; 2) through transscleral or intrascleral bleb outflow; or 3) through uveoscleral outflow (Figure 2.11B). Future studies with longer follow-up may clarify or reveal other mechanisms of DS outflow. For more information on DS, see Chapter 52.

Viscocanalostomy/Canaloplasty

Viscocanalostomy was described by Stegman in the late 1990s.[141] Although there is some variation among viscocanalostomy techniques, the procedure basically involves creation of a superficial and deep scleral flap, excision of the deep scleral flap, and unroofing of SC.

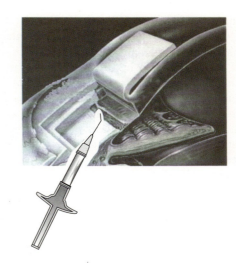

FIGURE 2.12 **Schematic of viscocanalostomy surgery**. After making a superficial scleral flap and removing a deep scleral flap, viscoelastic is injected into Schlemm's canal. (With permission of STAAR® Surgical Company, Monrovia, California)

After SC is entered, a high-viscosity viscoelastic is injected into both sides of SC, utilizing a delicate cannula to dilate part of SC (Figure 2.12). The superficial scleral flap is then closed with sutures.[141]

A variation of viscocanalostomy called canaloplasty uses a flexible microcatheter (iTrack 250A™ Canaloplasty Microcatheter, iScience Interventional™, Menlo Park, California), which is threaded into SC and dilates the full circumference of the canal while injecting viscoelastic substance during catheterization.[142] Therefore, a key difference between viscocanalostomy and canaloplasty is that canaloplasty opens the entire length of SC and not just one section of it. In canaloplasty, the SC is identified. The fiberoptic microcatheter then cannulates the entire length of SC under the guidance of an illuminated tip. Once the end of the catheter travels the full circumference of SC and reappears at the incision site, a 10–0 polypropylene suture is tied to the distal tip of the microcatheter. The microcatheter and attached suture are then withdrawn through the SC, as viscoelastic is simultaneously injected from the microcatheter to inflate the canal. After the suture is threaded 360 degrees through SC, the ends of the suture are tied using a slipknot. The intra-canalicular suture is ultimately meant to cinch and stretch the TM inwards in order to permanently open SC. Once the suture tension is adjusted to an appropriate amount of inward distention of TM, as confirmed by intraoperative UBM, locking knots are thrown.[142] The scleral flap and conjunctiva are then both tightly closed.

The intended goal of viscocanalostomy is to enlarge SC with viscoelastic and thereby enhance aqueous egress through the cut ends of SC and through previously non-functional areas of SC and aqueous collector channels.[104,110,129,138,141,143] In viscocanalostomy,

the partial-thickness scleral flap is also tightly sutured so that no aqueous outflow occurs through this flap. Enhanced out-flow occurs only through SC and its collector channels.[104,110,129,138,141]

Histology studies of both postmortem human eyes and monkey eyes have shown that injection of viscoelastic agents significantly increases the cross-sectional area of SC (Figure 2.13).[143,144] However, another study of monkey and human eyes demonstrated disruption of the wall and internal structures of SC after viscoelastic injection.[145] Disruption of these tissues by excessive dilation of SC may transiently enhance aqueous outflow, in that disruption of the posterior wall of SC

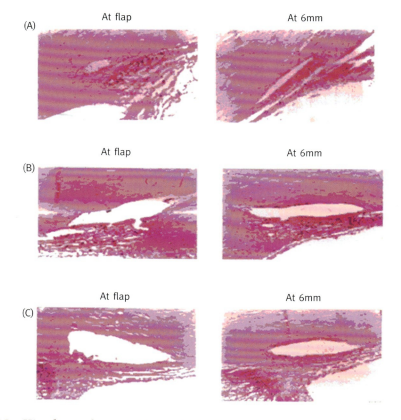

FIGURE 2.13 **Histologic changes of the Schlemm's canal with viscocanalostomy.** (A) Light photomicrographs of Schlemm's canal in normal postmortem human eyes without viscoelastic injection. The left column represents the eye at the site of the scleral flap, and the right column represents an area of Schlemm's canal 6 mm away from the flap site. (B) Light photomicrographs after injection of Healon GV® (Abbott Medical Optics, Inc., Santa Ana, California) and (C) Healon 5® (Abbott Medical Optics, Inc., Santa Ana, California). (From Wild et al 2001[143], with permission of Elsevier)

may provide direct communication between the lumen of SC and the tissues of the ciliary muscle and therefore enhance uveoscleral outflow.[145] In a pilot study of the iScience™ catheter in NPGS, better IOP control was achieved in the group undergoing dilation of 360 degrees of SC (80%) versus the group undergoing only one or 2 focal dilations of SC (63.6%).[146,145] Although the mechanism of canaloplasty is similar to that of viscocanalostomy, researchers have detected a trend toward improved IOP control with progressively greater lengths of the canal treated.[142,146] In addition, a tensioning suture placed within SC may potentially increase TM permeability.[142]

For more information on canaloplasty, see Chapter 51, and for more information on viscocanalostomy, see Chapter 52.

CONCLUSION

Angle glaucoma surgeries include goniotomy, trabeculotomy *ab externo*, trabeculodialysis, goniosynechiolysis, and *ab interno* trabeculectomy (Trabectome®). These procedures either incise trabecular tissue to reopen the pathway of aqueous into SC or remove iris-PAS tissue away from the TM face so that aqueous can better enter through TM into SC. As a result, outflow facility is increased, and IOP is decreased.

There are also 2 main forms of NPGS: DS and viscocanalostomy/canaloplasty. These 2 types of NPGS have different mechanisms for improving aqueous outflow. In DS, aqueous outflow initially occurs through the anterior TM and Descemet's membrane. The aqueous may then exit the eye through the subconjunctival filtering bleb, transscleral (or intrascleral bleb) outflow, or uveoscleral outflow. In viscocanalostomy or canaloplasty, however, aqueous outflow is enhanced through an enlarged SC and also possibly through previously nonfunctional aqueous collector channels. With canaloplasty, an additional tensioning suture may potentially increase TM permeability.

REFERENCES

1. Bill A, Phillips CI. Uveoscleral drainage of aqueous humour in human eyes. *Exp Eye Res.* Nov 1971;12(3):275–281.

2. Jocson VL, Sears ML. Experimental aqueous perfusion in enucleated human eyes. Results after obstruction of Schlemm's canal. *Arch Ophthalmol.* Jul 1971;86(1):65–71.

3. Inomata H, Bill A. Exit sites of uveoscleral flow of aqueous humor in cynomolgus monkey eyes. *Exp Eye Res.* Aug 1977;25(2):113–118.

4. Pederson JE, Gaasterland DE, MacLellan HM. Uveoscleral aqueous outflow in the rhesus monkey: importance of uveal reabsorption. *Invest Ophthalmol Vis Sci.* Nov 1977;16(11):1008–1007.

5. Stamper RL, Marc FL, MIchael VD. Developmental and childhood glaucoma. In: Stamper RL, Marc FL, Michael VD, eds. *Becker-Shaffer's Diagnosis and Therapy of the Glaucomas.* 7th ed. Beijing: Harcourt Asia & Mosby; 2001:361–412.

6. Lutjen-Drecoll E, Shimizu T, Rohrbach M, Rohen JW. Quantitative analysis of 'plaque material' in the inner- and outer wall of Schlemm's canal in normal- and glau-comatous eyes. *Exp Eye Res.* May 1986;42(5):443–455.

7. Rohen JW. Why is intraocular pressure elevated in chronic simple glaucoma? Anatomical considerations. *Ophthalmology.* Jul 1983;90(7):758–765.

8. Segawa K. Electron microscopic changes of the trabecular tissue in primary open-angle glaucoma. *Ann Ophthalmol.* Jan 1979;11(1):49–54.

9. Stamper RL, Marc FL, Michael VD. Primary open-angle glaucoma. In: Stamper RL, Marc FL, Michael VD, eds. *Becker-Shaffer's Diagnosis and Therapy of the Glaucomas.* 7th ed. Beijing: Harcourt Asia & Mosby; 2001:286–316.

10. Zimmerman LE. The outflow problem in normal and pathologic eyes. *Trans Am Acad Ophthalmol Otolaryngol.* Sept-Oct 1966;70(5):767–776.

11. Alvarado J, Murphy C, Juster R. Trabecular meshwork cellularity in primary open-angle glaucoma and nonglaucomatous normals. *Ophthalmology.* Jun 1984;91(6):564–579.

12. Allingham RR, de Kater AW, Ethier CR, Anderson PJ, Hertzmark E, Epstein DL. The relationship between pore density and outflow facility in human eyes. *Invest Ophthalmol Vis Sci.* Apr 1992;33(5):1661–1669.

13. Rohen JW, van der Zypen E. The phagocytic activity of the trabecularmeshwork endothelium. An electron-microscopic study of the vervet (Cercopithecus aethiops). *Albrecht Von Graefes Arch Klin Exp Ophthalmol.* 1968;175(2):143–160.

14. Shields MB. Classification of the glaucomas. *Textbook of Glaucoma*. 4th ed. Philadelphia, PA: Lippincott Williams & Wilkins; 2000:145–152.
15. Stamper RL, Marc FL, Michael VD. Angle-closure glaucoma with pupillary block. In: Stamper RL, Marc FL, Michael VD, eds. *Becker-Shaffer's Diagnosis and Therapy of the Glaucomas*. 7th ed. Beijing: Harcourt Asia & Mosby; 2001:216–246.
16. Barkan O. A new operation for chronic glaucoma. *Am J Ophthalmol*. 1936;19:951.
17. Barkan O. Operation for congenital glaucoma. *Am J Ophthalmol*. 1942;25:552–568.
18. Douglas DH. Reflections on buphthalmos and goniotomy. *Trans Ophthalmol Soc U K*. 1970;90:931–937.
19. Gramer E, Tausch M, Kraemer C. Time of diagnosis, reoperations and long-term results of goniotomy in the treatment of primary congenital glaucoma: a clinical study. *Int Ophthalmol*. 1996;20(1–3):117–123.
20. Moller PM. Goniotomy and congenital glaucoma. *Acta Ophthalmol (Copenh)*. Jun 1977;55(3):436–442.
21. Shaffer RN. Prognosis of goniotomy in primary infantile glaucoma (trabeculodysgenesis). *Trans Am Ophthalmol Soc*. 1982;80:321–325.
22. Freedman SF, Rodriguez-Rosa RE, Rojas MC, Enyedi LB. Goniotomy for glaucoma secondary to chronic childhood uveitis. *Am J Ophthalmol*. May 2002;133(5):617–621.
23. Ho CL, Walton DS. Goniosurgery for glaucoma secondary to chronic anterior uveitis: prognostic factors and surgical technique. *J Glaucoma*. Dec 2004;13(6):445–449.
24. Wallace DK, Plager DA, Snyder SK, Raiesdana A, Helveston EM, Ellis FD. Surgical results of secondary glaucomas in childhood. *Ophthalmology*. Jan 1998;105(1):101–111.
25. Chen TC, Walton DS. Goniosurgery for prevention of aniridic glaucoma. *Arch Ophthalmol*. Sept 1999;117(9):1144–1148.
26. Walton DS. Aniridic glaucoma: the results of gonio-surgery to prevent and treat this problem. *Trans Am Ophthalmol Soc*. 1986;84:59–70.
27. Broughton WL, Parks MM. An analysis of treatment of congenital glaucoma by gonio-tomy. *Am J Ophthalmol*. May 1981;91(5):566–572.
28. Draeger J, Wirt H, Ahrens V. [Long-term results following goniotomy in congenital glaucoma]. *Klin Monatsbl Augenheilkd*. Dec 1984;185(6):481–489.
29. Francois J, Van Oye R, Mendoza A, de Sutter E. [Goniotomy in congenital glaucoma]. *J Fr Ophtalmol*. 1982;5(11):661–664.
30. Promesberger H, Busse H, Mewe L. [Findings and surgical therapy in congenital glaucoma (author's transl)]. *Klin Monatsbl Augenheilkd*. Jan 1980;176(1):186–190.
31. Shields MB. Congenital glaucomas. *Shields' Textbook of Glaucoma*. 4th ed. Philadelphia, PA: Lippincott Williams & Wilkins; 2000:145–152.
32. Grant WM, Walton DS. Progressive changes in the angle in congenital aniridia, with development of glaucoma. *Am J Ophthalmol*. Nov 1974;78(5):842–847.
33. Barkan O. Goniotomy knife and surgical contact glass. *AMA Arch Ophthalmol*. Sept 1950;44(3):431–433.
34. Chen TC, Walton DS. Goniotomy. In: Chen TC, ed. *Surgical Techniques in Ophthalmology: Glaucoma Surgery*. Philadellphia, PD: Saunders Elsevier; 2008:153–163.
35. Hodapp E, Heuer DK. A simple technique for goniotomy. *Am J Ophthalmol*. Oct 1986;102(4):537.
36. Anderson DR. Pathology of the glaucomas. *Br J Ophthalmol*. Mar 1972;56(3):146–157.
37. Anderson DR. The development of the trabecular meshwork and its abnormality in primary infantile glaucoma. *Trans Am Ophthalmol Soc*. 1981;79:458–485.
38. Kupfer C, Kaiser-Kupfer MI. Observations on the development of the anterior chamber angle with reference to the pathogenesis of congenital glaucomas. *Am J Ophthalmol*. Sept 1979;88(3 Pt 1):424–426.
39. Maumenee AE. The pathogenesis of congenital glaucoma: a new theory. *Trans Am Ophthalmol Soc*. 1958;56:507–570.
40. Maumenee AE. Further observations on the pathogenesis of congenital glaucoma. *Am J Ophthalmol*. Jun 1963;55:1163–1176.
41. Maul E, Strozzi L, Munoz C, Reyes C. The outflow pathway in congenital glaucoma. *Am J Ophthalmol*. May 1980;89(5):667–673.
42. Sampaolesi R, Argento C. Scanning electron microscopy of the trabecular meshwork in normal and glucomatous eyes. *Invest Ophthalmol Vis Sci*. Apr 1977;16(4):302–314.
43. Smelser GK, Ozanics V. The development of the trabecular meshwork in primate eyes. *Am J Ophthalmol*. Jan 1971;1(1 Part 2):366–385.
44. Tawara A, Inomata H. Developmental immaturity of the trabecular meshwork in congenital glaucoma. *Am J Ophthalmol*. Oct 1981;92(4):508–525.
45. Rodrigues MM, Spaeth GL, Weinreb S. Juvenile glaucoma associated with goniodysgenesis. *Am J Ophthalmol*. Jun 1976;81(6):786–796.

46. Walton DS, Katsavounidou G. Newborn primary congenital glaucoma: 2005 update. *J Pediatr Ophthalmol Strabismus.* Nov-Dec 2005;42(6):333–341; quiz 365–336.

47. Azuara-Blanco A, Spaeth GL, Araujo SV, et al. Ultrasound biomicroscopy in infantile glaucoma. *Ophthalmology.* Jul 1997;104(7):1116–1119.

48. Dietlein TS, Engels BF, Jacobi PC, Krieglstein GK. Ultrasound biomicroscopic patterns after glaucoma surgery in congenital glaucoma. *Ophthalmology.* Jun 2000;107(6):1200–1205.

49. Stamper RL, Marc FL, Michael VD. Other outflow surgeries and surgical techniques. In: Stamper RL, Marc FL, Michael VD, eds. *Becker-Shaffer's Diagnosis and Therapy of the Glaucomas.* 7th ed. Beijing: Harcourt Asia & Mosby; 2001:662–676.

50. Allen L, Burian HM. Trabeculotomy ab externo. A new glaucoma operation: technique and results of experimental surgery. *Am J Ophthalmol.* Jan 1962;53:19–26.

51. Burian HM. A case of Marfan's syndrome with bilateral glaucoma. With description of a new type of operation for developmental glaucoma (trabeculotomy ab externo). *Am J Ophthalmol.* Dec 1960;50:1187–1192.

52. Smith R. A new technique for opening the canal of Schlemm. Preliminary report. *Br J Ophthalmol.* Jun 1960;44:370–373.

53. Smith R. Nylon filament trabeculotomy in glaucoma. *Trans Ophthalmol Soc U K.* 1962; 82:439–454.

54. Smith R. The comparison between a group of drainage operations and trabeculotomy, after a follow-up of five years. *Trans Ophthalmol Soc U K.* 1970;89:511–518.

55. Harms H, Dannheim R. Trabeculotomy 'ab externo'. *Trans Ophthalmol Soc U K.* 1970; 89:589–590.

56. Harms H, Dannheim R. Epicritical consideration of 300 cases of trabeculotomy 'ab externo'. *Trans Ophthalmol Soc U K.* 1970;89:491–499.

57. McPherson SD, Jr. Results of external trabeculotomy. *Am J Ophthalmol.* Dec 1973;76(6): 918–920.

58. Shrader CE, Clibis GW. External trabeculotomy. In: Thomas JV, Belcher CD, Simmons RJ, eds. *Glaucoma Surgery.* St. Louis, MO: Mosby Year Book; 1992:123–131.

59. Beck AD. Trabeculotomy. In: Chen TC, ed. *Surgical Techniques in Ophthalmology: Glaucoma Surgery.* Philadelphia, PD: Saunders Elsevier; 2008:165–178.

60. Tanihara H, Negi A, Akimoto M, et al. Surgical effects of trabeculotomy ab externo on adult eyes with primary open angle glaucoma and pseudoexfoliation syndrome. *Arch Ophthalmol.* Dec 1993;111(12):1653–1661.

61. Gimbel HV, Meyer D. Small incision trabeculotomy combined with phacoemulsification and intraocular lens implantation. *J Cataract Refract Surg.* Jan 1993;19(1):92–96.

62. Tanihara H, Negi A, Akimoto M, Nagata M. Long-term surgical results of combined trabeculotomy ab externo and cataract extraction. *Ophthalmic Surg.* Jul-Aug 1995; 26(4):316–324.

63. Grehn F. The value of trabeculotomy in glaucoma surgery. *Curr Opin Ophthalmol.* Apr 1995;6(2):52–60.

64. Becker B, Podos SM, Asseff CF. Symposium: microsurgery of the outflow channels. Clinical research. *Trans Am Acad Ophthalmol Otolaryngol.* Mar-Apr 1972;76(2):405–410.

65. Dannheim R, Barany EH. The effect of trabeculotomy in normal eyes of rhesus and cynomolgus monkeys studied by anterior chamber perfusion. *Doc Ophthalmol.* 1969;26: 90–107.

66. Ellingsen BA, Grant WM. Influence of intraocular pressure and trabeculotomy on aqueous outflow in enucleated monkey eyes. *Invest Ophthalmol.* Sept 1971;10(9):705–709.

67. Ellingsen BA, Grant WM. Trabeculotomy and sinusotomy in enucleated human eyes. *Invest Ophthalmol.* Jan 1972;11(1):21–28.

68. d'Epinay SL, Reme C. [Histopathological aspects of the surgical treatment of congenital glaucoma]. *Klin Monatsbl Augenheilkd.* Apr 1980;176(4):566–568.

69. Dellaporta A. The surgical separation of the corneoscleral trabeculum from its bed. I. Anterior trabeculodialysis. *Am J Ophthalmol.* Jun 1959;47(6):783–795.

70. Grant WM. Experimental aqueous perfusion in enucleated human eyes. *Arch Ophthalmol.* Jun 1963;69:783–801.

71. Johnson M, Shapiro A, Ethier CR, Kamm RD. Modulation of outflow resistance by the pores of the inner wall endothelium. *Invest Ophthalmol Vis Sci.* Apr 1992;33(5):1670–1675.

72. Maepea O, Bill A. Pressures in the juxtacanalicular tissue and Schlemm's canal in monkeys. *Exp Eye Res.* Jun 1992;54(6): 879–883.

73. Murphy CG, Johnson M, Alvarado JA. Juxtacanalicular tissue in pigmentary and primary open angle glaucoma. The hydrodynamic role of pigment and other constituents. *Arch Ophthalmol.* Dec 1992;110(12):1779–1785.

74. Herschler J, Davis EB. Modified goniotomy for inflammatory glaucoma. Histologic evidence for the mechanism of pressure reduction. *Arch Ophthalmol.* Apr 1980;98(4):684–687.

75. Hoskins HD, Hetherington J, Shaffer RN. Surgical management of the inflammatory glaucoma. *Perspect Ophthalmol.* 1977;1:173–181.

76. Kanski JJ, McAllister JA. Trabeculodialysis for inflammatory glaucoma in children and young adults. *Ophthalmology.* Jul 1985;92(7):927–930.

77. Walton DS. Goniotomy. In: Thomas JV, Belcher CD, Simmons RJ, eds. *Glaucoma Surgery.* St. Louis, MO: Mosby Year Book; 1992:107–122.

78. Williams RD, Hoskins HD, Shaffer RN. Trabeculodialysis for inflammatory glaucoma: a review of 25 cases. *Ophthalmic Surg.* Jan 1992;23(1):36–37.

79. Dellaporta A. The surgical separation of the corneoscleral trabeculum from its bed. II. Posterior trabeculodialysis. *Am J Ophthalmol.* Jul 1959;48(1, Part 1):15–21.

80. Dellaporta A. Evaluation of anterior and posterior trabeculodialysis. *Am J Ophthalmol.* Sept 1959;2 48(3), Part:294–309.

81. Campbell DG, Vela A. Modern goniosynechialysis for the treatment of synechial angle-closure glaucoma. *Ophthalmology.* Sept 1984;91(9):1052–1060.

82. Shingleton BJ, Chang MA, Bellows AR, Thomas JV. Surgical goniosynechialysis for angle-closure glaucoma. *Ophthalmology.* May 1990;97(5):551–556.

83. Tanihara H, Nishiwaki K, Nagata M. Surgical results and complications of goniosynechialysis. *Graefes Arch Clin Exp Ophthalmol.* 1992;230(4):309–313.

84. Yoshimura N, Iwaki M. Goniosynechialysis for secondary angle-closure glaucoma after previously failed filtering procedures. *Am J Ophthalmol.* Oct 1988;106(4):493.

85. Chen TC, RojanaPongpun P, Walton DS. Goniosynechialysis. In: Chen TC, ed. *Surgical Techniques in Ophthalmology: Glaucoma Surgery.* Philadellphia, PD: Saunders Elsevier; 2008:179–184.

86. Sharpe ED, Thomas JV, Simmons RJ. Goniosynechialysis. In: Thomas JV, Belcher CD, Simmons RJ, eds. *Glaucoma Surgery.* St. Louis, MO: Mosby Year Book; 1992:245–249.

87. Shaffer RN. Operating room gonioscopy in angle closure glaucoma surgery. *Trans Am Ophthalmol Soc.* 1957;55:59–64; discussion 64–56.

88. Canlas OA, Ishikawa H, Liebmann JM, Tello C, Ritch R. Ultrasound biomicroscopy before and after goniosynechialysis. *Am J Ophthalmol.* Oct 2001;132(4):570–571.

89. Chandler PA, Simmons RJ. Anterior chamber deepening for gonioscopy at time of surgery. *Arch Ophthalmol.* Aug 1965;74:177–190.

90. Harasymowycz PJ, Papamatheakis DG, Ahmed I, et al. Phacoemulsification and goniosynechialysis in the management of unresponsive primary angle closure. *J Glaucoma.* Jun 2005;14(3):186–189.

91. Lai JS, Tham CC, Chua JK, Lam DS. Efficacy and safety of inferior 180 degrees goniosynechialysis followed by diode laser peripheral iridoplasty in the treatment of chronic angle-closure glaucoma. *J Glaucoma.* Oct 2000;9(5):388–391.

92. Lai JS, Tham CC, Lam DS. The efficacy and safety of combined phacoemulsification, intraocular lens implantation, and limited goniosynechialysis, followed by diode laser peripheral iridoplasty, in the treatment of cataract and chronic angle-closure glaucoma. *J Glaucoma.* Aug 2001;10(4):309–315.

93. Baerveldt G, Chuck R, inventors; The Regents of the University of California, assignee. Minimally Invasive Glaucoma Surgical Instrument and Method. US patent 6,979,328. Dec. 27, 2005.

94. Minckler DS, Baerveldt G, Alfaro MR, Francis BA. Clinical results with the Trabectome for treatment of open-angle glaucoma. *Ophthalmology.* Jun 2005;112(6):962–967.

95. Francis BA, Minckler D, Dustin L, et al. Combined cataract extraction and trabeculotomy by the internal approach for coexisting cataract and open-angle glaucoma: initial results. *J Cataract Refract Surg.* Jul 2008;34(7):1096–1103.

96. Minckler D, Baerveldt G, Ramirez MA, et al. Clinical results with the Trabectome®, a novel surgical device for treatment of open-angle glaucoma. *Trans Am Ophthalmol Soc.* 2006;104:40–50.

97. Francis BA, See RF, Rao NA, Minckler DS, Baerveldt G. Ab interno trabeculectomy: development of a novel device (Trabectome) and surgery for open-angle glaucoma. *J Glaucoma.* Feb 2006;15(1):68–73.

98. Hirano K, Kobayashi M, Kobayashi K, Hoshino T, Awaya S. Age-related changes of microfibrils in the cornea and trabecular meshwork of the human eye. *Jpn J Ophthalmol.* 1991;35(2):166–174.

99. Nguyen QH. Trabectome®: a novel approach to angle surgery in the treatment of glaucoma. *Int Ophthalmol Clin*. Fall 2008;48(4):65–72.

100. Filippopoulos T, Rhee DJ. Novel surgical procedures in glaucoma: advances in penetrating glaucoma surgery. *Curr Opin Ophthalmol*. Mar 2008;19(2):149–154.

101. Gunderson E. Trabeculotomy Ab Interno, using the Trabectome®: a promising treatment for patients with open-angle glaucoma. *Insight*. Jan-Mar 2008;33(1):13–15.

102. Krasnov MM. [Sinusotomy in Glaucoma.]. *Vestn Oftalmol*. Mar-Apr 1964;77:37–41.

103. Krasnov MM. Externalization of Schlemm's canal (sinusotomy) in glaucoma. *Br J Ophthalmol*. Feb 1968;52(2):157–161.

104. Mermoud A. Sinusotomy and deep sclerectomy. *Eye*. Jun 2000;14 (Pt 3B):531–535.

105. Zimmerman TJ, Kooner KS, Ford VJ, et al. Trabeculectomy vs. nonpenetrating trabeculectomy: a retrospective study of two procedures in phakic patients with glaucoma. *Ophthalmic Surg*. Sept 1984;15(9):734–740.

106. Zimmerman TJ, Kooner KS, Ford VJ, et al. Effectiveness of nonpenetrating trabeculectomy in aphakic patients with glaucoma. *Ophthalmic Surg*. Jan 1984;15(1):44–50.

107. Gandolfi SA, Cimino L. Non-penetrating vs penetrating surgery of primary open-angle glaucoma. In: Grehn F, Stamper R, eds. *Glaucoma*. Berlin: Springer; 2004:209–215.

108. Fyodorov SN. Non-penetrating deep sclerectomy in open angle glaucoma. *Eye Microsurg*. 1989;1:52–55.

109. Koslov VI, Bagrov SN, Anisimova SY, et al. Nonpenetrating deep sclerectomy with collagen. *IRTC Eye Microsurg*. 1990;1(44–46).

110. Lachkar Y, Hamard P. Nonpenetrating filtering surgery. *Curr Opin Ophthalmol*. Apr 2002;13(2):110–115.

111. Demailly P, Lavat P, Kretz G, Jeanteur-Lunel MN. Nonpenetrating deep sclerectomy (NPDS) with or without collagen device (CD) in primary open-angle glaucoma. *Int Ophthalmol*. Jan 1996;20(1–3):131–140.

112. Karlen ME, Sanchez E, Schnyder CC, Sickenberg M, Mermoud A. Deep sclerectomy with collagen implant: medium term results. *Br J Ophthalmol*. Jan 1999;83(1):6–11.

113. Kershner RM. Nonpenetrating trabeculectomy with placement of a collagen drainage device. *J Cataract Refract Surg*. Nov 1995; 21(6):608–611.

114. Mermoud A, Schnyder CC, Sickenberg M, Chiou AG, Hediguer SE, Faggioni R. Comparison of deep sclerectomy with collagen implant and trabeculectomy in open-angle glaucoma. *J Cataract Refract Surg*. Mar 1999; 25(3):323–331.

115. Sanchez E, Schnyder CC, Sickenberg M, Chiou AGY, Mediguer SEA, Mermoud A. Deep sclerectomy: results with and without collagen implant. *Int Ophthalmol*. Jan 1996; 20(1–3):157–162.

116. Shaarawy T, Karlen M, Schnyder C, Achache F, Sanchez E, Mermoud A. Five-year results of deep sclerectomy with collagen implant. *J Cataract Refract Surg*. Nov 2001;27(11): 1770–1778.

117. Marchini G, Marraffa M, Brunelli C, Morbio R, Bonomi L. Ultrasound biomicroscopy and intraocular-pressure-lowering mechanisms of deep sclerectomy with reticulated hyaluronic acid implant. *J Cataract Refract Surg*. Apr 2001;27(4):507–517.

118. Sourdille P, Santiago PY, Villain F, et al. Reticulated hyaluronic acid implant in nonperforating trabecular surgery. *J Cataract Refract Surg*. Mar 1999;25(3):332–339.

119. Auer C, Mermoud A, Herbort CP. Deep sclerectomy for the management of uncontrolled uveitic glaucoma: preliminary data. *Klin Monatsbl Augenheilkd*. May 2004; 221(5):339–342.

120. Drolsum L. Conversion from trabeculectomy to deep sclerectomy. Prospective study of the first 44 cases. *J Cataract Refract Surg*. Jul 2003;29(7):1378–1384.

121. Ravinet E, Bovey E, Mermoud A. T-Flux® implant versus Healon GV® in deep sclerectomy. *J Glaucoma*. Feb 2004;13(1):46–50.

122. Devloo S, Deghislage C, Van Malderen L, Goethals M, Zeyen T. Non-penetrating deep sclerectomy without or with autologous scleral implant in open-angle glaucoma: medium-term results. *Graefes Arch Clin Exp Ophthalmol*. Dec 2005;243(12):1206–1212.

123. Mousa AS. Preliminary evaluation of nonpenetrating deep sclerectomy with autologous scleral implant in open-angle glaucoma. *Eye*. Sept 2007;21(9):1234–1238.

124. Russo V, Scott IU, Stella A, et al. Nonpenetrating deep sclerectomy with reticulated hyaluronic acid implant versus punch trabeculectomy: a prospective clinical trial. *Eur J Ophthalmol*. Sept-Oct 2008;18(5):751–757.

125. Hara T. Deep sclerectomy with Nd:YAG laser trabeculotomy ab interno: two-stage procedure. *Ophthalmic Surg*. Feb 1988;19(2): 101–106.

126. Vaudaux J, Mermoud A. Aqueous dynamics after deep sclerectomy. *Ophthalmol Practice.* 1998;16(5):204–209.

127. Spiegel D, Schefthaler M, Kobuch K. Outflow facilities through Descemet's membrane in rabbits. *Graefes Arch Clin Exp Ophthalmol.* Feb 2002;240(2):111–113.

128. Hamard P, Sourdille P, Valtot F, Baudouin C. [Evaluation of confocal microscopy in the analysis of the external trabecular membrane during deep nonpenetrating sclerectomy]. *J Fr Ophtalmol.* Jan 2001;24(1):29–35.

129. Shaarawy T, Flammer J. Pro: non-penetrating glaucoma surgery—a fair chance. *Graefes Arch Clin Exp Ophthalmol.* Sept 2003; 241(9):699–702.

130. Chiou AG, Mermoud A, Hediguer SE, Schnyder CC, Faggioni R. Ultrasound biomicroscopy of eyes undergoing deep sclerectomy with collagen implant. *Br J Ophthalmol.* Jun 1996;80(6):541–544.

131. Kazakova D, Roters S, Schnyder CC, et al. Ultrasound biomicroscopy images: long-term results after deep sclerectomy with collagen implant. *Graefes Arch Clin Exp Ophthalmol.* Nov 2002;240(11):918–923.

132. Allingham RR, Damji KF, Freedman S, Moroi SE, Shafranov G, Shields MB. Filtering surgery. *Shields' Textbook of Glaucoma.* 5th ed. Philadelphia: Lippincott Williams & Wilkins; 2005:568–609.

133. Benedikt O. [The effect of filtering operations (author's transl)]. *Klin Monatsbl Augenheilkd.* Jan 1977;170(1):10–19.

134. Galin MA, Baras I, McLean JM. How does a filtering bleb work? *Trans Am Acad Ophthalmol Otolaryngol.* Nov-Dec 1965;69(6): 1082–1091.

135. Kronfeld FC. The chemical demonstration of transconjunctival passage of aqueous after antiglaucomatous operations. *Am J Ophthalmol.* May 1952;35(5:2):38–45.

136. Teng CC, Chi HH, Katzin HM. Histology and mechanism of filtering operations. *Am J Ophthalmol.* Jan 1959;47(1 Part 1):16–33.

137. Delarive T, Rossier A, Rossier S, Ravinet E, Shaarawy T, Mermoud A. Aqueous dynamic and histological findings after deep sclerectomy with collagen implant in an animal model. *Br J Ophthalmol.* Nov 2003;87(11):1340–1344.

138. Goldsmith JA, Ahmed IK, Crandall AS. Nonpenetrating glaucoma surgery. *Ophthalmol Clin North Am.* Sept 2005;18(3):443–460, vii.

139. Mermoud A, Karlen ME, Schnyder CC, et al. Nd:Yag goniopuncture after deep sclerectomy with collagen implant. *Ophthalmic Surg Lasers.* Feb 1999;30(2):120–125.

140. Vuori ML. Complications of Neodymium: YAG laser goniopuncture after deep sclerectomy. *Acta Ophthalmol Scand.* Dec 2003;81(6): 573–576.

141. Stegmann R, Pienaar A, Miller D. Viscocanalostomy for open-angle glaucoma in black African patients. *J Cataract Refract Surg.* Mar 1999;25(3):316–322.

142. Lewis RA, von Wolff K, Tetz M, et al. Canaloplasty: circumferential viscodilation and tensioning of Schlemm's canal using a flexible microcatheter for the treatment of open-angle glaucoma in adults: interim clinical study analysis. *J Cataract Refract Surg.* Jul 2007;33(7):1217–1226.

143. Wild GJ, Kent AR, Peng Q. Dilation of Schlemm's canal in viscocanalostomy: comparison of 2 viscoelastic substances. *J Cataract Refract Surg.* Aug 2001;27(8):1294–1297.

144. Lundgren BO, Scampini G, Wickstrom K, Stegmann R. Histopathological evaluation in monkey eyes of the viscocanalostomy technique. ARVO abstract 438. *Invest Ophthalmol Vis Sci.* 2000;41(4):S83.

145. Smit BA, Johnstone MA. Effects of viscoelastic injection into Schlemm's canal in primate and human eyes: potential relevance to viscocanalostomy. *Ophthalmology.* Apr 2002;109(4):786–792.

146. Cameron B, Field M, Ball S, Kearney J. Circumferential viscodilation of Schlemm's canal with a flexible microcannula during non-penetrating glaucoma surgery. *Digit J Ophthalmol.* 2006;12(1).

147. Takanashi T, Masuda H, Tanito M, Nonoyama S, Katsube T, Ohira A. Scleral indentation optimizes visualization of anterior chamber angle during goniosynechialysis. *J Glaucoma.* Aug 2005;14(4):293–298.

PART TWO

WOUND HEALING IN GLAUCOMA

3

WOUND HEALING IN GLAUCOMA

KIMBERLY A. MANKIEWICZ, LEONARD K. SEIBOLD,
MALIK Y. KAHOOK AND MARK B. SHERWOOD

WOUND HEALING IN GLAUCOMA

The goal of wound healing in most surgeries is to bring the injured tissue back to its original state to prevent the wound from reopening. However, in glaucoma surgery, the goal is to have incomplete wound healing. Scar formation prevents the filtering mechanism and bleb from functioning properly, leading to poor pressure control and failure of the surgery. However, if there is too little wound healing, surgical failure may be marked by overfiltration and hypotony. Several modulators are currently used in conjunction with glaucoma surgery, and new targets are under investigation to improve our ability to control the healing process.

THREE PHASES OF WOUND HEALING

Normal wound healing occurs in 3 phases: the inflammatory phase, the proliferative/ repair phase, and the remodeling phase. In the inflammatory phase, blood cells and plasma proteins are released around the wound site. These proteins attract other wound healing factors, such as cytokines and growth factors. White blood cells are also recruited to the site, clearing out undesired cellular debris through phagocytosis. Additionally, platelet aggregation and fibrin clot formation occur. In the proliferative/repair phase, fibroblasts, crucial cells for tissue repair and scarring, begin reforming the extracellular matrix (ECM) and other components of connective tissue. Angiogenesis also occurs, and the wound begins to close. In the final phase, blood vessels are resorbed and fibroblasts disperse. Fibroblasts produce matrix metalloproteinases that, along with collagen and elastin, allowing for wound remodeling and scar formation. The modulators used in glaucoma surgery, as well as new agents in development, disrupt various aspects of this cycle.[1–5]

ANTI-INFLAMMATORIES

Corticosteroids

Use of topical corticosteroids in conjunction with filtering surgery is a routine part of postoperative management and has been for many decades. Corticosteroids blunt the wound healing response by altering the inflammatory phase through reducing the amount of inflammatory cells and cytokines that migrate to the wound site. Corticosteroids also prevent the complexing and conversion of inflammatory mediators, as well as reduce vascular permeability to limit mobility of wound healing factors to the wound site. All of these effects lead to reduced fibroblast activity and diminished scarring.[2,5,6]

Several studies have demonstrated that intraoperative and postoperative corticosteroids lead to higher success rates in filtering surgery. Addition of systemic corticosteroids provides no additional benefits.[6–10] Topical application is the most widely used and studied route,[6,7,9,10] while other routes have varied results.[11–13] Preoperative therapy may also be advantageous.[14–16] Reported complications of corticosteroid treatment include thin, cystic blebs, conjunctival thinning or melting, and increased scarring.[2,5,6] Cataract formation and infection are also known complications of corticosteroids.

Nonsteroidal anti-inflammatory drugs (NSAIDs)

NSAIDs operate by blocking cyclooxygenase conversion of arachidonic acid into inflammatory mediators and inhibiting platelet function and clotting.[6] Their use as an adjunct to filtering surgery has been suggested to be beneficial,[17] but further study is needed.

MITOMYCIN-C

Mitomycin-C (MMC) is a commonly used wound healing modulator in glaucoma filtration surgery (i.e., trabeculectomy). At the molecular level, MMC works by inhibiting DNA replication, mitosis, and protein synthesis, thereby preventing cell growth. Any phase of the cell cycle can be disrupted, and therefore MMC not only disrupts DNA replication but also protein synthesis.[1,2,6,18] At the cellular level, MMC has been shown to induce fibroblast apoptosis, thereby inhibiting fibroblast proliferation and migration. It also inhibits endothelial cell growth and replication and collagen contraction.[2,6,19] MMC has a half-life of 0.18–0.30 hours in the conjunctiva and 0.2–0.45 hours for sclera, with tissue levels minimal after 2–3 hours.[18] Despite the short half-life, MMC is extremely potent, with the effects on growth of cultured rabbit fibroblasts enduring at 1 month and chronic conjunctival tissue effects still observed many years later.[6,18]

MMC is extremely toxic, and its use can be associated with severe complications, which including thin-walled, avascular blebs, leading to increased transconjunctival filtration, with resultant lower intraocular pressure (IOP). However, taken to extremes, this morphology is also associated with hypotony, bleb leaks, and increased infection rates.[1,6,18,20–23] Toxicity effects can be seen on the conjunctival and episcleral vasculature, which has been hypothesized to cause the decreased vascularity of MMC-treated blebs.[1] Ciliary body toxicity,[1] scleritis,[24] scleromalacia,[25] and endothelial cell loss[26] have also been observed with MMC.

Despite these pitfalls, intraoperative MMC is an effective addition to filtering surgery. Its use is associated with lower IOP and a decreased need for IOP-lowering medications. In many trials, compared to procedures where no antifibrotic was used, MMC led to significantly better surgical success.[1,6,18,27]

5-FLUOROURACIL

5-fluorouracil (5-FU) is another wound healing modulator used in glaucoma filtering surgery. At the molecular level, 5-FU alters healing by inhibiting DNA synthesis though interfering with incorporation of thymine into DNA, resulting in cell death.[6,18,28] Unlike MMC, 5-FU's mechanism is cell cycle specific, only affecting S phase. 5-FU has also been shown to interfere with RNA synthesis, disrupt the actin cytoskeleton, and promote apoptosis of fibroblasts.[28] At the cellular level, 5-FU inhibits fibroblast proliferation. Fibroblasts are more sensitive to 5-FU than endothelial cells, while MMC is toxic to both. MMC is much more potent than 5-FU; in rabbit fibroblasts 5-FU has no effect after 7 days.[6]

5-FU is used currently intraoperatively or postoperatively.[29] Like MMC, 5-FU use can lead to serious complications. Corneal epithelial toxicity occurs due to 5-FU's effect on actively replicating tissue; changes are generally reversible. Bleb leaks, thin-walled and low resistance blebs, shallow anterior chamber, with all of their resultant sequelae (e.g., hypotony and endophthalmitis) can also occur with 5-FU use.[6,28,30–32]

Despite these complications, 5-FU use improves outcomes of glaucoma surgery. It has been shown to lower IOP and reduce the need for IOP-lowering medications. 5-FU has also been shown to improve success in cases of previously failed filtering surgery and in pseudophakic and aphakic eyes.[1,28,33] Overall, 5-FU use leads to lower failure rates, with the greatest benefit seen in the first 18 months.[34] After this initial period, the failure rate of filtering procedures with 5-FU occurs at a rate similar to cases where no antifibrotics are used, since fibrosis continues beyond the time of effect.[28,34]

MMC vs. 5-FU

Due to heterogeneity and differing patient populations, clinical trials for MMC and 5-FU are difficult to compare. Even so, these trials show a benefit to using MMC and 5-FU as adjuncts to filtering surgery.

One study determined that MMC was better in terms of IOP control and need for IOP-lowering medications; another found 5-FU to be better with normal tension glaucoma patients at a high risk of hypotony. MMC was also found to have better success in primary filtering surgeries. Complications are similar with both agents. No evidence currently in the literature definitely concludes which, or whether, one is better than the other. Each should be evaluated on a case-by-case basis.[1,18,28] However, because MMC is more potent and durable,[19,35,36] a single intraoperative application is usually adequate, whereas additional injections are occasionally required with intraoperative 5-FU.

WOUND HEALING MODULATORS IN TUBE SHUNTS

Antifibrotics, such as MMC and 5-FU, are not commonly used with tube shunt surgery, and therefore the literature is lacking on their use in this setting. However, based on the limited data, neither MMC nor 5-FU alter the outcome of tube shunt surgery.[6,18,28]

NEW WOUND HEALING MODULATORS

While MMC and 5-FU are the standard modulators used currently in glaucoma surgery, they are far from perfect. Because they are nonspecific inhibitors, these chemicals exert effects not only on those cells involved in wound healing but also on healthy cells. Additionally, the complications are often severe. New agents are being investigated in an attempt to decrease complications (thereby increasing surgical success) and find modulators targeted to only the desired cells in the healing process.

Anti-vascular Endothelial Growth Factor (VEGF) Agents

The wound healing process progresses due to fibroblast activity and angiogenesis. Vascular endothelial growth factor (VEGF) is present in large amounts after filtering surgery and plays a role in the healing process.[4,37] Bevacizumab (Avastin®, Genentech, Inc., South San Francisco, California) is a recombinant monoclonal immunoglobulin G1 antibody that inhibits VEGF activity. It is approved by the FDA for treatment of metastatic colorectal and breast cancer.[38] It is used off-label to treat eye conditions such as age-related macular degeneration, diabetic macular edema, neovascular glaucoma, and other diseases.[39,40] Ranibizumab (Lucentis®, Genentech, Inc., South San Francisco, California) is a higher affinity monoclonal antibody fragment (Fab) derived from bevacizumab and approved by the FDA for the treatment of age-related macular degeneration.[40]

Bevacizumab affects the migration and proliferation of blood vessels, as well as decreasing cytokine flow into the bleb during the inflammatory phase of wound healing. It also induces fibroblast apoptosis.[38,39] Additionally, because of its antiangiogenic properties, bevacizumab is hypothesized to affect the wound healing process by decreasing growth of new blood vessels, leading to a healthier bleb with less scarring.[39]

Elevated levels of VEGF have been found in the aqueous of eyes with primary open-angle glaucoma and also in the bleb and aqueous of post-trabeculectomy eyes. Upregulated levels of VEGF were found to stimulate fibroblast proliferation, suggesting that it is involved in the scarring process. Bevacizumab disrupted fibroblast proliferation and reduced angiogenesis and collagen deposition.[4,39] Postoperative injection of bevacizumab in rabbits increased survival time and improved morphology of trabeculectomy blebs.[41] Bevacizumab has also been reported to have a synergistic effect with 5-FU that leads to longer bleb survival in rabbits.[39,42]

Small studies in humans (fewer than 12 participants) have investigated the use of anti-VEGF agents as wound healing modulators. Subconjunctival bevacizumab was effective in lowering IOP after bleb needling and decreasing vascularization after bleb needling and cataract surgery.[43,44] Preoperative intravitreal bevacizumab before combined vitrectomy/trabeculectomy was reported to prevent intraoperative bleeding in eyes with neovascular glaucoma.[45] As an intraoperative adjunct, in conjunction with MMC, for high risk trabeculectomy in diabetic patients, this combination resulted in functioning filtering blebs with reduced IOP and no additional medications at 6 months.[46] In another study, primary trabeculectomy with bevacizumab as the only antifibrotic addition other than topical corticosteroids resulted in lowered IOP with a desirable bleb morphology and no adverse events.[47] In the first reported comparison of ranibizumab and MMC as adjuncts to filtration surgery, no difference in IOP was seen between the 2 groups (although both treatments lowered IOP), but bleb height and vascularity were significantly reduced in the ranibizumab group. No adverse events were reported with either treatment.[48] Anti-VEGF agents show promise as wound healing modulators, but further study is needed to investigate how to best utilize their properties.

Transforming Growth Factor-β (TGF-β) and Connective Tissue Growth Factor (CTGF)

TGF-β is a crucial regulator and stimulator of scarring in the eye. It plays a role in the synthesis and accumulation of ECM proteins (collagen, elastin, etc.) and is a potent chemoattractant for immune response cells. TGF-β also stimulates the activity of fibroblasts by its involvement in collagen contraction and fibroblast proliferation and migration.[2,49] Increased levels of TGF-β have been observed in many human fibrotic diseases in other organs (kidneys, liver, lungs, etc.).[50]

TGF-β has been hypothesized to increase ECM deposition in the trabecular meshwork. Additionally, TGF-β expression has been shown to be increased at the optic nerve head and hypothesized to be responsible for ECM remodeling at the lamina cribosa; it, therefore, may be potentially involved in optic disc cupping. Results of animal experiments have demonstrated that TGF-β is an important mediator of fibrosis. Of all the isoforms, TGF-β2 levels have been shown to be increased in glaucomatous eyes. TGF-β2 has also been shown to be expressed in the conjunctiva and appears to be a regulator of healing in the cornea. Treatment of skin incisions with TGF-β2 in rats promoted scar formation.[49,50]

CTGF has also been shown to be a regulator of scar formation as a mitogenic and chemoattractant for fibroblasts and a stimulator of ECM protein production in fibroblasts. CTGF has been found in cornea, conjunctiva, sclera, and uveal tissues. As with TGF-β, levels of CTGF are also increased in many fibrotic diseases.[51-53]

In observations of bleb tissue in rabbits with trabeculectomies, CTGF and TGF-β2 levels were found to be increased; these increased levels were found to be localized to the bleb and without elevated levels 180° away from the bleb.[54] Additionally, when CTGF and TGF-β2 were introduced to MMC-treated blebs, they increased the rate of bleb failure.[50] These studies further the conclusion that CTGF and TGF-β are important factors in the scarring process after filtering surgery.

The TGF-β and CTGF systems appear to be connected. Production of CTGF is induced by TGF-β, and antibodies/antisense oligo-nucleotides to CTGF block proliferation of fibroblasts mediated by TGF-β and increase synthesis of ECM proteins. Based on these observations, it appears that CTGF may be a downstream mediator for the TGF-β wound healing processes.[55] It has been hypothesized CTGF may control ECM deposition, a major contributor to wound healing, in a more direct fashion than TGF-β, making it a possible target for reducing scarring after glaucoma surgery.[50]

Research into how best to use TGF-β as a wound healing modulator is in the early stages. Initial studies in rabbits showed that neutralizing antibodies or antisense oligonucleotides to TGF-β resulted in longer bleb survival through reducing scar tissue and contraction of the bleb.[56] Similar results were also seen in other experimental studies.[57,58] A Phase I/IIa trial compared subconjunctival injections of TGF-β2 antibody preoperatively and postoperatively to placebo injections in patients at risk of bleb failure. This study showed no difference in complication rates between the 2 groups and no serious adverse events at 1 year of follow-up. The TGF-β2 blebs also appeared diffuse, noncystic, and avascular.[59] However, a Phase III study in patients undergoing primary trabeculectomy concluded there were no statistically significant differences in terms of IOP reduction, bleb failure, and bleb anatomical features with TGF-β2 injections as compared to placebo injections.[60]

Matrix Metalloproteinases (MMPs)

MMPs are a group of enzymes capable of cleaving ECM proteins. They are involved in fibroblast-mediated bleb contraction. Subconjunctival injections of ilomastat, a synthetic inhibitor of MMPs, significantly improved bleb survival and IOP in rabbits as compared to phosphate-buffered saline controls. Histology also showed reduced scarring.[61] When compared to MMC, ilomastat use resulted in a similar IOP, but ilomastat-treated tissues had more normal appearing conjunctiva. Bleb survival was also similar.[62] These studies show that MMPs are not only an important component of the wound healing process after filtering surgery, but they have the potential to be developed into wound healing modulators. As with TGF-β and CTGF,

further investigations are needed to elucidate their potential role in glaucoma surgery.

Suramin

Suramin is a growth factor inhibitor shown to have effects on platelet-derived growth factor, fibroblast growth factor, and TGF-β, among others.[63] Studies in rabbits showed increased bleb survival and decreased collagen synthesis and fibrosis.[64,65] One trial on 10 patients with advanced or complex glaucoma concluded that eyes treated with suramin had similar outcomes to MMC and superior outcomes compared to placebo. Hyperemic adverse events were an issue. However, due to the small sample size, safety could not be adequately assessed,[66] and there has been little recently published work on this agent.

Tranilast

Tranilast was first characterized as a histamine-release inhibitor and was subsequently found to inhibit growth factors and fibroblast stimulators.[67] Investigations in rabbits showed that tranilast decreased fibroblast numbers in Tenon's capsule and the cornea and also reduced collagen production.[68] In a pilot human study, topical postoperative use in patients undergoing primary trabeculectomy with MMC resulted in lower IOP and no difference in complications from controls.[69]

Photodynamic Therapy

In photodynamic therapy, a light-sensitive compound is injected into the eye and activated using a wavelength specific for the agent. This technique may potentially offer a way to modulate wound healing in a very selective tissue area. Small studies in humans have found that photodynamic therapy can improve surgical success with no complications reported,[70,71] but there has been little recent research reported on this area of wound healing modulation.

β-radiation

β-radiation is one potential technique being investigated as an alternative to the use of pharmacologic agents. Use of β-radiation has been found to have antiproliferative effects on Tenon's fibroblasts, obstruct cell growth, and change extracellular matrix production.[72–75] Some studies have shown a positive effect in terms of increased surgical success,[75,76] while others have shown no effect,[77,78] but comparison is difficult due to varying doses and populations of patients. Potential complications include cataract development and keratopathy.

CONCLUSION

Wound healing modulators improve surgical success in trabeculectomy. The use of MMC and/or 5-FU results in the incomplete wound healing state desired in glaucoma surgery. Although their application increases surgical success, it also increases the risk of complications. New modulators targeted specifically to different parts of the wound healing process are currently being investigated, but more research is needed to determine how best to utilize their properties. Bringing these agents to the market is expensive, and over the past 2 decades many have languished in development for lack of support for this limited clinical use.

Dr. Mankiewicz was supported by a Challenge Grant from Research to Prevent Blindness to The University of Texas Medical School at Houston and the Hermann Eye Fund. Dr. Sherwood was supported by an Unrestricted Grant from Research to Prevent Blindness to the University of Florida and additional research support from BioVascular, Inc. and Lpath, Inc.

REFERENCES

1. Atreides SP, Skuta GL, Reynolds AC. Wound healing modulation in glaucoma filtering surgery. *Int Ophthalmol Clin.* Spring 2004;44(2):61–106.
2. Chang L, Crowston JG, Cordeiro MF, Akbar AN, Khaw PT. The role of the immune system in conjunctival wound healing after glaucoma surgery. *Surv Ophthalmol.* Jul-Aug 2000;45(1):49–68.
3. Dahlmann AH, Mireskandari K, Cambrey AD, Bailly M, Khaw PT. Current and future prospects for the prevention of ocular fibrosis. *Ophthalmol Clin North Am.* Dec 2005;18(4):539–559.
4. Li Z, Van Bergen T, Van de Veire S, et al. Inhibition of vascular endothelial growth factor reduces scar formation after glaucoma filtration surgery. *Invest Ophthalmol Vis Sci.* Nov 2009;50(11):5217–5225.
5. Skuta GL, Parrish RK, 2nd. Wound healing in glaucoma filtering surgery. *Surv Ophthalmol.* Nov-Dec 1987;32(3):149–170.
6. Lama PJ, Fechtner RD. Antifibrotics and wound healing in glaucoma surgery. *Surv Ophthalmol.* May-Jun 2003;48(3):314–346.
7. Araujo SV, Spaeth GL, Roth SM, Starita RJ. A ten-year follow-up on a prospective, randomized trial of postoperative corticosteroids after trabeculectomy. *Ophthalmology.* Dec 1995; 102(12):1753–1759.
8. Azuara-Blanco A, Spaeth GL, Augsburger JJ. Oral prednisone in guarded filtration procedures supplemented with antimetabolites. *Ophthalmic Surg Lasers.* Feb 1999;30(2):126–132.
9. Roth SM, Spaeth GL, Starita RJ, Birbillis EM, Steinmann WC. The effects of postoperative corticosteroids on trabeculectomy and the clinical course of glaucoma: five-year follow-up study. *Ophthalmic Surg.* Dec 1991;22(12): 724–729.
10. Starita RJ, Fellman RL, Spaeth GL, Poryzees EM, Greenidge KC, Traverso CE. Short- and long-term effects of postoperative corticosteroids on trabeculectomy. *Ophthalmology.* Jul 1985;92(7):938–946.
11. Kahook MY, Camejo L, Noecker RJ. Trabeculectomy with intraoperative retrobulbar triamcinolone acetonide. *Clin Ophthalmol.* 2009;3:29–31.
12. Tham CC, Li FC, Leung DY, et al. Intrableb triamcinolone acetonide injection after bleb-forming filtration surgery (trabeculectomy, phacotrabeculectomy, and trabeculectomy revision by needling): a pilot study. *Eye.* Dec 2006;20(12):1484–1486.
13. Yuki K, Shiba D, Kimura I, Ohtake Y, Tsubota K. Trabeculectomy with or without intraoperative sub-tenon injection of triamcinolone acetonide in treating secondary glaucoma. *Am JOphthalmol.* Jun 2009;147(6):1055–1060, 1060 e1051–e1052.
14. Breusegem C, Spielberg L, Van Ginderdeuren R, et al. Preoperative nonsteroidal anti-inflammatory drug or steroid and outcomes after trabeculectomy: a randomized controlled trial. *Ophthalmology.* Jul 2010;117(7): 1324–1330.
15. Giangiacomo J, Dueker DK, Adelstein E. The effect of preoperative subconjunctival triamcinolone administration on glaucoma filtration. I. Trabeculectomy following sub-

conjunctival triamcinolone. *Arch Ophthalmol.* Jun 1986;104(6):838–841.

16. Broadway DC, Grierson I, Sturmer J, Hitchings RA. Reversal of topical antiglaucoma medication effects on the conjunctiva. *Arch Ophthalmol.* Mar 1996;114(3):262–267.

17. Kent AR, Dubiner HB, Whitaker R, et al. The efficacy and safety of diclofenac 0.1% versus prednisolone acetate 1% following trabeculectomy with adjunctive mitomycin-C.*Ophthalmic Surg Lasers.* Jul 1998;29(7):562–569.

18. Abraham LM, Selva D, Casson R, Leibovitch I. Mitomycin: clinical applications in ophthalmic practice. *Drugs.* 2006;66(3):321–340.

19. Smith S, D'Amore PA, Dreyer EB. Comparative toxicity of mitomycin C and 5-fluorouracil in vitro. *Am J Ophthalmol.* Sept 15 1994; 118(3):332–337.

20. Greenfield DS, Liebmann JM, Jee J, Ritch R. Late-onset bleb leaks after glaucoma filtering surgery. *Arch Ophthalmol.* Apr 1998; 116(4):443–447.

21. Jampel HD, Quigley HA, Kerrigan-Baumrind LA, et al. Risk factors for late-onset infection following glaucoma filtration surgery. *Arch Ophthalmol.* Jul 2001;119(7):1001–1008.

22. Soltau JB, Rothman RF, Budenz DL, et al. Risk factors for glaucoma filtering bleb infections. *Arch Ophthalmol.* Mar 2000;118(3):338–342.

23. Suner IJ, Greenfield DS, Miller MP, Nicolela MT, Palmberg PF. Hypotony maculopathy after filtering surgery with mitomycin C. Incidence and treatment. *Ophthalmology.* Feb 1997;104(2):207–214; discussion 214–205.

24. Fourman S. Scleritis after glaucoma filtering surgery with mitomycin C. *Ophthalmology.* Oct 1995;102(10):1569–1571.

25. Akova YA, Koc F, Yalvac I, Duman S. Scleromalacia following trabeculectomy with intraoperative mitomycin C. *Eur J Ophthalmol.* Jan-Mar 1999;9(1):63–65.

26. Storr-Paulsen T, Norregaard JC, Ahmed S, Storr-Paulsen A. Corneal endothelial cell loss after mitomycin C-augmented trabeculectomy. *J Glaucoma.* Dec 2008;17(8):654–657.

27. Wilkins M, Indar A, Wormald R. Intraoperative Mitomycin C for glaucoma surgery. *Cochrane Database Syst Rev.* 2005, Issue 4. Art No.: CD002897. DOI: 10.1002/14651858.CD00 2897. pub2.

28. Abraham LM, Selva D, Casson R, Leibovitch I. The clinical applications of fluorouracil in ophthalmic practice. *Drugs.* 2007;67(2):237–255.

29. Joshi AB, Parrish RK, 2nd, Feuer WF. 2002 survey of the American Glaucoma Society:

practice preferences for glaucoma surgery and antifibrotic use. *J Glaucoma.* Apr 2005;14(2):172–174.

30. Lattanzio FA, Jr., Sheppard JD, Jr., Allen RC, Baynham S, Samuel P, Samudre S. Do injections of 5-fluorouracil after trabeculectomy have toxic effects on the anterior segment? *J Ocul Pharmacol Ther.* Jun 2005;21(3):223–235.

31. Shapiro MS, Thoft RA, Friend J, Parrish RK, Gressel MG. 5-Fluorouracil toxicity to the ocular surface epithelium. *Invest Ophthalmol Vis Sci.* Apr 1985;26(4):580–583.

32. Wolner B, Liebmann JM, Sassani JW, Ritch R, Speaker M, Marmor M. Late bleb-related endophthalmitis after trabeculectomy with adjunctive 5-fluorouracil. *Ophthalmology.* Jul 1991;98(7):1053–1060.

33. Wormald R, Wilkins M, Bruce C. Postoperative 5-Fluorouracil for glaucoma surgery. *Cochrane Database Syst Rev.* 2001;(3):CD001132. DOI: 10.1002/14651858.CD001132.

34. Five-year follow-up of the Fluorouracil Filtering Surgery Study. The Fluorouracil Filtering Surgery Study Group. *Am J Ophthalmol.* Apr 1996;121(4):349–366.

35. Jampel HD. Effect of brief exposure to mitomycin C on viability and proliferation of cultured human Tenon's capsule fibroblasts. *Ophthalmology.* Sept 1992;99(9):1471–1476.

36. Khaw PT, Sherwood MB, MacKay SL, Rossi MJ, Schultz G. Five-minute treatments with fluorouracil, floxuridine, and mitomycin have long-term effects on human Tenon's capsule fibroblasts. *Arch Ophthalmol.* Aug 1992; 110(8):1150–1154.

37. Asahara T, Bauters C, Zheng LP, et al. Synergistic effect of vascular endothelial growth factor and basic fibroblast growth factor on angiogenesis in vivo. *Circulation.* Nov 1 1995;92(9)(suppl):II365–371.

38. Mathew R, Barton K. Anti-vascular endothelial growth factor therapy in glaucoma filtration surgery. *Am J Ophthalmol.* Jul 2011;152(1):10–15 e12.

39. Horsley MB, Kahook MY. Anti-VEGF therapy for glaucoma. *Curr Opin Ophthalmol.* Mar 2010;21(2):112–117.

40. Abouammoh M, Sharma S. Ranibizumab versus bevacizumab for the treatment of neovascular age-related macular degeneration. *Curr Opin Ophthalmol.* May 2011;22(3):152–158.

41. Memarzadeh F, Varma R, Lin LT, et al. Postoperative use of bevacizumab as an antifibrotic agent in glaucoma filtration surgery in the rabbit. *Invest Ophthalmol Vis Sci.* Jul 2009;50(7):3233–3237.

42. How A, Chua JL, Charlton A, et al. Combined treatment with bevacizumab and 5-fluorouracil attenuates the postoperative scarring response after experimental glaucoma filtration surgery. *Invest Ophthalmol Vis Sci.* Feb 2010;51(2):928–932.

43. Coote MA, Ruddle JB, Qin Q, Crowston JG. Vascular changes after intra-bleb injection of bevacizumab. *J Glaucoma.* Oct-Nov 2008;17(7):517–518.

44. Kahook MY, Schuman JS, Noecker RJ. Needle bleb revision of encapsulated filtering bleb with bevacizumab. *Ophthalmic Surg Lasers Imaging.* Mar-Apr 2006;37(2):148–150.

45. Miki A, Oshima Y, Otori Y, Kamei M, Tano Y. Efficacy of intravitreal bevacizumab as adjunctive treatment with pars plana vitrectomy, endolaser photocoagulation, and trabeculectomy for neovascular glaucoma. *Br J Ophthalmol.* Oct 2008;92(10):1431–1433.

46. Cornish KS, Ramamurthi S, Saidkasimova S, Ramaesh K. Intravitreal bevacizumab and augmented trabeculectomy for neovascular glaucoma in young diabetic patients. *Eye.* Apr 2009;23(4):979–981.

47. Grewal DS, Jain R, Kumar H, Grewal SP. Evaluation of subconjunctival bevacizumab as an adjunct to trabeculectomy a pilot study. *Ophthalmology.* Dec 2008;115(12):2141–2145 e2142.

48. Kahook MY. Bleb morphology and vascularity after trabeculectomy with intravitreal ranibizumab: a pilot study. *Am J Ophthalmol.* Sept 2010;150(3):399–403 e391.

49. Cordeiro MF. Beyond Mitomycin: TGF-beta and wound healing. *Prog Retin Eye Res.* Jan 2002;21(1):75–89.

50. Tuli S, Esson D, Sherwood MB, Schultz GS. Biological drivers of postoperative scarring. In: Shaarawy TM, Sherwood MB, Hitchings RA, Crowston JG, eds. *Glaucoma.* Vol 2. London: Elsevier; 2009:557–564.

51. Grotendorst GR. Connective tissue growth factor: a mediator of TGF-beta action on fibroblasts. *Cytokine Growth Factor Rev.* Sept 1997;8(3):171–179.

52. Brigstock DR. The connective tissue growth factor/cysteine-rich 61/nephroblastoma over-expressed (CCN) family. *Endocri Rev.* Apr 1999;20(2):189–206.

53. Moussad EE, Brigstock DR. Connective tissue growth factor: what's in a name? *Mol Genet Metab.* Sept-Oct 2000;71(1–2):276–292.

54. Esson DW, Neelakantan A, Iyer SA, et al. Expression of connective tissue growth factor after glaucoma filtration surgery in a rabbit model. *Invest Ophthalmol Vis Sci.* Feb 2004;45(2):485–491.

55. Duncan MR, Frazier KS, Abramson S, et al. Connective tissue growth factor mediates transforming growth factor beta-induced collagen synthesis: down-regulation by cAMP. *FASEB J.* Oct 1999;13(13):1774–1786.

56. Cordeiro MF, Gay JA, Khaw PT. Human anti-transforming growth factor-beta2 antibody: a new glaucoma anti-scarring agent. *Invest Ophthalmol Vis Sci.* Sept 1999;40(10):2225–2234.

57. Blobe GC, Schiemann WP, Lodish HF. Role of transforming growth factor beta in human disease. *N Engl J Med.* May 4 2000;342(18):1350–1358.

58. Border WA, Noble NA. Transforming growth factor beta in tissue fibrosis. *NEngl J Med.* Nov 10 1994;331(19):1286–1292.

59. Siriwardena D, Khaw PT, King AJ, et al. Human antitransforming growth factor beta(2) monoclonal antibody—a new modulator of wound healing in trabeculectomy: a randomized placebo controlled clinical study. *Ophthalmology.* Mar 2002;109(3):427–431.

60. C. A. T. Trabeculectomy Study Group, Khaw P, Grehn F, et. al. A phase III study of subconjunctival human anti-transforming growth factor beta(2) monoclonal antibody (CAT-152) to prevent scarring after first-time trabeculectomy. *Ophthalmology.* Oct 2007;114(10):1822–1830.

61. Wong TT, Mead AL, Khaw PT. Matrix metalloproteinase inhibition modulates postoperative scarring after experimental glaucoma filtration surgery. *Invest Ophthalmol Vis Sci.* Mar 2003;44(3):1097–1103.

62. Wong TT, Mead AL, Khaw PT. Prolonged antiscarring effects of ilomastat and MMC after experimental glaucoma filtration surgery. *Invest Ophthalmol Vis Sci.* Jun 2005; 46(6):2018–2022.

63. Stein CA. Suramin: a novel antineoplastic agent with multiple potential mechanisms of action. *Cancer Res.* May 15 1993;53(10) (suppl):2239–2248.

64. Akman A, Bilezikci B, Kucukerdonmez C, Demirhan B, Aydin P. Suramin modulates wound healing of rabbit conjunctiva after trabeculectomy: comparison with mitomycin C. *Curr Eye Res.* Jan 2003;26(1):37–43.

65. Mietz H, Chevez-Barrios P, Feldman RM, Lieberman MW. Suramin inhibits wound healing following filtering procedures for glaucoma. *Br J Ophthalmol.* Jul 1998;82(7):816–820.

66. Mietz H, Krieglstein GK. Suramin to enhance glaucoma filtering procedures: a clinical comparison with mitomycin. *Ophthalmic Surg Lasers*. Sept-Oct 2001;32(5):358–369.

67. Suzawa H, Kikuchi S, Ichikawa K, Koda A. Inhibitory action of tranilast, an anti-allergic drug, on the release of cytokines and PGE2 from human monocytes-macrophages. *Jpn J Pharmacol*. Oct 1992;60(2):85–90.

68. Oshima T, Kurosaka D, Kato K, et al. Tranilast inhibits cell proliferation and collagen synthesis by rabbit corneal and Tenon's capsule fibroblasts. *Curr Eye Res*. Apr 2000;20(4): 283–286.

69. Chihara E, Dong J, Ochiai H, Hamada S. Effects of tranilast on filtering blebs: a pilot study. *J Glaucoma*. Apr 2002;11(2):127–133.

70. Diestelhorst M, Grisanti S. Photodynamic therapy to control fibrosis in human glaucomatous eyes after trabeculectomy: a clinical pilot study. *Arch Ophthalmol*. Feb 2002;120(2): 130–134.

71. Jordan JF, Diestelhorst M, Grisanti S, Krieglstein GK. Photodynamic modulation of wound healing in glaucoma filtration surgery. *Br J Ophthalmol*. Jul 2003;87(7):870–875.

72. Constable PH, Crowston JG, Occleston NL, Cordeiro MF, Khaw PT. Long term growth arrest of human Tenon's fibroblasts following single applications of beta radiation. *Br J Ophthalmol*. Apr 1998;82(4):448–452.

73. Constable PH, Crowston JG, Occleston NL, Khaw PT. The effects of single doses of beta radiation on the wound healing behaviour of human Tenon's capsule fibroblasts. *Br J Ophthalmol*. Feb 2004;88(2):169–173.

74. Kastan MB, Onyekwere O, Sidransky D, Vogelstein B, Craig RW. Participation of p53 protein in the cellular response to DNA damage. *Cancer Res*. Dec 1 1991;51(23 Pt 1): 6304–6311.

75. Kirwan JF, Cousens S, Venter L, et al. Effect of beta radiation on success of glaucoma drainage surgery in South Africa: randomised controlled trial. *BMJ*. Nov 4 2006;333(7575):942.

76. Lai JS, Poon AS, Tham CC, Lam DS. Trabeculectomy with beta radiation: long-term follow-up. *Ophthalmology*. Sept 2003;110(9): 1822–1826.

77. Barnes RM, Mora JS, Best SJ. Beta radiation as an adjunct to low-risk trabeculectomy. *Clin Experiment Ophthalmol*. Aug 2000;28(4):259–262.

78. Rehman SU, Amoaku WM, Doran RM, Menage MJ, Morrell AJ. Randomized controlled clinical trial of beta irradiation as an adjunct to trabeculectomy in open-angle glaucoma. *Ophthalmology*. Feb 2002;109(2): 302–306.

PART THREE

FILTERING SURGERY COMPLICATIONS

A. INTRAOPERATIVE COMPLICATIONS

4

CONJUNCTIVAL BUTTONHOLES

MISHA F. SYED

CONJUNCTIVAL BUTTONHOLES

A conjunctival buttonhole is a defect in the conjunctival tissue that occurs during manipulation of the conjunctival flap where the underlying Tenon's capsule may or may not remain intact. Buttonholes during glaucoma filtering surgery have been reported in 3% of fornix-based conjunctival flaps[1] and approximately 1% of limbus-based conjunctival flaps.[2] Recognition of conjunctival defects is important since infections can occur if the microbial surface flora get into the bleb, and hypotony can result from excessive egress of filtered aqueous. Furthermore, if the bleb flattens, fibrous adhesions may compromise filtration. A conjunctival buttonhole presents a unique challenge intraoperatively during trabeculectomy surgery because the usual surgical approach must be revised, and the repair strategy depends on the location of the buttonhole.

HISTORICAL BACKGROUND

Conjunctival buttonholes are well-documented potential intraoperative complications during glaucoma surgery. Sugar was among the first to report their occurrence in the 1960s, when he described a conjunctival hood procedure for repairing buttonholes in a fornix-based flap. A conjunctival flap was dissected from Tenon's capsule after opening the conjunctiva at the limbal margin and then pulled down onto the peripheral cornea and sutured into place. Tincture of iodine was applied to the bleb surface, and the corneal margin was abraded.[3]

Grady and Forbes, among others, began reporting the use of tissue adhesive in the closure of ophthalmic surgical wounds. They suggested the novel use of alkyl 2-cyanoacrylate glue because the temporary nature of the adhesive was particularly well suited to repairing conjunctival buttonholes:

"Tissue adhesives serve to stop the continuous external flow of aqueous humor, thereby allowing the conjunctival wound to heal; after healing has occurred, the persistence of adhesive is no longer necessary or desirable."[4] These authors also mentioned other popular surgical repair options common at that time, including the rolling of a conjunctival flap over the buttonhole, suturing of the torn edge of conjunctiva into a corneal groove, or closing the buttonhole with a tissue patch of conjunctiva harvested from another area.[4] Interestingly, many of these same options are used today.

In the late 1970s, a new "atraumatic" needle emerged and was reported to improve treatment of intraoperative conjunctival buttonholes. Originally, the delicate atraumatic taper tip needle was developed for nerve anastomosis in neurosurgery and orthopedic surgery. Petursson and Fraunfelder authored a paper in 1979 that suggested this new taper point needle could sew atrophic or thinned conjunctival tissue without causing new leaks around the needle track, a common problem with previous ophthalmic needles. The authors advocated using a "shoestring" type of closure, taking wide bites to encompass the entire thin-walled area in a circumscribed manner. If the buttonhole occurred near the limbus, the taper point needle was used to apply a mattress suture onto the cornea.[5] Petursson and Fraunfelder's paper described the first reported use of this type of needle to accomplish a direct closure of conjunctival buttonholes, as up to this point, more complicated, time-consuming, and trauma-inducing methods of conjunctival closure had been recommended. Previously, using a regular spatulated needle often resulted in leaks along the needle track, rendering the buttonhole repair ineffective. The availability of a taper point needle was a great improvement in surgical repair.

ETIOLOGY OF CONJUNCTIVAL BUTTONHOLES

Conjunctival buttonholes may occur for a variety of reasons: thin and fragile tissue, conjunctival scarring from previous surgery, rough handling or manipulation of tissue, use of suboptimal surgical instruments, and conjunctival contact with antimetabolite (especially mitomycin-C [MMC]). Careful preoperative evaluation of patients can prepare the surgeon for possible intraoperative challenges. Elderly patients often have more delicate, friable, and thinner conjunctiva compared to other patient groups. Also, patients with a previous history of ocular surgery, particularly previous filtration surgery, may have compromised tissue integrity with scarring and increased likelihood of intraoperative conjunctival tears or breaks. Consideration of the patient's medical history is also important. Systemic connective tissue disease can affect ocular tissue, including the conjunctiva.

During surgery, it is imperative to use proper surgical instrumentation and techniques to handle fragile conjunctival tissue. Toothed forceps must be avoided in holding the conjunctiva; nontoothed forceps should be used only on incision edges. Pearse nontoothed conjunctival forceps with rounded tips are very useful in handling the conjunctiva with minimal trauma and can be ordered with a tying platform (Figure 4.1). The grasp on the tissue must be gentle, avoiding pulling or stretching with excessive force. However, toothed forceps may be used on Tenon's capsule, being careful to avoid the conjunctiva. When trimming tissue with Westcott or Vannas scissors, one must constantly evaluate the anterior and posterior

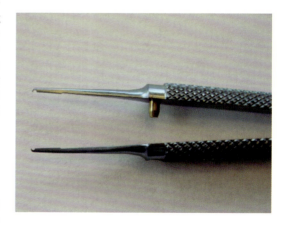

FIGURE 4.1   Tips of Pearse forceps with tying platform.

edges of tissue to be sure that inadvertent cuts are not made in other areas of conjunctiva. If tears or buttonholes are noted intraoperatively, immediate closure with a taper point vascular needle on a 9–0 or 10–0 nylon or polyglactin 910 (Vicryl™, Ethicon, Inc., Somerville, New Jersey) suture should prevent enlargement of the defect despite continued manipulation.

Although the use of MMC has in many ways revolutionized the trabeculectomy, one must be cautious in its application during surgery. While placing MMC on the sclera, the edge of the conjunctival wound must be held away from the area of treatment. Often pieces of sponges are used to place the MMC. However, these sponges can swell with moisture and make placement of the sponge more difficult under the conjunctiva and Tenon's capsule, possibly leading to exposure of the conjunctival edge to the antimetabolite. Occasionally, the sponge may even have a sharp edge and tear the conjunctiva. Cut pieces of tear strip test paper soaked in MMC work well to slide underneath conjunctiva and Tenon's capsule against the sclera with minimal elevation and do not disintegrate as sponge pieces occasionally can. Pieces of sponge have been also been reported to be inadvertently left behind.[6] Pooling of MMC at wound edges should also be avoided, as this may reduce the ability of fibroblasts to adequately heal, with a resulting ischemic leaking bleb.[7]

MANAGEMENT OF BUTTONHOLES

Despite the surgeon's best efforts, conjunctival buttonholes may still develop during glaucoma filtration surgery. Historically, closure of buttonholes sometimes required extensive surgical revision; however, the optimal treatment for this complication has evolved. More recently, use of purse-string sutures on a taper point needle has simplified repair, as described previously.

Generally, buttonholes that occur near the limbus during a fornix-based trabeculectomy are best repaired with excision and suturing of the anterior conjunctival edge to the limbus with a mattress suture, after epithelial debridement of the edge. Smaller buttonholes

located more posteriorly from the limbus may be closed with an interrupted or purse-string 10–0 nylon suture on a vascular (taper point) needle, incorporating Tenon's capsule when possible.[8] An absorbable suture on a taper point needle, such as a 9–0 polyglactin 910, can offer an advantage in repair since the suture will not need to be removed later and is the same size as the hole made by the needle. Other options for small buttonhole repair include light bipolar cautery or tissue adhesives, but both techniques are less reliable than suturing. Alkyl 2-cyanoacrylate glue can also cause patient discomfort due to the irregular surface created once the adhesive dries and possible further conjunctival tissue damage when the glue falls off. If a large buttonhole occurs early in the operation, it may be best to close the defect and select an adjacent site for the surgery. If a buttonhole occurs near the conjunctival wound in a limbus-based flap, it can be incorporated into the normal wound closure.

Various novel techniques have also been developed for dealing with buttonholes. Higashide et al reported the use of the viscoelastic sodium hyaluronate 2.3% (Healon5®; Abbot Medical Optics; Santa Ana, California) to repair intraoperative buttonholes (Figure 4.2). They suggest that this technique is especially useful when the buttonhole is located close to the scleral flap and involves thin conjunctiva likely to tear further with suturing. Healon5® is a superviscous cohesive viscoelastic, which in this small case series proved useful in sealing intraoperative small leaks secondary to buttonholes. No leakage, scarring, or inflammation in the early postoperative period were noted with Healon5® use in these cases.[9]

More recently, amniotic membrane transplantation (AMT) has been suggested as a conjunctival repair method intraoperatively during trabeculectomy with mitomycin-C. A retrospective case series reported use of AMT to close fragile conjunctiva in cases of intraoperative buttonholes. The amniotic membrane graft was placed epithelial side up, after being cut in a rectangular shape, up to 4 mm anterior to the closure site and 2 mm posterior to it, with a length approximately 10–12

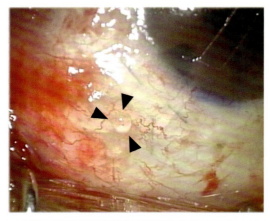

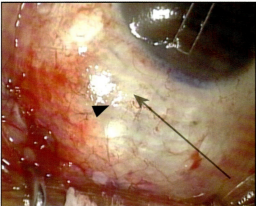

FIGURE 4.2 Intraoperative conjunctival break during trabeculectomy (top photo, A) and appearance following postsubconjunctival injection of Healon5® under area of buttonhole (bottom photo, D). Arrowheads indicate conjunctival break. Arrow indicates direction of 27-gauge needle advancement subconjunctivally for injection of Healon5®. Reprinted from Higashide et al[9] with permission from Elsevier.

mm horizontally along the wound. The anterior portion of the bleb, 0–4 mm posterior to the limbus, was not covered. A combination of techniques was used for application of the graft. Most cases employed the use of 8–0 polyglactin 910 on a BV needle with the posterior border of the graft sutured to underlying conjunctiva. Tissue glue was used in one case as well for attachment of the graft. All cases resulted in well-formed blebs without early

or late postoperative bleb leakage. Intraocular pressure control was achieved without medications in all cases.[10]

Early postoperative repair

This discussion focuses on *intraoperative* repair of conjunctival buttonholes; however, it is worth mentioning some *early postoperative* techniques for repair as well. In the case of a single, pinpoint bleb leak due to a small buttonhole postoperatively, a large bandage contact lens may allow for closure. However, if bleb shallowing is present, it is best to perform surgical repair of the leak to avoid subconjunctival-to-episcleral fibrosis, adhesion, and subsequent bleb failure.

The argon laser is another treatment modality for conjunctival buttonholes noted postoperatively. Theoretically, the argon laser may have an advantage in sealing small leaks as it causes focal thermal injury and conjunctival shrinkage, yet leaves other portions of the bleb unaffected. A prospective, nonrandomized, uncontrolled case series treating early- and late-onset buttonholes, along with other types of conjunctival defects, found that laser treatment could often effectively close the buttonholes, especially in early postoperative cases when the conjunctiva was more vascular and thickened.[11] An increase in the inflammatory response helped to close the leak. The laser settings used to attempt closure of buttonholes were a 500-μm spot size, 0.1 s duration, and 500–1800 mW power (usually less than 1000 mW was sufficient). Excessive power was noted to cause pitting or fenestration of the conjunctiva, which occurred in 3 patients. Laser spots were applied to the conjunctiva to cause a mild shriveling and browning of the tissue, which then forced the 2 conjunctival sides together and formed a coagulum over the hole. Enough applications were applied to close the defect, and then a second row of burns was placed surrounding the first to cause more conjunctival irritation and healing.[11] The benefit of using an argon laser to treat postoperative buttonhole leaks includes rapidity and relative painlessness of the procedure. A return to the operating room may also be avoided if the laser is successful.

CONCLUSION

Conjunctival buttonholes are a relatively uncommon but potentially serious complication of filtering surgery. Detection of a leak at the time of surgery is crucial in optimizing clinical outcomes and avoiding postoperative complications such as infection, hypotony, and bleb scarring with eventual surgical failure. Many varied methods of conjunctival buttonhole closure exist, but with careful patient selection, prudent use of antimetabolite, and gentle surgical technique, the occurrence of this intraoperative complication can be greatly minimized.

Dr. Syed was supported by an Unrestricted Grant from Research to Prevent Blindness to the University of Texas Medical Branch.

COMMENTARY
PAUL J. HARASYMOWYCZ

When faced with a thin conjunctiva that is prone to tear and form conjunctival buttonholes, it is important to diminish early aqueous filtration during a glaucoma procedure. This may involve opting for a nonpenetrating procedure (Chapter 52), adding extra sutures on the scleral flap in trabeculectomy, or tying off a tube shunt in order to facilitate a more rapid healing of the conjunctiva (Chapter 35). It may also be necessary to decrease aqueous production with topical drops, as well as avoid using nonsteroidal antiinflammatory drops (NSAIDS) or steroidal drops; they may impair proper healing.[12] When waiting for conjunctival healing after buttonhole formation, if the glaucoma filtration procedure shows signs of failure, it may also be necessary to needle under the scleral flap to increase subconjunctival filtration (Chapter 28).

Dr. Harasymowycz was supported by the Quebec Glaucoma Foundation.

COMMENTARY
MARK B. SHERWOOD

The key issues in deciding how to manage a conjunctival buttonhole are location of the hole, tissue quality (tissue thickness and vascularity at the hole and mobility of the surrounding conjunctival tissue), and time of discovery of the hole. As excellently described in the text, if the hole is close to the incision line in either a fornix- or limbal-based conjunctival flap, it can generally just be included in the routine closure. For both a limbal-based and fornix-based approach, pulling a small, tight conjunctival flap anteriorly using one or more mattress sutures to the peripheral cornea generally best closes a hole near the limbus. When the hole is in the body of the bleb, particularly if it overlies the scleral flap area, then a two-layer closure of Tenon's capsule using a running suture from underneath followed by a separate running or purse-string suture to the conjunctiva from its superficial surface is recommended. The closure should be Seidel tested by irrigating balanced salt solution from beneath the conjunctival flap at the leak site, after painting the external tissue with a fluorescein strip. With buttonholes discovered postoperatively or for very peripheral temporal or nasal holes that are hard to reach from an internal approach, an external, single layer conjunctival closure using a dissolvable polyglactin 910 suture with a taper point needle can be successful. If there is still a significant Seidel positive leak on testing after an external single layer conjunctival closure, then as a final resort the conjunctiva/Tenon's capsule can be sutured directly to the superficial sclera at the hole. This flattens and sacrifices an area of bleb but can help achieve a Seidel negative closure.

Dr. Sherwood was supported by an Unrestricted Grant from Research to Prevent Blindness to the University of Florida.

REFERENCES

1. Allingham RR, Damji KF, Freedman S, Moroi SE, Shafranov G, Shields MB. Filtering surgery. *Shields' Textbook of Glaucoma*. 5th ed. Philadephia, PA: Lippincott Williams & Wilkins; 2005:568–609.
2. Jampel HD, Musch DC, Gillespie BW, Lichter PR, Wright MM, Guire KE. Perioperative complications of trabeculectomy in the Collaborative Initial Glaucoma Treatment Study (CIGTS). *Am J Ophthalmol*. Jul 2005;140(1):16–22.
3. Sugar HS. Complications, repair and reoperation of antiglaucoma filtering blebs. *Am J Ophthalmol*. Apr 1967;63(4):825–833.
4. Grady FJ, Forbes M. Tissue adhesive for repair of conjunctival buttonhole in glaucoma surgery. *Am J Ophthalmol*. Oct 1969;68(4):656–658.
5. Petursson GJ, Fraunfelder FT. Repair of an inadvertent buttonhole or leaking filtering bleb. *Arch Ophthalmol*. May 1979;97(5):926–927.
6. Al-Shahwan S, Edward DP. Foreign body granulomas secondary to retained sponge fragment following mitomycin C trabeculectomy. *Graefes Arch Clin Exp Ophthalmol*. Feb 2005; 243(2):178–181.
7. Mattox C. Therapeutics and Techniques and Glaucoma Care Updates: Management of the Leaking Bleb. *JGlaucoma*. October 1995;4(5): 370–374.
8. Kolker AE. Filtration surgery. In: Morrison JC, Pollack IP, eds. *Glaucoma: Science and Practice*. New York, NY: Theime Medical Publishers; 2003:458–470.
9. Higashide T, Tagawa S, Sugiyama K. Intraoperative Healon5® injection into blebs for small conjunctival breaks created during trabeculectomy. *J Cataract Refract Surg*. Jul 2005;31(7):1279–1282.
10. Li G, O'Hearn T, Yiu S, Francis BA. Amniotic membrane transplantation for intraoperative conjunctival repair during trabeculectomy with mitomycin C. *J Glaucoma*. Sept 2007;16(6): 521–526.
11. Hennis HL, Stewart WC. Use of the argon laser to close filtering bleb leaks. *Graefes Arch Clin Exp Ophthalmol*. 1992;230(6):537–541.
12. Arey ML, Sullivan BR, Reinert CG, McCulley JP. Impaired corneal wound healing associated with ketorolac 0.5% after uncomplicated extracapsular cataract extraction. *Cornea*. Dec 2007;26(10):1159–1164.

5

INTRAOPERATIVE HYPHEMA

EDNEY R. MOURA FILHO AND ARTHUR J. SIT

INTRAOPERATIVE HYPHEMA

Hemorrhage is a common complication in trabeculectomy. Hyphema can be a manifestation of an intraoperative hemorrhage and has numerous potential causes. Although generally self-limited, severe complications are possible due to intraoperative hyphemas, and effort should be made to prevent or minimize their occurrence.

PREVALENCE AND RISK FACTORS

Large clinical trials suggest that intraoperative hyphema is a common complication of filtration surgery. In the Advanced Glaucoma Intervention Study (AGIS), the investigators found a 13% prevalence of intraoperative anterior chamber bleeding in eyes treated with trabeculectomy (67 of 513 eyes).[1] Similarly, the Collaborative Initial Glaucoma Treatment Study (CIGTS) found a hyphema prevalence of 8% in eyes (37 of 465 eyes) treated surgically.[2] More recently, the Tube Versus Trabeculectomy Study reported an intraoperative hyphema rate of 3% (3 of 105 eyes) in the trabeculectomy arm of the trial.[3]

Ocular risk factors for an intraoperative hyphema include elevated intraocular pressure (IOP), a sudden drop in IOP as a result of filtration surgery, and surgical trauma, particularly an iridectomy.[4,5] Additionally, the fragile rubeotic iris vessels that may be present in neovascular and inflammatory glaucomas may make those eyes especially susceptible to intraoperative (or postoperative) hyphema. Moreover, patients undergoing glaucoma surgery are often older and have multiple risk factors for intraoperative hemorrhage, including systemic hypertension and vasculopathy, as well as chronic oral anticoagulation therapy (ACT) or antiplatelet therapy (APT).

CAUSES AND PREVENTION OF INTRAOPERATIVE HYPHEMA

Anterior chamber bleeding leading to a hyphema can occur at multiple stages of filtration surgery. Intraoperative bleeding tends to happen most commonly when cutting the iridectomy, due to direct incision of the major arterial circle of the iris or from damage to the adjacent highly vascular ciliary processes. Hemorrhage also may occur while excising the sclerostomy or following the creation of the paracentesis (especially if there is a large drop in IOP with consequent rupture of fragile rubeotic vessels). During dissection of the partial thickness scleral flap, aqueous or episcleral veins may be cut. If hemorrhage from these vessels is not adequately cauterized, blood may eventually flow into the anterior chamber.

Possible surgical modifications to minimize the risk of hemorrhagic complications in the anterior chamber include careful cauterization of the scleral vessels prior to flap dissection, meticulous dissection of the episclera from the sclera, undermining of the flap anteriorly to the clear cornea, construction of the sclerostomy anterior to the scleral spur, and avoiding iridectomy in patients with a high risk of hemorrhage.

If the block of tissue removed during the sclerostomy construction is too far posterior and incises Schlemm's canal, reflux of blood into the anterior chamber may occur.[6] The cut edges of Schlemm's canal can be difficult to cauterize because of their fixed position within the sclera. "Needle tip" (23-gauge) cautery is most helpful in these situations. If minimal cautery is inadequate, application of a cotton swab or sponge to the site followed by gentle pressure for 1–2 minutes is usually effective in stopping bleeding.

Patients with glaucoma secondary to elevated episcleral venous pressure are also at risk for intraoperative reflux of blood from Schlemm's canal when IOP is lowered. Backflow through the trabecular meshwork may occur circumferentially. Since no focal bleeding source is present, cautery is not helpful. Tamponade of bleeding can be achieved by filling the anterior chamber with viscoelastic material to raise the IOP.

Excision of a "too posterior" iridectomy is likely to result in trauma to the ciliary tissue. Care must be taken to avoid excessive traction on the iris root so as to only pull iris and not pull ciliary processes, which will not be visible until the iridectomy is created. If ciliary body injury does occur, it may be helpful to fill the anterior chamber with a viscoelastic agent to both tamponade the broken vessel and to direct the blood out of the incision, rather than allowing it to drain inward.

Special Considerations for Neovascular Glaucoma. Neovascular glaucoma presents special challenges and risks for hyphema, where bleeding during or after trabeculectomy can be a frequent occurrence. In a study of neovascular glaucoma and trabeculectomy, Elgin et al aimed to reduce the risk of intraoperative and postoperative bleeding from the new vessels at the peripheral iridectomy site by performing trabeculectomy combined with direct cauterization of the peripheral iris, in addition to cauterization of the sclera. Minimal anterior chamber bleeding occurred in only 3 eyes (4.2% of 72 total eyes), a rate lower than that found in CIGTS or AGIS. Hyphema occurred in 15 eyes (20.8%) in the first postoperative week; however, most cases were transient and resolved spontaneously. From these results, Elgin et al proposed that cauterization of the iris before iridectomy effectively reduces the rate of postoperative hyphema in cases of neovascular glaucoma.[7]

Although preoperative intraocular injection of anti-VEGF (vascular endothelial growth factor) medication (i.e., bevacizumab or ranibizumab) may also temporarily decrease the caliber of the rubeotic vessels and limit the risk of intraoperative bleeding, conclusive studies are lacking in the literature. However, preoperative injection of bevacizumab has been shown to reduce the risk of early postoperative hyphema.[8,9]

COMPLICATIONS FROM INTRAOPERATIVE HYPHEMA

In most cases, hyphema is self-limited, and no specific therapy is indicated. A temporary decrease in visual acuity is the most common adverse effect of hyphema. However, in some cases, severe, large hyphema may cause corneal staining or spillover into the vitreous, resulting in more prolonged visual deficits.

Corneal bloodstaining can occur early if there is corneal endothelial cell dysfunction, with extremely elevated pressures. However, corneal bloodstaining is unlikely to occur in a healthy cornea before 5 days at an IOP less than 40 mm Hg or before 3 days at an IOP of 50 mm Hg.[10]

Intraocular blood may also occlude the sclerostomy site (or the lumen of the tube of aqueous shunting devices such as the EX-PRESS™ Glaucoma Filtration Device [Alcon Laboratories, Inc., Fort Worth, Texas]), compromising aqueous outflow and allowing scleral flap fibrosis and possible permanent filtration failure. Complete obstruction usually results in a severe IOP elevation as the trabecular meshwork, already dysfunctional from underlying disease and a low-flow state from early filtration, becomes clogged. Obstruction may result from red blood cells themselves or a macrophage response elicited by red blood cell breakdown products, a condition known as hemolytic glaucoma.[11] The presence of a functioning filtering bleb should protect the eye from elevated IOP in the event of such trabecular obstruction, but if a dense blood clot blocks the sclerostomy, the IOP is likely to rise. Intraoperative bleeding can also interfere with the desired wound healing reaction in trabeculectomy and diminish, or negate, the effects of antifibrotic regimens. Increased vigilance in antifibrosis therapy is warranted.

RISK REDUCTION AND TREATMENT OF INTRAOCULAR HYPHEMA

Intraoperative bleeding can generally be avoided with careful surgical technique and tissue handling. If intraoperative bleeding does occur, it can usually be controlled by tamponading the anterior chamber with a large air bubble or viscoelastic for a few minutes. Direct pressure with a sponge or the application of epinephrine can also be helpful. If a large hyphema occurs, washout of the anterior chamber can be performed at the time of surgery, but rebleeding is common.

Discontinuation/modification of ACT/APT therapy prior to surgery is one option to prophylactically reduce the risk of bleeding. In a retrospective case control study by Law et al, chronic ACT/APT was associated with a statistically significant higher rate of hemorrhagic complications, while perioperative ACT and a high preoperative IOP were found to be potential risk factors for hemorrhagic complications in patients undergoing glaucoma surgery.[12] On the other hand, if the patient is discontinued from ACT/APT therapy, serious systemic sequelae, such as stroke or myocardial infarction, could occur. Any decision to modify or discontinue ACT/APT therapy should be made with great care and in conjunction with the patient's primary care physician. For more information on ACT/APT therapy and hyphema, see Chapter 23. Lowering a high IOP gradually before surgery, or slowly via paracentesis at the time of surgery, may be effective in decreasing the risk of intraoperative bleeding.

If anterior chamber hemorrhage was adequately controlled in the operating room, but is present again on the first postoperative day, the eye is at risk for elevated IOP and failure of the trabeculectomy as discussed earlier in this chapter. For management options of early postoperative bleeding, please refer to Chapter 23.

CONCLUSION

Intraoperative hyphema is a known risk of trabeculectomy and usually resolves satisfactorily in the operating room with meticulous cautery or tamponade. However, if hemorrhage persists into the postoperative period, it can be accompanied by a rise of IOP or lead to failure of the trabeculectomy. Conservative management can usually control the IOP until the blood clears, but some cases require more aggressive intervention. To maximize long-term outcomes, every effort should be made to minimize the risks of intraoperative bleeding.

COMMENTARY

MISHA F. SYED

The authors have provided a well-written chapter that gives not only a basic overview of the topic of intraoperative hyphema but also excellent suggestions as to how to manage this complication. The authors mention that iridectomy should be avoided in patients with a high risk of hemorrhage. Patients that would fall into this category include those with thrombocytopenia, bleeding diathesis (i.e., hemophilia), and those on chronic ACT that cannot be discontinued for surgery. Secondly, in addition to the other treatments suggested for intraoperative hyphema, I would also like to mention that increased steroid treatment, topical and/or systemic, can also be used to manage this complication. Walton et al recommend using a topical corticosteroid (e.g., prednisolone acetate 1%, 4 times daily) to reduce intraocular inflammation, the risk of secondary hemorrhage, and the risk of formation of peripheral anterior and posterior synechiae. If the patient is using systemic corticosteroids, topical steroids are probably not necessary.[13]

Dr. Syed was supported by an Unrestricted Grant from Research to Prevent Blindness to the University of Texas Medical Branch.

COMMENTARY

SHAN C. LIN

Moura Filho and Sit have written a detailed and comprehensive review of the causes, prevention, complications, and treatment of intraoperative hyphema. The many potential sources of bleeding, including reflux from Schlemm's canal, damage to iris and ciliary vessels, and tracking from episcleral and conjunctival sources, are described well. The authors also have excellent suggestions for preventing hyphema, which should assist the reader when performing trabeculectomy or other filtering procedures.

In the section on *Special Considerations for Neovascular Glaucoma*, the authors present the work of Elgin et al,[7] in which cauterization of the iris was an effective method for preventing hyphema with iridectomy in these high-risk cases of glaucoma. In addition, they mention the potential of anti-VEGF treatment for reducing hyphema risk. Although assumed as general knowledge, it should be emphasized that preoperative treatment with panretinal photocoagulation (PRP) is still the mainstay of therapy for the neovascular disease in the majority of cases. PRP should be performed prior to filtering surgery to help prevent hyphema. PRP may not be possible in the early postoperative period due to poor visualization of the retina related to intraoperative or postoperative bleeding or excessive inflammation common in these eyes.

Dr. Lin was supported by an Unrestricted Grant from Research to Prevent Blindness to the University of California at San Francisco, National Eye Institute grant P30EY002162, and That Man May See, Inc.

REFERENCES

1. The Advanced Glaucoma Intervention Study (AGIS): 11. Risk factors for failure of trabeculectomy and argon laser trabeculoplasty. *Am J Ophthalmol.* Oct 2002;134(4):481–498.

2. Jampel HD, Musch DC, Gillespie BW, Lichter PR, Wright MM, Guire KE. Perioperative complications of trabeculectomy in the Collaborative Initial Glaucoma Treatment Study (CIGTS). *Am J Ophthalmol.* Jul 2005;140(1):16–22.

3. Gedde SJ, Herndon LW, Brandt JD, Budenz DL, Feuer WJ, Schiffman JC. Surgical complications in the Tube Versus Trabeculectomy Study during the first year of follow-up. *Am J Ophthalmol.* Jan 2007;143(1):23–31.

4. Cobb CJ, Chakrabarti S, Chadha V, Sanders R. The effect of aspirin and warfarin therapy in trabeculectomy. *Eye.* May 2007;21(5):598–603.

5. Jampel H. Glaucoma surgery in the patient undergoing anticoagulation. *J Glaucoma.* Aug 1998;7(4):278–281.

6. Namba H. Blood reflux into anterior chamber after trabeculectomy. *Jpn J Ophthalmol.* 1983; 27(4):616–625.

7. Elgin U, Berker N, Batman A, Simsek T, Cankaya B. Trabeculectomy with mitomycin C combined with direct cauterization of peripheral iris in the management of neovascular glaucoma. *J Glaucoma.* Oct 2006;15(5):466–470.

8. Takihara Y, Inatani M, Kawaji T, et al. Combined intravitreal bevacizumab and trabeculectomy with mitomycin C versus trabeculectomy with mitomycin C alone for neovascular glaucoma. *J Glaucoma.*.Mar 2011;20(3):196–201.

9. Saito Y, Higashide T, Takeda H, Ohkubo S, Sugiyama K. Beneficial effects of preoperative intravitreal bevacizumab on trabeculectomy outcomes in neovascular glaucoma. *Acta Ophthalmol.* Feb 2010;88(1):96–102.

10. Read J, Goldberg MF. Comparison of medical treatment for traumatic hyphema. *Trans Am Acad Ophthalmol Otolaryngol.* 1974; 78:799–815.

11. Fenton RH, Zimmerman LE. Hemolytic glaucoma. An unusual cause of acute open-angle secondary glaucoma. *Arch Ophthalmol.* Aug 1963;70:236–239.

12. Law SK, Song BJ, Yu F, Kurbanyan K, Yang TA, Caprioli J. Hemorrhagic complications from glaucoma surgery in patients on anticoagulation therapy or antiplatelet therapy. *Am J Ophthalmol.* Apr 2008;145(4): 736–746.

13. Walton W, Von Hagen S, Grigorian R, Zarbin M. Management of traumatic hyphema. *Surv Ophthalmol.* Jul-Aug 2002;47(4):297–334.

6

CHOROIDAL EFFUSION AND HEMORRHAGE

RONALD L. FELLMAN

CHOROIDAL EFFUSION AND HEMORRHAGE

Every intraocular surgery carries risk of a serious complication. One of the most worrisome is an intraoperative suprachoroidal hemorrhage. For a variety of reasons, especially hypotony, these hemorrhages occur more frequently in glaucoma patients, may develop at any time during the perioperative period, and may cause considerable visual loss. When a severe choroidal hemorrhage does occur, it can be visually devastating and may be very painful. A large perioperative choroidal effusion is also worrisome because it may be the initiating factor that precipitates a choroidal hemorrhage. Even after a "simple bleb needling" or postoperative suture lysis[1] for uncontrolled intraocular pressure (IOP), a suprachoroidal hemorrhage may develop, leading to catastrophic visual loss. In spite of best efforts, choroidal events will still occur and should be managed in a highly expeditious fashion. Proper prevention and management of a choroidal event is the best chance for saving vision.

DEFINITION

An intraoperative choroidal event is typically a spontaneous collection of either fluid and/or blood in the suprachoroidal space. This potential space is located between the choroid and the sclera. The fluid within a chronic choroidal effusion typically has a straw color due to the accumulation of proteins. Choroidal events are most common following glaucoma surgery, and choroidal hemorrhage or effusion may lead to complicated surgery with resulting visual loss.

A spontaneous intraoperative choroidal effusion may initiate a shallow anterior chamber and a firm eye. The mechanisms are complex and variable.[2] A spontaneous collection of blood into the suprachoroidal space may occur when the IOP is low, as seen during filtration surgery. Severe bleeding that breaks through into the vitreous is typically associated with a poor prognosis, as are bleeds that reach the optic nerve head. These eyes commonly end up with a pale optic disc and poor visual function. Every attempt is made to avoid these situations (see Table 6.1); nevertheless, the surgeon must remain calm during such an event and immediately close the eye to minimize visual harm.

PREVALENCE AND RISK FACTORS

Intraoperative choroidal events are rare in routine cases. In the Collaborative Initial Glaucoma Treatment Study (CIGTS), a multicenter, randomized clinical trial comparing trabeculectomy to medications as the initial treatment for glaucoma, the incidence of intraoperative choroidal effusion was 0.4%, and there were no reported cases of an intraoperative suprachoroidal hemorrhage. However, rates were definitely higher in the postoperative period, at 11% for serous choroidal effusion and 0.7% for localized suprachoroidal hemorrhages.[3] In the Tube Versus Trabeculectomy (TVT) study, another multicenter, randomized clinical trial evaluating the safety and efficacy of nonvalved tube shunt surgery versus trabeculectomy with mitomycin-C, there were no recorded intraoperative choroidal events associated with trabeculectomy, but in the postoperative period, choroidal effusion was noted in 19% of patients and suprachoroidal hemorrhage in 3%.[4] Another study found a mean incidence of 1.6% for perioperative suprachoroidal hemorrhage after filtration surgery.[5]

Multiple risk factors for choroidal hemorrhage are worrisome and require enhanced perioperative vigilance by the ophthalmic surgeon. For example, a patient who is aphakic, vitrectomized, diabetic, myopic, has uncontrolled hypertension, and also develops a large postoperative choroidal effusion is a choroidal hemorrhage waiting to happen. Such a scenario requires additional thought processes far different than for the normal postoperative patient. This patient likely requires drainage of the choroidal effusion in order to prevent an almost certain choroidal hemorrhage. A review of the essential steps associated with choroidal drainage is noted in Figure 6.1.

PREVENTION

Choroidal events are like earthquakes; they may be so subtle they are barely noticed or devastating and visually catastrophic. Early recognition and skillful management of an intraoperative suprachoroidal hemorrhage or effusion may be sight saving. It behooves the surgeon to know beforehand who is at greatest risk for a choroidal event, and with that knowledge, to select a procedure that minimizes the likelihood of such an event and also preoperatively determine a path to mitigate the damage if the hemorrhage occurs.[6] For example, a patient at high risk for a choroidal hemorrhage requiring drainage surgery may do best with a 2-stage procedure tube shunt rather than a trabeculectomy. In the first operation, the device is placed in the appropriate quadrant, and the tube tucked away. Six weeks later, during the second stage of the procedure, the tube is placed in the eye with a very controlled postoperative IOP course, avoiding hypotony. This 2-stage procedure is preferable to the untimed dissolution of a tube ligature as seen with a single stage procedure with associated hypotonous events. Other alternative techniques to avoid postoperative hypotony, such as total occlusion of the tube with an obturator suture with a nonabsorbable external ligature surrounding the tube, may also be effective.

Patients who are at high risk for a choroidal event require a team approach to prevent and minimize complications. Anticipation is the key to success. For example, the primary care physician may need to modify anticoagulants, the surgeon may alter the usual surgical procedure, and caretakers must adjust to accommodate the patient's postoperative needs. The entire process may become quite involved.

Mindful surgeons recognize risk factors preoperatively (Table 6.2) and minimize surgical risks through tireless, case by case efforts. Table 6.1 lists 26 approaches for decreasing the likelihood of a choroidal hemorrhage.

Table 6.1. Preoperative, Intraoperative, and Postoperative Factors for Reducing the Risk of a Suprachoroidal Hemorrhage

HOW TO REDUCE THE RISK OF A SUPRACHOROIDAL HEMORRHAGE

Preoperative Factors

- Aggressive IOP reduction in the preoperative holding area with intravenous carbonic anhydrase inhibitors such as acetazolamide and/or hyperosmotic agents including mannitol (1–2 g/kg)
- Aggressive preoperative control of systemic blood pressure
- Correction of any bleeding diathesis (platelet transfusion, vitamin K, etc.;   replacement of coumadin with shorter acting anticoagulants); coordinate with primary care provider
- Discontinuation of antiplatelet agents and vitamin E (if possible) 1–2 weeks prior to surgery
- Preoperative stool softeners if history of constipation

Intraoperative Factors

- Slow paracentesis to normalize IOP at beginning of case
- If cataract surgery is required, use small incision techniques
- Preplace scleral flap sutures in order to rapidly close the eye
- Fashion a large enough flap to adequately cover the stoma
- Minimize surgical time
- Avoid collapse of the globe during surgery; use an anterior chamber maintainer if necessary
- If vitrectomy is required, avoid low IOP during vitrectomy
- Prophylactic sclerostomy (Sturge-Weber and nanophthalmos)
- Superb monitoring and control of systemic blood pressure during surgery
- Prevention of postoperative hypotony by placing extra sutures in the trabeculectomy flap at the time of filtration surgery
- Avoid excessive concentration or duration of antimetabolites
- Protect the blood-aqueous barrier by preventing excessive inflammation with generous postoperative topical and, if necessary, oral corticosteroids

Postoperative Factors

- Recognition of vigorous treatment of postoperative choroidal effusions, knowing that these choroidal effusions are often the triggering event for hemorrhage and may require drainage in high-risk eyes
- Counseling patients not to do anything that mimics a Valsalva maneuver
- Use stool softeners; encourage liquid intake
- Use bandage contact lenses to tamponade the bleb and prevent hypotony
- Consider return to surgery to place additional scleral flap sutures if postoperative IOP is lower than anticipated
- Injection of viscoelastic into anterior chamber at any time to increase IOP if needed
- In very high-risk eyes, inject a gas bubble into the vitreous cavity
- Avoid premature release of sutures in the scleral flap
- If worried it is too early to release or cut a suture, use focal massage next to the bleb and determine how low the IOP drops; if excessive, wait to cut or release sutures

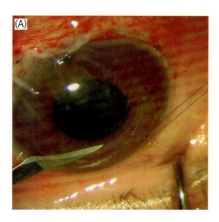

FIGURE 6.1A **Exposure and corneal paracentesis.** An inferior corneal traction suture is in place to gain exposure to the inferior quadrants. A temporal paracentesis track is created for placement of the anterior chamber maintainer. The eye should be firm and the anterior chamber maintained at all times during drainage of the choroidal effusion, decreasing the likelihood of further choroidal events during drainage.

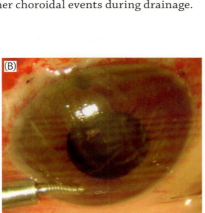

FIGURE 6.1B **Insertion of anterior chamber maintainer.** The maintainer facilitates adequate IOP during drainage of the effusion and protects the anterior chamber from collapse. The key is to make sure the maintainer is all the way into the anterior chamber before infusing. At the end of the procedure, turn the infusion off before removing.

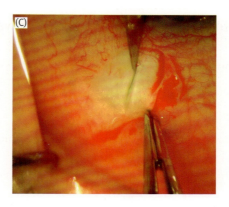

FIGURE 6.1C **Scleral cut down.** Use a super sharp or similar instrument to carefully dissect, layer by layer, down through the scleral fibers until arriving at the suprachoroidal space. The location of the cut down should be planned by viewing the fundus preoperatively to decide the best quadrant for drainage.

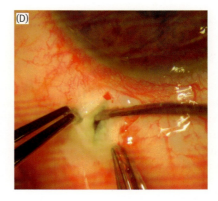

FIGURE 6.1D **Drainage with cyclodialysis spatula.** Carefully dissect the last few scleral fibers over the suprachoroidal space. Once down to the suprachoroidal space, slide the blunt end of a cyclodialysis spatula into the opening created by the scleral incision, carefully avoiding the vascular, spongy choroidal tissue and simultaneously lifting the scleral tissue away from the choroidal space. This maneuver is repeated several times in different directions to facilitate drainage.

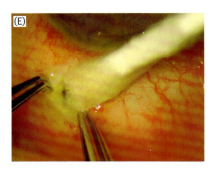

FIGURE 6.1E **Drainage with sponge.** A wedge-shaped surgical sponge is useful to soak up the choroidal fluid as it drains from the suprachoroidal space. The constant pressure from the anterior chamber maintainer helps the fluid continue to drain.

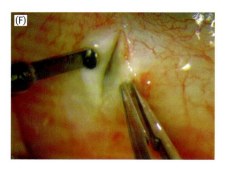

FIGURE 6.1F **Punch in position.** Some investigators recommend, as do I, to use a punch to remove a small piece of sclera to facilitate continued drainage of the site for a few days. The wound rapidly heals over, but continued drainage for a few days may be highly beneficial.

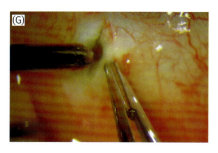

FIGURE 6.1G **Removal of scleral tissue with punch.** Place the punch just below the scleral lip, slide it into position, and remove a small piece of sclera from the lip of the cut down, leaving a very small segment of uveal tissue exposed for drainage.

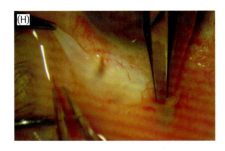

FIGURE 6.1H **Coverage of drainage site.** A bridge of Tenon's capsule is very useful to cover the sclerostomy site and allows continued drainage of the site with adequate coverage. Tack this down with two sutures.

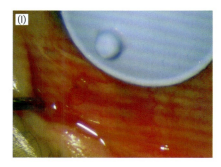

FIGURE 6.1I **Closure of conjunctiva.** Close the conjunctiva carefully over the layer of Tenon's capsule.

MANAGEMENT

Spontaneous intraoperative choroidal effusions are more common in patients with fragile vessels, diabetes, uveal effusion syndrome, short axial lengths[7] (such as in nanophthalmos), and other disorders related to scleral permeability. Spontaneous effusion may also occur with positive venous pressure and other Valsalva maneuvers. When these events occur and fluid accumulates in the anterior suprachoroidal space, an annular choroidal effusion may develop with ciliolenticular block,[8] mimicking aqueous misdirection syndrome. If recognized intraoperatively, treatments include cycloplegics, immediate closure of the eye, and aqueous suppressants. The eye gradually responds to therapy, becomes less firm, and the case may be completed. If the condition was severe, the choroidal space could be tapped to reduce the fluid volume in the suprachoroidal space.

Table 6.2 Risk Factors for Choroidal Events

RISK FACTORS FOR CHOROIDAL EVENTS

- Aphakia
- Previous or simultaneous vitrectomy
- High myopia
- Uncontrolled systemic hypertension
- High flow arterial—venous shunts
- Very high preoperative IOP, >30–40 mm Hg
- Sturge-Weber syndrome
- Osler-Rendu-Weber syndrome
- Short axial length and uveal effusion syndrome
- Intraoperative or postoperative Valsalva maneuver
- Use of anticoagulant and/or antiplatelet medications
- Blood dyscrasias associated with leukemia and aplastic anemia
- Thrombocytopenia
- Advanced age
- Buphthalmic eyes

Intraoperative choroidal events may occur posteriorly with a large choroidal effusion. Subsequently, the chamber usually flattens in conjunction with a firm eye. The eye should immediately be closed to reduce the size of the effusion, and aqueous suppressants should be administered. A choroidal effusion in an eye with normal IOP may resolve rapidly. If the IOP stays low for a couple of weeks, the choroidal effusion may persist but will resolve over several weeks as the IOP returns to a more normal range. These effusions rarely require drainage. In the postoperative period, if the anterior chamber is flat, the choroidal effusions are in apposition ("kissing"), or the patient has pain, the effusion should be drained (Figure 6.1). Typically, drainage of a choroidal effusion is highly successful and visual recovery excellent.[9]

Suprachoroidal hemorrhage is a far more devastating event than a choroidal effusion. It is a painful complication of ocular surgery and occurs most commonly in glaucoma patients. It may occur intraoperatively[10] or postoperatively. The major predisposing factor for all choroidal events is hypotony. Hypotony is exacerbated in patients with vascular anomalies[11] and is worsened by the Valsalva maneuver.[12] Antiplatelet therapy and anticoagulation therapy also complicate and worsen the situation.[13] Choroidal hemorrhages occur most frequently in glaucoma patients with aphakic, vitrectomized eyes undergoing filtration surgery.[14-20] Suprachoroidal hemorrhage is also more likely to occur in highly myopic, hypertensive patients with long-standing glaucoma and high IOP or may even occur at the time of cataract extraction. Visual loss may be severe or mild depending on preservation of intraocular contents, especially retinal tissue. Much of this vision loss is dependent on how long it takes to reestablish ocular integrity and close the eye during surgery. Immediate injection of a viscoelastic may help elevate the IOP and tamponade the blood.[21] Intraoperatively, the signs and symptoms of a suprachoroidal hemorrhage include shallowing of the anterior chamber, a firm eye, a shadow emerging over the red reflex, pain, and elevated blood pressure. Vitrectomized eyes may only show the shadow obscuring the red reflex as the initial sign of impending danger.[22] Proper technique is critical, especially in high-risk eyes.[23] For example, additional flap sutures, as noted in Table 6.1, are an important technique modification to help prevent postoperative hypotony.

Postoperative suprachoroidal hemorrhages typically occur during the first 2 weeks after trabeculectomy, especially following premature suture lysis or release, and their management is controversial.[24] A choroidal effusion develops as a result of hypotony, and as the choroidal effusion increases in size, the long ciliary artery stretches and breaks, spilling blood into the suprachoroidal space.[25] Surgeons should never be timid in returning to the operating room to drain a choroidal effusion, especially in high-risk monocular patients.

CONCLUSION

Fortunately, intraoperative choroidal events are uncommon. Surgeons should continue to be ever vigilant to reduce the incidence of this dreadful surgical complication. Should it occur, expeditious closure of the eye along with close observation may save vision for many patients.

COMMENTARY
STEVEN R. SARKISIAN, Jr.

Preparing for and preventing choroidal effusion and hemorrhage is a key component of the surgical treatment of glaucoma and demands careful attention. In fact, it is the fear of these potentially devastating complications, among other things, that has fueled surgical innovation to move to more precise, smaller incision filtration surgery (EX-PRESS™ Glaucoma Drainage Device; Alcon Laboratories, Inc., Fort Worth, Texas) or to nonpenetrating types of procedures (canaloplasty). Moreover, increased attention is being paid to *ab interno* procedures that can be performed at the time of cataract extraction in which choroidal effusions and choroidal hemorrhages are not an issue. These include endoscopic cyclophotocoagulation, Trabectome® (NeoMedix Corporation, Tustin, California; see Chapter 50), the iStent® Trabecular Micro-bypass (Glaukos® Corporation, Laguna Hills, California), and the SOLX® Gold shunt (SOLX®, Inc., Waltham, Massachusetts).

Dr. Fellman's chapter on choroidal effusion and hemorrhage is concise and complete. I would only submit one nuance to Dr. Fellman's excellent chapter. Regarding his technique for drainage of choroidal fluid, I would perform the procedure in the identical fashion with one minor exception of minimal consequence. I typically perform 2 cut downs in the inferior quadrants; however, rather than use a scleral punch to keep the incisions open for postoperative drainage, I use a 23-gauge pointed cautery tip and apply for the length of the incision to spread the external opening of the cut down and prevent it from appositional closure after the surgery.

Dr. Sarkisian was supported by an Unrestricted Grant from Research to Prevent Blindness to the University of Oklahoma College of Medicine and is a consultant for Alcon.

COMMENTARY
ANASTASIOS P. COSTARIDES

Intraoperative choroidal effusion and hemorrhage are the result of the reduction of IOP that occurs during glaucoma surgery. One of the most visually devastating complications of glaucoma surgery is a suprachoroidal hemorrhage, which is believed to be the result of a rapid reduction in eye pressure.

During glaucoma surgery, steps should be undertaken to reduce both the time and degree of hypotony. The author recommends the preplacement of scleral flap sutures. I preplace at least 2 sutures in the scleral flap during trabeculectomy. This significantly reduces the time it takes to close the scleral flap and re-establish eye pressure to a physiologic level. In patients who are at high risk for a suprachoroidal hemorrhage, the intracameral administration of viscoelastic prior to the filtering procedure is another method that should reduce the pressure differential when the eye is open. It is reasonable to leave some viscoelastic in the eye even after the scleral flap is closed in eyes at high risk as described by Dr. Fellman.

I recommend that scleral flaps be tied tightly. I routinely place an extra suture in a flap beyond what I believe it takes to control flow through the flap. The reasoning for this is that it reduces hypotony risk during conjunctival closure as well as decreasing risk of hypotony with suture removal in the early postoperative period. I believe more is better when suturing flaps.

Rapid closure of the eye as described by Dr. Fellman is imperative when a choroidal event takes place intraoperatively. The elevation of IOP may limit the extent of the effusion or hemorrhage. One approach for increasing the IOP is injecting viscoelastic into the anterior chamber. The pressure should remain elevated until expansion of the choroidal event has ceased. With a hemorrhage, keeping the pressure elevated for minutes beyond the cessation of the extension of the choroidal event is a way of ensuring that a clot has formed. Clot formation limits the extent of the hemorrhage. With an effusion, elevating IOP may be all that is necessary to reverse the process.

No consensus exists for the management of a choroidal hemorrhage once the blood extension has stopped.[24] One approach is to wait to drain the blood 7–10 days after the event, allowing time for clot dissolution. This approach reduces the risk of a rebleed but may leave the eye with a precariously elevated IOP with medical management as the only option. Another approach is the placement of a scleral window minutes after hemorrhaging has stopped, as described by Dr. Fellman. A clot is invariably present, but it is usually accompanied by a serosanguinous effusate that will drain readily through a scleral window. This drainage will promote the reformation of the anterior chamber and limit extension of the choroidal event once the clot begins to dissolve.

Various approaches for the management of choroidal hemorrhage are necessary because of the frequent difficulty in controlling these bleeds. Full recovery is possible with a limited hemorrhage while complete loss of vision may occur with extensive bleeds.

REFERENCES

1. Sathyan P, Singh G, Eong KG, Raman GV, Prashanth S. Suprachoroidal hemorrhage following removal of releasable suture after combined phacoemulsification-trabeculectomy. *J Cataract Refract Surg.* Jun 2007;33(6): 1104–1105.

2. Quigley HA, Friedman DS, Congdon NG. Possible mechanisms of primary angle-closure and malignant glaucoma. *J Glaucoma.* Apr 2003; 12(2):167–1180.

3. Jampel HD, Musch DC, Gillespie BW, Lichter PR, Wright MM, Guire KE. Perioperative complications of trabeculectomy in the Collaborative Initial Glaucoma Treatment Study (CIGTS). *Am J Ophthalmol.* Jul 2005; 140(1):16–122.

4. Gedde SJ, Herndon LW, Brandt JD, Budenz DL, Feuer WJ, Schiffman JC. Surgical complications in the Tube Versus Trabeculectomy Study during the first year of follow-up. *Am J Ophthalmol.* Jan 2007;143(1):23–131.

5. Givens K, Shields MB. Suprachoroidal hemorrhage after glaucoma filtering surgery. *Am J Ophthalmol.* May 15 1987;103(5): 689–1694.

6. Chu TG, Green RL. Suprachoroidal hemorrhage. *Surv Ophthalmol.* May-Jun 1999; 43(6):471–1486.

7. Wladis EJ, Gewirtz MB, Guo S. Cataract surgery in the small adult eye. *Surv Ophthalmol.* Mar-Apr 2006;51(2):153–161.

8. Fellman RL. Cataract surgical problem. *J Cataract Refract Surg .* 2007;33:944–947.

9. WuDunn D, Ryser D, Cantor LB. Surgical drainage of choroidal effusions following glaucoma surgery. *J Glaucoma.* Apr 2005;14(2): 103–108.

10. Iaccarino G, Rosa N, Romano M, Capasso L, Romano A. Expulsive hemorrhage before phacoemulsification. *J Cataract Refract Surg.* Jun 2002;28(6):1074–1076.

11. Mahmoud TH, Deramo VA, Kim T, Fekrat S. Intraoperative choroidal hemorrhage in the Osler-Rendu-Weber syndrome. *Am J Ophthalmol.* Feb 2002;133(2):282–284.

12. Pollack AL, McDonald HR, Ai E, et al. Massive suprachoroidal hemorrhage during pars plana vitrectomy associated with Valsalva maneuver. *Am J Ophthalmol.* Sept 2001;132(3):383–387.

13. Law SK, Song BJ, Yu F, Kurbanyan K, Yang TA, Caprioli J. Hemorrhagic complications from glaucoma surgery in patients on anticoagulation therapy or antiplatelet therapy. *Am J Ophthalmol.* Apr 2008;145(4):736–746.

14. Cantor LB, Katz LJ, Spaeth GL. Complications of surgery in glaucoma. Suprachoroidal expulsive hemorrhage in glaucoma patients undergoing intraocular surgery. *Ophthalmology.* Sept 1985;92(9):1266–1270.

15. Ruderman JM, Harbin TS, Jr., Campbell DG. Postoperative suprachoroidal hemorrhage following filtration procedures. *Arch Ophthalmol.* Feb 1986;104(2):201–205.

16. Haynes JH, Payne JW, Green WR. Clinicopathologic study of eyes obtained postmortem from a patient 6 and 2 years after operative choroidal hemorrhage. *Ophthalmic Surg.* Sept 1987;18(9):667–671.

17. Welch JC, Spaeth GL, Benson WE. Massive suprachoroidal hemorrhage. Follow-up and outcome of 30 cases. *Ophthalmology.* Sept 1988;95(9):1202–1206.

18. Speaker MG, Guerriero PN, Met JA, Coad CT, Berger A, Marmor M. A case-control study of risk factors for intraoperative suprachoroidal expulsive hemorrhage. *Ophthalmology*. Feb 1991;98(2): 202–209; discussion 210.

19. Canning CR, Lavin M, McCartney AC, Hitchings RA, Gregor ZJ. Delayed suprachoroidal haemorrhage after glaucoma operations. *Eye*. 1989;3(Pt 3):327–331.

20. Spaeth GL, Baez KA. Long-term prognosis of eyes having had operative suprachoroidal expulsive hemorrhage. *Ger J Ophthalmol*. May 1994;3(3): 159–163.

21. Vold SD, Rylander N. Healon5 in the management of intraoperative expulsive hemorrhage. *J Cataract Refract Surg*. Mar 2007; 33(3):545–547.

22. Wong KK, Saleh TA, Gray RH. Suprachoroidal hemorrhage during cataract surgery in a vitrectomized eye. *J Cataract Refract Surg*. Jun 2005;31(6):1242–1243.

23. Fellman RL. Trabeculectomy. In: Yanoff M, Duker JS, eds. *Ophthalmology*. 2nd ed. St. Louis: Mosby; 2004:1586–1595.

24. Healey PR, Herndon L, Smiddy W. Management of suprachoroidal hemorrhage. *J Glaucoma*. Sept 2007;16(6):577–579.

25. Bellows AR, Chylack LT, Jr., Hutchinson BT. Choroidal detachment. Clinical manifestation, therapy and mechanism of formation. *Ophthalmology*. Nov 1981;88(11):1107–1115.

7

VITREOUS PROLAPSE AND LENS INJURY

PAUL J. HARASYMOWYCZ

VITREOUS PROLAPSE AND LENS INJURY

During trabeculectomy, when a sclerostomy and iridectomy are performed, the structures immediately posterior to the iris, namely the zonules, lens capsule, ciliary processes, and anterior hyaloid face may be violated, resulting in a variety of intraoperative and postoperative complications. Lens injury, including cataract formation, and vitreous prolapse are 2 of the complications that may occur intraoperatively.

LENS INJURY

Cataract

Cataract formation is one of the most common occurrences after trabeculectomy, reported in approximately 50%[1-3] of cases. While development of the cataract is usually a slow process, it occurs more frequently in patients with a history of diabetes, postoperative flat anterior chambers, or intraocular inflammation,[1] as well as in a patient with a negative spherical equivalent (preoperative lens status) and pseudoexfoliation syndrome.[4] Older age is a risk factor,[1] since natural cataract development may be accelerated; however, cataracts may develop in up to 25% of younger (<55 years of age) patients undergoing trabeculectomy.[5] The utilization of postoperative steroids has also been implicated in the development of posterior subcapsular opacities.[6]

Although not a common occurrence, cataracts may also develop soon after surgery due to direct intraoperative surgical trauma to the lens.[7] If the opacity is focal and does not encroach on or obstruct the visual axis, no further action may be needed. If there is obvious rupture of the lens capsule causing clinically significant inflammation that may compromise bleb development, urgent lens extraction should be performed. If the clinical situation permits, it is desirable to wait at least 3 months until the bleb matures.

Rapidly forming cataracts may also develop due to prolonged contact between the lens and the cornea, such as occurs intraoperatively if forceps inadvertently indent the cornea while retracting the conjunctiva during a limbus-based trabeculectomy. Similarly, the lens may opacify if the anterior chamber is flat for an extended period of time before the scleral flap sutures are adequately tied. Likewise, postoperative hypotony with a flat anterior chamber may lead to cataract formation (see Chapter 10).

In patients who already have cataractous lens opacities, a lower threshold for lens removal may be warranted, as extraction can be performed in combination with a trabeculectomy. Additionally, lens changes may be involved in the pathology of elevated intraocular pressure (i.e., phacomorphic), and combined surgery would reduce the likely need for additional surgery.

Lens dislocation

During creation of the sclerostomy and iridectomy, damage may occur to the lens zonules, resulting in subluxation of the crystalline lens or intraocular lens (IOL).[8] The haptics of IOLs in pseudophakic patients may also be inadvertently bent or cut, which potentially results in IOL decentration. Particular care must be taken with lenses that are not in the capsular bag, such as anterior chamber IOLs and sulcus-fixated lenses.[9] As suture fixation of IOLs to the posterior side of the iris gains popularity, the glaucoma surgeon must be certain that one of these sutures is not cut while excising tissue for an iridectomy.

Careful preoperative examination may reveal phacodonesis or pseudophacodonesis and should note IOL haptic position; this information should be used to determine site of surgery and filtration technique. In patients with higher preoperative posterior pressure, oral or intravenous carbonic anhydrase inhibitors and/or osmotic diuretics may be administered before surgery to dehydrate the vitreous, reducing the likelihood of damage to anterior structures.

VITREOUS PROLAPSE

Vitreous prolapse may also occur at the site of iridectomy[10] and may not necessarily be indicative of poor technique but rather high pressure in the vitreous cavity, as may result from aqueous (or infusion) misdirection syndrome,[11] choroidal effusion, or hemorrhage. These conditions occur more frequently in patients with angle closure glaucoma, Sturge-Weber syndrome,[12] or nanophthalmos.[9]

When operating on a pseudophakic eye, if the integrity of the posterior capsule is not certain or if it is known to be open, the trabeculectomy surgeon must be vigilant looking for vitreous prolapse into the anterior chamber and to the sclerostomy. Occasionally, glaucoma filtering surgery is performed in a patient who previously had a complicated cataract extraction, and vitreous may already be present in the anterior chamber. Regardless of the lens status, if the sclerostomy is created too far posteriorly, what is believed to be an iridectomy may actually be removal of a piece of ciliary body, and the sclerostomy may be communicating with the posterior segment rather than the anterior chamber. If the clear fluid that presents to the sclerostomy is gelatinous rather than aqueous, vitreous, unfortunately, has been found.

Once vitreous has been identified, prompt removal should be done to prevent the sclerostomy from being blocked postoperatively. A single port pars plana approach may be useful, with infusion into the anterior chamber in pseudophakic eyes. In any case, the newer technology phacoemulsification machines have high cut rates on the anterior vitrectomy settings. The infusion cannula should be inserted into the anterior chamber through a separate side port to avoid further disruption of the vitreous. Alternatively, the vitrectomy can be performed using a dry or viscoelastic assisted technique through the sclerostomy, especially if vitreous prolapse is limited.

Intracameral triamcinolone may help in visualizing vitreous strands and additionally decrease postoperative inflammation. Smaller gauge (23 or 25) posterior vitrectomy may also be useful in these settings. In patients with vitreous loss and higher posterior pressure, hemorrhagic choroidal complications are more frequent; therefore, the scleral flap should be closed as rapidly as possible, especially in patients who may be older, aphakic, and/or anticoagulated. In these patients, the scleral flap should be sutured tightly to prevent hypotony and postoperative shallowing of the anterior chamber. Consideration could be given to using IOP-lowering agents in the immediate postoperative period, in order to wait for the vitreous to "shrink back." Suture lysis or removal of releasable or adjustable sutures should be performed judiciously for the same reasons. For more information on vitreous prolapse, see Chapter 32.

CONCLUSION

In most cases, disturbance of structures posterior to the iris is limited and prolapse or damage to those structures rare. Careful preoperative planning and meticulous surgical technique can help make these complications unusual but not totally avoidable. If isolated, vitreous prolapse or cataract formation can be managed with good outcomes.

Dr. Harasymowycz was supported by the Quebec Glaucoma Foundation.

COMMENTARY
RONALD L. GROSS

This is an excellent discussion of the topic. The risk of an increased rate of cataract formation following trabeculectomy is well demonstrated in several excellent trials (see above), to the extent that it should be included in the routine preoperative discussion with phakic patients. It is important to point out that in the vast majority of cases, a relative acceleration of the development of lens opacification occurs over years. It is more likely that an eye that has undergone trabeculectomy will require cataract extraction sooner than an eye that has not. As to whether a combined trabeculectomy and cataract extraction should be performed given this increased risk of cataract formation, in most cases the increased rate of opacification is relatively slow, and the patient's visual needs at the time of trabeculectomy determine the appropriateness of lens extraction.

Luckily, vitreous presentation or lens injury during glaucoma filtration surgery are rare, but represents one of those times when a deep breath and checking your own pulse may be appropriate. Preoperative evaluation is the key to prevention. As is pointed out, seeing lens instability or identifying vitreous in the posterior chamber preoperatively allows the surgeon to be prepared to address these complications with a plan rather than on the fly in the high stress of the moment. The discussion on management is excellent. In an eye where there is concern that vitreous may be in the posterior chamber and that a peripheral iridotomy would be best avoided, the use of an EX-PRESS™ shunt (Alcon Laboratories, Inc., Fort Worth, Texas) as a component of the trabeculectomy may be considered. This provides the additional benefit of minimizing the shallowing of the anterior chamber intraoperatively that could potentially cause anterior movement of vitreous. This may also be used in eyes with large posterior capsulotomies where vitreous behind the IOL could move forward during surgery. Alternatively, a viscoelastic agent (OVD) can be used to maintain the anterior chamber during surgery. When removed, however, there is risk of abruptly shallowing the anterior chamber. Alternatively, leaving it in place makes checking flow difficult and may increase the risk of an elevated IOP postoperatively.[1,4,13]

Dr. Gross is a consultant for Alcon and has received honoraria and research funding from Alcon.

REFERENCES

1. The Advanced Glaucoma Intervention Study: 8. Risk of cataract formation after trabeculectomy. *Arch Ophthalmol.* Dec 2001; 119(12):1771–1779.

2. Husain R, Liang S, Foster PJ, et al. Cataract surgery after trabeculectomy: the effect on trabeculectomy function. *Arch Ophthalmol.* Feb 2012;130(2):165–170.

3. Gedde SJ, Schiffman JC, Feuer WJ, Herndon LW, Brandt JD, Budenz DL. Three-year follow-up of the tube versus trabeculectomy study. *Am J Ophthalmol.* Nov 2009;148(5):670–684.

4. Musch DC, Gillespie BW, Niziol LM, et al. Cataract extraction in the collaborative initial glaucoma treatment study: incidence, risk factors, and the effect of cataract progression and extraction on clinical and quality-of-life outcomes. *Arch Ophthalmol.* Dec 2006; 124(12):1694–1700.

5. Adelman RA, Brauner SC, Afshari NA, Grosskreutz CL. Cataract formation after initial trabeculectomy in young patients. *Ophthalmology.* Mar 2003;110(3):625–629.

6. Husain R, Aung T, Gazzard G, et al. Effect of trabeculectomy on lens opacities in an East Asian population. *Arch Ophthalmol.* Jun 2006;124(6):787–792.

7. Lin JC, Katz LJ, Spaeth GL, Klancnik JM, Jr. An "exploding cataract" following Nd:YAG laser iridectomy. *Ophthalmic Surg Lasers Imaging.* Jul-Aug 2003;34(4):310–311.

8. Sagara N, Kimura A, Arimura K, Yonemura M, Tanihara H. Lens luxation and prolapse into the surgical wound region during trabeculectomy. *Acta Ophthalmol Scand.* Aug 2003;81(4):409–411.

9. Wu W, Dawson DG, Sugar A, et al. Cataract surgery in patients with nanophthalmos: results and complications. *J Cataract Refract Surg.* Mar 2004;30(3):584–590.

10. Loewenthal LM. Trabeculectomy as treatment for glaucoma: a preliminary report. *Ann Ophthalmol.* Sept 1977;9(9):1179–1186.

11. Realini T, Vaphiades MS. Infusion misdirection syndrome during trabeculectomy for primary trabeculodysgenesis. *Am J Ophthalmol.* Jan 2002;133(1):138–139.

12. Agarwal HC, Sandramouli S, Sihota R, Sood NN. Sturge-Weber syndrome: management of glaucoma with combined trabeculotomy-trabeculectomy. *Ophthalmic Surg.* Jun 1993;24(6):399–402.

13. Comparison of glaucomatous progression between untreated patients with normal-tension glaucoma and patients with therapeutically reduced intraocular pressures. Collaborative Normal-Tension Glaucoma Study Group. *Am J Ophthalmol.* Oct 1998;126(4): 487–497.

8

DESCEMET'S MEMBRANE DETACHMENT

MALIK Y. KAHOOK

DESCEMET'S MEMBRANE DETACHMENT

Corneal injury resulting from glaucoma surgery has been well described.[1] Causes of injury can range from direct mechanical manipulation to the often more subtle pharmacologically induced injuries that occur with use of anti-fibrotic medications. Descemet's membrane detachment (DMD) occurs uncommonly during or after intraocular surgery and has been linked with a variety of procedures ranging from simple clear cornea cataract extraction to deep lamellar keratoplasty.[2,3] The corneal endothelium, which rests upon Descemet's membrane, functions as a pump to keep the stroma from becoming swollen. Therefore, DMD results in focal corneal edema and possibly bullous keratopathy. If detachment of Descemet's membrane extends far enough centrally, visual acuity may become sufficiently compromised to necessitate corneal transplantation surgery (either full-thickness penetrating keratoplasty [PKP] or Descemet's stripping with automated endothelial keratoplasty [DSAEK]). In glaucoma surgery, DMD often results from the mechanical manipulation that occurs with creation of the corneal-trabecular meshwork opening. Knowing how to accurately diagnose and treat DMD can prevent disastrous consequences and preserve vision.

CLASSIFICATION OF DESCEMET'S MEMBRANE DETACHMENT

Mackool and Holtz proposed separating DMD into 2 categories, planar and nonplanar, depending on the distance of separation between Descemet's membrane and the posterior corneal stroma.[4] Planar DMD involves less than 1 mm separation of Descemet's membrane from the corneal stroma and may be limited to the periphery or extend from the periphery to central regions. Nonplanar DMD involves greater than 1 mm separation of Descemet's membrane from the corneal stroma and may also be categorized as limited to the periphery or extending to central regions. The significance of this classification was the belief that planar DMD was more likely to spontaneously resolve while nonplanar DMD required surgical intervention. Assia and colleagues also split DMD into 2 categories: DMD with scrolling of tissue and DMD without scrolling of tissue. They believed this classification more accurately described potential for spontaneous resolution in that nonscrolled DMD was more likely to resolve without surgical intervention, even if its location was >1mm from the posterior corneal stroma.[5] While useful as a general guide, these classification systems are not foolproof, and each case of DMD should be viewed independently. See Table 8.1 for a breakdown of classifications of DMD.

DIAGNOSING DESCEMET'S MEMBRANE DETACHMENT

DMD may be noted during dissection of the scleral flap and entry into the anterior chamber with traditional trabeculectomy. The surgeon should also exercise caution when injecting balanced salt solution or viscoelastic

Table 8.1 Classifications of Descemet's Membrane Detachment

CLASSIFICATIONS OF DESCEMET'S MEMBRANE DETACHMENT

1. A) Planar: Less than 1 mm separation between Descemet's membrane and stroma
   B) Nonplanar: More than 1 mm separation between Descemet's membrane and stroma
2. A) Scrolled: Exhibits a rolled edge
   B) Nonscrolled: No rolled edge
3. A) Peripheral: Does not involve the visual axis
   B) Peripheral with central involvement

*author: Andrew C. Crichton and Ahmed Al-Ghoul

material through a paracentesis wound. With viscocanalostomy or canaloplasty, the cannula used to inject viscoelastic into Schlemm's canal may be misdirected into the cornea. Subsequent injection of the viscoelastic can lead to limited or diffuse DMD with viscoelastic rather than aqueous or balanced salt solution in the interface.

In the acute phase of limited DMD, the corneal tissue remains clear, and the subtle separation of tissue planes can be hard to recognize. In the case of large intraoperative DMD encroaching on the visual axis, the surgeon might appreciate very subtle signs such as mild corneal edema, early stromal folds, and/or a dulling of the corneal light reflex overlying the DMD that may not be noticed intraoperatively. Consequently, DMD is often appreciated only in the postoperative phase, even by the seasoned glaucoma surgeon.

During the postoperative phase, diagnosis of DMD may be limited by the existence of significant corneal edema. Suspicion should arise when localized edematous corneal tissue is seen adjacent to the anterior chamber entry site, in cases of traditional filtration surgery, or beginning at the limbal margin, as is the case with nonpenetrating surgery. It is not unusual to see sharp demarcation lines of edema corresponding to the border of the DMD from the posterior corneal stroma. However, if retained viscoelastic occupies the space between the detached Descemet's membrane and the stroma, edema may not develop until the viscoelastic dissipates, thereby delaying the diagnosis of DMD. Blood intermixed with the fluid or viscoelastic occupying the DMD space may allow for better visualization and alert the examiner to the existence of the pathology.

When these findings are present, ultrasound biomicroscopy (UBM) and/or anterior segment optical coherence tomography (ASOCT) are very helpful in bypassing corneal haze to qualify and quantify DMD.[6–8] ASOCT can reveal even subclinical DMD (Figure 8.1) and has a higher resolution than UBM, making it a particularly valuable tool in diagnosing this pathology. The clinician should look for a small band of hyper-reflective tissue (representing the DMD) underlying the corneal

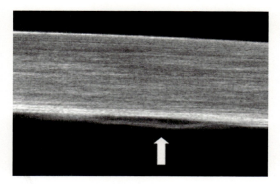

FIGURE 8.1 Anterior Segment Optical Coherence Tomography image of a limited Descemet's membrane detachment (arrow).

stroma with an intervening hypo-reflective band (representing fluid or viscoelastic). While valuable for diagnosis, these modalities can also be used for postoperative follow-up to ensure resolution of the pathology or to investigate suspected recurrences.

TREATING DMD

In hopes of avoiding a second surgical intervention, a "watch and wait" approach may be appropriate for small planar and/or non-scrolled DMD that are not encroaching on the visual axis and not limiting the patient's visual function. Even when spontaneous reattachment occurs, it can take weeks to months and leave affected patients with significant morbidity. For this reason, most surgeons now advocate for early intervention in cases with visually significant DMD, even when classified as planar or nonscrolled. Methods for repair include manual repositioning, repositioning under viscoelastic agents or air, direct suturing of Descemet's membrane to the peripheral cornea, as well as use of intracameral gases such as sulfur hexafluoride (SF_6) and perfluoropropane (C_3F_8) for long-standing tamponade of Descemet's membrane to the corneal stroma.[9–17]

If limited DMD is noted intraoperatively, it is important to avoid further manipulation of tissue at the surgical site, if possible, and to leave an air tamponade at the site of tissue dissection. Use of sutures, viscoelastic, or gas

tamponade is often not needed in this situation, and prognosis is excellent.

In cases of persistent visually significant DMD, my preferred intervention is use of long-acting SF_6 gas tamponade.[18,19] First, a cohesive viscoelastic is injected into the anterior chamber through a side port paracentesis while ensuring that the viscoelastic is directed posterior to Descemet's membrane. The viscoelastic should be used to elevate the DMD as much as possible so as to avoid the need for direct contact between the endothelium and a blunt instrument while reapproximating the tissue. Even so, a cyclodialysis spatula is often needed to smooth out the DMD against the posterior corneal stroma, especially along the periphery where Descemet's membrane reaches the limbus. Once the detached tissue has been repositioned onto the stroma, SF_6 gas should be injected through the side port incision. For best results and to avoid complications, a 20% mixture of SF_6 gas with air should be used. This mixture will not expand in the anterior chamber. The bubble should remain in the anterior chamber for 1–2 weeks, giving the endothelium time to recover and transport fluid appropriately to allow for adhesion to the corneal stroma.

Once repair has been completed, the surgeon should be aware that postoperative complications after use of SF_6 gas may include increased intraocular pressure (IOP) from an expanding bubble (improperly mixed), pupillary block, and loss of tissue apposition to the corneal stoma due to escape of gas from the surgical wound. For these reasons, frequent postoperative follow-up is needed to quickly diagnose these complications and intervene. In the case of SF_6 failure, it may be necessary to reinject a gas bubble and/or suture the DMD to the corneal stroma using interrupted 10–0 nylon sutures with 100% thickness bites.

CONCLUSION

DMD is an uncommon complication of filtration surgery more often seen with nonpenetrating procedures. Intraoperative diagnosis of DMD is uncommon due to the often limited nature of the pathology and the absence of edema to signal presence of the dissected tissue. Postoperative diagnosis may be hindered by the presence of significant corneal edema. DMD should be considered in the differential diagnosis of nonresolving corneal edema following filtration surgery. Recognition may be improved with use of sensitive imaging devices such as UBM and/or ASOCT. In the case of visually significant and/or large DMD, use of SF_6 gas for long-term tamponade may allow for resolution and visual rehabilitation. Alternative treatments may also include manual repositioning with a blunt cannula or spatula, injection of air rather than long acting gases, and/or direct suturing of the detached tissue to restore normal anatomical relationships.

While surgical intervention is a main cause for DMD, it is important to note that nonsurgical factors such as trauma,[20,21] corneal edema,[22] corneal ectasia,[23,24] and elevated IOP[25,26] have all been noted to increase the risk of or cause DMD. Extra intraoperative care should be taken in patients who have these conditions as manipulation of limbal and corneal tissue is more likely to lead to Descemet's membrane pathology.

COMMENTARY

FRANCISCO E. FANTES† AND MICHAEL R. BANITT

The causes of Descemet's membrane detachments during trabeculectomy are outlined in the chapter. Contact with instruments or the inadvertent injection of fluid or viscoelastic anterior to Descemet's membrane are the most common causes. Detachments can occur at either the paracentesis or trabeculectomy sites. Intraoperative diagnosis is not always possible but should be suspected in the early postoperative course when corneal edema is focal or persists near a wound. When DMD is suspected, ASOCT is our diagnostic tool of choice. In general, focal, peripheral detachments may be left untreated. Larger detachments, particularly those involving the visual axis, may require intervention.

Our standard technique involves injecting air through the limbus into the anterior chamber with a 30-gauge needle kept parallel to the iris. With a small air bubble already in the anterior chamber, folded or poorly placed segments of Descemet's membrane can be repositioned with a reverse Sinsky hook. We typically avoid the use of ophthalmic viscoelastic devices (OVD) in doing this as OVD can get into the interface and prevent or significantly delay reattachment. The peripheral iridectomy made during the trabeculectomy permits a full anterior chamber air fill. Administering dilating drops at the end of the case and leaving an air bubble that clears the inferior pupillary border with the patient upright will reduce the risk of pupillary block.

Patients with central detachments should remain supine for 1–2 hours. Patients with peripheral detachments should remain on their right or left sides to maximize contact between the air bubble and the detached tissue. A slit-lamp exam can be performed an hour after surgery to check for pupillary block. Although not frequently necessary, full-thickness venting slits made with a paracentesis blade held perpendicular to the surface of the eye can be made in the area of the detachment. Fluid in the interface can often be expressed by torquing these wounds intraoperatively or postoperatively. Incompletely resolved Descemet's membrane detachments can be observed for weeks as spontaneous reattachment can sometimes occur. Alternatively, the eye can be rebubbled with air or a nonexpansile concentration (20%) of SF_6.

Dr. Banitt was supported by National Eye Institute grant R01EY014957, National Eye Institute grant P30EY014801, Department of Defense grant W81XWH-09-1-0675, and an Unrestricted Grant from Research to Prevent Blindness to Bascom Palmer Eye Institute, Miller School of Medicine, University of Miami.

COMMENTARY

ANDREW C. CRICHTON AND AHMED AL-GHOUL

In Descemet's membrane detachment, it is important to recognize that endothelial function is not compromised as cells derive nourishment from aqueous. The cells, therefore, remain viable for an extended period of time. The diagnosis can be difficult to make intraoperatively, but it can be recognized during surgery by a movement of the detached Descemet's membrane during intracameral fluid injection. Small Descemet's membrane detachments are more commonly seen during cataract surgery with clear corneal wounds, and this movement is easily recognized.

As is always the situation regarding treatment, the benefits must be weighed against the risks of further intervention. Any manipulation to Descemet's membrane intraoperatively as well as use of intracameral gases will induce endothelial damage. As such, repairing Descemet's membrane detachments should be done cautiously and only in cases deemed to benefit from further intervention.[27,28]

REFERENCES

1. Hau S, Barton K. Corneal complications of glaucoma surgery. *Curr Opin Ophthalmol.* Mar 2009;20(2):131–136.

2. Marcon AS, Rapuano CJ, Jones MR, Laibson PR, Cohen EJ. Descemet's membrane detachment after cataract surgery: management and outcome. *Ophthalmology.* Dec 2002; 109(12):2325–2330.

3. Sugita J, Kondo J. Deep lamellar keratoplasty with complete removal of pathological stroma for vision improvement. *Br J Ophthalmol.* Mar 1997;81(3):184–188.

4. Mackool RJ, Holtz SJ. Descemet membrane detachment. *Arch Ophthalmol.* Mar 1977;95(3): 459–463.

5. Assia EI, Levkovich-Verbin H, Blumenthal M. Management of Descemet's membrane detachment. *J Cataract Refract Surg.* Nov 1995; 21(6):714–717.

6. Morinelli EN, Najac RD, Speaker MG, Tello C, Liebmann JM, Ritch R. Repair of Descemet's membrane detachment with the assistance of intraoperative ultrasound biomicroscopy. *Am J Ophthalmol.* Jun 1996;121(6):718–720.

7. Mendrinos E, Mermoud A, Shaarawy T. Nonpenetrating glaucoma surgery. *Surv Ophthalmol.* Nov-Dec 2008;53(6):592–630.

8. Behrens A, Stark WJ, Pratzer KA, McDonnell PJ. Dynamics of small-incision clear cornea wounds after phacoemulsification surgery using optical coherence tomography in the early postoperative period. *J Refract Surg.* Jan 2008; 24(1):46–49.

9. Sparks GM. Descemetopexy. Surgical reattachment of stripped Descemet's membrane. *Arch Ophthalmol.* Jul 1967;78(1):31–34.

10. Hagan JC, 3rd. Treatment of progressive Descemet's membrane detachment. *Ophthalmic Surg.* Sept 1992;23(9):641; author reply 642.

11. Donzis PB, Karcioglu ZA, Insler MS. Sodium hyaluronate (Healon®) in the surgical repair of Descemet's membrane detachment. *Ophthalmic Surg.* Nov 1986;17(11):735–737.

12. Jurgens I. Repair of Descemet's membrane detachment with sulfur hexafluoride. *Cornea.* Jul 1996;15(4):439–440.

13. Zeiter HJ, Zeiter JT. Descemet's membrane separation during five hundred forty-four intraocular lens implantations. 1975–1982. *J Am Intraocul Implant Soc.* Winter 1983;9(1): 36–39.

14. Makley TA, Jr., Keates RH. Detachment of Descemet's membrane with insertion of an intraocular lens. *Ophthalmic Surg.* Aug 1980; 11(8):492–494.

15. Walland MJ, Stevens JD, Steele AD. Repair of Descemet's membrane detachment after intraocular surgery. *J Cataract Refract Surg.* May 1995;21(3):250–253.

16. Shah M, Bathia J, Kothari K. Repair of late Descemet's membrane detachment with perfluoropropane gas. *J Cataract Refract Surg.* Jun 2003;29(6):1242–1244.

17. Macsai MS, Gainer KM, Chisholm L. Repair of Descemet's membrane detachment with perfluoropropane (C3F8). *Cornea.* Mar 1998; 17(2):129–134.

18. Ellis DR, Cohen KL. Sulfur hexafluoride gas in the repair of Descemet's membrane detachment. *Cornea.* Jul 1995;14(4):436–437.

19. Kremer I, Stiebel H, Yassur Y, Weinberger D. Sulfur hexafluoride injection for Descemet's membrane detachment in cataract surgery.

J Cataract Refract Surg. Dec 1997;23(10): 1449–1453.

20. Yuen HK, Yeung BY, Wong TH, Wu WK, Lam DS. Descemet membrane detachment caused by hydrogen peroxide injury. *Cornea.* May 2004; 23(4):409–411.

21. Najjar DM, Rapuano CJ, Cohen EJ. Descemet membrane detachment with hemorrhage after alkali burn to the cornea. *Am J Ophthalmol.* Jan 2004;137(1):185–187.

22. Mahmood MA, Teichmann KD, Tomey KF, al-Rashed D. Detachment of Descemet's membrane. *J Cataract Refract Surg.* Jun 1998; 24(6):827–833.

23. Bezzina MA, Bianchi PE, Rosso R, Barone C. Detachment of Descemet's membrane in a case of keratoconus. *Annals of Ophthalmology: Glaucoma.* 1995;27(5):278–282.

24. Ezra DG, Mehta JS, Allan BD. Late corneal hydrops after penetrating keratoplasty for keratoconus. *Cornea.* Jun 2007;26(5): 639–640.

25. Calladine D, Tanner V. Optical coherence tomography of the effects of stromal hydration on clear corneal incision architecture. *J Cataract Refract Surg.* Aug 2009;35(8):1367–1371.

26. Allingham RR, Damji KF, Freedman S, Moroi SE, Shafranov G, Shields MB. Congenital glaucomas. *Shields' Textbook of Glaucoma.* 5th ed. Philadelphia, PA: Lippincott Williams & Wilkins; 2005:235–251.

27. Eiferman RA, Wilkins EL. The effect of air on human corneal endothelium. *Am J Ophthalmol.* Sept 1981;92(3):328–331.

28. Foulks GN, de Juan E, Hatchell DL, McAdoo T, Hardin J. The effect of perfluoropropane on the cornea in rabbits and cats. *Arch Ophthalmol.* Feb 1987;105(2):256–259.

9

SCLERAL FLAP DEHISCENCE

JEFF MALTZMAN AND SILVIA D. ORENGO-NANIA

SCLERAL FLAP DEHISCENCE

Following its introduction by Cairns in 1968,[1] trabeculectomy quickly became the procedure of choice for the management of elevated intraocular pressure (IOP) inadequately controlled by medications, and it remains the gold standard today. This procedure's popularity stemmed from dissatisfaction with the existing practices of the time, which typically involved full-thickness sclerectomy. Although quite effective at IOP reduction, an unguarded sclerectomy invited severe and often prolonged hypotony, with the associated risks of a flat anterior chamber, maculopathy, and suprachoroidal hemorrhage, to name but a few. Placement of the sclerectomy beneath a partial thickness scleral flap added much needed control to filtering surgery. Indeed, proper construction and suturing of the scleral flap are vital to preventing scleral flap dehiscence and promoting further surgical success, as the

scleral "valve" provides the majority of the resistance to initial aqueous outflow, limiting the risk of early hypotony.

CONSTRUCTION OF THE SCLERAL FLAP

There is no consensus on the size or shape of scleral flap required to produce effective IOP control.[2] Surgeon preference is generally what was taught during training, with square, rectangular, trapezoidal, and triangular flaps all commonly employed. Although scleral flap shape is probably unimportant, the flap should be at least one-half to two-thirds scleral thickness to avoid tearing or avulsing the tissue and to prevent "cheese wiring" by sutures.[3] Most surgeons prefer to hinge the flap as far forward as possible to ensure that the sclerectomy is created anterior to the scleral spur, avoiding the ciliary body. Extending the sides of the flap too far beyond the limbus, however, may result in excessive filtration and early hypotony.[4] Recently, some have advocated leaving the sides of the flap short, not extending fully to the limbus, in order to force aqueous posteriorly and create a more diffuse bleb.[5] In this case a wider flap may assist with proper anterior placement of the sclerectomy.

PREVENTING SCLERAL FLAP COMPLICATIONS

In many cases, complications involving the scleral flap can be avoided by attention to risk factors preoperatively and careful handling of tissue intraoperatively. The most important risk factor for scleral complications is previous ocular surgery performed at the intended trabeculectomy site,[6] particularly extracapsular cataract extraction. At times, wound gape or irregular scarring may be visible transconjunctivally. Even in the absence of these signs, the pattern of extracapsular wound healing is uncertain, and attempts to dissect a scleral flap of proper depth and form can be difficult. Unanticipated tissue planes may be encountered, leading to thin flaps with irregular margins, or the flap may tear along the prior incision line, sometimes avulsing completely. Although these complications can be managed successfully, many surgeons prefer to avoid such problems altogether, opting against trabeculectomy and favoring a tube shunt or other procedure in such patients. If a trabeculectomy is performed, extreme care must be taken with the scleral dissection, which should proceed with very gentle traction on the flap.

Other conditions in which abnormal sclera might be encountered should be considered prior to surgery. High myopia is known to be associated with significant scleral thinning,[7,8] and scleral flap depth must be reduced to avoid dissecting too deeply. A thin flap is more susceptible to intraoperative damage, and caution must be taken to avoid inadvertently tearing the tissue or macerating the margins.

Less commonly encountered conditions that may affect the scleral thickness or elasticity include scleritis and associated autoimmune inflammatory disorders,[9,10] as well as genetic disorders of tissue structure such as Ehlers-Danlos and Marfan's syndromes.[11,12]

Once again, extreme care must be exercised when creating the scleral flap, with slow, meticulous dissection, attempting to avoid areas of obvious thinning. Alternative procedures, such as tube shunt implantation, might also be considered.

MANAGEMENT OF SCLERAL FLAP COMPLICATIONS

As noted previously, a number of problems may occur during construction of the scleral flap. The flap may be dissected too thin either inadvertently or, in the case of known scleral thinning, purposefully. A buttonhole may develop within the flap, or an edge may tear or avulse. In the most extreme case, the entire flap may become detached, as may occur with excessive traction following prior extracapsular cataract surgery. Each of these situations requires careful evaluation and repair in order to achieve the necessary restriction of aqueous outflow and avoid postoperative hypotony.

Should a scleral flap complication develop prior to entry into the anterior chamber, the surgeon might consider simply abandoning the surgical site and moving to another scleral location to create a new flap. This option may not always be practical, however, due to scarring from prior surgery or to other physical constraints. In this case a tube shunt would be the next option.

Loss of a relatively small portion of the posterior flap edge may be managed by simply mobilizing the flap a bit farther into the cornea and performing a slightly more anterior sclerostomy. Relatively tight anterior flap sutures can be placed for adequate support and restriction of flow, followed by laser suture lysis if necessary.

Thin Flap

A thin flap, while perhaps not a major complication itself, must be handled carefully. The flap should be manipulated as little as possible with nontoothed, noncrushing forceps. Suture tracts should be longer than usual, and tension on sutures must be minimized to avoid "cheese wiring." Should the flap prove too thin to adequately restrict aqueous flow and maintain IOP, a patching technique (described below) must be employed to achieve stability.

Although relatively uncommon, a scleral flap buttonhole is most likely to develop in the presence of a thin flap, particularly in patients with a history of prior scleral surgery. A flap hole can be repaired with a patch graft of pericardium or sclera, possibly using a small autologous graft taken from adjacent sclera. One author reported the use of overlying Tenon's tissue incorporated in a purse-string fashion with 10–0 nylon on a vascular needle into such a defect with good results.[13]

Patch Graft Repair

Complete scleral flap dehiscence is most likely to occur in eyes that have undergone prior extracapsular cataract surgery. If the tissue is found to be otherwise healthy, the dehisced flap may be repaired primarily. Two 9–0 or 10–0 nylon sutures placed in horizontal mattress fashion through the flap base, under the limbus, and out through clear cornea can be used to re-anchor the flap and achieve a watertight hinge, allowing surgery to proceed normally.[14] While the flap may then be sutured back in standard fashion, additional interrupted sutures may be necessary to prevent excessive flow. A partial tear in the base of the flap can be repaired in a similar manner, with a single horizontal mattress suture anchoring the torn edge, bolstered by additional interrupted sutures if necessary.

Following repair the flap may remain incompetent, with inadequate resistance to aqueous flow. Alternatively, primary repair of a torn or otherwise damaged scleral flap may not be possible due to excessively thin or friable tissue. In such cases a new flap must be fashioned out of available graft materials. While little has been published regarding grafting for scleral flap complications during trabeculectomy,[15] a number of authors have addressed the issue of patch grafts for the management of post-surgical hypotony due to overfiltration.[16–21] Furthermore, the management of other scleral defects with patch grafts of various types has been well documented.[22–24]

Traditionally, sclera has been the most commonly used patch material for the repair of scleral defects. Human sclera for grafting is available from eye banks, preserved by freezing or ethanol fixation, or from commercial sources, preserved by dehydration in glycerin, acetone (Tutoplast®, IOP, Inc, Costa Mesa, California), or by freeze-drying.[25] Scleral autografting is another option,[22] with tissue taken from a suitable location on the operated or fellow eye. Successful scleral flap reconstruction has been achieved using either partial-thickness[16] or full-thickness[15,18,21,22] donor sclera, with 9–0 or 10–0 nylon sutures placed in interrupted and/or mattress fashion. Anchoring the graft tightly along the anterior margin is recommended to avoid wound leaks and focal, avascular blebs.

In recent years, pericardial patch grafts have become popular for coverage of the subconjunctival portion of the tube in tube shunt surgery.[26,27] Reports have indicated successful use of pericardium to revise trabeculectomies with incompetent scleral flaps and hypotony,[20] though no published record of pericardium used to repair a thin or damaged flap during primary filtering surgery could be found. Nonetheless, given the known qualities of commercially available preparations of pericardium, the material likely would serve as well as sclera for this purpose. Use of double or even triple-thickness tissue is recommended,[27] fixated with simple interrupted or horizontal mattress sutures as indicated. Other tissues, such as cornea[17] or fascia lata,[28] would most likely serve well for scleral flap repair; however, these materials are less likely to be routinely available to the surgeon, particularly when an unexpected intraoperative complication occurs.

Tissue Adhesives

In some cases, despite the placement of multiple sutures, either a primarily repaired flap or a graft may fail to adequately restrict aqueous flow and maintain chamber depth. This scenario is mostly likely to occur with thin or irregular tissue. The placement of additional sutures may only serve to further distort tissue, exacerbating the problem and potentially causing astigmatism.[29] In such situations, one might consider using tissue adhesives as a means of temporary wound closure. The most commonly used product is fibrin-based. Fibrin-based adhesives have been found to be biocompatible, inducing little cytotoxicity or inflammation.[30,31] The seal created by these adhesives is temporary, dissolving over a period of several days to a week.[32] They have been used effectively in trabeculectomy for closure of both the conjunctival and scleral flaps.[33] Fibrin glue has also been used to manage bleb leaks[34] and temporarily tamponade the scleral flap in cases of posttrabeculectomy hypotony.[35] The biocompatibility and transient adhesion offered by these products may allow them to serve as perfect adjuncts to sutures in cases of scleral flap incompetence, providing necessary resistance to outflow initially and later allowing a progressive increase in flow as healing progresses. Placement of viscoelastic agents in the anterior chamber of the eye will also temporarily maintain the anterior chamber depth and decrease flow through the sclerostomy, allowing the healing process to increase resistance to outflow.

CONCLUSION

The paucity of reports in the medical literature concerning intraoperative scleral flap complications during trabeculectomy suggests that these problems are relatively infrequent. Nonetheless, every surgeon performing filtering surgery will most likely encounter some difficulty with scleral flap construction during his or her career. Being prepared and understanding the options available can turn a potentially serious complication into a fairly standard case.

COMMENTARY

MARK B. SHERWOOD

This complication's full-blown form, in which the scleral flap is completely avulsed, occurs uncommonly, but the partial tear along a flap edge or buttonhole of the flap, often along a suture track, is less infrequent. The 2 major reasons for this to happen are either with tissues that have undergone previous surgery (generally a scleral incision extracapsular cataract surgery or a previous trabeculectomy that is being revised) or cases in which the surgeon creates a superficial scleral flap that is too thin.

If the anterior chamber has not been entered, it is generally best to select a new site for the trabeculectomy. If the sclerectomy has already been made, a viscoelastic should be injected to help maintain the anterior chamber while the dehisced flap is resutured or a partial tear in the scleral flap is repaired. Interrupted, mattress, purse-string, and/or running sutures can be used. They should be partial thickness and relatively long passes in order to reduce the risk of "cheese wiring", with the aim being to achieve an almost watertight closure and minimal flow of aqueous. In many cases the tissues are thin, boggy, and fragile, leading to the creation of further holes in the flap. If, after flap repair, there is still excessive aqueous flow on reforming the anterior chamber with balanced salt solution via the paracentesis track, then an additional reinforcing donor pericardial or scleral patch graft can be sutured over the scleral flap area and viscoelastic left in the anterior chamber at the end of the procedure. It may be difficult to titrate the postoperative IOP in these latter cases by laser suture lysis, but sometimes they achieve a good long-term pressure. The alternative of a tube shunt procedure is still available should the bleb fail.

Dr. Sherwood was supported by an Unrestricted Grant from Research to Prevent Blindness to the University of Florida.

COMMENTARY

STEVEN J. GEDDE

Few intraoperative complications evoke more anxiety than dehiscence of a scleral flap during a trabeculectomy. In its extreme form, a trabeculectomy (or guarded filtration procedure) is converted into a full-thickness procedure. Full-thickness procedures were abandoned for the surgical management of glaucoma because of their high rate of hypotony-related complications. The presence of a partial thickness scleral flap provides resistance to aqueous outflow through the filtration site and allows the surgeon to titrate the level of IOP intraoperatively and post-operatively. Drs. Maltzman and Orengo-Nania have provided an excellent discussion of techniques to address partial or complete dehiscence of a scleral flap during glaucoma filtering surgery.

Careful preoperative planning can minimize the risk of scleral flap dehiscence. Cases of scleral thinning (whether secondary to high myopia, congenital glaucoma with buphthalmos, or ectatic diseases of the sclera) may preclude the dissection of a scleral flap of adequate thickness. As discussed by the authors, patients who have undergone previous extracapsular cataract extraction may develop dehiscence of the scleral flap at the old cataract incision. I prefer to place a tube shunt in these clinical situations. The Tube Versus Trabeculectomy (TVT) Study provides strong evidence to support the use of tube shunts in patients with prior cataract surgery. This multicenter, randomized clinical trial prospectively enrolled patients with medically uncontrolled glaucoma who had previous cataract extraction with intraocular lens implantation and/or failed filtering surgery and randomized them to surgical treatment with a 350-mm^2 Baerveldt® glaucoma implant or a trabeculectomy with mitomycin-C (MMC).[36] Patients who underwent tube shunt surgery had a higher rate of surgical success compared with those who had undergone trabeculectomy with MMC after 3 years of follow-up. Similar mean IOP, adjunctive medical therapy use, and rates of serious postoperative complications were observed with both surgical procedures at 3 years. Interestingly, the subgroup of patients who showed the greatest difference in success rates favoring tube shunts were those who had undergone only prior cataract surgery at the time of enrollment in the TVT Study.

Dr. Gedde was supported by National Eye Institute grant P30EY014801, Department of Defense Grant W81XWH-09-1-0675, and an Unrestricted Grant from Research to Prevent Blindness to Bascom Palmer Eye Institute, Miller School of Medicine, University of Miami.

REFERENCES

1. Cairns JE. Trabeculectomy. Preliminary report of a new method. *Am J Ophthalmol.* Oct 1968;66(4):673–679.

2. Kimbrough RL, Stewart RH, Decker WL, Praeger TC. Trabeculectomy: square or triangular scleral flap? *Ophthalmic Surg.* Sept 1982; 13(9):753.

3. Allingham RR. Filtering surgery in the management of glaucoma. In: Epstein MJ, Allingham RR, Schuman JS, eds. *Chandler and Grant's Glaucoma.* 4th ed. Baltimore: Williams and Wilkins; 1997:516–537.

4. Birchall W, Wakely L, Wells AP. The influence of scleral flap position and dimensions on intraocular pressure control in experimental trabeculectomy. *J Glaucoma.* Aug 2006;15(4):286–290.

5. Jones E, Clarke J, Khaw PT. Recent advances in trabeculectomy technique. *Curr Opin Ophthalmol.* Apr 2005;16(2):107–113.

6. Rockwood EJ. II. Advantages of trabeculectomy with an antimetabolite. *Survey of Ophthalmology.* Nov-Dec 2001;46(3):276–279.

7. Curtin BJ, Teng CC. Scleral changes in pathological myopia. *Trans Am Acad Ophthalmol Otolaryngol.* Nov-Dec 1958;62(6):777–788; discussion 788–790.

8. Curtin BJ, Iwamoto T, Renaldo DP. Normal and staphylomatous sclera of high myopia. An electron microscopic study. *Arch Ophthalmol.* May 1979;97(5):912–915.

9. Messmer EM, Foster CS. Destructive corneal and scleral disease associated with rheumatoid arthritis. Medical and surgical management. *Cornea.* Jul 1995;14(4):408–417.

10. Watson PG, Young RD. Scleral structure, organisation and disease. A review. *Exp Eye Res.* Mar 2004;78(3):609–623.

11. Cameron JA. Corneal abnormalities in Ehlers-Danlos syndrome type VI. *Cornea.* Jan 1993;12(1):54–59.

12. Maumenee IH. The eye in the Marfan syndrome. *Trans Am Ophthalmol Soc.* 1981;79:684–733.

13. Brown SV. Management of a partial-thickness scleral-flap buttonhole during trabeculectomy. *Ophthalmic Surg.* Nov-Dec 1994;25(10): 732–733.

14. Riley SF, Smith TJ, Simmons RJ. Repair of a disinserted scleral flap in trabeculectomy. *Ophthalmic Surg.* May 1993;24(5):349–350.

15. Riley SF, Lima FL, Smith TJ, Simmons RJ. Using donor sclera to create a flap in glaucoma

filtering procedures. *Ophthalmic Surg.* Feb 1994;25(2):117–118.

16. Clune MJ, Shin DH, Olivier MM, Kupin TH. Partial-thickness scleral-patch graft in revision of trabeculectomy. *Am J Ophthalmol.* Jun 15 1993;115(6):818–820.

17. Rumelt S, Rehany U. A donor corneal patch graft for an incompetent scleral flap following trabeculectomy. *Ophthalmic Surg Lasers.* Oct 1996;27(10):878–880.

18. Kosmin AS, Wishart PK. A full-thickness scleral graft for the surgical management of a late filtration bleb leak. *Ophthalmic Surg Lasers.* Jun 1997;28(6):461–468.

19. Mistlberger A, Biowski R, Grabner G. Repair of a late-onset filtering bleb leak using a corneal graft shaped with an excimer laser. *Ophthalmic Surg Lasers.* Sept-Oct 2001;32(5):428–431.

20. Tannenbaum DP, Hoffman D, Greaney MJ, Caprioli J. Outcomes of bleb excision and conjunctival advancement for leaking or hypotonous eyes after glaucoma filtering surgery. *Br J Ophthalmol.* Jan 2004;88(1):99–103.

21. Harizman N, Ben-Cnaan R, Goldenfeld M, Levkovitch-Verbin H, Melamed S. Donor scleral patch for treating hypotony due to leaking and/or overfiltering blebs. *J Glaucoma.* Dec 2005;14(6):492–496.

22. Gopal L, Badrinath SS. Autoscleral flap grafting: a technique of scleral repair. *Ophthalmic Surg.* Jan-Feb 1995;26(1):44–48.

23. Ti SE, Tan DT. Tectonic corneal lamellar grafting for severe scleral melting after pterygium surgery. *Ophthalmology.* Jun 2003; 110(6):1126–1136.

24. Sangwan VS, Jain V, Gupta P. Structural and functional outcome of scleral patch graft. *Eye.* Jul 2007;21(7):930–935.

25. Frota AC, Lima Filho AA, Dias AB, Lourenco AC, Antecka E, Burnier MN, Jr. Freeze-drying as an alternative method of human sclera preservation. *Arq Bras Oftalmol.* Mar-Apr 2008;71(2):137–141.

26. Raviv T, Greenfield DS, Liebmann JM, Sidoti PA, Ishikawa H, Ritch R. Pericardial patch grafts in glaucoma implant surgery. *J Glaucoma.* Feb 1998;7(1):27–32.

27. Lankaranian D, Reis R, Henderer JD, Choe S, Moster MR. Comparison of single thickness and double thickness processed pericardium patch graft in glaucoma drainage device surgery: a single surgeon comparison of outcome. *J Glaucoma.* Jan-Feb 2008;17(1):48–51.

28. Tanji TM, Lundy DC, Minckler DS, Heuer DK, Varma R. Fascia lata patch graft in glaucoma tube surgery. *Ophthalmology.* Aug 1996; 103(8):1309–1312.

29. Claridge KG, Galbraith JK, Karmel V, Bates AK. The effect of trabeculectomy on refraction, keratometry and corneal topography. *Eye.* 1995;9(Pt 3):292–298.

30. Forseth M, O'Grady K, Toriumi DM. The current status of cyanoacrylate and fibrin tissue adhesives. *J Long Term Eff Med Implants.* 1992; 2(4):221–233.

31. Chen WL, Lin CT, Hsieh CY, Tu IH, Chen WY, Hu FR. Comparison of the bacteriostatic effects, corneal cytotoxicity, and the ability to seal corneal incisions among three different tissue adhesives. *Cornea.* Dec 2007; 26(10):1228–1234.

32. Bahar I, Weinberger D, Lusky M, Avisar R, Robinson A, Gaton D. Fibrin glue as a suture substitute: histological evaluation of trabeculectomy in rabbit eyes. *Curr Eye Res.* Jan 2006;31(1):31–36.

33. Bahar I, Lusky M, Gaton D, Robinson A, Avisar R, Weinberger D. The use of fibrin adhesive in trabeculectomy: a pilot study. *Br J Ophthalmol.* Nov 2006;90(11):1430.

34. Seligsohn A, Moster MR, Steinmann W, Fontanarosa J. Use of Tisseel fibrin sealant to manage bleb leaks and hypotony: case series. *J Glaucoma.* Jun 2004;13(3):227.

35. Grewing R, Mester U. Fibrin sealant in the management of complicated hypotony after trabeculectomy. *Ophthalmic Surg Lasers.* Feb 1997;28(2):124–127.

36. Gedde SJ, Schiffman JC, Feuer WJ, Herndon LW, Brandt JD, Budenz DL. Three-year follow-up of the tube versus trabeculectomy study. *Am J Ophthalmol.* Nov 2009;148(5): 670–684.

B. EARLY POSTOPERATIVE COMPLICATIONS

10

HYPOTONY

HÉCTOR J. VILLARRUBIA AND NICHOLAS P. BELL

HYPOTONY

The overall goal of glaucoma filtering surgery is to lower the intraocular pressure (IOP) to a level where further optic nerve damage is prevented. There is a narrow therapeutic index for IOP that results in a delicate equilibrium between slowing and preventing progression of glaucoma while maintaining good visual function. Reaching that balance with glaucoma filtering surgery can be challenging, even in the best of hands performing uncomplicated surgery.

In some patients the IOP becomes so low after trabeculectomy that damage to other ocular structures occurs, leading to impaired visual function. This condition is known as ocular hypotony and generally occurs at IOPs less than 6 mm Hg; however, we have seen cases of clinical hypotony with IOP as high as 12 mm Hg. The use of antifibrotics during trabeculectomy has greatly increased the success

of trabeculectomy, but has also increased the risk of hypotony.[1–4]

Most glaucoma specialists refer to early postoperative hypotony as that which occurs within a period of 2 months or less after surgery regardless of its mechanism. Early postoperative hypotony occurs via 2 mechanisms: 1) *decreased aqueous production*, due to inflammation, ciliochoroidal or retinal detachment, or use of aqueous suppressants; or 2) *excessive aqueous outflow*, due to overfiltration, bleb leak, or a cyclodialysis cleft.[5–8] Fortunately, most cases of early postoperative hypotony do not last longer than a few weeks and improve with conservative management.

RISK FACTORS

Although it is impossible to predict preoperatively which patient will develop early postoperative hypotony, preventative measures can be effective. Preventing and managing postoperative hypotony depends heavily upon operative and postoperative technique. Care should be taken in preoperative planning and intraoperative execution to avoid overfiltration and punctures of the conjunctival bleb that may turn into leaks. The use of nontoothed conjunctival forceps is essential.

If the IOP remains too low for too long, the eye may develop hypotony maculopathy (see Chapter 22), a complication in which the macula develops choroidal folds due to chronically low IOP. Young age, primary filtering surgery, and myopia have all been shown to be risk factors for developing hypotony maculopathy.[9,10] One study has also proposed that elevated preoperative IOP can be associated with hypotony maculopathy.[11] Although demographic risk factors cannot be controlled, they should be identified so the patient can be appropriately counseled and the surgeon can be prepared to deal with hypotony.

PREVENTION AND MANAGEMENT

A systematic and meticulous approach is needed for successful diagnosis and management. Careful attention should be given to the IOP, visual acuity, anterior chamber depth, lid function (blepharospasm), medication use, and the presence of choroidal effusions or maculopathy. If the anterior chamber is not deep, the grading system in Table 10.1 can be used to document shallowing.[12,13] A peripherally flat chamber can be easily managed with long acting topical cycloplegics, such as atropine, which rotate the lens-iris diaphragm posteriorly. More severe flattening with lens-to-cornea apposition may require reformation, drainage of choroidal effusions, and urgent repair of the underlying cause of overfiltration

Table 10.1. Anterior Chamber Depth Grading System

Grade I	Peripheral iris-cornea apposition
Grade II	Pupillary border-cornea apposition
Grade III	Lens-cornea apposition

if cycloplegics fail to deepen the chamber. To minimize the risk of suprachoroidal hemorrhage and subsequent profound visual loss, *all* postoperative patients with hypotony must be instructed to restrict activity (no heavy lifting, bending, or straining), not to rub the operative eye, to use a protective shield when sleeping, and to avoid conditions causing Valsalva maneuvers. Using short times and low concentrations of intraoperative antifibrotic agents may also reduce the risk of hypotony, but particular times and concentrations are very patient-dependent.[14]

Bleb morphology is also important in determining the etiology of early postoperative hypotony. If the bleb is flat, there is either a bleb leak, cyclodialysis cleft, or reduced aqueous production. Seidel testing may assist in determining etiology; however, a false negative result may be obtained if the IOP is so low that there is no flow or that leaks occur only with blinking. The etiology of the hypotony will dictate the proper therapeutic intervention. Early hypotony with a deep anterior chamber and an intact, elevated bleb might only require close observation and no alteration of routine postoperative management,[15] except possibly increased surveillance. Low IOP on the first postoperative day might also simply result from inadequate re-inflation of the anterior chamber at the completion of the surgery; this condition will quickly resolve without intervention. Unfortunately, many cases are not so simply managed.

Bleb leaks

A hypotonous eye with a low bleb is often the result of overfiltration due to a bleb leak occurring from a conjunctival buttonhole or a wound leak. Wound leaks are common with fornix-based conjunctival flaps and unusual with limbus-based flaps.[16–18] If a leak is identified, its management will depend on the size of the leak and whether or not the anterior chamber is formed. Use of intraoperative antimetabolites to inhibit the fibroblast healing response, such as 5-fluorouracil and mitomycin-C, during the original trabeculectomy procedure may make treatment more challenging.

If a small leak is present in the early postoperative period, it can be managed by observation, as long as the anterior chamber and bleb remain formed. A temporary reduction in the frequency of topical steroids may allow the normal postoperative inflammatory response to assist in closing the leak. Aqueous suppression may also be utilized to decrease the flow through the defect, allowing natural closure. The patient on this regimen should be seen frequently until the leak stops. As soon as closure occurs, a return to more frequent dosing of topical steroids is indicated as well as discontinuation of the topical aqueous suppressant to prevent excessive episcleral fibrosis. Prophylactic topical antibiotics should be continued until the leak is resolved. Even a small leak managed this way is a risk for failure of the trabeculectomy and should be avoided by using meticulous surgical technique during the trabeculectomy procedure to avoid any buttonholes or wound leaks. Surgery should not be considered complete until all leaks are closed.

Nonresponsive small conjunctival leaks, whether from wound leaks or buttonholes, may respond to other conservative measures used in combination with the previously described method. Pressure patching the eyelid closed up to a few days may stop the flow and allow the defect to heal. Other surgeons prefer the use of a large diameter soft bandage contact lens, which is generally kept in place for at least a week. Patients instructed to wear a contact lens around the clock for numerous days must use prophylactic topical antibiotics and be monitored closely for corneal infection. Other approaches have been advocated with variable success, including use of cyanoacrylate or fibrin tissue glue to cover the leak[19-22] and injection of the bleb with autologous blood (Table 10.2).[23,24] Autologous blood injection, however, may have serious complications, and when used early in the postoperative period, may lead to long-term bleb failure; therefore it is not recommended.

If the conjunctival leak persists despite the above measures, surgical closure is indicated to prevent bleb failure. Leaks associated with shallow or flat anterior chambers should also be managed surgically to maintain the bleb and prevent other complications, such as synechiae, endothelial cell loss, and cataracts.[15,25]

Overfiltration without leaks

When the eye is hypotonous with an intact, large, diffuse bleb, overfiltration is the problem.

Table 10.2. Autologous blood injection into bleb

AUTOLOGOUS BLOOD INJECTION INTO BLEB

- The procedure can be done at the slit lamp under topical anesthesia.
- Apply a topical antibiotic to the conjunctiva, eyelid margins, eyelashes, and eyelids before starting the procedure. Povidone-iodine 5% solution may also be applied to the same areas prior to the procedure.
- Place the lid speculum.
- To minimize postinjection hyphema, fill the anterior chamber with viscoelastic material (optional).
- Draw approximately 1.0 mL of venous blood from the patient's arm with a 23-gauge butterfly needle and a 1.0 mL syringe.
- Use a 25-gauge or 27-gauge needle (5/8 inch) to promptly inject blood into the bleb. Prompt injection is necessary to prevent blood coagulation.
- Injection: insert the needle into the conjunctiva 6–8 mm away from the filtering site and advance the needle toward the bleb.
- Inject 0.1–0.2 mL of blood into the center of the bleb.
- Apply topical antibiotics postoperatively.

This scenario can be encountered during the first week after the trabeculectomy procedure and can also occur following modification of the scleral flap by suture lysis,[26–28] removal of releasable sutures,[29,30] or needle revision.[31,32] Overfiltration usually will resolve with routine postoperative care. A more rapid than usual reduction in antiinflammatory agents may help the bleb to shrink by allowing more wound healing of the scleral flap. Similarly, using aqueous suppressant medications may decrease the flow through the sclerostomy and facilitate resolution of overfiltration. However, if there is a shallow anterior chamber, aqueous suppression is not indicated, and bleb reduction using a large diameter soft contact lens,[33] a Simmons shell,[34,35] or a symblepharon ring[36] may be indicated. These techniques approximate the scleral flap to its bed, thereby decreasing the aqueous flow and allowing fibrosis. Ultimately, some cases will require a bleb revision with resuturing of the scleral flap.[37,38] See Chapter 27 for more information on overfiltration.

Ciliary body shutdown

If the anterior chamber is formed and there is a flat bleb *with no identifiable leaks*, ciliary body dysfunction ("shutdown") is the likely cause and is probably related to an inflammatory response to the surgical procedure. If aqueous production drops to less than 10% of normal, hypotony may result.[39] Aqueous hyposecretion may result in the development of choroidal effusions, which may exacerbate the aqueous hypoproduction, perpetuating continued hypotony.[40] Treatment consists of inhibiting inflammation, usually with frequent topical or systemic steroids. Cycloplegics may also be useful. Typically, the ciliary body function returns once inflammation resolves and IOP returns to normal levels. Ophthalmic viscoelastic devices may be injected into the anterior chamber to elevate the IOP and potentially break the cycle of decreased aqueous production and choroidal detachment. If the visual axis becomes obstructed by choroidal detachments or if the retinal tissue is in apposition ("kissing choroidals"), drainage of the effusions may become necessary.[12] For

a technique on draining a choroidal effusion, see Chapter 6.

Cyclodialysis cleft

A cyclodialysis cleft may cause hypotony with or without a concurrent filtering bleb. The cleft may be caused by previous trauma,[41,42] surgical injury,[43–45] or from previous surgery (e.g., cataract surgery) and reopened during decompression of the trabeculectomy. These clefts can be identified gonioscopically if the chamber is formed but may be difficult to find in a soft eye. Use of an ophthalmic viscoelastic device to deepen the chamber may make visualization and diagnosis possible.[46] Ultrasound biomicroscopy is also useful in making this diagnosis.[47,48] See Chapter 21 for more information about diagnosis of a cyclodialysis cleft.

Repair of a cyclodialysis cleft can performed by laser cyclopexy followed by cycloplegia if less than one clock hour is involved,[45,46,49–51] but larger clefts require direct cyclopexy with suture as described by Kuchle and Naumann. With their technique, after injection of viscoelastic into the anterior chamber, a two-thirds thickness scleral flap is created 4 mm posterior from the limbus and 2 mm in length. After elevating the flap, a second full-thickness incision is then made 1.5 mm posterior and parallel to the limbus that enters the cyclodialysis cleft and releases aqueous. Direct visualization of the cyclodialysis of the cleft should now be possible. The ciliary body is then directly sutured to the sclera with interrupted 10–0 nylon loop sutures, with each suture going through the anterior lip of the sclera into the scleral spur space, through the ciliary muscle, and then exiting through the posterior lip of the scleral flap.[46,52]

Blepharospasm

Often overlooked as a cause of postoperative hypotony is blepharospasm, a condition where tight squeezing of the eyelids results in a "massage" of the filtering bleb and overfiltration. The cause of the blepharospasm should be determined and treated. If blepharospasm is present preoperatively, injection of the orbicularis oculi muscle with botulinum toxin may be useful to reduce the spasm and prevent this issue.[53]

Hypotony with a flat anterior chamber

When facing a grade III flat anterior chamber (Table 10.1) from any etiology, urgent resolution is needed to prevent corneal decompensation, iridocorneal adhesions, and acceleration of cataract formation. A rapid approach in the office setting can be to reform the anterior chamber with air, balanced saline solution, or an ophthalmic viscoelastic device. Reforming the chamber is likely a temporary solution used to gain time to get the patient into the operating room. Drainage of choroidal effusions is generally required. If there is only irido-corneal touch, it may be wise to treat conservatively with cycloplegics and corticosteroids. If at 1–2 weeks postoperatively the shallow chamber persists or if at any point there is lens-cornea touch or corneal decompensation, measures to reform the anterior chamber and drain the choroidal effusions should be employed.

CONCLUSION

Early hypotony is a fairly common complication after glaucoma filtering surgery. Careful operative technique will go a long way toward preventing hypotony. Fortunately, most cases can be resolved with only close observation and topical medications. However, more involved methods to treat bleb leaks, overfiltration, blepharospasm, and ciliary body shutdown may need to be used to resolve the cause of the hypotony. If hypotony persists, surgical treatment may be required.

COMMENTARY

DONALD L. BUDENZ

The proper evaluation and management of the patient with hypotony soon after a trabeculectomy is critical for the success of surgery and prevention of further complications. In order to manage this problem properly, the cause of the hypotony should be determined. Bleb leak, overfiltration, and choroidal effusion are the most common causes of early postoperative hypotony, and, if absent, should prompt investigations for less common causes such as annular choroidal effusions (often seen only on ultrasound), cyclodialysis cleft, or retinal detachment.

Cause-specific treatment of the above conditions is essential. Immediate intervention is necessary in cases of lens-corneal touch since this condition will result in irreversible damage to the lens (cataract) and cornea (edema and scarring). As a temporizing maneuver, a viscoelastic device can be injected in the clinic for lens-corneal touch, but definitive management should be planned for the near future.

An additional technique for managing overfiltration is transconjunctival suturing of the sclera flap as described by Eha et al. In this technique, the flap is resutured by going through the conjunctiva. A 10–0 nylon suture on a cutting needle is used. Remarkably, the holes that the needles create close spontaneously. This technique resulted in resolution of hypotony maculopathy in all 16 of the original cases described and there was no wound leakage long-term.[54]

Dr. Bell was supported by a Challenge Grant from Research to Prevent Blindness to The University of Texas Medical School at Houston and the Hermann Eye Fund.

REFERENCES

1. Zacharia PT, Deppermann SR, Schuman JS. Ocular hypotony after trabeculectomy with mitomycin C. *Am J Ophthalmol.* Sep 15 1993; 116(3):314–326.

2. Costa VP, Moster MR, Wilson RP, Schmidt CM, Gandham S, Smith M. Effects of topical mitomycin C on primary trabeculectomies and combined procedures. *Br J Ophthalmol.* Nov 1993;77(11):693–697.

3. Tsai JC, Chang HW, Kao CN, Lai IC, Teng MC. Trabeculectomy with mitomycin C versus trabeculectomy alone for juvenile primary open-angle glaucoma. *Ophthalmologica*. Jan-Feb 2003;217(1):24–30.

4. Kupin TH, Juzych MS, Shin DH, Khatana AK, Olivier MM. Adjunctive mitomycin C in primary trabeculectomy in phakic eyes. *Am J Ophthalmol*. Jan 1995;119(1):30–39.

5. Azuara-Blanco A, Katz LJ. Dysfunctional filtering blebs. *Surv Ophthalmol*. Sept-Oct 1998; 43(2):93–126.

6. Liebmann JM, Ritch R. Complications of glaucoma filtering surgery. In: Ritch R, Shields MB, Krupin T, eds. *The Glaucomas*. Vol 3: Glaucoma Therapy. 2nd ed. St. Louis: Mosby; 1996:1703–1736.

7. Simmons RJ. Filtering operations. In: Epstein DL, ed. *Chandler and Grant's Glaucoma*. Philadelphia: Lea & Febiger; 1986.

8. Schubert HD. Postsurgical hypotony: relationship to fistulization, inflammation, chorioretinal lesions, and the vitreous. *Surv Ophthalmol*. Sept-Oct 1996;41(2):97–125.

9. Stamper RL, McMenemy MG, Lieberman MF. Hypotonous maculopathy after trabeculectomy with subconjunctival 5-fluorouracil. *Am J Ophthalmol*. Nov 15 1992;114(5):544–553.

10. Suner IJ, Greenfield DS, Miller MP, Nicolela MT, Palmberg PF. Hypotony maculopathy after filtering surgery with mitomycin C. Incidence and treatment. *Ophthalmology*. Feb 1997;104(2):207–214; discussion 214–205.

11. Jampel HD, Pasquale LR, Dibernardo C. Hypotony maculopathy following trabeculectomy with mitomycin C. *Arch Ophthalmol*. Aug 1992;110(8):1049–1050.

12. Orengo-Nania S. Anterior and posterior chambers, iris and pupil, and lens. In: Gross RL, ed. *Clinical Glaucoma Management: Critical Signs in Diagnosis and Therapy*. Philadelphia: W.B. Saunders Company; 2001:347–363.

13. Herndon LWJr. Shallow or flat anterior chamber. In: Spaeth GL, ed. *Ophthalmic Surgery: Principles and Practice*. 3rd ed: Philadelphia, PA: Saunders; 2003:369–377.

14. Lee SJ, Paranhos A, Shields MB. Does titration of mitomycin C as an adjunct to trabeculectomy significantly influence the intraocular pressure outcome? *Clin Ophthalmol*. 2009;3:81–87.

15. Allingham RR, Damji KF, Freedman S, Moroi SE, Shafranov G, Shields MB. Filtering surgery. *Shields' Textbook of Glaucoma*. 5th ed. Philadelphia: Lippincott Williams & Wilkins; 2005:568–609.

16. Kohl DA, Walton DS. Limbus-based versus fornix-based conjunctival flaps in trabeculectomy: 2005 update. *Int Ophthalmol Clin*. Fall 2005;45(4):107–113.

17. Shuster JN, Krupin T, Kolker AE, Becker B. Limbus- v fornix-based conjunctival flap in trabeculectomy. A long-term randomized study. *Arch Ophthalmol*. Mar 1984;102(3): 361–362.

18. Batterbury M, Wishart PK. Is high initial aqueous outflow of benefit in trabeculectomy? *Eye (Lond)*. 1993;7(Pt 1):109–112.

19. Aminlari A, Sassani JW. Tissue adhesive for closure of wound leak in filtering operations. *Glaucoma*. 1989;11:86–89.

20. Asrani SG, Wilensky JT. Management of bleb leaks after glaucoma filtering surgery. Use of autologous fibrin tissue glue as an alternative. *Ophthalmology*. Feb 1996;103(2):294–298.

21. Grady FJ, Forbes M. Tissue adhesive for repair of conjunctival buttonhole in glaucoma surgery. *Am J Ophthalmol*. Oct 1969;68(4):656–658.

22. Graham SL, Murray B, Goldberg I. Closure of fornix-based posttrabeculectomy conjunctival wound leaks with autologous fibrin glue. *Am J Ophthalmol*. Aug 15 1992;114(2):221–222.

23. Smith MF, Magauran RG, 3rd, Betchkal J, Doyle JW. Treatment of postfiltration bleb leaks with autologous blood. *Ophthalmology*. Jun 1995;102(6):868–871.

24. Smith MF, Magauran R, Doyle JW. Treatment of postfiltration bleb leak by bleb injection of autologous blood. *Ophthalmic Surg*. Sept-Oct 1994;25(9):636–637.

25. Fiore PM, Richter CU, Arzeno G, et al. The effect of anterior chamber depth on endothelial cell count after filtration surgery. *Arch Ophthalmol*. Nov 1989;107(11):1609–1611.

26. Kapetansky FM. Laser suture lysis after trabeculectomy. *J Glaucoma*. Aug 2003; 12(4):316–320.

27. Bardak Y, Cuypers MH, Tilanus MA, Eggink CA. Ocular hypotony after laser suture lysis following trabeculectomy with mitomycin C. *Int Ophthalmol*. 1997;21(6):325–330.

28. Morinelli EN, Sidoti PA, Heuer DK, et al. Laser suture lysis after mitomycin C trabeculectomy. *Ophthalmology*. Feb 1996;103(2):306–314.

29. Simsek T, Citirik M, Batman A, Mutevelli S, Zilelioglu O. Efficacy and complications of releasable suture trabeculectomy and standard trabeculectomy. *Int Ophthalmol*. Feb-Apr 2005;26(1–2):9–14.

30. Raina UK, Tuli D. Trabeculectomy with releasable sutures: a prospective, randomized

pilot study. *Arch Ophthalmol.* Oct 1998;116(10): 1288–1293.

31. Chang SH, Hou CH. Needling revision with subconjunctival 5-fluorouracil in failing filtering blebs. *Chang Gung Med J.* Feb 2002;25(2): 97–103.

32. Mardelli PG, Lederer CM, Jr., Murray PL, Pastor SA, Hassanein KM. Slit-lamp needle revision of failed filtering blebs using mitomycin C. *Ophthalmology.* Nov 1996;103(11):1946–1955.

33. Smith MF, Doyle JW. Use of oversized bandage soft contact lenses in the management of early hypotony following filtration surgery. *Ophthalmic Surg Lasers.* Jun 1996;27(6):417–421.

34. Simmons RJ, Kimbrough RL. Shell tamponade in filtering surgery for glaucoma. *Ophthalmic Surg.* Sept 1979;10(9):17–34.

35. Simmons RJ, Singh OS. Shell tamponade technique in glaucoma surgery. *Symposium on Glaucoma: Transactions of the New Orleans Academy of Ophthalmology.* St. Louis: CV Mosby; 1981:266–279.

36. Hill RA, Aminlari A, Sassani JW, Michalski M. Use of a symblepharon ring for treatment of over-filtration and leaking blebs after glaucoma filtration surgery. *Ophthalmic Surg.* Oct 1990;21(10):707–710.

37. Nuyts RM, Greve EL, Geijssen HC, Langerhorst CT. Treatment of hypotonous maculopathy after trabeculectomy with mitomycin C. *Am J Ophthalmol.* Sept 15 1994;118(3):322–331.

38. Maruyama K, Shirato S. Efficacy and safety of transconjunctival scleral flap resuturing for hypotony after glaucoma filtering surgery. *Graefes Arch Clin Exp Ophthalmol.* Dec 2008;246(12):1751–1756.

39. Bellows AR, Chylack LT, Jr., Hutchinson BT. Choroidal detachment. Clinical manifestation, therapy and mechanism of formation. *Ophthalmology.* Nov 1981;88(11):1107–1115.

40. Pederson JE. Ocular hypotony. In: Ritch R, Shields MB, Krupin T, eds. *The Glaucomas.* Vol 1: Basic Sciences. 2nd ed. St. Louis: Mosby; 1996:385–395.

41. Malandrini A, Balestrazzi A, Martone G, Tosi GM, Caporossi A. Diagnosis and management of traumatic cyclodialysis cleft. *J Cataract Refract Surg.* Jul 2008;34(7):1213–1216.

42. Garcia-Serrano JL, Cabello-Aparicio C. [Filtering bleb after surgical cyclodialysis]. *Arch Soc Esp Oftalmol.* Oct 2006;81(10):591–594.

43. Aminlari A, Callahan CE. Medical, laser, and surgical management of inadvertent cyclodialysis cleft with hypotony. *Arch Ophthalmol.* Mar 2004;122(3):399–404.

44. Mushtaq B, Chiang MY, Kumar V, Ramanathan US, Shah P. Phacoemulsification, persistent hypotony, and cyclodialysis clefts. *J Cataract Refract Surg.* Jul 2005;31(7):1428–1432.

45. Ioannidis AS, Barton K. Cyclodialysis cleft: causes and repair. *Curr Opin Ophthalmol.* Mar 2010;21(2):150–154.

46. Motuz Leen M, Mills RP. Low postoperative intraocular pressure. In: Spaeth GL, ed. *Ophthalmic Surgery: Principles and Practice.* 3rd ed. Philadelphia: Saunders; 2003:379–387.

47. Hwang JM, Ahn K, Kim C, Park KA, Kee C. Ultrasonic biomicroscopic evaluation of cyclodialysis before and after direct cyclopexy. *Arch Ophthalmol.* Sept 2008;126(9):1222–1225.

48. Gentile RC, Pavlin CJ, Liebmann JM, et al. Diagnosis of traumatic cyclodialysis by ultrasound biomicroscopy. *Ophthalmic Surg Lasers.* Feb 1996;27(2):97–105.

49. Harbin TS, Jr. Treatment of cyclodialysis clefts with argon laser photocoagulation. *Ophthalmology.* Sept 1982;89(9):1082–1083.

50. Bauer B. Argon laser photocoagulation of cyclodialysis clefts after cataract surgery. *Acta Ophthalmol Scand.* Jun 1995;73(3):283–284.

51. Joondeph HC. Management of postoperative and post-traumatic cyclodialysis clefts with argon laser photocoagulation. *Ophthalmic Surg.* Mar 1980;11(3):186–188.

52. Kuchle M, Naumann GO. Direct cyclopexy for traumatic cyclodialysis with persisting hypotony. Report in 29 consecutive patients. *Ophthalmology.* Feb 1995;102(2):322–333.

53. Kenney C, Jankovic J. Botulinum toxin in the treatment of blepharospasm and hemifacial spasm. *J Neural Transm.* 2008;115(4):585–591.

54. Eha J, Hoffmann EM, Wahl J, Pfeiffer N. Flap suture—a simple technique for the revision of hypotony maculopathy following trabeculectomy with mitomycin C. *Graefes Arch Clin Exp Ophthalmol.* Jun 2008;246(6):869–874.

11

ELEVATED IOP WITH A FLAT ANTERIOR CHAMBER

DAVID G. GODFREY

ELEVATED IOP WITH A FLAT ANTERIOR CHAMBER

A flat anterior chamber following filtering surgery has many etiologies. Included in the differential diagnosis are overfiltration, wound leak, choroidal effusions/hemorrhage, and pupillary block; however, the key is the central anterior chamber depth. If the intraocular pressure (IOP) is normal to high, the anterior chamber shallow centrally, and choroidal effusions/hemorrhage ruled out, then the likely diagnosis is aqueous misdirection syndrome.

Aqueous misdirection syndrome (AMS), previously referred to as malignant glaucoma, was first described by von Graefe in 1869 as an unusual complication of eye surgery, in the presence of a patent peripheral iridectomy, with elevated IOP and a flat anterior chamber.[1] This condition has been referred to as ciliary block glaucoma because the ciliary processes may be in apposition to the anterior

vitreous or lens, with the lens moving into the ciliary sulcus.[2] Diversion of aqueous posteriorly into the vitreous cavity, thus increasing the volume of the vitreous, is considered the main mechanism in the development of AMS. This diversion pushes the lens forward, leaving the central as well as the peripheral anterior chamber shallow or even flat (Figure 11.1).[3] Once a diagnosis is made, treatment is effective at resolving the problem.

PREVALENCE

Filtering surgery, either alone or in combination with another surgery, has been shown to be the inciting event for AMS in 10 of 24 cases (42%) reported in a series from Harbour.[4] Tsai et al reported 12 of 19 cases (63%) with AMS followed filtering surgery.[5] One case of AMS among 105 (1%) trabeculectomy procedures was reported by Gedde et al in the Tube Versus Trabeculectomy (TVT) Study.[6]

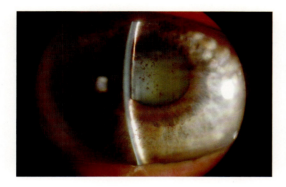

FIGURE 11.1 Axial length shallowing can be seen in this eye with aqueous misdirection syndrome (AMS). This eye had previously undergone a trabeculectomy with mitomycin-C and presented with an IOP of 60 mm Hg and a flat anterior chamber. Choroidal effusions/hemorrhages were ruled out by ultrasonography.

Two instances of AMS out of 465 (0.4%) trabeculectomy procedures were reported in the Collaborative Initial Glaucoma Treatment Study (CIGTS).[7] The rates from these studies of open-angle glaucoma patients may not apply to other populations in which angle closure glaucoma (a known risk factor for AMS) is more prevalent.[8]

Typically, AMS develops within the first few weeks of filtering surgery. Ten of 13 cases reported by Harbour et al occurred within the first month after trabeculectomy.[4] Little is known about the impact of using antimetabolites on the development of AMS. AMS can also occur several months after surgery, often with a slowly developing shallow central anterior chamber. Again, little published data is available regarding this situation.

RISK FACTORS

Multiple ocular factors seem to predispose for AMS. The most common anatomic feature associated with AMS is a narrow iridocorneal angle, as found in both acute and chronic angle closure.[4,9,10] Pseudoexfoliation is also associated with narrow angles and has been reported in cases of AMS.[4,7] Furthermore, use of topical or systemic miotics, vitritis, retinopathy of prematurity, and aphakia have all been implicated in cases with AMS.[8]

Additionally, I have observed presumed spontaneous cases of misdirection, and presumed cases of unilateral AMS have also been reported.[11,12] Occasionally, postoperative shallowing of the anterior chamber from another mechanism, such as wound leak or choroidal effusions, can precede an AMS-type presentation. Usually these patients have shallow chambers, and high IOP develops after the antecedent event resolves. The differential diagnosis for this presentation includes annular choroidal effusions, which may present identically and can only be differentiated by ultrasound biomicroscopy (UBM).

DIAGNOSIS

AMS is a diagnosis of exclusion, and pupillary block glaucoma must first be ruled out, by either creating and/or observing a patent peripheral iridotomy. One can often clinically rule out pupillary block as the central anterior chamber is usually moderately deep, as opposed to in AMS where the central anterior chamber is more likely to be shallow or even flat. Additionally, IOP is usually high in pupillary block; in contrast, IOP may be in a "normal" range in AMS, especially in the earlier stages of the process. In eyes with a history of inflammatory glaucoma, the observer should be highly suspicious of a fibrinous membrane spanning a seemingly patent iridotomy/iridectomy. The presence of iris bombé would also suggest a possible pupillary block mechanism. Again, the key is the careful examination of the central anterior chamber depth.

Another diagnostic pearl is to assess the depth of the posterior chamber. There is virtually no space between the iris and the lens nor between the lens and the vitreous (when visible) in an eye with AMS.

Choroidal effusions must also be ruled out before making the diagnosis of AMS. Usually, the clinician can make the diagnosis at the slit lamp or with indirect ophthalmoscopy. However, if the view to the posterior segment is poor, one can use ultrasound techniques to confirm this diagnosis.[13,14] Occasionally, one must make this decision in the operating room, as a scleral cut-down is performed to attempt drainage of the effusion. Choroidal hemorrhage may also mimic the presentation of AMS, but one would expect a more sudden onset and severe pain with hemorrhage. When available, UBM can detect choroidal effusions that cannot be seen with a B-scan ultrasound.

Etiologies of ciliary body rotation and edema must also be ruled out before diagnosing AMS. Medications (especially sulfa compounds), scleral buckling procedures, panretinal photocoagulation, viral infections, and other mechanisms should be considered.

Finally, one must make sure there is no evidence of a wound leak or overfiltration decreasing the anterior chamber volume. These conditions would likely cause a low IOP; however, occasionally one can still have a normal-to-high IOP with these problems.

TREATMENT

Medical

Treatments for AMS and choroidal effusions are similar, with the initial institution of cycloplegics and topical steroids. B-scan ultrasonography and/or UBM can assist in differentiating between these 2 diagnoses.

Medical therapy with steroids and cycloplegics may be effective in treating AMS. Steroids are used to stabilize the blood-aqueous barrier within the ciliary processes. Cycloplegics relax the ciliary muscle and cause a posterior rotation of the ciliary body/iris complex,[15] which typically results in deepening of the central anterior chamber in AMS.

Topical and oral aqueous suppressants are instituted to decrease the amount of aqueous being pumped into the vitreous within the posterior segment and to lower the IOP as needed. The clinician should use these agents at least until the IOP normalizes and the anterior chamber deepens. Previous reports show that 50% of cases of AMS are relieved within 5 days of using this medical method.[16,17] If there is grade III shallowing of the anterior chamber centrally (pupillary margin in contact with the corneal endothelium),[18,19] one may not be able to wait long enough for medical therapy to be effective. However, if the IOP has normalized,

gonioscopy should be performed, and the status of the angle can help decide whether stopping topical IOP-lowering medications should be attempted. A trial of discontinuing cycloplegics should be attempted next, but with close observation of the patient over the next several days, weeks, and months. Careful examination of the involved eye(s), including central anterior chamber depth and IOP, should be included. If the eye fails the suspension of therapy, long-term use of cycloplegics may be indicated.

When medical therapy fails to control IOP or restore anatomy or cessation of therapy fails, the next step is surgical intervention, either with a laser or incisional methods (Figure 11.2).

Laser

Disruption of the anterior hyaloid face is usually the initial laser procedure in AMS.[20-23] The anterior hyaloid face can be disrupted either centrally or peripherally. Because of the lack of a posterior chamber in AMS, this disruption can be easily obtained. Nd:YAG laser treatment of the posterior capsule accomplishes the central disruption and is useful in pseudophakic and aphakic eyes. An attempt to disrupt the anterior face should be made peripherally to the intraocular lens (IOL) optic. In my experience, this technique can relieve AMS in some patients, but often they will still need to be chronically dilated as the egress of fluid cannot get around the IOL.

Next, disruption of the peripheral anterior hyaloid face through a peripheral iridotomy can be attempted. The physician must initially create, or enlarge, a laser iridotomy (or surgical iridectomy). Nd:YAG laser bursts are aimed at the anterior hyaloid face and often one can see fluid egress. Again, this procedure would be difficult in phakic patients as there is the risk of disrupting the lens capsule. It is also difficult due to the iris being in apposition with the cornea. Typically, topical steroids are continued for 4–5 days following this procedure.

All of these procedures require careful attention postoperatively to the anterior chamber depth and the IOP. If central anterior

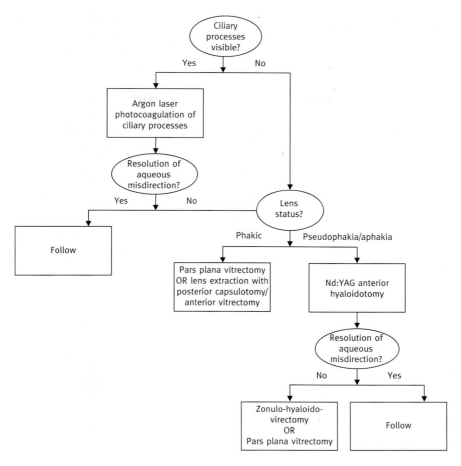

FIGURE 11.2 Algorithm for the surgical management of aqueous misdirection. (Used with permission from Reference 8: Ramulu PY, Gedde SJ. Aqueous misdirection. In: Shaarawy TM, Sherwood MB, Crowston JG, Hitchings RA, eds. *Glaucoma Medical Diagnosis and Therapy.* Vol 2. London: Saunders; 2009:211–221.)

chamber depth improves and the IOP is more controlled, then cycloplegics can be discontinued slowly. In some cases, discontinuation of cycloplegics will answer the question of whether or not the AMS has been sufficiently treated with laser therapy. Even with adequate laser treatment, the physician should watch the patient carefully over the ensuing months, as the AMS can return to pretreatment status.

Incisional Surgery

Francis and Wong reported using a needling procedure at the slit lamp to disrupt the anterior hyaloid face similar to what is attempted with the Nd:YAG laser.[24]

Pars plana vitrectomy has become the main treatment for AMS not rapidly responsive to medical and laser therapy. The surgeon must be adept at removing the anterior vitreous, often a difficult task if the eye is phakic. In some cases, a pars plana lensectomy must be combined with the vitrectomy.[4] The key to these cases is to create a passage from the posterior to anterior chamber. From my personal experience, if this passage is not made, there is a high percentage of recurrence of AMS.

The pars plana vitrectomy maneuver discussed above is similar to an

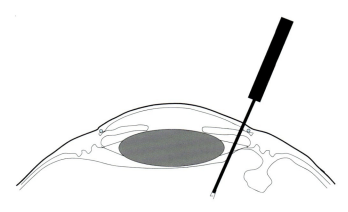

FIGURE 11.3 Schematic of vitreo-zonuloido-vitrectomy, in which vitreous is removed through an anterior approach, through the iris (or an iridectomy), zonules, and anterior hyaloid. (Used with permission from Reference 8: Ramulu PY, Gedde SJ. Aqueous misdirection. In: Shaarawy TM, Sherwood MB, Crowston JG, Hitchings RA, eds. *Glaucoma Medical Diagnosis and Therapy.* Vol2 London: Saunders; 2009: 211–221.)

anterior chamber approach known as a zonulo-hyaloido-vitrectomy. In this procedure, a vitreous cutter is placed in the anterior chamber through a limbal paracentesis wound, and by either creating or moving the cutter through an existing peripheral iridotomy, a zonulectomy, hyaloid disruption, and anterior vitrectomy is performed (Figure 11.3).[25] With either the anterior or the posterior approach, one can often see an immediate deepening of the anterior chamber and proper positioning of the lens once communication is established between the anterior and posterior chambers.

Another option, which I use more frequently, is an approach not yet reported in the literature and appropriately named an iridocyclovitrectomy. The goal of this procedure is to break the AMS by creating a passageway for aqueous between the anterior chamber, posterior chamber, and vitreous cavity. This procedure is similar to the published anterior approach discussed above,[25] but it uses a scleral incision similar to that used in a trabeculectomy. The procedure starts by opening conjunctiva in a fornix-based manner, creating a partial thickness scleral flap hinged at the limbus, removing a block of trabecular tissue, and creating a large basal iridectomy. Then, one or 2 ciliary

body processes are cauterized, rotated posteriorly, and removed. This removal exposes an intact hyaloid face, the site of obstruction in AMS. The hyaloid face is then pierced with an MVR blade. Irrigation is achieved through a pars plana incision, and a vitrector is used to remove zonules and any vitreous that moves anteriorly through the "trabeculectomy" site. A thorough anterior vitrectomy is also performed. At this stage, the anterior chamber usually dramatically deepens, essentially connecting the anterior chamber, posterior chamber, and vitreous cavity and effectively allowing aqueous to communicate from the vitreous cavity to the anterior chamber and out normal drainage pathways or through the trabeculectomy flap. Use of antifibrotics (before creation of the scleral flap) and the tension of the flap closure can be titrated based on the risk of future glaucomatous damage.

On occasion, the AMS will not dissipate or will return despite surgical treatment of the disorder. A more thorough pars plana vitrectomy, as discussed above, will likely be needed, along with zonular disruption.

Little published information exists regarding the success of filtering surgery once AMS has been treated. In my experience, trabeculectomy success is significantly lowered once surgical treatment is needed. One could consider placing a pars plana tube shunt at the same time as the vitrectomy, especially in those patients with gonioscopically proven angle closure.[26] Theoretically, tube placement could prevent an increase in vitreous volume and pressure, providing long-term IOP control.[8] Alternatively, once the AMS is proven to be under somewhat longer term surgical control, if the IOP remains elevated, a tube shunt can be placed in a subsequent surgery.

CONCLUSION

With the approaches discussed in this chapter, the successful recognition and management of AMS following filtering surgery can be attained. However, one must be constantly aware of central anterior chamber depth changes, with or without elevation of IOP, and be ready to alter treatment patterns, even years after the initial problem. Careful planning must ensue if the contralateral eye requires glaucoma surgery.

COMMENTARY
DETLEV SPIEGEL

I agree totally with the author's management suggestions for aqueous misdirection syndrome (AMS). In my experience, AMS is increasing in frequency, not only in eyes with the classic risk factors described but also in eyes with pseudoexfoliation. As the author stated, the initial filtering procedure is more likely to fail in eyes that require additional surgery for AMS. To manage eyes at high risk for AMS, I prefer to combine early cataract extraction (even though it may also induce AMS) with the iStent® (Glaukos® Corporation, Laguna Hills, California) surgery if anatomically feasible. This may provide at least a temporary IOP reduction and makes AMS treatment (if necessary later) in a pseudophakic eye simpler. In addition, I discuss the risk of AMS preoperatively with high risk patients. This simplifies acceptance of further treatment if needed.

When AMS occurs, I follow a rigid management regimen to limit its duration. As the authors suggest, during the first hour I also apply atropine 1% drops 4 times, followed by hourly applications for the first 2 days, with intravenous acetazolamide 500 mg, then 250 mg 3 times daily orally; a topical beta blocker twice daily; as well as hourly application of topical steroids.

If under this management the anterior chamber does not deepen during the next 1–2 days, I perform a 2-port pars plana vitrectomy. In order to minimize conjunctival trauma, I position the incision for the infusion line in an inferior quadrant with the second port at 9-o'clock for a 23-gauge cutter. An extensive anterior vitrectomy (with high cutting rates up to 2500/min) should be performed and connect the posterior chamber to the vitreous cavity through the zonulae, capsule of the lens, and iris resulting in a unicameral eye. Once the eye is functionally unicameral, the anterior chamber will immediately deepen.

COMMENTARY
JEFFREY S. SCHULTZ

Aqueous misdirection syndrome (AMS) is probably a misnomer as it implies a mechanism that is not completely understood and might not be entirely accurate. AMS is used to describe a group of clinical entities that share the clinical characteristics of marked anterior shallowing (both centrally and peripherally) and elevated intraocular pressure in the absence of supra-choroidal fluid or blood (though small choroidal effusions may be present). There may be causal factors including zonular laxity, altered vitreous fluid dynamics, altered permeability of the vitreous face and choroidal expansion. While there are other entities that mimic AMS, such as angle closure seen after pan retinal photocoagulation or topiramate, what make this entity different is the persistence of the angle closure and malignant course without definitive intervention.

Medical treatment can be successful, but it involves prolonged use of strong cycloplegic agents and aqueous suppressants along with systemic hyperosmotic agents. As oral hyperosmotic agents are no longer commercially available, this significantly limits the efficacy of this approach. Laser treatment tends to have limited success in phakic patients but better success in pseudophakic patients. Thermal treatment of the ciliary processes has limited success. However laser disruption of the hyloid face can be quite effective in aphakic and pseudophakic cases. The key to success in these eyes is that the hyloid needs to be incised in a location where it has direct contact to the anterior chamber such as a peripheral iridectomy or a positioning hole in an intraocular lens optic (with a dilated pupil). These eyes don't respond with immediate deepening as we see with iridotomies for pupillary block, but deepen slowly over a period of 30–60 minutes.

With the advent of modern vitreous surgery, surgical intervention often falls into the hands of the vitreo-retinal surgeon. As Dr. Godfrey has stated, the key to success is removing the anterior vitreous along with the hyloid face. Core vitrectomy alone with anterior chamber reformation will often lead to recurrence. Persistent cases may require more aggressive treatment, such as lensectomy and/or focal zonulectomy creating a unicameral eye, to definitively break the attack.

REFERENCES

1. von Graefe A. Beitrage zur pathologie und therapie des glaucoms. [Contributions to the pathology and therapy of the glaucomas.] *Arch Ophthalmol.* 1869;15:108–252.
2. Weiss DI, Shaffer RN. Ciliary block (malignant) glaucoma. *Trans Am Acad Ophthalmol Otolaryngol.* Mar-Apr 1972;76(2):450–461.
3. Epstein DL. The malignant glaucoma syndromes. In: Epstein DL, Allingham RR, Schuman JS, eds. *Chandler and Grant's Glaucoma.* 4th ed. Baltimore, MD: Williams & Wilkins; 1997:285–303.
4. Harbour JW, Rubsamen PE, Palmberg P. Pars plana vitrectomy in the management of phakic and pseudophakic malignant glaucoma. *Arch Ophthalmol.* Sept 1996;114(9):1073–1078.
5. Tsai JC, Barton KA, Miller MH, Khaw PT, Hitchings RA. Surgical results in malignant glaucoma refractory to medical or laser therapy. *Eye.* 1997;11(Pt 5):677–681.
6. Gedde SJ, Herndon LW, Brandt JD, Budenz DL, Feuer WJ, Schiffman JC. Surgical complications in the Tube Versus Trabeculectomy Study during the first year of follow-up. *Am J Ophthalmol.* Jan 2007;143(1):23–31.
7. Jampel HD, Musch DC, Gillespie BW, Lichter PR, Wright MM, Guire KE. Perioperative complications of trabeculectomy in the Collaborative Initial Glaucoma Treatment Study (CIGTS). *Am J Ophthalmol.* Jul 2005; 140(1):16–22.
8. Ramulu PY, Gedde SJ. Aqueous misdirection. In: Shaarawy TM, Sherwood MB, Hitchings RA, Crowston JG, eds. *Glaucoma: Medical Diagnosis and Therapy.* Vol 2. London: Saunders; 2009:211–221.
9. Lowe RF. Malignant glaucoma related to primary angle closure glaucoma. *Aust J Ophthalmol.* 1979;7:11–18.
10. Greenfield DS, Tello C, Budenz DL, Liebmann JM, Ritch R. Aqueous misdirection after glaucoma drainage device implantation. *Ophthalmology.* May 1999;106(5):1035–1040.
11. Fanous S, Brouillette G. Ciliary block glaucoma: malignant glaucoma in the absence of a history of surgery and of miotic therapy. *Can J Ophthalmol.* Oct 1983;18(6):302–303.
12. Schwartz AL, Anderson DR. Malignant glaucoma in an eye with no antecedent operation or miotics. *Arch Ophthalmol.* May 1975;93(5):379–381.
13. Dugel PU, Heuer DK, Thach AB, et al. Annular peripheral choroidal detachment simulating aqueous misdirection after glaucoma surgery. *Ophthalmology.* Mar 1997;104(3):439–444.
14. Trope GE, Pavlin CJ, Bau A, Baumal CR, Foster FS. Malignant glaucoma. Clinical and ultrasound biomicroscopic features. *Ophthalmology.* Jun 1994;101(6):1030–1035.

15. Wang T, Liu L, Li Z, Hu S, Yang W, Zhu X. Ultrasound biomicroscopic study on changes of ocular anterior segment structure after topical application of cycloplegia. *Chinese Medl J.* Mar 1999;112(3):217–220.

16. Chandler PA, Simmons RJ, Grant WM. Malignant glaucoma. Medical and surgical treatment. *Am J Ophthalmol.* Sept 1968;66(3):495–502.

17. Simmons RJ. Malignant glaucoma. *Br J Ophthalmol.* Mar 1972;56(3):263–272.

18. Orengo-Nania S. Anterior and posterior chambers, iris and pupil, and lens. In: Gross RL, ed. *Clinical Glaucoma Management: Critical Signs in Diagnosis and Therapy.* Philadelphia: W.B. Saunders Company; 2001:347–363.

19. Herndon LW Jr. Shallow or flat anterior chamber. In: Spaeth GL, ed. *Ophthalmic Surgery: Principles and Practice.* 3rd ed: Philadelphia, PA: Saunders; 2003:369–377.

20. Brown RH, Lynch MG, Tearse JE, Nunn RD. Neodymium-YAG vitreous surgery for phakic and pseudophakic malignant glaucoma. *Arch Ophthalmol.* Oct 1986;104(10):1464–1466.

21. Halkias A, Magauran DM, Joyce M. Ciliary block (malignant) glaucoma after cataract extraction with lens implant treated with YAG laser capsulotomy and anterior hyaloidotomy. *Br J Ophthalmol.* Sept 1992;76(9):569–570.

22. Lockie P. Ciliary-block glaucoma treated by posterior capsulotomy. *Aust N Z J Ophthalmol.* Aug 1987;15(3):207–209.

23. Risco JM, Tomey KF, Perkins TW. Laser capsulotomy through intraocular lens positioning holes in anterior aqueous misdirection. Case report. *Arch Ophthalmol.* Nov 1989;107(11):1569.

24. Francis BA, Wong RM, Minckler DS. Slit-lamp needle revision for aqueous misdirection after trabeculectomy. *J Glaucoma.* Jun 2002;11(3):183–188.

25. Lois N, Wong D, Groenewald C. New surgical approach in the management of pseudophakic malignant glaucoma. *Ophthalmology.* Apr 2001;108(4):780–783.

26. Azuara-Blanco A, Katz LJ, Gandham SB, Spaeth GL. Pars plana tube insertion of aqueous shunt with vitrectomy in malignant glaucoma. *Arch Ophthalmol.* Jun 1998;116(6):808–810.

12

ELEVATED IOP WITH A DEEP ANTERIOR CHAMBER

ANNIE K. BAIK AND JAMES D. BRANDT

ELEVATED IOP WITH A DEEP ANTERIOR CHAMBER

Early postoperative elevation of intraocular pressure (IOP) in the setting of a deep anterior chamber following trabeculectomy can generally be attributed to either mechanical obstruction or underfiltration. A careful clinical exam will almost always reveal the cause of elevated IOP and guide the clinician to logical, step-wise management.

IDENTIFYING THE CAUSES OF ELEVATED INTRAOCULAR PRESSURE

First, one should confirm that the anterior chamber is deep and the conjunctival wound is intact. Further investigation is directed by clinical signs, such as blood or fibrin in the anterior chamber, the pupil configuration, the appearance of the filtering bleb, internal obstruction of the sclerostomy, blood under the scleral flap, or subconjunctival hemorrhage. In the absence of such findings, underfiltration is most likely due to an inadequately sized sclerostomy, tight sutures on the scleral flap, or early fibrosis of the external sclerostomy site.

Gonioscopy, in conjunction with anterior segment slit-lamp examination, is crucial in the evaluation of elevated IOP in the early postoperative period. Although adequate flow may have been established at the time of surgery, continued patency of the trabeculectomy should be confirmed to distinguish between underfiltration and obstruction. Obstruction of the sclerostomy site by blood, fibrin, vitreous, iris tissue, or fragments of Descemet's membrane should be visible on gonioscopy examination.

If the trabeculectomy site appears internally patent, examination of the scleral flap may further demonstrate causes for elevated IOP. Intraoperative or postoperative bleeding may lead to development of subconjunctival hemorrhage. Even in the absence of subconjunctival hemorrhage, blood and fibrin can occlude the trabeculectomy flap. If there is no evidence of physical obstruction, intrinsic properties of the trabeculectomy itself (such as ostium size and/or tension on the scleral flap sutures) may be contributing to elevated IOP.

INTERVENTIONS TO ENCOURAGE FILTRATION OR ALLEVIATE EXTERNAL OBSTRUCTION OF THE FILTERING SITE

Gentle massage or digital manipulation serves both diagnostic and therapeutic purposes. If gonioscopy has not yet been performed and the bleb is unresponsive to digital manipulation, an internal obstruction may be present. Since internal obstruction of the ostium may not be readily apparent on routine slit-lamp examination, the threshold for gonioscopy should be low.

Digital manipulation may dislodge blood and/or fibrin obstructing the trabeculectomy flap. The goal of ocular massage is to increase IOP and force flow through the site of lowest resistance, the trabeculectomy site. Our method consists of asking the patient to look inferiorly as gentle, transient digital pressure is applied just posterior to the scleral flap, through the upper eyelid. Direct observation at the slit lamp will immediately confirm if digital manipulation has been successful and allow monitoring of anterior chamber depth. In the very early postoperative period, repeat Seidel testing should be performed after digital manipulation if there is any concern about bleb rupture or iatrogenic disruption of the conjunctiva.

Another method involves asking the patient to look superiorly while applying constant pressure, fluctuating in intensity, to the inferior aspect of the globe through the eyelid for a few seconds. Reliable patients may be taught how to independently perform ocular massage using this technique. Application of pressure to the inferior globe may help to avoid inadvertent injury to the filtering bleb when the patient massages at home. Correct technique should be confirmed by direct observation of the patient in an office setting. Patients should be cautioned against prolonged application of pressure to the globe, as IOP may rise significantly with digital manipulation.

The cotton-tipped maneuver, also known as the Carlo Traverso Maneuver (CTM) after the clinician who first described it,[1] consists of focal application of pressure under topical anesthesia using an anesthetic-moistened cotton-tipped applicator. The cotton-tipped applicator is placed just posterior or adjacent to the margins of the scleral flap. The goal is to encourage outflow not by simply increasing IOP, but by deforming the surgical wound to enable aqueous flow. The application of local pressure near the margins of the trabeculectomy flap is proposed to be a more effective and less forceful method of promoting filtration.[1] If sutures in particular regions of the flap are noted to be tied loosely at the time of surgery, the efficacy of CTM may be enhanced.

Early application of massage or CTM may often relieve obstruction with blood or fibrin, with subsequent successful filtration. However, some patients may remain refractory to such manipulation. Rechecking the IOP 15–30 minutes after such manipulations will indicate whether massage was successful in flushing fibrin or blood from under the flap and if additional interventions are indicated. It is worth noting the direction in which the bleb forms during such interventions; for example, a bleb that expands only nasally with massage indicates that releasing the nasal-most flap suture is most likely to result in sustained IOP lowering.

Gonioscopy after massage should be considered, as manipulation itself may promote internal occlusion of the ostium (e.g., by iris tissue). If there is no evidence of occlusion and digital manipulation does not lower IOP or create inflation of the bleb, selective release of flap sutures is indicated. Suture release can be performed by argon laser suture lysis (ALSL) or through the use of releasable sutures.

Both techniques permit early postoperative intervention in the setting of an underfiltering bleb.

Noting the relative suture tensions in the operative report may help with postoperative planning for ALSL. We use a Ritch or Hoskins lens with a green or red laser to perform suture lysis (Ritch Nylon Suture Laser Lens, Ocular Instruments, Bellevue, Washington; Hoskins Nylon Suture Lens, Ocular Instruments, Bellevue, Washington). If neither of these lenses is available, the flat portion between the mirrors of a Zeiss-style 4-mirror gonioprism can usually be employed to flatten the conjunctiva sufficiently to visualize the sutures. If necessary, topical phenylephrine 2.5% can be applied to promote blanching of conjunctival and episcleral vessels for enhanced visualization of sutures.[2] Red laser wavelengths may also be employed if subconjunctival hemorrhage is present, although a diode laser may be preferred.[3] Our initial settings are 50 µM spot size, 500–600 mW, 0.10 s duration, with appropriate adjustment as needed. Gentle ocular massage may be employed after suture lysis to facilitate bleb elevation and to assess whether additional suture lysis is necessary. If poor response to ALSL and digital manipulation is observed, gonioscopy should be repeated.

As with digital manipulation or ocular massage, ALSL can result in disruption of the conjunctiva. When substantial subconjunctival blood is present, green wavelengths can generate enough heat to create a Seidel-positive full-thickness burn through the conjunctiva overlying the suture. Such small thermal burns usually heal quickly. Early suture lysis carries a risk of hypotony, and patients will require additional postoperative instructions after routine suture lysis to reduce the risk of complications such as choroidal effusion or hemorrhage.

INTERVENTIONS TO ALLEVIATE INTERNAL OBSTRUCTION OF THE FILTERING SITE

Gonioscopic examination may reveal obstruction of the internal ostium. Continued internal obstruction of the trabeculectomy can rapidly lead to adhesion of the conjunctiva to the surgical site with fibrosis of the bleb and should be addressed expeditiously.

Argon or Nd:YAG laser with a gonioscopic lens, such as a Goldmann lens, can be used to remove blood, vitreous, iris tissue, fragments of Descemet's membrane, or fibrin to reestablish patency of the ostium.[4] The presence of atrophic iris tissue may predispose patients to internal obstruction with iris tissue. Advance planning for a larger peripheral iridectomy may prevent occlusion from occurring.[5] If iris or tissue fragments continue to plug the trabeculectomy site, a surgical approach with internal sweeping of the angle or washout of the anterior chamber may ultimately be required.

Bleeding during surgical manipulation or in the postoperative period promotes the development of fibrin at the surgical site. Tissue plasminogen activator (tPA; Activase®, Genentech, San Francisco, California), injected subconjunctivally (25 µg)[6] or intracamerally (15 µg and 25 µg),[7] has been reported to lead to successful lowering of IOP and reestablishment of filtration. In doses of 6–25 µg, it may also be administered to facilitate resolution of subconjunctival hemorrhage that is obscuring the view to the trabeculectomy flap and sutures; lower doses of 6–12.5 µg have been shown to be as effective as the higher doses but less likely to cause hyphema.[8] Administration of tPA to disrupt clotting at the trabeculectomy site may also promote rebleeding and hyphema by dissolving clots elsewhere.[8] For more information on intraoperative hyphema, see Chapter 5.

Vascular endothelial growth factor (VEGF) is thought to modulate ocular angiogenesis and vascular permeability in both pathologic and physiologic contexts.[9] The anti-VEGF antibody bevacizumab (Genentech, San Francisco, California) has been reported to decrease bleb vascularity when administered subconjunctivally in trabeculectomy patients.[10,11] Although bevacizumab has been described as a surgical adjuvant for trabeculectomy,[12] its efficacy in this capacity or in the very early postoperative period remains unknown.

A FINAL WORD ON PREVENTING UNDERFILTRATION AND OBSTRUCTION

Preoperative planning and intraoperative flexibility are two important considerations in achieving success with filtering surgery. Examination of the conjunctiva, vasculature, and sclera before selecting the trabeculectomy site can prevent postoperative complications. As patients may not recall all surgical procedures they have had and may have undergone surgery by other ophthalmologists with unknown surgical approach, careful slit-lamp examination is critical.

Evidence of prior surgical interventions, including cataract extraction with superior scleral tunnel, pterygium repair with superior conjunctival autograft harvest, or retinal detachment repair (either with placement of a scleral buckle or by 3-port pars plana vitrectomy), should be noted in the preoperative examination. In some cases, subconjunctival scarring may not be readily apparent. In such cases, at the time of surgery we sometimes find it useful to use a 30-gauge needle to inject balanced salt solution or 2% lidocaine with epinephrine subconjunctivally, posterior to the area of the planned surgery, and employ a muscle hook or cotton-tipped applicator to massage the fluid towards the limbus. This procedure often reveals areas of scarring that were not obvious preoperatively. Should an alternate procedure become necessary, the surgeon should ensure that all equipment and materials are readily available. Given the results of the Tube versus Trabeculectomy (TVT) Study, the threshold for a change of plan to a tube shunt should be low.[13]

It is often useful to reexamine patients under the operating microscope just before initiating the initial incision. This examination may reveal penetrating vessels near the intended trabeculectomy site (Figure 12.1). Avoiding the transection of penetrating vessels while fashioning the scleral flap will both reduce intraoperative bleeding and help prevent common causes of early obstruction of the filtration site, such as rebleeding

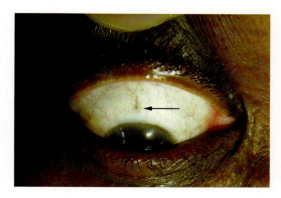

FIGURE 12.1 It is our custom to create the trabeculectomy flap at the 12-o'clock meridian. In this case, examination under the microscope revealed a large penetrating vessel (arrow) in this area, and we altered our surgical plan to create the scleral flap more nasally. By doing so, we avoided a source of intraoperative bleeding and reduced the likelihood of bleeding beneath the scleral flap in the early postoperative period.

or fibrin formation under the scleral flap. Although electrocautery may be employed to achieve hemostasis during surgery, it often leads to shrinkage of the scleral tissue that supports these penetrating vessels. Cautery only provides temporary hemostasis of these vessels, and they often rebleed in the first few days after surgery. Gentle abrasion of the scleral bed after applying cautery may provoke rebleeding and reveal vessels that are likely to continue to ooze during the procedure or in the early postoperative period.

In creating the scleral flap, dissection should be extended to the peripheral clear cornea in order to prevent a more posterior sclerostomy, injury to the ciliary body, and consequent presentation of vitreous or hemorrhage.[5] Similarly, care should be taken when fashioning the iridectomy, as posterior extension may cause injury to the ciliary body, lens, or iris root, or promote vitreous prolapse.[5] As intraoperative bleeding from the ciliary body or iris can result in hyphema and exuberant postoperative inflammation with fibrin formation, avoidance of excessively posterior entry and iridectomy is vital.

One other cause of elevated IOP following trabeculectomy should be mentioned. When viscoelastic is utilized to deepen the anterior chamber, care should be taken to remove as much of the viscoelastic as possible before completion of the procedure. This action will prevent early elevation of IOP with a deep chamber and retained viscoelastic within the bleb. Furthermore, the presence of viscoelastic may impede accurate assessment of aqueous flow prior to conjunctival closure.

CONCLUSION

Elevated IOP may be considered a normal part of postoperative trabeculectomy care when the surgeon plans to perform postoperative scleral flap suture lysis or release. While good surgical technique can often prevent unanticipated pressure elevation, with appropriate diagnostic evaluation, the cause of elevated IOP in the setting of a deep chamber usually can be managed to provide excellent results.

COMMENTARY

JONATHAN S. MYERS

Release of flap sutures following trabeculectomy, whether by removal of externalized sutures or by laser suture lysis, can dramatically reduce intraocular pressures. Suture release is typically performed 1–4 weeks after surgery. The timing is quite important: premature release, before there is some conjunctival healing, may result in hypotony or leaks. (Leaks may be more common with fornix-based conjunctival flaps.) Later, after further episcleral fibrosis, suture release may prove ineffective. Optimal timing depends greatly on patient factors, such as conjunctival thickness and speed of healing, and on surgical choices. Thinner flaps, sclerostomy placement near flap edges, and higher doses of mitomycin-C all tend to prolong the potential window of effectiveness for suture release. However, these factors also increase the potential for hypotony.

Laser suture lysis is an effective tool for the release of sutures in patients with inadequate filtration. Subconjunctival hemorrhage may increase the risk of burns, buttonholes, or failure to lyse the suture. Burns and buttonholes are much more likely with increased energy, but fortunately almost always close after a course of observation or aqueous suppressants. A red laser (e.g., krypton) may better penetrate a hemorrhage with less blood-marked conjunctival uptake and therefore less burn potential than a green laser, such as the argon laser. Compression of the tissue may allow a clearer view and access, as may sliding an adjacent area of conjunctiva without hemorrhage over the suture. In some cases, suture release may need to be delayed.

The Blumenthal lens (Volk Optical, Inc., Mentor, Ohio) has a smaller tip than the Hoskins (Ocular Instruments, Bellevue, Washington) or Ritch (Ocular Instruments, Bellevue, Washington) lenses, allowing greater compression of the tissue and better visualization of sutures in eyes with thick tissue; this may allow laser suture release in cases where it was otherwise not possible. However, this smaller tip may be less comfortable for some patients, and care should be used in tissue manipulation.

External releasable sutures can be used to avoid these issues. There are many techniques of releasable sutures, each with its own strengths and weaknesses.[14] Some techniques are more likely to be associated with irritation or astigmatism. Suture abscess is a rare complication of sutures that are left long-term in the cornea, even if epithelialized.

COMMENTARY

PETER A. NETLAND

Drs. Baik and Brandt have thoroughly reviewed causes and management of elevated intraocular pressure during the immediate postoperative period. Surgeons often suture the trabeculectomy flap tightly to prevent overfiltration and its associated complications, such as anterior chamber shallowing, choroidal effusion, suprachoroidal hemorrhage, and hypotony maculopathy. Thus, mild elevation of intraocular pressure is a frequent occurrence after trabeculectomy and is often treated with laserable or releasable sutures. Laser suture lysis provides control of intraocular pressure during the postoperative period, as described by the authors of this chapter. This technique produces consistent results and is the preferred approach of many surgeons.

An alternative approach is the releasable suture technique.[15-17] This approach does not require use of a laser and may be less time consuming during the postoperative period (depending on the location of the laser). In the presence of subconjunctival hemorrhage, thick scarring in Tenon's capsule, or a noncooperative patient, releasable sutures may be more effective compared with laser suture lysis. Several different techniques have been described in detail,[16] all of which use a slip-knot that is released by pulling on a suture that may be grasped at the slit lamp with forceps. Complications are uncommon, but include infection, wicking of aqueous and hypotony along the suture tract, and breakage of or failure to release the suture.[16] Timing of laser suture lysis or release of suture has been described as at least 3–5 days and, ideally 2–3 weeks postoperatively. When using the EX-PRESS™ Glaucoma Filtration Device (Alcon Laboratories, Inc., Fort Worth, Texas), we have been more aggressive with laser suture lysis, cutting sutures earlier in the postoperative period. When intraoperative conjunctival buttonholes occur, testing for watertight closure can be performed by releasing a small amount of aqueous into the subconjunctival space as described by the authors of this chapter. During the postoperative period, sutures can be released as needed when buttonholes are water tight. If water-tight closure cannot be achieved, suture lysis should be delayed as long as possible, to allow wound healing and closure of the buttonhole.

If fibrosis of the external sclerostomy site does occur during the early or intermediate postoperative period, needling can be considered.[18] Needling can be performed easily at the slit lamp using topical anesthesia. Balanced salt solution can be injected into the subconjunctival space adjacent to the bleb to separate the conjunctiva from the sclera, which may minimize the chance of trauma to the conjunctiva. Injection of balanced salt solution, however, may reduce visualization of aqueous flow when the site of resistance to aqueous flow is identified. For good visualization during the procedure, use of an eyelid speculum and patient cooperation are important. A 27-gauge needle is introduced under the conjunctiva, 5–10 mm away from the bleb. After passing the needle under the partial-thickness scleral flap, a gentle lifting or side-to-side motion can reestablish flow in some cases. After the needling, topical antibiotics are administered, and the needle track is checked for excessive aqueous flow. Although rarely necessary, a suture may be used to close the needle track opening. In the intermediate and late postoperative period, elevated intraocular pressure with a deep anterior chamber is often encountered with encapsulated blebs or failing blebs, which can be managed with conservative therapy, needling, surgical revision, or alternative glaucoma procedures.[18]

As described in this chapter, prompt evaluation and treatment can avoid further problems and maintain bleb function. As pointed out by the Drs. Baik and Brandt, meticulous intraoperative surgical technique and vigilance during the early postoperative period may improve outcomes when patients develop elevated intraocular pressure with a deep anterior chamber.

REFERENCES

1. Traverso CE, Greenidge KC, Spaeth GL, Wilson RP. Focal pressure: a new method to encourage filtration after trabeculectomy. *Ophthalmic Surg.* Jan 1984;15(1):62–65.
2. Trope GE. *Glaucoma Surgery*. Boca Raton, FL: Taylor & Francis Group; 2005.
3. Spaeth GL. Laser suture lysis. In: Spaeth GL, ed. *Ophthalmic Surgery: Principles and Practice*. 3rd ed. Philadelphia: Saunders; 2003.
4. Allingham RR. Filtering surgery in the management of glaucoma. In: Epstein DL, Allingham RR, Schuman JS, eds. *Chandler and Grant's Glaucoma*. 4th ed. Baltimore, MD: Williams & Wilkins; 1997.

5. Jones LS, Shetty RK, Spaeth GL. Trabeculectomy. In: Chen TC, ed. *Surgical Techniques in Ophthalmogy: Glaucoma Surgery*. Philadelphia, PA: Saunders; 2008.

6. Piltz JR, Starita RJ. The use of subconjunctivally administered tissue plasminogen activator after trabeculectomy. *Ophthalmic Surg*. Jan 1994;25(1):51–53.

7. Tripathi RC, Tripathi BJ, Park JK, et al. Intracameral tissue plasminogen activator for resolution of fibrin clots after glaucoma filtering procedures. *Am J Ophthalmol*. Feb 15 1991;111(2):247–248.

8. Lundy DC, Sidoti P, Winarko T, Minckler D, Heuer DK. Intracameral tissue plasminogen activator after glaucoma surgery. Indications, effectiveness, and complications. *Ophthalmology*. Feb 1996;103(2):274–282.

9. Schlingemann RO, van Hinsbergh VW. Role of vascular permeability factor/vascular endothelial growth factor in eye disease. *Br J Ophthalmol*. Jun 1997;81(6):501–512.

10. Kahook MY, Schuman JS, Noecker RJ. Needle bleb revision of encapsulated filtering bleb with bevacizumab. *Ophthalmic Surg Lasers Imaging*. Mar-Apr 2006;37(2):148–150.

11. Coote MA, Ruddle JB, Qin Q, Crowston JG. Vascular changes after intra-bleb injection of bevacizumab. *J Glaucoma*. Oct-Nov 2008; 17(7):517–518.

12. Grewal DS, Jain R, Kumar H, Grewal SP. Evaluation of subconjunctival bevacizumab as an adjunct to trabeculectomy a pilot study. *Ophthalmology*. Dec 2008;115(12):2141–2145 e2142.

13. Gedde SJ, Schiffman JC, Feuer WJ, Herndon LW, Brandt JD, Budenz DL. Three-year follow-up of the Tube versus Trabeculectomy study. *Am J Ophthalmol*. Nov 2009;148(5):670–684.

14. Wanner JB, Katz LJ. Releasable suture techniques for trabeculectomy: an illustrative review. *Ophthalmic Surg Lasers Imaging*. Nov-Dec 2004;35(6):465–474.

15. Cohen JS, Osher RH. Releasable scleral flap suture. *Ophthalmology Clinics of North America*. 1988;1:187–197.

16. de Barros DS, Gheith ME, Siam GA, Katz LJ. Releasable suture technique. *J Glaucoma*. Aug 2008;17(5):414–421.

17. Kolker AE, Kass MA, Rait JL. Trabeculectomy with releasable sutures. *ArchOphthalmol*. Jan 1994;112(1):62–66.

18. Lupinacci APC, Netland PA. Bleb-related problems after glaucoma filtering surgery. *Contemporary Ophthalmology*. 2008;7(13):1–8.

13

EARLY EXCESSIVE IRITIS

KUNDANDEEP S. NAGI

EARLY EXCESSIVE IRITIS

Inflammation in the early postoperative period after filtration surgery generally resolves quickly; however, there are certain underlying conditions that may produce more than the usual degree of iritis. Uveitis or iritis after glaucoma surgery may often be more severe and longer lasting than the minimal postoperative inflammation common after some other intraocular surgeries. Recognizing excessive inflammation may allow steps to be taken to prevent permanent adverse sequelae.

DIABETES

Lacy vacuolization of the iris stroma and pigment epithelium is often present in diabetic patients.[1] Manipulation of this abnormal iris may cause excessive, recalcitrant postoperative inflammation believed to be due to instability of the iris and/or iris pigment epithelium and a fragile blood aqueous barrier. Patients with diabetes are also at increased risk of developing endophthalmitis after intraocular surgery.[2] Unless infectious in nature, this excessive iritis can generally be controlled with aggressive topical corticosteroid therapy.

ACUTE ENDOPHTHALMITIS

With prophylactic pre- and perioperative application of antibiotics, wound infections are rare, and the risk of early endophthalmitis following trabeculectomy remains small.[3] However, bacterial endophthalmitis may develop months to years after routine trabeculectomy. A retrospective review of 988 trabeculectomies performed over 5 years reported only one case of early bleb-related endophthalmitis, due to *Morganella morganii*.[4] Host flora is usually responsible for early cases, *Staphylococcus epidermidis* being the most common organism.[5] Papaconstantinou and colleagues reported a case of acute-onset *Lactobacillus* endophthalmitis occurring 10 days after trabeculectomy with the OloGen™ (OculusGen Biomedical Inc. Taipei, Taiwan) implant in the absence of antimetabolite.[5]

Severe iritis that represents endophthalmitis may present acutely after filtering surgery. The clinical picture is that of acute endophthalmitis, but the etiology is noninfectious. Subjective complaints of pain and decreased vision combined with objective findings of anterior and posterior inflammation are common. [6] For more information on endophthalmitis, see Chapters 24 and 42.

TOXIC ANTERIOR SEGMENT SYNDROME (TASS)

Excessive inflammation that is not responsive to routine therapy may represent toxic anterior segment syndrome (TASS), an acute, postoperative inflammatory disorder that may occur after anterior segment surgery. TASS is a sterile inflammatory reaction that is typically seen at the first postoperative visit. It is believed to be due to introduction of a toxic substance into the anterior chamber during surgery. Diffuse corneal edema is a classic finding. Breakdown of the blood-aqueous barrier with fibrin deposition across the anterior chamber and a sterile hypopyon are also hallmark findings. Iris ischemia may result in pigment release.

Cases of TASS tend to occur more commonly after cataract surgery, perhaps due to the greater degree of intraocular manipulation and more substances and instruments entering the eye. However, it should be suspected in cases of diffuse limbus-to-limbus corneal edema and excessive anterior segment inflammation after any anterior segment surgery. Perhaps the low frequency of TASS in filtration surgery may be explained by the fact that routine glaucoma filtering surgery is mostly limited to sclera, conjunctiva, and external structures with few devices or solutions entering the anterior chamber. TASS has been described after uneventful cataract surgery,[7]

intravitreal anti-VEGF (vascular endothelial growth factor) injections,[8] penetrating keratoplasty,[9] and vitreous surgery.[10] We have seen 2 cases after trabeculectomy.

TASS is believed to result from the entry of toxic substances into the anterior chamber. A variety of materials have been implicated. The Task Force on Ophthalmic Sterilization has organized these agents into 3 categories.[11] First, extraocular substances that enter the anterior chamber unintentionally during surgery; for example, talcum powder from surgical gloves,[12] ophthalmic ointment,[13] or topical antiseptic agents.[14] Second, substances or devices inserted into the anterior chamber as part of the procedure; for example, anesthetic agents such as lidocaine,[15] preservatives such as benzalkonium chloride,[16] inappropriately reconstituted intraocular preparations, mitomycin-C,[17] intraocular lenses,[18] and contaminated irrigating solutions. Category 3 consists of contaminants that have accumulated on the surfaces of intraocular surgical instruments as a result of insufficient or inappropriate cleaning. Examples are denatured viscoelastic, enzymatic detergents, bacterial contamination of ultrasound water bath cleaners,[19] and impurities of the autoclave steam.[20,21]

Aggressive treatment with topical steroids is required for resolution. However, long-term sequelae may develop, such as permanent corneal edema, glaucoma from trabecular meshwork damage, iris synechiae (anterior and/or posterior), and iris atrophy. The most important treatment of TASS is prevention, a course that is dependent on the entire surgical team's knowledge of the surgical procedure and the agents appropriate for ocular use.

UNDERLYING UVEITIS

A severe and recalcitrant iritis may manifest after glaucoma surgery and may be the initial presentation of a dormant, underlying predisposition to uveitis. Aggressive steroid therapy eventually leads to resolution. Laboratory work-up to discern the etiology of such iritis may be indicated if it responds abnormally to treatment, is chronic, or recurs. For more information on uveitis, see Chapter 20.

SYMPATHETIC OPHTHALMIA

Sympathetic ophthalmia (SO) is a rare, bilateral granulomatous panuveitis that occurs after trauma to the eye. An insidious or acute postoperative anterior uveitis with classical mutton-fat keratic precipitates in which both eyes are affected may lead to this diagnosis.[22] As this disease is thought to represent a T-cell mediated autoimmune attack on choriodal melanocytes,[22] the entire eye is affected, not only the anterior structures. This feature can be used to discriminate it from other disease entities.

Cases of SO have been described after glaucoma surgery, the risk being higher in eyes with advanced stage of disease, regardless of the type of surgery performed.[23] Clinical presentation is an insidious or acute anterior uveitis with mutton-fat keratic precipitates. The posterior segment manifests moderate to severe vitritis, usually accompanied by multiple yellowish-white choroidal lesions. Diagnosis is based on clinical findings and a history of previous ocular trauma or surgery. Other causes of granulomatous panuveitis (e.g., Vogt-Koyanagi-Harada disease, sarcoidosis, tuberculosis, syphilis) should be considered.

Treatment of SO consists of systemic anti-inflammatory agents, with high dose oral corticosteroid as the drug of choice. However, if the inflammation cannot be controlled, other systemic immunosuppression should be considered. The role of enucleation after the diagnosis of sympathetic ophthalmia remains controversial. For more information on sympathetic ophthalmia, see Chapter 20.

EPITHELIAL DOWNGROWTH

Epithelial downgrowth is a well-known complication after cataract surgery,[24] penetrating keratoplasty, and lamellar keratoplasty. It has also been reported following tube shunt surgery[25] and following surgery for congenital glaucoma.[26]

Epithelial downgrowth most commonly results from delayed closure of a corneal or scleral wound, with migrating epithelial cells gaining entry site through a persistent opening. It has even been seen entering along a full-thickness needle track. Downgrowth may be associated with a variable degree of cells and flare disproportionate to ciliary flush or symptoms.[27] The iritis is unusual in that the aqueous contains large clumps of cellular material, rather than fine particles. These cells may represent epithelial cells rather than true inflammatory cells. Laser photocoagulation may be used as a diagnostic tool to delineate borders and differentiate it from other entities, causing fluffy whitening of the epithelial membrane when applied to affected areas. It is important to recognize epithelial downgrowth as it is rare with significant morbidity. Treatment is difficult and may require peeling of the membrane combined with intracameral 5-fluorouracil, followed by later keratoplasty.

MASQUERADE SYNDROMES

Various malignancies may present with iritis after intraocular surgery. Masquerade syndromes such as leukemia, other tumors, and peripheral retinal detachments may present similarly. Therefore, a complete ocular examination should be performed with any fulminant iritis that responds atypically to medical treatment.

CONCLUSION

Fulminant noninfectious iritis can sometimes present early in the postoperative period after glaucoma surgery. The patient may be predisposed to this by underlying systemic conditions, most commonly diabetes. Other times, an aggressive inflammatory response after filtering surgery is the first manifestation of a local underlying inflammatory eye disease. Unusual responses to treatment should prompt suspicion of underlying malignancies or posterior chamber disorders. Lastly, TASS can occur after almost any intraocular intervention. Prevention, when possible, and aggressive antiinflammatory treatment generally result in a favorable outcome.

COMMENTARY
MAHMOUD A. KHAIMI

This is an excellent review of unexpected early iritis. I would like to emphasize that on rare occasions intraocular surgery unmasks a patient's dormant predisposition to uveitis. Although the patient may not have had a prior episode of iridocyclitis, this should be considered if the inflammatory response to the surgical procedure is more substantial and persists longer than usual. On a similar note, if routine postoperative inflammation is inadequately controlled, the response may smolder for weeks to months longer than expected, especially if topical corticosteroids are tapered too rapidly.

Dr. Khaimi was supported by an Unrestricted Grant from Research to Prevent Blindness to the Dean McGee Eye Institute, University of Oklahoma College of Medicine.

COMMENTARY
NICK MAMALIS

Mild inflammation in the early postoperative period following filtration surgery is common and resolves relatively quickly. Excessive early anterior segment inflammation following uncomplicated filtering surgery is less frequent, but may be severe and should be recognized early and treated aggressively to avoid complications.

Patients who are prone to breakdown of the blood-aqueous barrier may be predisposed to excessive early inflammation of the anterior segment. Patients with a history of uveitis should be well controlled prior to any kind of filtering surgery. However, in patients who require surgery acutely, it is necessary to aggressively treat any postoperative inflammation in patients with pre-existing uveitis. The most common systemic factor involved with excessive postoperative inflammation is diabetes. These patients are prone to excessive and prolonged breakdown of the blood aqueous barrier, as well as to increased liberation of pigment following anterior segment filtering surgery.

Toxic anterior segment syndrome (TASS) is an acute, sterile anterior segment inflammation following any anterior segment surgery. TASS is seen most commonly in patients who have undergone cataract surgery or combined cataract and trabeculectomy surgery. TASS is relatively uncommon following a simple glaucoma filtering surgery.

The etiology of TASS is very broad and may occur secondary to any materials that gain access to the anterior chamber of the eye during surgery.[28] A recent study evaluated data from questionnaires and onsite visits to surgical centers and hospitals that had experienced TASS. It found that issues related to the cleaning and sterilization of instruments were the most common factor in causing TASS. Issues identified included inadequate cleaning and flushing of ophthalmic instruments and handpieces, as well as the use of enzyme detergents and ultrasound water baths.[29,30] The likeliest factor for the infrequent occurrence of TASS among patients undergoing straight filtration surgery is the fact that ultrasound and irrigation/aspiration handpieces are not used during the procedure, and there is limited entry into the anterior chamber of not only instruments, but also fluids and medications implicated in the etiology of TASS.

Acute endophthalmitis is much less common than delayed-onset endophthalmitis following filtering surgery. If excessive anterior segment inflammation is present during the first week following filtering surgery, it is important to have a high index of suspicion for the possibility of an infectious endophthalmitis. Care must also be taken to rule out an infectious etiology in these cases of increased inflammation that are usually sterile with a noninfectious etiology.

Great care should be taken when using antimetabolites such as mitomycin-C or 5-fluorouracil during filtering surgery to ensure that these agents do not gain access into the anterior chamber of the eye, as they are potentially toxic and could lead to an excessive early postoperative iritis. Fortunately, proper use of antifibrotics during surgery can help eliminate this possibility.

Dr. Mamalis was supported by an Unrestricted Grant from Research to Prevent Blindness to the University of Utah.

REFERENCES

1. Yanoff M, Fine BS, Berkow JW. Diabetic lacy vacuolation of iris pigment epithelium; a histopathologic report. *Am J Ophthalmol.* Feb 1970;69(2):201–210.

2. Doft BH, Wisniewski SR, Kelsey SF, Fitzgerald SG. Diabetes and postoperative endophthalmitis in the Endophthalmitis Vitrectomy Study. *Arch Ophthalmol.* May 2001;119(5):650–656.

3. Bindlish R, Condon GP, Schlosser JD, D'Antonio J, Lauer KB, Lehrer R. Efficacy and safety of mitomycin-C in primary trabeculectomy: five-year follow-up. *Ophthalmology.* Jul 2002; 109(7):1336–1341; discussion 1341–1332.

4. Kuang TM, Lin YC, Liu CJ, Hsu WM, Chou CK. Early and late endophthalmitis following trabeculectomy in a Chinese population. *Eur J Ophthalmol.* Jan-Feb 2008;18(1):66–70.

5. Papaconstantinou D, Georgalas I, Karmiris T, Ladas I, Droutsas K, Georgopoulos G. Acute onset lactobacillus endophthalmitis after trabeculectomy: a case report. *J Med Case Reports.* 2010;4:203.

6. Sternberg P Jr., Martin DF. Management of endophthalmitis in the post-Endophthalmitis Vitrectomy Study era. *Arch Ophthalmol.* May 2001;119(5):754–755.

7. Kim SY, Park YH, Kim HS, Lee YC. Bilateral toxic anterior segment syndrome after cataract surgery. *Can J Ophthalmol.* Jun 2007; 42(3):490–491.

8. Sato T, Emi K, Ikeda T, et al. Severe intraocular inflammation after intravitreal injection of bevacizumab. *Ophthalmology.* Mar 2010;117(3):512–516, 516 e511–e512.

9. Maier P, Birnbaum F, Bohringer D, Reinhard T. Toxic anterior segment syndrome following penetrating keratoplasty. *Arch Ophthalmol.* Dec 2008;126(12):1677–1681.

10. Andonegui J, Jimenez-Lasanta L, Aliseda D, Lameiro F. [Outbreak of toxic anterior segment syndrome after vitreous surgery]. *Arch Soc Esp Oftalmol.* Aug 2009;84(8):403–405.

11. Hellinger WC, Bacalis LP, Edelhauser HF, Mamalis N, Milstein B, Masket S. Recommended practices for cleaning and sterilizing intraocular surgical instruments. *J Cataract Refract Surg.* Jun 2007;33(6):1095–1100.

12. Sellar PW, Sparrow RA. Are ophthalmic surgeons aware that starch powdered surgical gloves are a risk factor in ocular surgery? *Int Ophthalmol.* 1998;22(4):247–251.

13. Werner L, Sher JH, Taylor JR, et al. Toxic anterior segment syndrome and possible association with ointment in the anterior chamber following cataract surgery. *J Cataract Refract Surg.* Feb 2006;32(2):227–235.

14. Liu H, Routley I, Teichmann KD. Toxic endothelial cell destruction from intraocular benzalkonium chloride. *J Cataract Refract Surg.* Nov 2001;27(11):1746–1750.

15. Kim T, Holley GP, Lee JH, Broocker G, Edelhauser HF. The effects of intraocular lidocaine on the corneal endothelium. *Ophthalmology.* Jan 1998;105(1):125–130.

16. Eleftheriadis H, Cheong M, Sandeman S, et al. Corneal toxicity secondary to inadvertent use of benzalkonium chloride preserved viscoelastic material in cataract surgery. *Br J Ophthalmol.* Mar 2002;86(3):299–305.

17. Fukuchi T, Hayakawa Y, Hara H, Abe H. Corneal endothelial damage after trabeculectomy with mitomycin C in two patients with glaucoma with cornea guttata. *Cornea.* Apr 2002;21(3): 300–304.

18. Moshirfar M, Whitehead G, Beutler BC, Mamalis N. Toxic anterior segment syndrome after Verisyse iris-supported phakic intraocular lens implantation. *J Cataract Refract Surg.* Jul 2006;32(7):1233–1237.

19. Richburg FA, Reidy JJ, Apple DJ, Olson RJ. Sterile hypopyon secondary to ultrasonic cleaning solution. *J Cataract Refract Surg.* May 1986;12(3):248–251.

20. Hellinger WC, Hasan SA, Bacalis LP, et al. Outbreak of toxic anterior segment syndrome following cataract surgery associated with impurities in autoclave steam moisture. *Infect Control Hosp Epidemiol.* Mar 2006;27(3): 294–298.

21. Whitby JL, Hitchins VM. Endotoxin levels in steam and reservoirs of table-top steam sterilizers. *J Refract Surg.* Jan-Feb 2002;18(1): 51–57.

22. Damico FM, Kiss S, Young LH. Sympathetic ophthalmia. *Semin Ophthalmol.* Jul-Sept 2005; 20(3):191–197.

23. Shammas HF, Zubyk NA, Stanfield TF. Sympathetic uveitis following glaucoma surgery. *Arch Ophthalmol.* Apr 1977;95(4):638–641.

24. Vargas LG, Vroman DT, Solomon KD, et al. Epithelial downgrowth after clear cornea phacoemulsification: report of two cases and review of the literature. *Ophthalmology.* Dec 2002;109(12):2331–2335.

25. Sidoti PA, Minckler DS, Baerveldt G, Lee PP, Heuer DK. Epithelial ingrowth and glaucoma drainage implants. *Ophthalmology.* May 1994; 101(5):872–875.

26. Giaconi JA, Coleman AL, Aldave AJ. Epithelial downgrowth following surgery for congenital glaucoma. *Am J Ophthalmol.* Dec 2004;138(6):1075–1077.

27. Feder RS, Krachmer JH. The diagnosis of epithelial downgrowth after keratoplasty. *Am J Ophthalmol.* Jun 15 1985;99(6):697–703.

28. Mamalis N, Edelhauser HF, Dawson DG, Chew J, LeBoyer RM, Werner L. Toxic anterior segment syndrome. *J Cataract Refract Surg.* Feb 2006;32(2):324–333.

29. Mamalis N. Toxic anterior segment syndrome update. *J Cataract Refract Surg.* Jul 2010; 36(7):1067–1068.

30. Cutler Peck CM, Brubaker J, Clouser S, Danford C, Edelhauser HE, Mamalis N. Toxic anterior segment syndrome: common causes. *J Cataract Refract Surg.* Jul 2010;36(7):1073–1080.

14

EARLY VISION LOSS AFTER TRABECULECTOMY

ROBERT D. FECHTNER AND ALBERT S. KHOURI

EARLY VISION LOSS AFTER TRABECULECTOMY

"This surgery is designed to help you preserve the vision you have. If we are completely successful, you will not see worse once we are done."

Hardly an encouraging message we give to patients needing glaucoma surgery. An experienced glaucoma surgeon knows that aqueous diversion procedures are fraught with complications, including the ever terrifying loss of vision. Early complications of trabeculectomy that can lead to vision loss can be categorized as refractive, inflammatory/infectious, hemorrhagic, and other. It is important to recognize these complications promptly and understand the appropriate time to intervene. Thoughtful preoperative planning, meticulous technique,

and a dose of good luck can help prevent these complications. It is the ability to anticipate, avoid, and manage complications that distinguishes the successful and satisfied glaucoma surgeon from a frustrated one.

REFRACTIVE COMPLICATIONS

Induced refractive error

Trabeculectomy may induce new spherical and cylindrical aberrations.[1] When intraocular pressure (IOP) is reduced, and particularly if there is overfiltration, the lens-iris diaphragm moves forward, and the anterior chamber shallows. These combined actions usually induce a spherical refractive error (myopic shift).[2] The clinical signs of a myopic shift will be a shallow anterior chamber and visual acuity that will improve with a pinhole occluder or refraction. Interestingly, should the overfiltration be accompanied by macular edema, the myopic effect may be counteracted by a hyperopic shift due to macular elevation and shortening of axial length,[3] and the patient may not have any change in refraction or may even have a hyperopic shift. For more information about axial length and changes in refraction, including after trabeculectomy, see Chapter 41.

Astigmatic shift can have several origins. If a trabeculectomy flap is dissected too far anteriorly into the peripheral cornea and not sutured securely back to its origin, "against the rule" astigmatism can be induced. If a superiorly located flap is sutured with too much tension, astigmatism can be induced along the axis of the tightest suture(s), usually "with the rule." (See Chapter 26.) Additionally, uneven suture tension in the conjunctival closure (whether limbus- or fornix-based) can affect the degree of postoperative astigmatism.

Management. Shifts in spherical correction can be expected to resolve as IOP stabilizes, as long as chronic hypotony does not ensue. If hypotony persists, it can lead to hypotony maculopathy (see Chapter 22); of note, macular thickening may manifest with induced hyperopia. Astigmatism due to a poorly constructed flap is difficult to correct, but fortunately it is rarely severe enough that a change of refractive correction is not adequate. Sometimes astigmatism induced by a tight flap can be relieved by release of flap sutures. If IOP is at the target, it is best to wait a few months before releasing tight flap sutures. The surgeon must be cautious because late release of sutures can lead to elevation of the flap with a loss of resistance and additional outflow in eyes that have received antifibrotics (particularly mitomycin-C). Astigmatism induced by uneven suturing of the conjunctiva and Tenon's layer at the limbus will usually improve when these sutures are removed or dissolve (usually 1–2 months after surgery).

INFLAMMATORY/INFECTIOUS

Iritis

Trabeculectomy is mostly an extraocular procedure. It is uncommon to see substantial intraocular inflammation in the immediate postoperative period following trabeculectomy, unless the eye is predisposed to uveitis. Success rates in high-risk eyes can be improved with the use of more frequent or stronger topical corticosteroids.[4,5] A practical clinical approach for an eye that is at risk for inflammation is to treat preoperatively with topical and/or oral steroids. Prednisolone acetate, 1% can be administered 4 times daily for a week prior to surgery. Oral prednisone can be started a few days before surgery, typically at a dose between 40 and 60 mg per day, and should be tapered relatively rapidly over the first few postoperative weeks.

Management. When intraocular inflammation is significant enough to interfere with vision, it should be managed aggressively with steroids and nonsteroidal antiinflammatory agents. The surgeon should have a very high index of suspicion for endophthalmitis, but toxic anterior segment syndrome should also be considered (see Chapter 13). Intraocular inflammation can be associated with elevated IOP, which can lead to corneal edema and blurred vision. For more information about iritis, see Chapter 13.

Cystoid Macular Edema

Cystoid macular edema (CME) can occur following any ocular surgery. It is not clear whether any unique mechanisms are associated with CME following trabeculectomy.[6]

Management. Usually, CME will resolve after trabeculectomy. Patients should be maintained on topical antiinflammatory treatment. In the setting of hypotony, suspect hypotony maculopathy[7] (see Chapter 22).

Endophthalmitis

Despite meticulous surgical technique, endophthalmitis can be an early or late severe complication.[8] Therefore, every surgeon must entertain a high level of suspicion for endophthalmitis. There is nothing unique about the presentation of endophthalmitis following trabeculectomy. Classic findings of a red, painful eye with decreased vision and anterior chamber or vitreous cells should be evaluated promptly and treated appropriately.[9,10] For more information on endophthalmitis, including prevention and management, see Chapters 24 and 42.

HEMORRHAGIC COMPLICATIONS

Hyphema

During trabeculectomy the eye is entered only for a paracentesis, creation of the ostium, and iridectomy, if needed. Meticulous intraoperative technique can minimize the chances of a visually significant hyphema in the early postoperative period. Still, hyphema remains one of the common postoperative complications encountered after trabeculectomy.[11]

Vessels in the bed of the trabeculectomy flap should be cauterized. However, one must be careful not to cauterize along the edge of the bed of the flap, as it will distort the anatomy and alter the amount of aqueous flow through the flap. The sclerostomy site can also bleed, particularly if the dissection of the flap is not anterior enough.

Another common site for bleeding is at the cut edge of the iridectomy. More significant bleeding can occur if a ciliary process is inadvertently amputated. The most common cause of this injury is creation of the iridectomy too far posteriorly. During iridectomy the ciliary process can be captured along with the iris when it is grabbed. In order to avoid this event, we recommend engaging the iris under the anterior edge of the sclerostomy when externalizing it for iridectomy.

An isolated vitreous hemorrhage is an uncommon complication of trabeculectomy. The most likely source would be an unrecognized injury to a ciliary process flowing posteriorly. An unexplained vitreous hemorrhage should prompt an investigation for a possible retinal break or detachment.

Management. Observe the eye throughout surgery and at the end of the case. Any active bleeding should be addressed in the operating room with cautery and/or tamponade by viscoelastics. Postoperatively, a small hyphema can be observed without intervention. Once aqueous is flowing through the sclerostomy, the blood will often flow out if it has not clotted.

If the chamber is largely filled with blood, it may be worth returning to the operating room to wash it out. If a vessel is actively bleeding (e.g., ciliary process), it might be necessary to open the surgical site for hemostasis, a rare occurrence for patients not on anticoagulation therapy. A limited vitreous hemorrhage can be observed. Ultrasonography may be appropriate to rule out retinal detachment. For more information about hyphema after trabeculectomy, see Chapter 23.

Decompression Retinopathy

Decompression retinopathy has been described with a constellation of findings, typically including preretinal and intraretinal hemorrhages (some with white centers).[12] To some observers, it appears similar to a central retinal vein occlusion. Decompression retinopathy tends to occur in eyes that have very high IOP preoperatively that are then rapidly decompressed intraoperatively. The underlying mechanism remains unclear. Decompression retinopathy has a dramatic appearance, but usually does not effect postoperative visual acuity significantly, except when a macular hemorrhage occurs. Spontaneous resolution is the norm. However, when there is macular involvement there may be residual scotoma or preretinal fibrosis, resulting in a permanently decreased vision.

Management. The usual management for decompression retinopathy is observation. Significant vitreous hemorrhage associated with decompression retinopathy is rare.

Suprachoroidal Hemorrhage

The most devastating condition associated with early vision loss following glaucoma surgery is suprachoroidal hemorrhage.[13] When a suprachoroidal hemorrhage occurs intraoperatively with an open globe, it is referred to as an expulsive hemorrhage. In the setting of the relatively small ostium created with trabeculectomy, one would expect to see iris and perhaps vitreous prolapse (see Chapter 7) at the time of intraoperative suprachoroidal hemorrhage.

More commonly, a suprachoroidal hemorrhage occurs one to several days following surgery. IOP has been lowered by the surgery, and a choroidal vessel ruptures. It typically does not occur in a high-pressure eye, but rather once the pressure is lowered. Risk factors for suprachoroidal hemorrhage include advanced age,[14,15] higher preoperative IOP,[16] and anticoagulation therapy.[17] The hemorrhage usually has an acute onset, often associated with a Valsalva maneuver, highly elevated IOP, immediate severe pain, and rapid loss of vision. Usually the patients can remember exactly what they were doing, often activities involving some straining. A limited suprachoroidal hemorrhage may have a favorable visual outcome, but a massive suprachoroidal hemorrhage usually results in permanent (and possibly total) vision loss.

Management. The best management for suprachoroidal hemorrhage is prevention. Unfortunately it is not always possible to prevent these hemorrhages. In consultation with the primary care provider, stop anticoagulation therapy if possible. For patients with constipation or chronic cough, stool softeners and cough suppressant in the perioperative period may be helpful. The patient should also avoid lifting, bending, or straining in the early postoperative period.

A high index of suspicion can help with prompt intraoperative management of a suprachoroidal hemorrhage. Iris prolapse is not unusual when performing trabeculectomy in a phakic eye. However, vitreous prolapse after iridectomy in a phakic eye or an eye that had uncomplicated cataract surgery should raise the suspicion of increased posterior pressure. Quickly assess the presence of a red reflex whenever vitreous presents through the sclerostomy. A loss of the red reflex is often an early indication of intraoperative suprachoroidal hemorrhage. If you suspect intraoperative suprachoroidal hemorrhage, close the scleral flap immediately in a watertight fashion. This factor is one reason why it may be useful to preplace at least 2 flap sutures prior to entering the eye and creating the sclerostomy. If the anterior chamber has not collapsed, some balanced salt solution or viscoelastic can be added through the paracentesis to help tamponade the hemorrhage. If there is definitive intraoperative suprachoroidal hemorrhage,

immediate drainage is not possible, as either there will be continued bleeding due to lack of a clot or nothing will drain from a sclerostomy. Some surgeons perform radial sclerostomies without attempting drainage after closure of the trabeculectomy to assist later drainage and possibly reduce postoperative pain. Unfortunately, there is little else you can or should do at this point.

Initial management for a delayed postoperative suprachoroidal hemorrhage is usually observation. These patients often need strong analgesics, possibly to the point of hospital admission and pain team consultation. Cycloplegia can be helpful in relieving pain associated with ciliary spasm. IOP will often be elevated and should be treated medically, but the surgeon should avoid the inclination to reduce IOP by tapping the paracentesis as additional bleeding may be initiated.

Sometimes the outcome of a significant suprachoroidal hemorrhage can be improved by evacuating the blood. Although there are no hard and fast rules, the blood typically is clotted shortly after the hemorrhage; however, evacuation of a large clot can be very difficult. Drainage of suprachoroidal hemorrhage is most successful after 1–2 weeks, when the clot lyses. Clot lysis is indicated by the aqueous acquiring a yellow tinge. For more information on suprachoroidal hemorrhages, see Chapter 6.

OTHER CAUSES OF EARLY VISION LOSS AFTER TRABECULECTOMY

Choroidal Effusion

The sudden lowering of IOP that follows trabeculectomy can result in a serous choroidal effusion. Small choroidal effusions probably accompany many trabeculectomies and have only a limited impact on vision. Large choroidal effusions typically accumulate over a few days. They occur in low-pressure eyes and might develop initially or after release of a flap suture. The accumulation of fluid in the potential suprachoroidal space causes a ballooning inward of the retina and choroid with a resulting shadow cast upon the posterior retina. In some patients the fluid accumulation is sufficient for the nasal and temporal retina to touch, called "kissing choroidals." These occurrences may necessitate prompt intervention to prevent retinal adhesions.[18]

Management. Opinions vary about when and whether the surgeon should intervene for serous choroidal detachments. Conservative treatment can consist of topical steroid, cycloplegia, and watchful waiting. Resolution starts as the pressure in the eye begins to rise, but choroidal effusions can persist for several weeks.

In some clinical situations it makes sense to consider early surgical drainage of the choroidals. These include "kissing choroidals," a monocular patient in whom there is need to rapidly restore vision, and a patient who requires more rapid rehabilitation of the eye due to imminent surgery in the fellow eye.[19,20] For more information on choroidal effusions, see Chapter 6.

Sudden Visual Loss (Snuff Out Syndrome)

Sudden and complete loss of central vision postoperatively is perhaps the most dreaded unanticipated complication of uncomplicated glaucoma surgery. It is painless and permanent. Reportedly, the more advanced the optic neuropathy, the higher the risk of loss of fixation.[21] While uncommon, patients with visual field defects close to or splitting fixation are at increased risk for this loss. The pathophysiology and triggers of this catastrophic cascade in "snuff out syndrome" are not clearly understood. Many patients with advanced glaucoma do well after trabeculectomy and maintain their "island" of vision.[22,23] Others with apparently less advanced glaucoma come out of surgery with loss of central vision. Multiple ocular and possibly systemic factors may determine the degree of optic nerve vulnerability.

Management. Predicting patients who might "snuff out" after trabeculectomy is impossible. Performing surgery on eyes with advanced progressive visual field loss encroaching on fixation is a choice between the risk of progression and the risk of snuff; thus, counseling patients on this possibility is always prudent. As described above, high-risk cases include eyes with advanced disease and visual field loss encroaching on fixation. Some suggestions to minimize risk include avoiding retrobulbar anesthesia and not using anesthetic with epinephrine. Slow intraoperative decompression of the globe may be helpful. For eyes in which central fixation is threatened, it might be useful to check IOP 4–6 hours after surgery to detect and manage early postoperative IOP spike.

CONCLUSIONS

For patients with glaucoma who have chronic, progressive vision loss, trabeculectomy offers the possibility of slowing this loss, but not without risk. Disclosing the risks of glaucoma and the risks of glaucoma surgery is a difficult but necessary discussion to have with the patient. When offered only 2 unattractive options, the best approach is to decide which seems worse and pick the other.

Drs Fechtner and Khouri were supported by an Unrestricted Grant from Research to Prevent Blindness to the New Jersey Medical School, University of Medicine and Dentistry of New Jersey and the Glaucoma Research and Education Foundation, Inc.

COMMENTARY
RONALD L. FELLMAN

As the authors note in this well-written chapter, early vision loss after trabeculectomy is common. It is therefore incumbent on the physician and staff to adequately emphasize to the patient and family what I call the "glaucoma surgery preamble." Failure to perform this task is an added complication of surgery.

Society today is conditioned to expect a quick fix for their eye problems. Word travels fast about superb vision after uncomplicated cataract surgery. In addition, there is a constant media bombardment from eye surgeons who advertise about the miracles of eye surgery. This cultural scenario of visual perfection is a setup for a medical-legal disaster for glaucoma patients because they have similar expectations. Unfortunately, the filtration experience requires a different mindset. Preoperative counseling mandates an uphill battle approach for filtration surgery, the foundation of the glaucoma surgery preamble.

Glaucoma patients need to know that there are no quick surgical fixes and lowering IOP without associated visual acuity loss is a difficult task that requires not only surgical expertise, but a great deal of effort by the patient to come to the office for frequent postoperative visits. This requires a glaucoma mindset that differs from routine eye surgery. Patients who are not committed to this are not good candidates for filtration surgery because postoperative fine-tuning is essential to success. For these patients, determine another procedure that will benefit their particular situation.

Glaucoma patients must understand that glaucoma surgery is high risk. This is evident from all the complications listed in this chapter. The chair time associated with this discussion is significant. Patients need to know that their vision will be blurry for several weeks after surgery. The glaucoma surgery preamble must be thoroughly understood and documented by the patient prior to surgery. Be especially careful with patients who are spectacle-free prior to glaucoma surgery, for they may be surprised and disappointed that they now have to wear glasses to see optimally.

The authors have put together an excellent review of factors that cause early vision loss after trabeculectomy. In addition to the factors they recited, I would emphasize the problems related to postoperative flap suture lysis. Under this scenario, the patient may see fairly well after trabeculectomy and be stable at one week, but the surgeon then decides to use laser to lyse one or more sutures to increase flow through the flap; hypotony with decreased vision may ensue. From the patient's viewpoint, things were doing well after surgery until suture lysis, and now vision is impaired. This special situation must be spelled out to the patient so they don't think something went wrong.

All of the above points constitute the glaucoma surgery preamble. A skilled surgeon will tailor the surgery to the patient's individual needs, wait to cut sutures until the opportune moment, and select patients who are the best candidates for successful filtration surgery. Every surgical step should revolve around perfection in order to avoid damaging eye pressures, either too high or too low.

A confident physician will convey his/her concerns regarding the glaucoma preamble but will deliver the message in an upbeat manner to instill confidence during this uphill battle against blindness.

COMMENTARY
RONALD L. GROSS

This is an excellent discussion of the all too common concern of decreased vision following glaucoma filtration surgery. The alternative view might be that with this surgery although there may be risks to short-term, or rarely long-term, vision, the alternative is to not perform surgery and for disease to continue to progress. Intervention at least brings the real possibility of maintaining current visual function. The authors present a very logical discussion of the important etiologies for vision loss in the early postoperative period. By far, the most common reason is refractive. Luckily, most of the refractive effects of the uncomplicated trabeculectomy diminish within 1–2 weeks after surgery.[1] Another cause not mentioned is the use of cycloplegia postoperatively. While deepening the anterior chamber, this will affect the refractive status of the eye.[24] Additionally, induced astigmatism can be reduced by decreasing the size of the scleral flap, similarly to what occurs with cataract wounds.

In eyes with a known high risk of substantial postoperative inflammation, particularly if recurrent, the use of a tube shunt might be considered. In resolving hypotony maculopathy from CME, the use of Optical Coherence Tomography (OCT) is invaluable to determine the proper treatment. Hyphema can also occur after suture lysis or removal when elevation of the bleb causes a bleed that can flow directly into the anterior chamber. Hyphemas do not doom successful filtration, but close observation to increase flow may be necessary as the blood components may increase healing and scarring in the subconjunctival space as the hyphema clears through the filter.

If the preoperative IOP is very high, rapid complete decompression should be avoided to decrease the risk of decompression retinopathy and choroidal effusions. This may include preoperative medications (oral carbonic anhydrase inhibitors and osmotic agents) and placing the paracentesis very early in the procedure and slowly bringing down the IOP over time before the sclerostomy. A similar strategy can be used when performing suture lysis or release in the early postoperative period. By having multiple sutures and only opening one at a time, the profound rapid decrease in IOP can be minimized, particularly in those patients at greatest risk.

Lastly, in the presence of a choroidal effusion, aqueous production is reduced. Therefore another indication to drain the choroidal is a failing bleb. Removing the supraciliary fluid results in increased aqueous production, allowing greater flow through the sclerostomy.

Overall, as the authors pointed out, by recognizing the cause and addressing it, the quality of life for both patient and surgeon will be markedly enhanced.

REFERENCES

1. Dietze PJ, Oram O, Kohnen T, Feldman RM, Koch DD, Gross RL. Visual function following trabeculectomy: effect on corneal topography and contrast sensitivity. *J Glaucoma*. Apr 1997; 6(2):99–103.

2. Cunliffe IA, Dapling RB, West J, Longstaff S. A prospective study examining the changes in factors that affect visual acuity following trabeculectomy. *Eye (Lond)*. 1992;6(Pt 6): 618–622.

3. Cashwell LF, Martin CA. Axial length decrease accompanying successful glaucoma filtration surgery. *Ophthalmology*. Dec 1999; 106(12):2307–2311.

4. Roth SM, Spaeth GL, Starita RJ, Birbillis EM, Steinmann WC. The effects of postoperative corticosteroids on trabeculectomy and the clinical course of glaucoma: five-year follow-up study. *Ophthalmic Surg*. Dec 1991; 22(12):724–729.

5. Starita RJ, Fellman RL, Spaeth GL, Poryzees EM, Greenidge KC, Traverso CE. Short- and long-term effects of postoperative corticosteroids on trabeculectomy. *Ophthalmology*. Jul 1985;92(7):938–946.

6. Karasheva G, Goebel W, Klink T, Haigis W, Grehn F. Changes in macular thickness and depth of anterior chamber in patients after filtration surgery. *Graefes Arch Clin Exp Ophthalmol*. Mar 2003;241(3):170–175.

7. Bashford KP, Shafranov G, Shields MB. Bleb revision for hypotony maculopathy after trabeculectomy. *J Glaucoma*. Jun 2004;13(3): 256–260.

8. Katz LJ, Cantor LB, Spaeth GL. Complications of surgery in glaucoma. Early and late bacterial endophthalmitis following glaucoma filtering surgery. *Ophthalmology*. Jul 1985; 92(7):959–963.

9. Results of the Endophthalmitis Vitrectomy Study. A randomized trial of immediate vitrectomy and of intravenous antibiotics for the treatment of postoperative bacterial endophthalmitis. Endophthalmitis Vitrectomy Study Group. *Arch Ophthalmol*. Dec 1995; 113(12):1479–1496.

10. Doft BH, Barza M. Optimal management of postoperative endophthalmitis and results of the Endophthalmitis Vitrectomy Study. *Curr Opin Ophthalmol*. Jun 1996;7(3):84–94.

11. Jampel HD, Musch DC, Gillespie BW, Lichter PR, Wright MM, Guire KE. Perioperative complications of trabeculectomy in the Collaborative Initial Glaucoma Treatment Study (CIGTS). *Am J Ophthalmol*. Jul 2005; 140(1):16–22.

12. Fechtner RD, Minckler D, Weinreb RN, Frangei G, Jampol LM. Complications of glaucoma surgery. Ocular decompression retinopathy. *Arch Ophthalmol*. Jul 1992;110(7):965–968.

13. Reynolds MG, Haimovici R, Flynn HW Jr., DiBernardo C, Byrne SF, Feuer W. Suprachoroidal

hemorrhage. Clinical features and results of secondary surgical management. *Ophthalmology.* Apr 1993;100(4):460–465.

14. Frenkel RE, Shin DH. Prevention and management of delayed suprachoroidal hemorrhage after filtration surgery. *Arch Ophthalmol.* Oct 1986;104(10):1459–1463.

15. Gressel MG, Parrish RK 2nd, Heuer DK. Delayed nonexpulsive suprachoroidal hemorrhage. *Arch Ophthalmol.* Dec 1984;102(12):1757–1760.

16. Risk factors for suprachoroidal hemorrhage after filtering surgery. The Fluorouracil Filtering Surgery Study Group. *Am J Ophthalmol.* May 15 1992;113(5):501–507.

17. Jeganathan VS, Ghosh S, Ruddle JB, Gupta V, Coote MA, Crowston JG. Risk factors for delayed suprachoroidal haemorrhage following glaucoma surgery. *Br J Ophthalmol.* Oct 2008;92(10):1393–1396.

18. Bellows AR, Chylack LT Jr., Hutchinson BT. Choroidal detachment. Clinical manifestation, therapy and mechanism of formation. *Ophthalmology.* Nov 1981;88(11):1107–1115.

19. Altan C, Ozturker C, Bayraktar S, Eren H, Ozturker ZK, Yilmaz OF. Post-trabeculectomy choroidal detachment: not an adverse prognostic sign for either visual acuity or surgical success. *Eur J Ophthalmol.* Sept-Oct 2008;18(5):771–777.

20. WuDunn D, Ryser D, Cantor LB. Surgical drainage of choroidal effusions following glaucoma surgery. *J Glaucoma.* Apr 2005;14(2):103–108.

21. Costa VP, Smith M, Spaeth GL, Gandham S, Markovitz B. Loss of visual acuity after trabeculectomy. *Ophthalmology.* May 1993;100(5):599–612.

22. Martinez JA, Brown RH, Lynch MG, Caplan MB. Risk of postoperative visual loss in advanced glaucoma. *Am J Ophthalmol.* Mar 15 1993;115(3):332–337.

23. Topouzis F, Tranos P, Koskosas A, et al. Risk of sudden visual loss following filtration surgery in end-stage glaucoma. *Am J Ophthalmol.* Oct 2005;140(4):661–666.

24. Orengo-Nania S, El-Harazi SM, Oram O, Feldman RM, Chuang AZ, Gross RL. Effects of atropine on anterior chamber depth and anterior chamber inflammation after primary trabeculectomy. *J Glaucoma.* Aug 2000;9(4):303–310.

C. LATE POSTOPERATIVE COMPLICATIONS

15

LATE BLEB FAILURE

PETER T. CHANG

LATE BLEB FAILURE

The goal of filtering surgery is to create a filtering bleb to lower intraocular pressure (IOP). A successful bleb can be characterized by subconjunctival elevation, moderate avascularity, and microcystic appearance of the bleb. Failure of the filtering bleb may occur in the late postoperative period, leading to inadequate control of glaucoma. (Figure 15.1) Prevention and management of late postoperative bleb failure are important in maintaining the success of the trabeculectomy.

RISK FACTORS FOR LATE BLEB FAILURE

Bleb failure may occur months to years following an initial filtering surgery. Some risk factors for bleb failure include young age, high preoperative IOP, African or Hispanic ethnicity, multiple prior conjunctival procedures, long-term therapy with topical glaucoma medications, and secondary glaucomas, such as uveitic and neovascular glaucoma. Male gender and aphakia also increase the risk of late bleb failure.[1-6]

PREVENTION AND MANAGEMENT OF LATE BLEB FAILURE

Structurally, bleb failure may be due to numerous causes, including obstruction of the internal ostium, episcleral fibrosis, and conjunctival scarring. Evaluation of the etiology of the failure requires careful slit-lamp biomicroscopy and gonioscopy.

Obstruction of the ostium

Although obstruction of the internal ostium typically occurs during the early postoperative period, materials such as blood and fibrin may block the ostium years after the surgery.

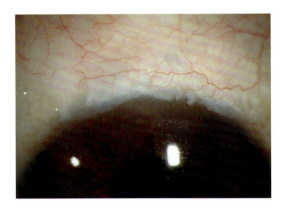

FIGURE 15.1   Low, underfiltering bleb approximately 2 years following trabeculectomy

Therefore, gonioscopy should be performed in all suspected cases of late bleb failure. Retained lens material and ophthalmic viscoelastic devices can occlude the ostium following a cataract surgery in a previously filtered eye. In cases of Axenfeld-Rieger syndrome and iridocorneal endothelial (ICE) syndrome, iris or other aberrant tissue may also cause obstruction of the internal ostium, leading to a higher rate of bleb failure.[7, 8] Physical manipulation using a 30-gauge needle, laser contracture (with argon or diode) or obliteration (with Nd:YAG),[9] or topical pharmacological intervention with pilocarpine and phenylephrine may be attempted to dislodge incarcerated iris from the internal ostium. Blood clots or fibrin can be dissolved with intracameral injection of tissue plasminogen activator (tPA)[10] (see Chapter 5).

Episcleral Fibrosis

Despite the use of adjunctive antimetabolites with filtration surgeries, conjunctival scarring and episcleral fibrosis around the scleral flap remain the primary causes of late bleb failure. Histopathology of a scarred filtration site shows abundant fibroblasts with contractile intracellular proteins and deposition of new collagen fibers.[11] Intraoperative application of mitomycin-C (MMC) has led to an increase in the success rate of filtration

surgery, but at the cost of higher rates of complications, including overfiltration, hypotony, bleb leak, and intraocular infection.[12-14] Use of 5-fluorouracil may improve surgical outcomes with lower risk profile than MMC in eyes with less chance of scarring.[14] In situations when the bleb appears threatened, some have proposed the use of oral antiinflammatory suppression of fibrosis with prednisone (2.5–10 mg, 3 times daily), a nonsteroidal anti-inflammatory agent (diclofenac sustained release 100 mg daily or 50 mg 3 times daily), and colchicine (0.2–0.3 mg 3 times daily) to improve the long term success of filtration surgery.[15] More recently, efforts have been directed at inhibition of vascular endothelial growth factor (VEGF) to reduce scar formation after filtration surgery.[16, 17] Subconjunctival bevacizumab given postoperatively has been reported to dramatically reduce bleb vascularity, associated with scarring of filtration surgery.[18]

Bleb Needling

Besides a full surgical revision of a scarred bleb or creation of another sclerostomy, bleb needling may be attempted to revive a failing bleb. The external needling procedure may be augmented with subconjunctival or sub-Tenon's injection of 5-fluorouracil, MMC, or bevacizumab. Success rates ranging from 45% to 71% at 1-year have been reported in the literature. Low IOP immediately following the needling procedure has been associated with favorable outcomes, while higher preneedling pressure, multiple prior conjunctival surgeries, and repeat needle revisions were associated with lower success rates. Reported complications from a needling procedure include hypotony, choroidal effusion, bleb leak, aqueous misdirection, and blebitis.[19-28] For more information, see Chapter 28.

CONCLUSION

Despite advances in surgical techniques and use of antimetabolites, late bleb failure remains an undesired but sometimes unavoidable complication of trabeculectomy. Further understanding of individual wound healing responses and methods of modulation should lead to an enhancement of surgical outcomes.

COMMENTARY

ALFRED M. SOLISH

Filtration surgery creates an unnatural opening between the anterior chamber and the subconjunctival space. Mechanisms within the human body will try to close that opening, the sclera not being amenable to holes in its substance. It is therefore remarkable that filtration surgery is ever successful. Even years after a successful sclerostomy and filtering bleb have been achieved, any activation of the inflammatory system can begin the cascade that ends with scar formation.

Materials, both natural and artificial, may obstruct the internal opening as well. In addition to the substances elaborated by Dr. Chang, vitreous can obstruct the sclerostomy following cataract surgery, capsulotomy, or trauma.

As failure of the filtration operations may occur at any time, eyes that have undergone glaucoma surgery require constant vigilance to ensure continued function and pressure control.

COMMENTARY

JAMES C. TSAI

While topical steroids and antiproliferative agents (e.g., MMC) have improved the surgical success rates of filtering surgery, late bleb failure is still too common a clinical outcome. As noted in the chapter, clinical gonioscopy is an essential diagnostic technique and should be performed in all suspected cases to rule out obstruction of the internal ostium vs. episcleral fibrosis/conjunctival scarring. In my own experience, bleb needling provides greater long-term success in patients who have encapsulated filtering blebs rather than flat blebs with episcleral fibrosis (see Chapter 28). Another useful technique is the intracameral insertion of a cyclodialysis spatula (through corneal paracentesis) to dissect away any fibrosis near the internal ostium and/or subconjunctival space. This internal bleb revision technique has the inherent advantage of not creating an external needle track hole (i.e., conjunctival bleb leak), thus allowing more aggressive and early postprocedure addition of subconjunctival antimetabolite therapy (e.g., 5-fluorouracil).

To minimize the risk of late bleb failure, I advocate early and aggressive modulation of the postoperative healing phase. This should include early removal of a releasable flap suture (my preference) and/or laser suture lysis. Any conjunctival leak should be treated quickly to ensure the long-term sustainability of the filtering bleb. Judicious use of subconjunctival antimetabolite injections should be employed. In certain patients I will prescribe daily bleb massage as a prophylactic measure; in others, I will slowly taper the steroids therapy. I also believe that exciting novel approaches such as subconjunctival and/or topical bevacizumab should be explored and studied further.

Dr. Tsai was supported by a Departmental Challenge Grant from Research to Prevent Blindness, Inc.

REFERENCES

1. Stavrou P, Murray PI. Long-term follow-up of trabeculectomy without antimetabolites in patients with uveitis. *Am J Ophthalmol.* Oct 1999;128(4):434–439.
2. Schwartz AL, Van Veldhuisen PC, Gaasterland DE, Ederer F, Sullivan EK, Cyrlin MN. The Advanced Glaucoma Intervention Study (AGIS): 5. Encapsulated bleb after initial trabeculectomy. *Am J Ophthalmol.* Jan 1999;127(1):8–19.
3. Ceballos EM, Beck AD, Lynn MJ. Trabeculectomy with antiproliferative agents in uveitic glaucoma. *J Glaucoma.* Jun 2002;11(3):189–196.
4. Rockwood EJ, Parrish RK 2nd, Heuer DK, et al. Glaucoma filtering surgery with 5-fluorouracil. *Ophthalmology.* Sept 1987;94(9):1071–1078.
5. Five-year follow-up of the Fluorouracil Filtering Surgery Study. The Fluorouracil Filtering Surgery Study Group. *Am J Ophthalmol.* Apr 1996;121(4):349–366.
6. Borisuth NS, Phillips B, Krupin T. The risk profile of glaucoma filtration surgery. *Curr Opin Ophthalmol.* Apr 1999;10(2):112–116.
7. Wright MM, Grajewski AL, Cristol SM, Parrish RK. 5-Fluorouracil after trabeculectomy and the iridocorneal endothelial syndrome. *Ophthalmology.* Mar 1991;98(3):314–316.
8. Mandal AK, Prasad K, Naduvilath TJ. Surgical results and complications of mitomycin C-augmented trabeculectomy in refractory developmental glaucoma. *Ophthalmic Surg Lasers.* Jun 1999;30(6):473–480.
9. Dailey RA, Samples JR, Van Buskirk EM. Reopening filtration fistulas with the neodymium-YAG laser. *Am J Ophthalmol.* Oct 15 1986;102(4):491–495.
10. Lundy DC, Sidoti P, Winarko T, Minckler D, Heuer DK. Intracameral tissue plasminogen activator after glaucoma surgery. Indications, effectiveness, and complications. *Ophthalmology.* Feb 1996;103(2):274–282.
11. Mietz H, Arnold G, Kirchhof B, Diestelhorst M, Krieglstein GK. Histopathology of episcleral fibrosis after trabeculectomy with and without mitomycin C. *Graefes Arch Clin Exp Ophthalmol.* Jun 1996;234(6):364–368.
12. Casson R, Rahman R, Salmon JF. Long term results and complications of trabeculectomy augmented with low dose mitomycin C in patients at risk for filtration failure. *Br J Ophthalmol.* Jun 2001;85(6):686–688.
13. Mermoud A, Salmon JF, Murray AD. Trabeculectomy with mitomycin C for refractory glaucoma in blacks. *Am J Ophthalmol.* Jul 15 1993;116(1):72–78.
14. Membrey WL, Poinoosawmy DP, Bunce C, Hitchings RA. Glaucoma surgery with or without adjunctive antiproliferatives in normal tension glaucoma: 1 intraocular pressure control and complications. *Br J Ophthalmol.* Jun 2000;84(6):586–590.
15. Fuller JR, Bevin TH, Molteno AC, Vote BJ, Herbison P. Anti-inflammatory fibrosis suppression in threatened trabeculectomy bleb failure produces good long term control of intraocular pressure without risk of sight threatening complications. *Br J Ophthalmol.* Dec 2002;86(12):1352–1354.
16. Memarzadeh F, Varma R, Lin LT, et al. Postoperative use of bevacizumab as an antifibrotic agent in glaucoma filtration surgery in the rabbit. *Invest Ophthalmol Vis Sci.* Jul 2009;50(7):3233–3237.
17. Grewal DS, Jain R, Kumar H, Grewal SP. Evaluation of subconjunctival bevacizumab as an adjunct to trabeculectomy a pilot study. *Ophthalmology.* Dec 2008;115(12):2141–2145 e2142.
18. Coote MA, Ruddle JB, Qin Q, Crowston JG. Vascular changes after intra-bleb injection of bevacizumab. *J Glaucoma.* Oct-Nov 2008; 17(7):517–518.
19. Kapasi MS, Birt CM. The efficacy of 5-fluorouracil bleb needling performed 1 year or more posttrabeculectomy: a retrospective study. *J Glaucoma.* Feb 2009;18(2): 144–148.
20. Anand N, Khan A. Long-term outcomes of needle revision of trabeculectomy blebs with mitomycin C and 5-fluorouracil: a comparative safety and efficacy report. *J Glaucoma.* Sept 2009;18(7):513–520.
21. Feldman RM, Tabet RR. Needle revision of filtering blebs. *J Glaucoma.* Oct-Nov 2008;17(7):594–600.
22. Kahook MY, Schuman JS, Noecker RJ. Needle bleb revision of encapsulated filtering bleb with bevacizumab. *Ophthalmic Surg Lasers Imaging.* Mar-Apr 2006;37(2):148–150.
23. Rotchford AP, King AJ. Needling revision of trabeculectomies bleb morphology and long-term survival. *Ophthalmology.* Jul 2008; 115(7):1148–1153 e1144.
24. Greenfield DS, Miller MP, Suner IJ, Palmberg PF. Needle elevation of the scleral flap for failing filtration blebs after trabeculectomy with mitomycin C. *Am J Ophthalmol.* Aug 1996;122(2):195–204.

25. Broadway DC, Bloom PA, Bunce C, Thiagarajan M, Khaw PT. Needle revision of failing and failed trabeculectomy blebs with adjunctive 5-fluorouracil: survival analysis. *Ophthalmology.* Apr 2004;111(4):665–673.
26. Shin DH, Kim YY, Ginde SY, et al. Risk factors for failure of 5-fluorouracil needling revision for failed conjunctival filtration blebs. *Am J Ophthalmol.* Dec 2001;132(6):875–880.
27. Potash SD, Ritch R, Liebmann J. Ocular hypotony and choroidal effusion following bleb needling. *Ophthalmic Surg.* Apr 1993;24(4):279–280.
28. Ramanathan US, Kumar V, O'Neill E, Shah P. Aqueous misdirection following needling of trabeculectomy bleb. *Eye (Lond).* Apr 2003;17(3):441–442.

16

LATE BLEB LEAKS

PARUL KHATOR AND JONATHAN S. MYERS

LATE BLEB LEAKS

Glaucoma filtering surgery is an effective method to lower intraocular pressure (IOP).[1,2] However, as is the case with any interventional procedure, filtering surgery poses risks to the eye. At a reported incidence of 4.2%–10%, late leakage of filtering blebs is one of the most common and challenging complications encountered by glaucoma surgeons [3,4] Bleb leaks pose many sight-threatening risks to the eye, including inflammation, blebitis,[5] endophthalmitis,[6] hypotony[7] with its attendant risk of choroidal effusions and maculopathy,[8] flat chamber with corneal decompensation, cataractous changes, and suprachoroidal hemorrhage.[3] Additionally, allowing bleb leaks to persist risks failure of the filtration surgery.

ETIOLOGY AND RISK FACTORS FOR A LEAKING BLEB

Leaks can occur at any point in the life of the bleb, from months to years after surgery,[9] and late bleb leaks are commonly referred to as those occurring at least 2 months after surgery.[10] Unlike early bleb leaks, which are frequently located at incisions and suture tracks or are secondary to intraoperative surgical trauma (buttonholes), late bleb leaks can often be seen at the apex of a cystic, avascular bleb (Figure 16.1). These leaks arise from focal epithelial thinning, which eventually culminates in a conjunctival defect in the wall of the bleb.[11]

Bleb leaks occur for a variety of reasons, including trauma to the conjunctival bleb wall. Thin-walled, focal, cystic blebs are at a much

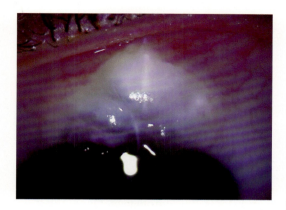

FIGURE 16.1   A thin-walled, avascular bleb that is likely to leak.

greater risk of leaking than diffuse, vascular blebs.[12] One important risk factor for development of thin-walled blebs is the use of antifibrotic agents, such as 5-fluorouracil and mitomycin-C (see Chapter 27).[13] Mechanical factors, such as eye rubbing, contact lenses, and giant papillary conjunctivitis, also increase the risk of bleb leaks by causing trauma to a focal area of susceptible conjunctiva. Although digital ocular compression is frequently performed and prescribed by ophthalmologists for management of encapsulated filtering blebs, one study from Japan showed that there is an increased risk of leak (3.1%–5.6%) with digital ocular bleb compression.[14] This risk was especially increased in blebs with a larger avascular area or a longer intraoperative duration of mitomycin-C. In addition, conditions that cause conjunctival exposure, such as thyroid ophthalmopathy or a large overhanging bleb, can also increase the chances of leakage. This scenario may be related to bleb desiccation. One review of bleb leaks found that age, sex, race, number of IOP-lowering medications, duration of mitomycin-C exposure, and total 5-fluorouracil dose were not associated risk factors.[4]

PREVENTION OF BLEB LEAKS

It is important to identify characteristics of a bleb that increase the risk of leak formation. These characteristics include blebs that are avascular, especially for a large (>4 mm^2)

area,[12] and transparent blebs with lobulated or cystic structures.[11] Blebs located far temporally or nasally without adequate eyelid coverage also are at greater risk. Next, consideration must be given to patient risk factors such as contact lens wear, allergic conjunctivitis with frequent eye rubbing, and the presence of ocular diseases that increase the chance of drying or conjunctival exposure, such as thyroid eye disease, orbital pseudotumor,[15] or other lid defects. Because leaks are not always constant, it is also important to screen for patient symptoms of intermittent leak and consequent hypotony, such as occasional heavy tearing with decreased vision, red eye, or eye ache. The associated tearing is most commonly noted by patients when going to sleep.

Preoperative, intraoperative, and postoperative considerations must be given to prevent leak formation. When planning the type and dose of antifibrotic to use, if the fellow eye has also had a filtering procedure, the duration of antifibrotic exposure and resulting bleb morphology should be considered. Careful examination of natural lid placement should be noted, and the bleb should be planned in an area that will afford greatest lid coverage. Intraoperatively, dissection and antifibrotic application should be as broad as possible to prevent focal, avascular bleb formation. If fragile conjunctiva is noted during dissection, the planned antifibrotic time should be minimized. In addition, avoiding contact between the antimetabolite and the conjunctival wound edges is prudent to minimize the risk of early wound leaks. Postoperatively, the signs and symptoms of bleb leaks and infection should be reviewed with the patient, especially in those situations with high-risk blebs. It is important to check for a leak when a patient complains of new tearing symptoms or if examination reveals an unexpected reduction in IOP. Associated exacerbating ocular risk factors (as discussed above) should be addressed.

TREATMENT OF BLEB LEAKS

The plethora of treatments available for bleb leaks reflects the diverse etiology of leaks as well as the lack of one definitively superior treatment. The nature of the defect causing the leak and whether it is conjunctival alone or associated with a scleral defect may help guide treatment. Leaks can result in a collapse of the conjunctival/Tenon's layer roof onto the scleral base of the bleb, leading to bleb failure secondary to scarring (adhesions). Although a known risk factor for development of bleb leaks, antifibrotics such as mitomycin-C can also help to prevent healing of the bleb in the event a leak does occur.[16]

In general, treatment should begin with conservative therapy, progressing to more interventional treatments as conservative measures fail. However, it should be noted that in one series, this conservative approach was associated with an increased incidence of infection, and for this reason some clinicians move quickly to surgical revision of leaks.[10] Favorable prognostic indicators for conservative therapy include healthy, vascularized conjunctiva surrounding the leak and smaller, slower leaks. Avascular tissue, higher flow rates, and blepharitis may be associated with reduced success and increased infection risk. Table 16.1 lists bleb and patient characteristics that may warrant earlier intervention.

From a practical perspective, we recommend that in those patients judged to have more favorable prognostic factors and who will be able to return emergently in case of signs or symptoms of infection, observation with a topical antibiotic and possibly an aqueous suppressant be tried for up to several weeks. The concern has been raised that prophylactic antibiotics may select for more virulent or resistant bacteria[17]; however, there is yet no definitive answer to this question.

If improvement with conservative therapy is not seen, further intervention should be considered. Highly avascular blebs with leaks do not usually respond to observation, pressure patching, or bandage contact lenses, and when they do, the leak often recurs later. The success rate for autologous blood injection is disappointing, and complications, such as hyphema or spillover into the posterior segment with prolonged impact on sight, are not rare.[18] Bleb needling with antimetabolites has been described to increase the area of filtration and divert fluid away from the area of leakage but has not been widely adopted.[19,20] Glue can be used successfully,[21–24] with a bandage contact lens to aid comfort, but when the glue dislodges the hole may reopen, and sometimes become larger. It is difficult to achieve water-tight closure of avascular tissue in long-standing blebs with direct suturing of the avascular tissue.

Most leaks can be managed definitively with sliding advancement of the conjunctiva, with or without Tenon's capsule, over the leaking, avascular area (see Figure 16.2) and may be done with or without excision of the underlying bleb.[25] If the underlying bleb is high,

Table 16.1 Characteristics Favoring Earlier Intervention

CHARACTERISTICS FAVORING EARLIER INTERVENTION

- Brisk leak
- Highly avascular tissue
- Large defect in conjunctiva
- Evidence of early bleb failure
- Blepharitis/poor lid hygiene
- History of prior leak
- Hypotony with reduced vision
- Patient inability to seek emergent care
- Monocular status

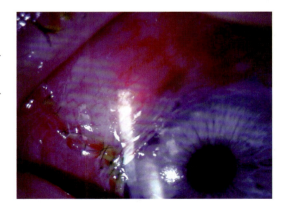

FIGURE 16.2   Bleb leak revised by conjunctival advancement.

which may make mobilization of the tissue to the limbus more difficult, then excision or reduction of the bleb with cautery may aid the procedure. If the prior bleb is left intact, the surface should still be denuded of epithelium with light cautery, scraping, or careful application of dehydrated 100% ethanol to prevent conjunctival inclusion cyst formation. The first step of the surgery is to outline the area of avascular bleb that will be covered with Vannas scissors or a knife. The vascular tissue is then extensively undermined to make sure that it can be advanced to the limbus with absolutely no tension. If adequate undermining and dissection are not performed, wound dehiscence, ptosis, and diplopia are significant risks. If the tissue is not able to be adequately mobilized, a posterior incision creating a "bucket handle" conjunctiva flap will allow mobilization. The posterior edge is then sutured to bare sclera. Alternatively, a free autologous conjunctival flap from another area, such as the inferior quadrant or the fellow eye, may be harvested and used.[26,27] Amniotic membrane grafts have also been employed.[28]

If overfiltration at the level of the scleral flap is present, the transscleral flow should also be lessened, as excessive hydrostatic pressure within the bleb may prevent timely healing of a leak by placing too much strain on the defective conjunctiva.[29] Numerous treatment modalities are listed in Table 16.2. Overfiltration may be corrected by directly suturing the scleral flap. However, intraoperative iatrogenic trauma from the initial filtering procedure or postoperative inflammatory or mechanical forces may leave the scleral flap tissue thin, macerated, or shredded. Additional suturing of the scleral flap may not be technically feasible, so a donor patch graft (pericardium, sclera, or cornea) may be useful.

Eyes that have bleb leaks generally do not require medications for IOP control. While surgical revision for leaking blebs has an excellent success rate,[10,13,30,31] some patients may require topical medications for pressure control. Unfortunately, complete filtration failure may occasionally occur.[32] Preoperative discussion with the patient must emphasize that bleb revision is necessary to prevent infection and

Table 16.2 Various Treatments for Late-Onset Bleb Leaks

VARIOUS TREATMENTS FOR LATE-ONSET BLEB LEAKS

Nonsurgical

- Observation ± antibiotics
- Aqueous suppressants[37]
- Decrease in frequency of steroids
- Pressure patching[10]
- Bandage contact lens[38]
- Collagen shield[39]
- Tamponade shell[40]

Office Procedures

- Glue (cyanoacrylate or fibrin)[23,24]
- Cautery
- Cryotherapy[41]
- Laser (ND:YAG or argon)[42,43]
- Autologous blood injection (topical or subconjunctival)[44,45]

Surgical Conjunctival Etiology

- Autologous blood injection
- Needling with antimetabolite
- Direct suturing of leaking margins[40]
- Conjunctival advancement with or without excision of the bleb[11,26,36]
- Autologous conjunctival patch[27]
- Amniotic membrane[28]

Conjunctival + Scleral Etiology

- Amniotic membrane to the sclera
- Autologous Tenon's capsule to the sclera[46]
- Patch graft (pericardium, sclera,[28]or cornea[46])

the negative sequelae of hypotony. To avoid unrealistic expectations and disappointment, the patient should understand that although every effort will be made to maintain IOP control, the possibility remains that medication or further surgery may be necessary.

CONCLUSION

Late bleb leak after trabeculectomy is an important complication to detect because of the risk it poses to the eye. Patient education, careful preoperative planning, and vigilant postsurgical examinations are key factors in preventing not only the bleb leak but also resultant hypotony and/or infection. If a bleb leak does occur, a variety of techniques for repair are at the ophthalmologist's disposal.

COMMENTARY
ANGELO P. TANNA

The key to reducing the risk of the late development of a bleb leak is to perform a trabeculectomy and manage the wound healing process so as to minimize the risk of the development of a small, localized bleb with a thin wall. Somewhat paradoxically, this balancing act centers around the use of sufficiently potent antifibrotic therapy to prevent the development of a cystic or otherwise limited bleb, while at the same time using the agent judiciously so as to prevent the development of an ischemic bleb. Appropriate titration of the antifibrotic therapy based on the characteristics of the patient (age, skin pigmentation, type of glaucoma, etc.) and the conjunctiva (scarred, thick or thin, etc.) is important.

Although intraoperative antifibrotic therapy should be avoided in a small minority of eyes due to the presence of thin conjunctiva in some elderly patients, in most cases, it is crucial to treat a large surface area of sclera with an antifibrotic agent at the time of surgery, and to supplement that, if necessary, with postoperative 5-fluorouracil injections. The use of a fornix-based conjunctival flap may also reduce the risk of the development of the so-called "ring of steel" subconjunctival fibrotic scar that often limits the extent of the bleb. If the bleb ultimately develops a small surface area, the force of the IOP in the anterior chamber will be spread over a smaller surface area of conjunctiva in the bleb, and the bleb wall will become thinner over time, increasing the risk of the development of a leak.

If a bleb leak does develop, as Drs. Khator and Myers point out, there are numerous options. However, there are few good options. If a leak is small, and occurs in an otherwise healthy-appearing bleb (well-vascularized and not thin-walled), conservative measures coupled with changes in patient behavior may result in long-term resolution. Conversely, if the conjunctival tissue is unhealthy (avascular and diffusely thin), surgical revision will likely be required.

Subconjunctival autologous blood injections seldom work in the setting of an active leak. Conversely, they do work to reverse hypotony in the setting of an overly exuberant, diffuse bleb with healthy conjunctival tissue.

In cystic, thin-walled, ischemic blebs, needle revision with the use of supplemental antifibrotic therapy has, surprisingly, been used successfully in the treatment of bleb leaks.[33] The rationale is that if the bleb can be expanded, the pressure in the bleb can be spread over a larger surface area of conjunctiva, and tissue remodeling can occur and allow sealing of the leak. This approach is particularly valuable if the leak is small, and the eye is not hypotonous. For more information on needling, see Chapter 28.

Epithelial removal followed by conjunctival advancement or the use of a conjunctival autograft (with or without the supplemental use of an allograft to reinforce the scleral flap) are the definitive options and usually result in preservation of bleb function.[34] The use of tissue adhesives such as TISSEEL (fibrin sealant; Baxter, Deerfield, Illinois) facilitates the surgical procedure, but does not obviate the need for a watertight suture closure.

Counseling patients about the signs and symptoms of a bleb-related infection and a plan of action should those symptoms develop is important (see Chapter 24). We give patients a laminated card with these instructions that can be presented to triage staff with the aim of shortening the time to the involvement of an ophthalmologist. It is also very important to counsel patients to avoid the use of makeup around the eye and to avoid other forms of mechanical trauma to the eye, including rubbing.

Dr. Tanna was supported by an Unrestricted Grant from Research to Prevent Blindness to Northwestern University.

COMMENTARY
MARTIN WAND

Drs. Khator and Myers have provided a concise and thorough review of late bleb leaks, a complication that all glaucoma surgeons face more often than they would like. They have summarized the multiple treatments advocated for this complication. The reason there are so many purported cures is because there is not a single treatment that works so much better than others that only one treatment needs to be reported and utilized.

Over my 35 years of practicing glaucoma, I have learned one very simple and conservative treatment that will cure many late bleb leaks without surgical intervention. Without question, there are more late bleb leaks since the widespread use of antimetabolites.[4] With the use of antimetabolites, there are more thin, avascular blebs prone to leakage either spontaneously, but more often physical or just increased dependent hydrostatic pressure can over time cause a very thin bleb to leak. When questioned about sleeping positions, patients often will relate that they sleep on the side of the leaking bleb. Furthermore, many patients have prominent orbits and/or are pillow huggers. In these cases direct mechanical pressure on the eye can contribute toward further thinning of the bleb and ultimately to leakage over time. Even without direct pressure on the eye, just sleeping with the head on the dependent side will appreciably increase the hydrostatic pressure within that eye. Furthermore, when questioned about how and how often a patient rubs his/her eyes, many will confess to rubbing with moderate or greater force on the lids.

If the bleb leak is small and without infection or a flat anterior chamber, I have found that an eye shield applied at bedtime with instructions not to rub the eye at any time, not to perform any activity with heavy exertion, or not to perform any activities with the head bent below the heart will often allow the epithelium to heal over a small leak with reformation of the anterior chamber and an increase in IOP. It will also often resolve any hypotony-related corneal problems and/or macular edema. Initially, I prescribe only broad spectrum antibiotic drops (fourth-generation fluoroquinolone); I refrain from a topical steroid until the leak is resolved. I follow the patient frequently and give detailed instructions on the signs of an infection and to call or come in if there are any signs of one. Even in eyes with early blebitis, I have treated in this conservative manner with more frequent topical antibiotics and with daily observation. Most patients would choose this alternative to surgery.

I have also seen asymptomatic eyes with thin, avascular blebs that have fine leaks detectable only with fluorescein, with IOPs in the low single digits with deep anterior chambers, and 20/20 vision. If these patients are reliable and maintain general good hygiene, I have followed them for years with no treatment except to have them wear a shield at bedtime forever and to report back at the first signs of infection or decreased vision. I do not prescribe topical antibiotics for chronic use because they do not prevent the pathogenic bacteria from colonizing the conjunctival flora.[35]

That said, there are, of course, late bleb leaks that are infected, have flat anterior chambers, and/or large leaks that do not respond to this conservative therapy. In these cases having tried all the treatments cited by Drs. Khator and Myers and found them unsatisfactory, I go directly to conjunctival advancement to repair the leaking blebs, aware that even then there will be some failures and complications.[36]

In conclusion, preventive medicine is always the best medicine. I have always given every patient who has had a glaucoma filtration operation an instruction sheet detailing the following: (1) signs and symptoms of an eye infection or leak; (2) warnings against rubbing the operated eye or engaging in activities that result in increased intrathoracic pressure; (3) instructions to call the office if there are any signs of infection or leaks; (4) an undated prescription for topical antibiotic drops; and (5) instructions to fill the prescription and start using the drops if an ophthalmologist is not immediately available.

REFERENCES

1. Fontana H, Nouri-Mahdavi K, Caprioli J. Trabeculectomy with mitomycin C in pseudophakic patients with open-angle glaucoma: outcomes and risk factors for failure. *Am J Ophthalmol.* Apr 2006;141(4):652–659.

2. Fontana H, Nouri-Mahdavi K, Lumba J, Ralli M, Caprioli J. Trabeculectomy with mitomycin C: outcomes and risk factors for failure in phakic open-angle glaucoma. *Ophthalmology.* Jun 2006;113(6):930–936.

3. DeBry PW, Perkins TW, Heatley G, Kaufman P, Brumback LC. Incidence of late-onset bleb-related complications following trabeculectomy with mitomycin. *Arch Ophthalmol.* Mar 2002; 120(3):297–300.

4. Greenfield DS, Liebmann JM, Jee J, Ritch R. Late-onset bleb leaks after glaucoma filtering surgery. *Arch Ophthalmol.* Apr 1998;116(4): 443–447.

5. Sharan S, Trope GE, Chipman M, Buys YM. Late-onset bleb infections: prevalence and risk factors. *Can J Ophthalmol.* Jun 2009; 44(3):279–283.

6. Song A, Scott IU, Flynn HW Jr., Budenz DL. Delayed-onset bleb-associated endophthalmitis: clinical features and visual acuity outcomes. *Ophthalmology.* May 2002;109(5):985–991.

7. Liebmann JM, Ritch R. Bleb related ocular infection: a feature of the HELP syndrome. Hypotony, endophthalmitis, leak, pain. *Br J Ophthalmol.* Dec 2000;84(12):1338–1339.

8. Costa VP, Arcieri ES. Hypotony maculopathy. *Acta Ophthalmol Scand.* Sept 2007;85(6):586–597.

9. Loane ME, Galanopoulos A. The surgical management of leaking filtering blebs. *Curr Opin Ophthalmol.* Apr 1999;10(2):121–125.

10. Burnstein AL, WuDunn D, Knotts SL, Catoira Y, Cantor LB. Conjunctival advancement versus nonincisional treatment for late-onset glaucoma filtering bleb leaks. *Ophthalmology.* Jan 2002;109(1):71–75.

11. Belyea DA, Dan JA, Stamper RL, Lieberman MF, Spencer WH. Late onset of sequential multifocal bleb leaks after glaucoma filtration surgery with 5-fluorouracil and mitomycin C. *Am J Ophthalmol.* Jul 1997;124(1):40–45.

12. Anand N, Arora S, Clowes M. Mitomycin C augmented glaucoma surgery: evolution of filtering bleb avascularity, transconjunctival oozing, and leaks. *Br J Ophthalmol.* Feb 2006;90(2):175–180.

13. Al-Shahwan S, Al-Torbak AA, Al-Jadaan I, Omran M, Edward DP. Long-term follow up of surgical repair of late bleb leaks after glaucoma filtering surgery. *J Glaucoma.* Oct 2006;15(5):432–436.

14. Hu CY, Matsuo H, Tomita G, et al. Clinical characteristics and leakage of functioning blebs after trabeculectomy with mitomycin-C in primary glaucoma patients. *Ophthalmology.* Feb 2003;110(2):345–352.

15. Luk FO, Leung DY, Yuen HK, Lam DS. Late leakage of filtering bleb in a patient with orbital pseudotumor. *Eur J Ophthalmol.* Jul-Aug 2006;16(4):611–613.

16. Alwitry A, Rotchford A, Patel V, Abedin A, Moodie J, King AJ. Early bleb leak after trabeculectomy and prognosis for bleb failure. *Eye (Lond).* Apr 2009;23(4):858–863.

17. Jampel HD, Quigley HA, Kerrigan-Baumrind LA, Melia BM, Friedman D, Barron Y. Risk factors for late-onset infection following glaucoma filtration surgery. *Arch Ophthalmol.* Jul 2001;119(7):1001–1008.

18. Flynn WJ, Rosen WJ, Campbell DG. Delayed hyphema and intravitreal blood following intrableb autologous blood injection after trabeculectomy. *Am J Ophthalmol.* Jul 1997;124(1):115–116.

19. Ares C, Kasner OP. Bleb needle redirection for the treatment of early postoperative trabeculectomy leaks: a novel approach. *Can J Ophthalmol.* Apr 2008;43(2):225–228.

20. Maeda H, Eno A, Nakamura M, Negi A. Safe management of a late-onset bleb leak with a needling technique. *Eye (Lond).* Oct 2000; 14(Pt 5):802–804.

21. Gammon RR, Prum BE, Jr., Avery N, Mintz PD. Rapid preparation of small-volume autologous fibrinogen concentrate and its same day use in bleb leaks after glaucoma filtration surgery. *Ophthalmic Surg Lasers.* Dec 1998;29(12):1010–1012.

22. Wright MM, Brown EA, Maxwell K, Cameron JD, Walsh AW. Laser-cured fibrinogen glue to repair bleb leaks in rabbits. *Arch Ophthalmol.* Feb 1998;116(2):199–202.

23. Asrani SG, Wilensky JT. Management of bleb leaks after glaucoma filtering surgery. Use of autologous fibrin tissue glue as an alternative. *Ophthalmology.* Feb 1996;103(2):294–298.

24. Zalta AH, Wieder RH. Closure of leaking filtering blebs with cyanoacrylate tissue adhesive. *Br J Ophthalmol.* Mar 1991;75(3):170–173.

25. Tannenbaum DP, Hoffman D, Greaney MJ, Caprioli J. Outcomes of bleb excision and conjunctival advancement for leaking or hypotonous eyes after glaucoma filtering surgery. *Br J Ophthalmol.* Jan 2004;88(1):99–103.

26. Harris LD, Yang G, Feldman RM, et al. Autologous conjunctival resurfacing of leaking filtering blebs. *Ophthalmology.* Sept 2000;107(9):1675–1680.

27. Schnyder CC, Shaarawy T, Ravinet E, Achache F, Uffer S, Mermoud A. Free conjunctival autologous graft for bleb repair and bleb reduction after trabeculectomy and nonpenetrating filtering surgery. *J Glaucoma.* Feb 2002;11(1):10–16.

28. Budenz DL, Barton K, Tseng SC. Amniotic membrane transplantation for repair of leaking glaucoma filtering blebs. *Am J Ophthalmol.* Nov 2000;130(5):580–588.

29. Kosmin AS, Wishart PK. A full-thickness scleral graft for the surgical management of a late filtration bleb leak. *Ophthalmic Surg Lasers.* Jun 1997;28(6):461–468.

30. Wadhwani RA, Bellows AR, Hutchinson BT. Surgical repair of leaking filtering blebs. *Ophthalmology.* Sept 2000;107(9):1681–1687.

31. Feldman RM, Altaher G. Management of late-onset bleb leaks. *Curr Opin Ophthalmol.* Apr 2004;15(2):151–154.

32. Myers JS, Yang CB, Herndon LW, Allingham RR, Shields MB. Excisional bleb revision to correct overfiltration or leakage. *J Glaucoma.* Apr 2000;9(2):169–173.

33. Solish AM. Is mitomycin really the culprit in leaking filtration blebs? Evidence from a clinical series of belb expansion as a treatment for leaking blebs. *Invest Ophthalmol Vis Sci* 2002; 43: E-Abstract 3350.

34. Radhakrishnan S, Quigley HA, Jampel HD, et al. Outcomes of surgical bleb revision for complications of trabeculectomy. *Ophthalmology.* Sept 2009;116(9):1713–1718.

35. Wand M, Quintiliani R, Robinson A. Antibiotic prophylaxis in eyes with filtration blebs: survey of glaucoma specialists, microbiological study, and recommendations. *J Glaucoma.* Apr 1995;4(2):103–109.

36. Budenz DL, Chen PP, Weaver YK. Conjunctival advancement for late-onset filtering bleb leaks: indications and outcomes. *Arch Ophthalmol.* Aug 1999;117(8):1014–1019.

37. Pederson JE. Ocular hypotony. In: Ritch R, Shields MB, Kruppin T, eds. *The Glaucomas.* St. Louis, MO: Mosby; 1996:385–395.

38. Shoham A, Tessler Z, Finkelman Y, Lifshitz T. Large soft contact lenses in the management of leaking blebs. *CLAO J.* Jan 2000;26(1): 37–39.

39. Fourman S, Wiley L. Use of a collagen shield to treat a glaucoma filter bleb leak. *Am J Ophthalmol.* Jun 15 1989;107(6):673–674.

40. Tomlinson CP, Belcher CD 3rd, Smith PD, Simmons RJ. Management of leaking filtration blebs. *Ann Ophthalmol.* Nov 1987;19(11): 405–408, 411.

41. Graham SL, Goldberg I. Cryotherapy to close a corneal subepithelial aqueous track after trabeculectomy. *Aust N Z J Ophthalmol.* May 1993;21(2):127–129.

42. Geyer O. Management of large, leaking, and inadvertent filtering blebs with the neodymium:YAG laser. *Ophthalmology.* Jun 1998;105(6):983–987.

43. Hennis HL, Stewart WC. Use of the argon laser to close filtering bleb leaks. *Graefes Arch Clin Exp Ophthalmol.* 1992;230(6):537–541.

44. Choudhri SA, Herndon LW, Damji KF, Allingham RR, Shields MB. Efficacy of autologous blood injection for treating overfiltering or leaking blebs after glaucoma surgery. *Am J Ophthalmol.* Apr 1997;123(4):554–555.

45. Matsuo H, Tomidokoro A, Tomita G, Araie M. Topical application of autologous serum for the treatment of late-onset aqueous oozing or point-leak through filtering bleb. *Eye (Lond).* Jan 2005;19(1):23–28.

46. Morris DA, Ramocki JM, Shin DH, Glover BK, Kim YY. Use of autologous Tenon's capsule and scleral patch grafts for repair of excessively draining fistulas with leaking filtering blebs. *J Glaucoma.* Dec 1998;7(6):417–419.

17

CATARACTS AND VISUAL AXIS OPACITIES

JOHN P. BERDAHL AND THOMAS W. SAMUELSON

CATARACTS AND VISUAL AXIS OPACITIES

Glaucoma surgery can result in worsened visual acuity.[1, 2] This worsening may result from alterations to the ocular structures in the visual axis during or following surgery. This outcome is often troublesome for advanced glaucoma patients with severely restricted visual fields as they are very dependent on the remaining central island of vision. In patients with less severe glaucoma, postsurgical loss of acuity may be their first symptom of glaucoma. Many conditions result in decreased visual acuity following glaucoma surgery, and appropriate management of these complications is important for maintaining visual acuity.

CATARACT

Etiologies of formation after filtering surgery

Cataract is the most common cause of decreased visual acuity after filtering surgery.[3–11] Filtering surgery increases the 5-year risk of developing a visually significant cataract by 78%.[12] The reason for cataract formation following trabeculectomy is unclear. The most accepted hypothesis is that aqueous dynamics are altered by trabeculectomy surgery. A surgical peripheral iridectomy is typically performed as part of a trabeculectomy, which permits aqueous to pass directly from the posterior chamber to the anterior chamber without first supplying nutrition to the anterior lens. This theory is consistent with the observation that cataracts are more common after laser peripheral iridotomy.[13] Inadvertent puncture of the lens capsule during trabeculectomy surgery is also a potential cause (see Chapter 7).

Another proposed cause of cataract formation is postoperative inflammation, although plausible, convincing evidence is lacking. Increased cataract formation has been observed with the use of mitomycin-C (MMC) and may be due either to increased aqueous outflow bypassing the lens or direct toxicity to the lens.[6] Surgical complications such as intraoperative or postoperative flat anterior chamber with lens-cornea touch increase the risk of cataract formation.[12, 14]

Additionally, postoperative medications, especially corticosteroids, are also known to be associated with cataract formation.[15, 16] The risk of cataract formation from topical ocular steroids is difficult to determine because of the many confounding variables.. However, the odds ratio of cataract formation from systemic and inhaled chronic corticosteroid use is approximately 1.5–2.0.[17, 18] The surgeon should bear potential steroid effects in mind during the postoperative period in phakic patients.

Cataract Surgery After Filtering Surgery

Cataract surgery after trabeculectomy is generally similar to standard cataract surgery with a few additional considerations. First, it is important to avoid the bleb when creating the main incision and any paracentesis. Avoiding the bleb is easily accomplished by altering the incision location and/or performing clear corneal incisions. We advocate clear corneal incisions to preserve as much conjunctiva as possible should the need for further glaucoma surgery be necessary. Routine suturing of clear corneal cataract incisions in eyes with prior trabeculectomy and high flow filters may be warranted to ensure a water-tight seal.

Second, the anterior chamber is occasionally less stable in post-trabeculectomy eyes, due to fluid flow through the filter. Strategically placing viscoelastic at the sclerostomy site to prevent excessive flow through the trabeculectomy may reduce outflow via the sclerostomy but is rarely necessary.

Third, glaucoma patients often have small pupils. Typical strategies can be employed as needed, including viscodilation,[19] lysis of posterior synechiae, intracameral epinephrine,[20] gentle bimanual pupil stretching techniques,[21] iris hooks,[22, 23] or other surgical devices,[19] such as the Malyugin ring.[24, 25]

Fourth, care should be taken to remove all viscoelastic from the eye to prevent a postoperative intraocular pressure (IOP) spike in an already glaucomatous eye.

Finally, postoperative inflammation should be aggressively managed to prevent fibrosis of the bleb. Controlling the inflammation may require more aggressive steroid administration than is typical. If cataract surgery should lead to fibrosis of the filter, a bleb needling procedure with MMC or 5-fluorouracil (5-FU) can be very effective at restoring filter function.[26, 27]

PUPILLARY MEMBRANE

Pupillary membranes can occur after filtering surgery and are usually the result of excessive inflammation, fibrin formation, and subsequent organization following glaucoma surgery.[28] Typically pupillary membranes decrease during the perioperative period with aggressive topical corticosteroid treatment.. However, they can persist after the perioperative inflammation has subsided. Dense pupillary membranes may require surgical removal by anterior vitrectomy. However, in aphakic and pseudophakic patients most pupillary membranes can be lysed with a Nd:YAG laser[29, 30] or removed with a forceps. The surgeon must keep in mind that the reason for the membrane formation was excessive perioperative inflammation. Aggressive topical corticosteroid treatment for at least 3 days prior to membrane removal and continued aggressive corticosteroid treatment in the immediate postoperative period, followed by a slow taper over a couple of months, may be required to prevent recurrence.

INTRAOCULAR LENS (IOL) OPACITIES IN PSEUDOPHAKIC EYES

Early generation silicone intraocular lenses (IOLs) and acrylic IOLs are more likely to have a proliferation of cellular debris comprised of residual lenticular epithelial cells or aggregations of inflammatory giant cells across the anterior IOL surface when compared to recent generation silicone IOLs.[31] This thin sheet of epithelial cells can give a smudged appearance to the lens. No conclusive studies have shown that an actual decrease in visual acuity or contrast sensitivity results from this anterior membrane.[32] The Nd:YAG laser can be used to remove the cells on the anterior lens surface if they are causing visual compromise.

POSTERIOR CAPSULAR OPACIFICATION

Posterior capsular opacification (PCO) is quite common after cataract surgery. No clear evidence exists that a trabeculectomy alone or phacoemulsification combined with trabeculectomy increases or decreases the risk of PCO.[32, 33] Recent animal studies have shown that MMC decreases the rate of PCO in rabbits.[34] However, when performing a trabeculectomy, great care is taken to prevent MMC from entering the anterior chamber, and MMC may or may not influence the rate of PCO formation.[35] If PCO is present prior to performing a trabeculectomy or implanting a tube shunt, we recommend waiting to perform capsulotomy until after the trabeculectomy has been completed to decrease the possibility of vitreous incarceration in the sclerostomy. Aggressive control of inflammation after capsulotomy is important to prevent bleb fibrosis.

ENDOTHELIAL CELL LOSS AND CORNEAL EDEMA

Endothelial cell loss occurs at low levels after a trabeculectomy.[36, 37] The adjunctive use of MMC or 5-FU postoperatively may contribute to a slightly increased endothelial cell loss, although the data are conflicting.[38–40] In patients with compromised endothelial function, trabeculectomy can lead to corneal edema and decreased vision. Additionally, intraoperative and/or postoperative hypotony can lead to folds in Descemet's membrane and endothelial cell loss (see Chapters 10 and 22). Conversely, a spike in IOP after trabeculectomy can overwhelm the ability of the endothelial cell to pump fluid out of the corneal stroma. Penetrating keratoplasty[41, 42] and endothelial keratoplasty have lower success rates in patients with prior glaucoma surgery.[42, 43] For these reasons, we recommend paying special attention to surgical techniques in patients with Fuchs' endothelial dystrophy, or other causes of low endothelial cell count, to prevent persistent corneal edema.

DELLEN

Dellen are focal areas of corneal thinning, adjacent to a local elevation of the cornea or perilimbal tissue, due to discontinuity of the tear film. Dellen may be painful or irritating and result in irregular astigmatism, corneal scarring, or, in severe cases, corneal perforation. Following trabeculectomy, a highly elevated filtering bleb can lead to an adjacent dellen.[44] Some clinicians believe a fornix-based conjunctival flap may create a lower lying bleb with posteriorly directed aqueous outflow and hence reduce the likelihood of dellen formation.[36] If bleb elevation results in chronic corneal pathology, bleb reduction surgery is indicated.[45]

DRY EYE SYNDROME

Ocular surface dryness has been estimated to affect up to 19% of glaucoma patients.[46] Patients with glaucoma may be particularly vulnerable because the ocular surface has typically been altered by the chronic use of ocular hypotensive drops.[46] Adjunctive use of 5-FU and MMC can also contribute to ocular surface irregularity.[38] Dryness typically does not result in scarring or significant visual decline; however, in severe cases visual disability can occur.[47, 48] Treatment is directed at the underlying cause, removal of the offending agent, control of blepharitis, artificial tear replacement, or use of anti inflammatory medications, such as topical cyclosporine or oral doxycycline.

DESCEMET'S MEMBRANE TEAR

Descemet's membrane tears are an uncommon complication of glaucoma surgery.[49, 50] Small localized tears rarely cause symptoms; however, a large tear can result in persistent corneal edema directly over the tear or throughout the cornea (see Chapter 8). Treatment can include hypertonic saline, injection of intraocular air to reappose Descemet's membrane, observation, or ultimately endothelial or penetrating keratoplasty.

BAND KERATOPATHY

Band keratopathy is the accumulation of calcium deposits in Bowman's membrane of the cornea. Band keratopathy can occur after glaucoma surgery[51, 52] and is likely caused by a chronic inflammatory process. Band keratopathy can range from mild and innocuous to quite severe, causing pain and decreased vision. Treatment of band keratopathy is guided by symptoms. Treatment is typically performed in the office or a minor procedure room. The corneal epithelium is debrided. A 0.05 to 0.2 M concentration of ethylenediaminetetraacetic acid (EDTA) is applied to the cornea with triangular surgical spear sponges.[53] After the area of band keratopathy has dissolved, a bandage contact lens is placed onto the eye, and the epithelium is allowed to heal.

CONCLUSIONS

Glaucoma surgeons should take steps to avoid visual axis opacities. Although numerous visual axis alterations can limit visual function after trabeculectomy, cataracts are the most common. Should visual axis opacities develop after glaucoma surgery, the surgeon should make every effort to minimize them since nearly all are treatable, at least to a degree.

COMMENTARY
RICHARD P. MILLS

Visual axis astigmatism is an additional cause of reduced vision following filtering surgery. Some surgeons employ flap compression sutures that may need to be tied tight intraoperatively to stem excessive aqueous flow. Even tight flap edge sutures may create corneal astigmatism and blurred vision, especially in a soft eye. Corneal topography is an excellent diagnostic aid. Suture release with knife or laser may need to be delayed if hypotony is present, but after a few months when flap healing is stable, the scleral flap sutures can be released with expected resolution of cylinder and return of vision.

An important goal of cataract surgery in the presence of a functioning filtration bleb is to preserve filter function. I agree with the authors that clear corneal incisions for the cataract surgery are preferable to limbal or scleral incisions because they seem to produce less bleb inflammation and scarring. Even so, within the first postoperative week following cataract surgery, it is my practice to give a single 2.5 mg subconjunctival 5-FU injection adjacent to the bleb in hopes of reducing local fibroblast proliferation. If inflammation persists in the anterior chamber or conjunctiva beyond a week or two, subconjunctival dexamethasone 2 mg can be given.

COMMENTARY
ALAN S. CRANDALL

In the discussion on cataract post-trabeculectomy, the authors comment that suturing a clear cornea incision routinely may be warranted. I agree, but feel it should always be done. It frees one up to manipulate the bleb if necessary and secures the wound to reduce the worry for endophthalmitis.

The chapter points out that antimetabolites can be used to restore filtration. This can be done at the time of the surgery or if one feels that the bleb is marginal at any time early in the postoperative period.

When using a Nd:YAG laser to remove cells on an IOL, it is important to use low energy and to deftly focus in front of the lens, letting the backward projection of energy clear the deposits to reduce the risk of pitting lenses, especially with silicone lenses.

When operating on patients with Fuchs' endothelial dystrophy or other corneal endothelial issues, special attention to the surgical technique is critical. In this setting, one should use a dispersive viscoelastic and a low flow technique. These are patients where the use of prechopping is indicated to reduce the energy and fluid necessary.

Finally, one other problem that can occur is significant astigmatism. The use of toric IOLs at the time of the cataract surgery may be helpful.

Dr. Crandall was supported by an Unrestricted Grant from Research to Prevent Blindness to the University of Utah.

REFERENCES

1. Gedde SJ, Schiffman JC, Feuer WJ, Herndon LW, Brandt JD, Budenz DL. Three-year follow-up of the Tube versus Trabeculectomy study. *Am J Ophthalmol*. Nov 2009;148(5):670–684.

2. Costa VP, Smith M, Spaeth GL, Gandham S, Markovitz B. Loss of visual acuity after trabeculectomy. *Ophthalmology*. May 1993; 100(5):599–612.

3. Beckers HJ, Kinders KC, Webers CA. Five-year results of trabeculectomy with mitomycin C. *Graefes Arch Clin Exp Ophthalmol*. Feb 2003; 241(2):106–110.

4. Borisuth NS, Phillips B, Krupin T. The risk profile of glaucoma filtration surgery. *Curr Opin Ophthalmol*. Apr 1999;10(2):112–116.

5. Costa VP, Moster MR, Wilson RP, Schmidt CM, Gandham S, Smith M. Effects of topical mitomycin C on primary trabeculectomies and combined procedures. *Br J Ophthalmol*. Nov 1993;77(11):693–697.

6. Daugeliene L, Yamamoto T, Kitazawa Y. Cataract development after trabeculectomy with mitomycin C: a 1-year study. *Jpn J Ophthalmol*. Jan-Feb 2000;44(1):52–57.

7. Hylton C, Congdon N, Friedman D, et al. Cataract after glaucoma filtration surgery. *Am J Ophthalmol*. Feb 2003;135(2):231–232.

8. Kook MS, Kim HB, Lee SU. Short-term effect of mitomycin-C augmented trabeculectomy on axial length and corneal astigmatism. *J Cataract Refract Surg*. Apr 2001;27(4):518–523.

9. Mermoud A, Schnyder CC, Sickenberg M, Chiou AG, Hediguer SE, Faggioni R. Comparison of deep sclerectomy with collagen implant and trabeculectomy in open-angle glaucoma. *J Cataract Refract Surg*. Mar 1999;25(3):323–331.

10. O'Brart DP, Rowlands E, Islam N, Noury AM. A randomised, prospective study comparing trabeculectomy augmented with antimetabolites with a viscocanalostomy technique for the management of open angle glaucoma uncontrolled by medical therapy. *Br J Ophthalmol*. Jul 2002;86(7):748–754.

11. Watson PG, Jakeman C, Ozturk M, Barnett MF, Barnett F, Khaw KT. The complications of trabeculectomy (a 20-year follow-up). *Eye*. 1990;4(Pt 3):425–438.

12. The Advanced Glaucoma Intervention Study: 8. Risk of cataract formation after trabeculectomy. *Arch Ophthalmol*. Dec 2001; 119(12):1771–1779.

13. Lim LS, Husain R, Gazzard G, Seah SK, Aung T. Cataract progression after prophylactic laser peripheral iridotomy: potential implications for the prevention of glaucoma blindness. *Ophthalmology*. Aug 2005;112(8):1355–1359.

14. Stewart WC, Shields MB. Management of anterior chamber depth after trabeculectomy. *Am J Ophthalmol*. Jul 15 1988;106(1):41–44.

15. Carnahan MC, Goldstein DA. Ocular complications of topical, peri-ocular, and systemic corticosteroids. *Curr Opin Ophthalmol*. Dec 2000;11(6):478–483.

16. Skalka HW, Prchal JT. Effect of corticosteroids on cataract formation. *Arch Ophthalmol*. Oct 1980;98(10):1773–1777.

17. Cumming RG, Mitchell P. Medications and cataract. The Blue Mountains Eye Study. *Ophthalmology*. Sept 1998;105(9):1751–1758.

18. Cumming RG, Mitchell P, Leeder SR. Use of inhaled corticosteroids and the risk of cataracts. *N Engl J Med*. Jul 3 1997;337(1):8–14.

19. Goldman JM, Karp CL. Adjunct devices for managing challenging cases in cataract surgery: pupil expansion and stabilization of the capsular bag. *Curr Opin Ophthalmol*. Feb 2007;18(1):44–51.

20. Liou SW, Chen CC. Maintenance of mydriasis with one bolus of epinephrine injection during phacoemulsification. *J Ocul Pharmacol Ther*. Jun 2001;17(3):249–253.

21. Akman A, Yilmaz G, Oto S, Akova YA. Comparison of various pupil dilatation

methods for phacoemulsification in eyes with a small pupil secondary to pseudoexfoliation. *Ophthalmology.* Sept 2004;111(9):1693–1698.

22. Novak J. Flexible iris hooks for phacoemulsification. *J Cataract Refract Surg.* Jul-Aug 1997;23(6):828–831.

23. Nichamin LD. Enlarging the pupil for cataract extraction using flexible nylon iris retractors. *J Cataract Refract Surg.* Nov 1993;19(6):793–796.

24. Agarwal A, Malyugin B, Kumar DA, Jacob S, Laks L. Modified Malyugin ring iris expansion technique in small-pupil cataract surgery with posterior capsule defect. *J Cataract Refract Surg.* May 2008;34(5):724–726.

25. Malyugin B. Small pupil phaco surgery: a new technique. *Ann Ophthalmol (Skokie).* Sept 2007;39(3):185–193.

26. Broadway DC, Bloom PA, Bunce C, Thiagarajan M, Khaw PT. Needle revision of failing and failed trabeculectomy blebs with adjunctive 5-fluorouracil: survival analysis. *Ophthalmology.* Apr 2004;111(4):665–673.

27. Iwach AG, Delgado MF, Novack GD, Nguyen N, Wong PC. Transconjunctival mitomycin-C in needle revisions of failing filtering blebs. *Ophthalmology.* Apr 2003;110(4):734–742.

28. Friedrich Y, Raniel Y, Lubovsky E, Friedman Z. Late pigmented-membrane formation on silicone intraocular lenses after phacoemulsification with or without trabeculectomy. *J Cataract Refract Surg.* Sept 1999;25(9):1220–1225.

29. Haynes WL, Alward WL. Control of intraocular pressure after trabeculectomy. *Surv Ophthalmol.* Jan-Feb 1999;43(4):345–355.

30. Virdi M, Beirouty ZA, Saba SN. Neodymium: YAG laser discission of postoperative pupillary membrane: peripheral photodisruption. *J Cataract Refract Surg.* Mar 1997;23(2):166–168.

31. Samuelson TW, Chu YR, Kreiger RA. Evaluation of giant-cell deposits on foldable intraocular lenses after combined cataract and glaucoma surgery. *J Cataract Refract Surg.* Jun 2000;26(6):817–823.

32. Ober MD, Lemon LC, Shin DH, Nootheti P, Cha SC, Kim PH. Posterior capsular opacification in phacotrabeculectomy: a long-term comparative study of silicone versus acrylic intraocular lens. *Ophthalmology.* Oct 2000;107(10):1868–1873; discussion 1874.

33. Tyson SL. Posterior capsular opacification in phacotrabeculectomy. *Evidence-Based Ophthalmology.* April 2001;2:98.

34. Haus CM, Galand AL. Mitomycin against posterior capsular opacification: an experimental study in rabbits. *Br J Ophthalmol.* Dec 1996;80(12):1087–1091.

35. Shin DH, Kim YY, Ren J, et al. Decrease of capsular opacification with adjunctive mitomycin C in combined glaucoma and cataract surgery. *Ophthalmology.* Jul 1998;105(7):1222–1226.

36. Fukuchi T, Hayakawa Y, Hara H, Abe H. Corneal endothelial damage after trabeculectomy with mitomycin C in two patients with glaucoma with cornea guttata. *Cornea.* Apr 2002;21(3):300–304.

37. Smith DL, Skuta GL, Lindenmuth KA, Musch DC, Bergstrom TJ. The effect of glaucoma filtering surgery on corneal endothelial cell density. *Ophthalmic Surg.* May 1991;22(5):251–255.

38. Dreyer EB, Chaturvedi N, Zurakowski D. Effect of mitomycin C and fluorouracil-supplemented trabeculectomies on the anterior segment. *Arch Ophthalmol.* May 1995;113(5):578–580.

39. Nuyts RM, Pels E, Greve EL. The effects of 5-fluorouracil and mitomycin C on the corneal endothelium. *Curr Eye Res.* Jun 1992; 11(6):565–570.

40. Sihota R, Sharma T, Agarwal HC. Intraoperative mitomycin C and the corneal endothelium. *Acta Ophthalmol Scand.* Feb 1998;76(1):80–82.

41. Yamagami S, Suzuki Y, Tsuru T. Risk factors for graft failure in penetrating keratoplasty. *Acta Ophthalmol Scand.* Dec 1996;74(6):584–588.

42. Kirkness CM, Steele AD, Ficker LA, Rice NS. Coexistent corneal disease and glaucoma managed by either drainage surgery and subsequent keratoplasty or combined drainage surgery and penetrating keratoplasty. *Br J Ophthalmol.* Mar 1992;76(3):146–152.

43. Vajaranant TS, Price MO, Price FW, Gao W, Wilensky JT, Edward DP. Visual acuity and intraocular pressure after Descemet's stripping endothelial keratoplasty in eyes with and without preexisting glaucoma. *Ophthalmology.* Sept 2009;116(9):1644–1650.

44. Budenz DL, Hoffman K, Zacchei A. Glaucoma filtering bleb dysesthesia. *Am J Ophthalmol.* May 2001;131(5):626–630.

45. La Borwit SE, Quigley HA, Jampel HD. Bleb reduction and bleb repair after trabeculectomy. *Ophthalmology.* Apr 2000;107(4):712–718.

46. Moss SE, Klein R, Klein BE. Prevalence of and risk factors for dry eye syndrome. *Arch Ophthalmol.* Sept 2000;118(9):1264–1268.

47. Puell MC, Benitez-del-Castillo JM, Martinez-de-la-Casa J, et al. Contrast sensitivity and disability glare in patients with dry eye. *Acta Ophthalmol Scand.* Aug 2006;84(4):527–531.

48. Goto E, Yagi Y, Matsumoto Y, Tsubota K. Impaired functional visual acuity of dry eye patients. *Am J Ophthalmol.* Feb 2002;133(2):181–186.

49. Kozobolis VP, Christodoulakis EV, Siganos CS, Pallikaris IG. Hemorrhagic Descemet's membrane detachment as a complication of deep sclerectomy: a case report. *J Glaucoma.* Dec 2001;10(6):497–500.

50. Ravinet E, Tritten JJ, Roy S, et al. Descemet membrane detachment after nonpenetrating filtering surgery. *J Glaucoma.* Jun 2002;11(3):244–252.

51. Law SK, Shih K, Tran DH, Coleman AL, Caprioli J. Long-term outcomes of repeat vs initial trabeculectomy in open-angle glaucoma. *Am J Ophthalmol.* Nov 2009;148(5):685–695 e681.

52. Esquenazi S, Rand W, Velazquez G, Grunstein L. Novel therapeutic approach in the management of band keratopathy using amniotic membrane transplantation with fibrin glue. *Ophthalmic Surg Lasers Imaging.* Sept-Oct 2008;39(5):418–421.

53. Najjar DM, Cohen EJ, Rapuano CJ, Laibson PR. EDTA chelation for calcific band keratopathy: results and long-term follow-up. *Am J Ophthalmol.* Jun 2004;137(6):1056–1064.

18

DYSESTHETIC BLEBS

JASON A. GOLDSMITH

DYSESTHETIC BLEBS

Mild, chronic ocular irritation following trabeculectomy is common and can manifest as a constant annoyance of bleb awareness with blinking[1,2]; however severe debilitating discomfort can also occur. Bleb-related dysesthesia is an ocular surface disorder where a glaucoma filtering bleb interferes with lid function and tear film distribution such that signs and symptoms similar to dry eye syndrome may result.[3,4] Proper prevention and management of dysesthetic blebs is crucial for success of a trabeculectomy.

REPORTING OF BLEB-RELATED DYSESTHESIA

Utilizing a self-report questionnaire, Budenz et al found that chronic ocular discomfort exists in a majority of patients with filtering blebs[2]; however, many patients do not disclose mild bleb dysesthesia unless specifically questioned because they have either adapted to the symptoms or because of ascertainment bias. Additionally, the symptoms associated with bleb dysesthesia may be attributed to other common ocular surface disorders. Treatment directed at those disorders may effectively relieve symptoms of dysesthesia, so that the physician underestimates prevalence of the true etiology.

ETIOLOGY OF BLEB-RELATED DYSESTHESIA

More symptomatic and disabling forms of bleb-related dysesthesia are generally associated with larger, dysmorphic blebs, including 1) markedly elevated, anteriorly located (Figure 18.1), and thin-walled, ischemic blebs limited in their lateral and posterior flow by circumferential conjunctival scarring ("ring of steel")[5,6]; 2) large and exuberant filtering blebs that extend into the interpalpebral fissure[2,4]

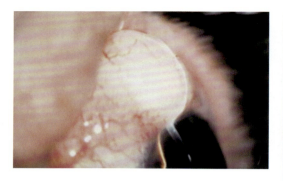

FIGURE 18.1 Markedly elevated and anterior located dysesthetic bleb. Reprinted with permission of Elsevier from Budenz DL, Hoffman K, Zacchei A. Glaucoma filtering bleb dysesthesia. *Am J Ophthalmol.* 2001; 131(5): 626–630.

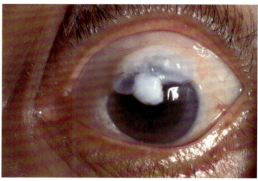

FIGURE 18.3 Dysesthetic bleb with corneal overhang. Photo courtesy of James Gilman, Ophthalmic Photographer, Moran Eye Center, University of Utah.

(Figure 18.2) and occasionally circumferentially[1]; and 3) blebs that overhang the cornea (Figure 18.3)[7,8]. These bleb dysmorphologies typically develop slowly over time as the result of scarring and tissue remodeling. Blebs that extend into the interpalpebral fissure generally occur in the early postoperative period and may or may not be related to overfiltration. Other factors that contribute to bleb-related dysesthesia include chronic irritation of the palpebral conjunctiva and exposure of the bulbar

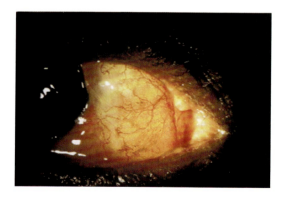

FIGURE 18.2 Large and exuberant dysesthetic bleb extending into interpalpebral space. Reprinted with permission of Lippincott Williams & Wilkins from El-Harazi SM, Fellman RL, Feldman RM, Dang YN, Chuang AZ. Bleb window cryopexy for the management of oversized, misplaced bleb. *J Glaucoma.* 2001;10(1):47–50.

conjunctiva protruding between the eyelids and rubbing on the lid margins.[4] Breakdown of the epithelium on the surface of ischemic blebs may result from altered tear film composition as aqueous passes across the bleb.

The formation of a semicircular wall of scar tissue limiting posterior flow may result in a high, dysesthetic bleb due to inflation, expansion, and thinning of the roof of the bleb. Although frequently associated with antimetabolite exposure because of the ischemic effect on the conjunctiva, dysesthetic blebs can also occur following trabeculectomy without antifibrotics because of a circumferential wall of scar tissue.[8,9] Various factors may contribute to this flow-restricting fibrosis, including 1) a limbus-based conjunctival incision placed too anteriorly; 2) insufficient sub-Tenon's surgical dissection posterior and lateral to the scleral flap; and 3) inadequate modulation of aqueous outflow in the early postoperative period.

"Ring of Steel" blebs

Dense subconjunctival scar tissue around a bleb ("ring of steel")[5] (Figure 18.4) may limit posterior and posterolateral flow,[6,10] causing the bleb to remain anterior and highly elevated. Ongoing localized barotrauma may contribute to progressive bleb thinning and elevation with resultant structural weakness and fatigue of the bleb wall.[11] These blebs may behave much like a balloon that has lost

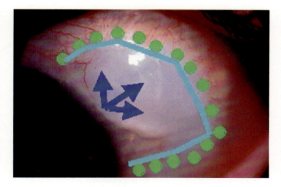

Large blebs extending into the interpalpebral fissure

While diffuse flow appears desirable, an extensive area of flow early during the postoperative period may extend into the interpalpebral space,[12] increasing the risk for dysesthesia. However, perilimbal extension usually resolves when fibrosis develops at any combination of the scleral flap, the sub-Tenon's space, or the bleb wall itself. Additionally, the bleb may decrease in size due to an increase in aqueous absorption through Tenon's layer and into conjunctival veins. On the other hand, tissue remodeling in the late postoperative period can result in bleb enlargement.[13–16] Long-term posterior flow may create chronic stress on the bleb wall and loss of tensile strength, finally resulting in lateral bleb extension (Figure 18.5). Such bleb changes can occur even if the bleb initially had an ideal morphology.

FIGURE 18.4 Ring of steel. Reprinted with permission of Lippincott Williams & Wilkins from Jones E, Clarke J, Khaw PT. Recent advances in trabeculectomy technique. *Curr Opin Ophthalmol.* 2005;16(2):107–113.

elasticity from material fatigue; they becomes easier to inflate over time. Avascularity, especially after treatment with antifibrotic agents, may limit bleb wall repair mechanisms, further reducing bleb wall tensile strength. These blebs are often described as localized and cystic, with thin external walls that ooze aqueous.

Overhanging Blebs

Another type of dysesthetic bleb is the overhanging bleb, which may develop as a result

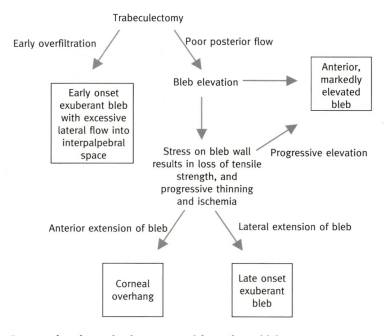

FIGURE 18.5 Proposed pathway for formation of dysesthetic blebs.

of downward bleb massage over the cornea with each eyelid blink.[17] Alternatively, posterior bleb wall fibrosis may result in fluid being directed anteriorly into the corneal stroma in a manner that causes the conjunctiva to overhang from the excessive weight of the bleb (Figure 18.5).[18]

RISK FACTORS FOR BLEB-RELATED DYSESTHESIA

Budenz et al found that some clinical factors were significantly associated with bleb dysesthesia: superonasal bleb location, poor lid coverage of the bleb (with the bleb extending into the interpalpebral space), bubbles in the tear film (which correlated with bleb angle and height), and younger age. Surgical approach, comparing fornix- and limbus-based techniques, and choice of antifibrotic agent were not related to the degree of bleb dysesthesia.[2]

Dellen formation and epithelial defects are also likely associated with highly elevated blebs and may result in discomfort. Dellen have been reported to occur in as frequently as 9% of trabeculectomy cases (9 of 97 cases).[19] Dellen likely result secondary to corneal drying anterior to the bleb, which results from abnormal wetting in a mechanism similar to the discomfort of dysesthesia. In extreme cases corneal ulceration may result.[19]

Bleb-related dysesthesia being more frequent in younger patients[2] suggests that despite the symptoms being similar to those experienced with dry eye, the etiology is not necessarily an exacerbation of an underlying tendency for dry eye. Although younger patients appear to be more predisposed to bleb-related dysesthesia, it may be that younger patients have a lower tolerance for discomfort because many older patients may be already accustomed to dry eye symptoms and do not report potential bleb-related discomfort as being unusual. Furthermore, many older patients with underlying dry eye syndrome are already being managed with topical lubrication. Additionally, older patients may be less likely to tell their physicians about pain,[20] resulting in underreporting of bleb-related dysesthesia.

PREVENTION OF BLEB-RELATED DYSESTHESIA

Anecdotal experience would suggest that patients with low profile blebs that are diffuse and appear normally vascularized are less likely to suffer from dysesthesia symptoms. Trabeculectomy techniques that result in low, diffuse, and normally vascularized blebs have been advocated (see Figure 18.6).[5,10,21,22] Central to this approach is (1) the use of fornix-based flaps to avoid the circumferential scarring that may be associated with the use of limbus-based flaps[5,10]; (2) the use of wide posterior and posterolateral sub-Tenon's dissection[5];

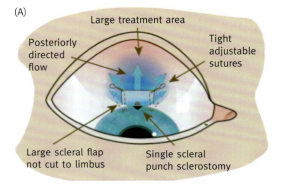

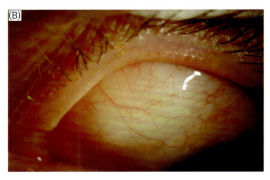

FIGURE 18.6 A) Features of trabeculectomy with a fornix-based flap, adjustable sutures, and posterior aqueous flow. Reprinted with permission of Lippincott Williams & Wilkins from Jones E, Clarke J, Khaw PT. Recent advances in trabeculectomy technique. *Curr Opin Ophthalmol* 2005;16(2):107–113. B) A healthy-appearing, well-vascularized bleb with good posterior and posterolateral flow situated in the superonasal quadrant without causing dysesthesia.

(3) the diffuse application of mitomycin-C[5,11,23]; (4) avoidance of antifibrotic agent contact with the incised conjunctival edges[5]; (5) design of the scleral flap to promote posterior flow[10]; (6) titration of tension on the scleral flap sutures in order to both avoid immediate postoperative hypotony[5] and to direct flow posteriorly[10]; (7) and finally, careful closure of the conjunctiva at the limbus in order to avoid leakage and thus promote diffuse bleb formation.[5]

Efforts should be undertaken intraoperatively and in the early postoperative period to direct aqueous flow posteriorly to prevent formation of the early exuberant bleb that extends perilimbally into the interpalpebral space. During surgery, the lateral scleral flap sutures should be tighter than the posterior sutures. Erring on the side of underfiltration for the first postoperative weeks (tighter sutures), followed by titrated suture release, may avoid early overfiltration and subsequent development of exuberant and dysesthetic blebs.

A higher rate of dysesthesia occurs with blebs located in the superonasal quadrant. Saunders et al found that 25% of 60 patients (5 patients) with superonasal blebs experienced discomfort, compared with 10% (2 patients) in superotemporal cases, and 0% (0 patients) in superior cases.[24] For this reason the superonasal location for trabeculectomy should probably be avoided, especially for initial surgery.

Budenz et al also found an association between dysesthesia and diffuse, but not necessarily highly elevated, blebs that extended into the interpalpebral space.[2] Exuberant blebs extending into the interpalpebral space may impair efficient blinking and disrupt the tear film layer similar to what occurs with markedly elevated blebs. These results would suggest that ptosis repair in patients with filtering blebs might cause or exacerbate dysesthesia; therefore, any surgical raising of the eyelid should not be too aggressive (see Chapter 25).

Highly localized antimetabolite application may enhance the likelihood of developing dysfunctional and dysesthetic blebs that expand in height and progressively become too thin. To prevent posterior limiting scars,

the conjunctival incision for a limbus-based technique should be far posterior with widespread antifibrotic application so that the conjunctival Tenon's incision does not adhere to sclera.

TREATMENT OF BLEB-RELATED DYSESTHESIA

There is generally a correlation between degree of bleb dysmorphia and severity of clinical symptoms. The most important component of managing bleb-associated dysesthesia is using surgical techniques aimed at preventing it. However, some patients report dysesthesia despite "ideal" bleb morphologies.[5]

A treatment approach to bleb-related dysesthesia is multifactorial and based on (1) the type of dysesthetic bleb, as summarized in Table 18.1; (2) the bleb morphology with respect to the likelihood of long-term function and risk for leakage/infection; (3) the underlying etiology of the dysesthetic bleb; (4) the target IOP; and (5) the overall clinical picture.

Conservative Approaches

If the IOP is well-controlled without significant bleb dysmorphology and not at high risk for infection, then surgery should be avoided. A conservative approach aimed at lubrication of the ocular surface should be adequate. As blebs remodel, most will become smaller and less symptomatic with conservative management,[25] especially if the bleb is relatively young and exuberant (as opposed to the longstanding ischemic/thin-walled variety). If a large and exuberant bleb forms in the early postoperative period, reduction or discontinuation of topical antiinflammatory agents should be considered to permit a degree of scarring.

The conservative approach includes aggressive lubrication with artificial tears and nighttime ointment. Punctal plugs may also be of benefit. Aqueous suppressants can be successful in lowering bleb height,[13,26] However, caution is advised in aqueous suppression due to the increased risk of failure of filtration.[27] Topical nonsteroidal antiinflammatory

Table 18.1 Types of Dysesthetic Blebs

DYSESTHETIC BLEB TYPE	MORPHOLOGY	ETIOLOGY
Markedly Elevated	Anteriorly located and elevated; often thin and ischemic	Circumferential scarring limits posterior flow, leading to bleb elevation; ongoing barotrauma results in progressive thinning, loss of tensile strength, and progressive elevation of bleb
Exuberant—Early Onset	Lateral extension of bleb, often into interpalpebral space or circumferentially	Overfiltration secondary to insufficient resistance at the scleral flap relative to the tensile strength of the bleb
Exuberant—Late Onset	Lateral extension of bleb, often into interpalpebral space or circumferentially	Extension of bleb secondary to loss of tensile strength of bleb wall
Overhanging Bleb	Bleb overhangs cornea, typically thin and ischemic	Extension of bleb secondary to loss of tensile strength of bleb wall; upper lid may massage bleb downwards

medications may alleviate discomfort,[2] but also may slow bleb remodeling.

Tear film bubbles are likely the result of poor lid approximation to the globe at the site of distorted blebs (see Figure 18.7). These large bubbles are associated with high blebs[2] and likely a direct cause of discomfort. Symptoms are generally intermittent and may occur with

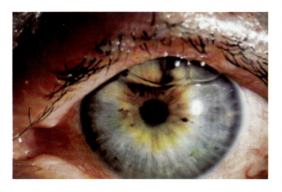

FIGURE 18.7 Bubble formation secondary to blinking over an elevated and dysesthetic bleb. Reprinted with permission of Elsevier from Budenz DL, Hoffman K, Zacchei A, Glaucoma filtering bleb dysesthesia. *Am J Ophthalmol.* 2001;131(5):626–630.

a popping sound from bubble bursting (hence the name bubble dysesthesia).[28] Bubble bursting may also cause temporary visual fluctuation. Artificial tears can be effective in reducing bubble formation.[29]

If conservative measures are inadequate or fail to resolve significant dysesthesia, then surgical intervention should be considered. One clinical factor that may indicate early intervention is dysesthesia combined with bleb dysfunction. For example, a dysesthetic bleb with a history of intermittent leakage would require an early definitive intervention. The presence of recalcitrant dellen, a risk factor for ulceration, also would favor surgical intervention. Patient reliability, compliance, and ready access to emergent, expert care may also factor in deciding upon a conservative versus interventional approach. Other aspects that may influence this decision include the stage of glaucoma and the status of the fellow eye.

Intermediate Approaches

Intermediate-risk procedures for the treatment of the elevated or exuberant dysesthetic bleb include strategies that bring episcleral and conjunctival/Tenon's tissues into apposition such that they partially fuse. Numerous procedures have been described that compress the bleb or induce inflammation and fibrosis, either within the bleb, on its surface, or both. If successful, the desired effect would lower the height of the elevated dysesthetic bleb or reduce the degree of circumferential bleb extension. The risk, however, is that the resultant increase in outflow resistance could reduce flow and increase IOP in the long-term. In the case of the dysesthetic bleb with concurrent overfiltration, this strategy makes sense, as the primary goal would be to increase resistance to outflow.

Bleb Compression. Bleb compression can be attempted with application of a large diameter bandage contact lens or a Simmons shell.[10,13] A compression patch alone or in combination with aqueous suppression can also be attempted.[13] Another strategy is to directly flatten the bleb by placing compression sutures.[30] The sutures may cause epiphora and discomfort but will eventually erode into the bleb.[31] The exuberant/circumferential bleb can be segmentally walled-off where needed with radial compression sutures. The goal is to induce adhesion of the conjunctival and Tenon's tissues to the underlying sclera at these positions and thus limit bleb size to a position underneath the upper eyelid. However, the success of this approach is controversial.

Autologous blood injection. Autologous blood injection can be used to induce fibrosis of the bleb,[9] but may create complications including hyphema,[32–37] IOP spikes,[32,37,38] bleb failure, corneal graft rejection, and corneal blood-staining.[32,37] (For more information on autologous blood injection, see Chapters 10 and 22.)

Trichloroacetic acid. Topical trichloroacetic acid has been applied to induce inflammation and scarring of large and symptomatic blebs,[10,39] but the results have generally been disappointing.[13]

Cryotherapy. Cryotherapy has also been to treat large overfiltering blebs.[40] A cryoprobe is applied directly to the bleb (but away from the scleral flap) in order to create a full thickness freeze and thus induce scarring down of exuberant filtering blebs. Although it has been used for many years, success is limited.[40–42]

Bleb window cryopexy. Bleb window cryopexy, a variation on the use of cryopexy for the treatment of oversized, misplaced dysesthetic blebs, has been reported.[43] In this technique, a 3 x 3 mm conjunctival window incision is made where the dysesthetic bleb needs to be lowered in a position located away from the scleral flap. Light cryopexy is then applied through the window directly to the sclera, followed by placement of a bandage contact lens until the edges of the conjunctival window are scarred-down to the sclera. All 9 patients in the reported study had successful outcomes and symptomatic relief with lowering of the bleb.[43] A more recent publication by the same group omitted the cryotherapy and applied tissue glue with similar results (*"bleb window"-pexy*).[44]

Laser. Laser approaches to the treatment of overfiltering, dysesthetic blebs also employ the strategy of inducing inflammation and scarring. Argon,[40,45,46] Nd:YAG,[40,47] THC:YAG (Holmium),[48] and Krypton green[49] lasers have all been used to remodel large blebs with mixed results.[7,31,40] The main concern is that even though short-term results may demonstrate shrinkage of the bleb surface (argon laser[40]), or internal bleb scarring with thermal spread to the surface (Nd:YAG laser[40] [Figure 18.8])—resulting in short-term positive

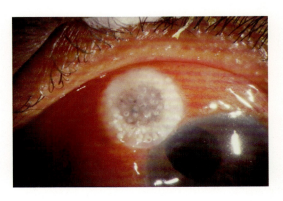

FIGURE 18.8   Treatment of overfiltering bleb with Nd:YAG laser. Photo courtesy of Mary Lynch, MD. Photography by James Gilman, Ophthalmic Photographer, Moran Eye Center, University of Utah.

effects—long-term, continued barotrauma may further thin the ischemic bleb wall with recurrent bleb dysmorphology and dysesthetic symptoms.[40] Holes and leaks are common complications of these laser procedures.

Needle revision. Needle revision of a dysesthetic bleb has also been described,[27] in which lysis of subconjunctival adhesions can be attempted in an effort to create a wider bleb that is lower in height. If the "ring of steel" is not too dense, an entrance can be made through healthy conjunctiva posterior to the fibrotic conjunctiva. A tunnel is then created through the fibrotic wall, disassembling the scar tissue as much as possible with the sharp side of the needle tip prior to entering the ischemic bleb. Once in the bleb, transconjunctival septae can be lysed. Entering from a posterior position should promote posterior flow (see Chapter 28).

Surgical Approaches

The surgical management of elevated and ischemic blebs with poor posterior flow secondary to a "ring of steel" can be challenging. Most literature that addresses the thin, ischemic bleb does so in the context of the leaking bleb. If the bleb is not leaking, but nevertheless thin, elevated, and dysesthetic, then the main goal has to be lowering of the bleb while maintaining good IOP control. Every effort should be made to establish a posterior flow pattern in order to prevent reformation of the thin and elevated perilimbal dysesthetic bleb.

Bleb excision is a technique commonly used. An advantage is that it allows exploration of the underlying scleral flap to address the etiology of the bleb dysmorphology and/or dysfunction. The surgeon can repair any potential defects, attempt to redirect flow posteriorly, and then advance healthy conjunctiva hopefully resulting in a bleb with better morphology.

However, the surgeon doesn't know *a priori* what will be discovered. Removal of long-standing thin, ischemic blebs may expose an underlying scleral flap that is so friable it is impossible to suture or one that has melted, exposing underlying uveal tissue. To repair exposed uveal tissue, a patch graft may be employed. The graft should be tightly secured to the anterior and lateral borders of host tissue with 10–0 nylon, leaving open the posterior border for aqueous flow.[50] Alternatively, all 4 edges can be closed, thus impeding outflow and requiring later suture lysis or possibly a later tube shunt. Placement of a first-stage tube shunt (plate) at this time may be useful if a future tube is likely to be needed. To cover the sclera, healthy posterior conjunctiva must be freed from the wall of circumferential fibrosis and advanced anteriorly to the limbus. My preferred closure is with 10–0 or 9–0 polyglactin 910 (Vicryl™, Ethicon, Inc., Somerville, New Jersey) on a vascular needle using a running horizontal mattress suturing technique. If the sutured conjunctiva/Tenon's layer is too tight to advance to the limbus, then a posterior conjunctival relaxing incision can be made. Alternatively, if inadequate superior conjunctiva is available for advancement, then a free conjunctival autograft[44,51] or rotational graft can be considered.

To lower the risk of postoperative hypotony when performing this repair, the surgeon may elect to only de-epithelialize the conjunctiva[52] and leave the deeper layers intact. A combination of alcohol and light cautery may be effective and also contract the bleb. A conjunctival flap can then be advanced anteriorly, which would not only replace thin ischemic conjunctiva with healthier tissue but also compress the elevated, dysesthetic bleb. Disadvantages of this approach include 1) the compression strategy might be ineffective, and the bleb would remain elevated with unresolved dysesthesia; 2) temporary flattening of the bleb and resolution of dysesthesia might be followed by recurrent thinning and elevation with a return of dysesthesia; and 3) long-term elevation of IOP with need to restart medications and potential loss of disease control. Furthermore, by performing a conjunctival advancement over an intact bleb, the surgeon would not be able to take advantage of the opportunity to perform a surgical exploration to repair any underlying problems and to redirect flow posteriorly. Precious conjunctiva that might be needed for a later surgery might also be depleted.

An entirely different approach to the thin, elevated, and dysesthetic (but not leaking nor hypotonous) bleb is to simply leave it alone and perform another trabeculectomy.[53,54] This approach may be easier and more successful than a large reconstruction of the ischemic bleb, as described above, and may provide greater assurance of postoperative pressure control. By redirecting flow to the new bleb, and thus lowering the pressure head in the ischemic dysesthetic bleb, the ischemic bleb will often decrease in size and height, alleviating the symptoms of dysesthesia.

The key to this approach is to direct the aqueous posteriorly and to be sure that there is no connection with the dysesthetic bleb. Placement of a tube shunt can also be effective in directing flow away from the ischemic bleb to allow bleb remodeling.

Overhanging bleb approaches

Although an overhanging bleb may be thin and ischemic, it is distinctly different and requires a different approach. The overhanging bleb is rarely amenable to conservative treatment options. It may be part of a larger bleb that has a functional component overlying the sclera. In this case, the portion that overhangs the cornea can be simply excised after blunt dissection from Bowman's membrane, with the remaining portion of the bleb that overlies the sclera left in place. Blebs dissecting anteriorly to Bowman's membrane (rather than dissecting into the cornea stroma) can be lifted off by blunt dissection and simply cut off. Mild leakage is expected and will resolve within a few days. Suture closure is rarely required. Overhanging blebs generally require no dissection to free them off the cornea and can also be simply excised with little risk of significant leakage as long as the main loculations of the bleb are not violated.[7,8,17]

The overfiltering and exuberant blebs that extend circumferentially into the interpalpebral fissure that do not resolve with conservative measures are amenable to bleb window cryopexy[43] or "bleb window"-pexy [44] as described above. If this is unsuccessful, then additional flap sutures may be indicated.

Loss of scleral flap integrity is unlikely to have occurred in the early postoperative period. More chronic, exuberant, and significantly dysesthetic blebs with good IOP control may require a surgical procedure aimed at limiting lateral flow. Again, a simple procedure such as bleb window cryopexy or "bleb window"-pexy is useful but others have been more aggressive. Rahman and Thaller describe the use of *bleb-limiting conjunctivoplasty*.[55] Radial incisions are made on either side of the trabeculectomy flap outside the main loculation of the bleb, down to sclera, limiting the bleb to the superior quadrant. Lloyd et all hypothesized that patients with exuberant blebs should also have subconjunctival scar tissue removed from the interpalpebral region[4] because this fibrotic connective tissue impairs adhesion of the conjunctiva to the underlying sclera, and its continued presence allows for accumulation of fluid in the interpalpebral space.

CONCLUSION

Despite good intraoperative and postoperative techniques, dysfunctional and dysesthetic blebs cannot be completely avoided. Despite the risk, many forms of dysesthetic and dysfunctional blebs require more aggressive and definitive surgical intervention in order to increase the likelihood of good long-term function along with minimal dysesthesia. Effective surgical techniques have been developed for the exuberant and corneal overhanging dysesthetic bleb types. Thin and ischemic dysesthetic blebs, however, continue to pose surgical challenges that are nevertheless surmountable with good preoperative planning and flexible intraoperative execution. Nonetheless, the etiology of dysesthetic blebs highlights the relationships between surgical techniques, modulation of the healing response, titration of aqueous outflow, and filtering surgery outcome. With modification of techniques to promote posterior flow, dysesthetic blebs and many other bleb-related complications may be largely avoidable.

Dr. Goldsmith was supported by an Unrestricted Grant from Research to Prevent Blindness to the University of Utah.

COMMENTARY
NICHOLAS P. BELL

Dr. Goldsmith's comprehensive and thorough review of the mechanisms and treatment options for various types of bleb dysmorphologies and dysesthesia is excellent. As he pointed out, this is probably under-recognized because patients may not report the symptoms to their surgeons unless specifically questioned. No physician wishes to place a patient in a position of chronic discomfort, especially following an ocular procedure we hope will produce effects lasting the remainder of the patient's life. Therefore, Dr. Goldsmith's recommendations for how to modify trabeculectomy technique to minimize the development of dysmorphological blebs should be seen as the central point of his review.

Unfortunately, all glaucoma surgeons have patients with overhanging blebs, blebs which extend into the interpalpebral fissure, and highly elevated, ischemic blebs. Not all of the patients are symptomatic, but when a complaint of burning, dryness, "popping," or epiphora is made, my first line of therapy is to lubricate with the more viscous, gel-based artificial tears. Often, the symptoms are improved but not completely alleviated.

In the event of continued discomfort, my patients have found relief from the "bleb window"-pexy (BWP) procedure that Dr. Goldsmith referenced.[44] By excising affected interpalpebral conjunctiva and Tenon's capsule, the offending portion of the bleb is eliminated. Fibrin tissue glue is applied to adhere the cut edges to the underlying sclera in a watertight seal. In my experience, the bleb has not grown back, and IOP remains controlled. This procedure can be performed under topical anesthesia in a minor procedure room or in the operating room.

One approach I have taken inadvertently was to treat one patient with a bleb that dissected into the corneal stroma superiorly (not to be confused with an overhanging, "beer-belly" bleb that has flopped over the cornea) by making a corneal paracentesis wound into the bleb when performing cataract extraction (through a temporal phacoemulsification wound). The bleb decompressed and never recurred.

Dr. Bell was supported by a Challenge Grant from Research to Prevent Blindness to The University of Texas Medical School at Houston and the Hermann Eye Fund.

COMMENTARY
CYNTHIA MATTOX

Dr. Goldsmith has provided a thorough and extensive description of the causes and treatment of dysesthetic filtration blebs. Blebs evolve through various stages in the early postoperative period, and many times a patient who has early complaints about the sensation of the bleb will develop tolerance to them as the weeks go on. Most likely, besides the tear film alterations, the patient's eyelid needs to adapt to the sensation of the new bleb structure on the surface of the eye. This simple explanation to the patient helps them understand the nature of their discomfort and encourages patience in allowing the adaption to occur.

Underlying ocular surface disease, dry eye, and meibomian gland dysfunction should all be treated vigorously, and treatments may succeed in reducing symptoms. Besides topical lubrication with drops and ointments, systemic omega-3 supplementation and topical cyclosporine drops may be useful.

One other clinical finding may explain why some patients are symptomatic from their blebs that extend into the interpalpebral space and others are not: look carefully for subtle "draping" of the conjunctiva onto the lower lid margin. In my experience these patients are more symptomatic, because with each blink, the small amount of conjunctiva is compressed between the lid margins, causing discomfort. In such cases, tightening or "tacking down" the interpalpebral conjunctiva to the underlying sclera with a nonabsorbable suture has, in my experience, been very successful.

Ultimately, clinically relevant bleb dysesthesia almost always occurs in eyes in which the surgeon is pleased with the IOP control, but the patient is dissatisfied with the comfort level of the eye. The risks and benefits of additional surgical maneuvers to correct bleb dysesthesia must be fully discussed with the patient, because the most devastating consequence to the surgeon and patient is the loss of IOP control that had been attained by the original surgery.

REFERENCES

1. Anis S, Ritch R, Shihadeh W, Liebmann J. Surgical reduction of symptomatic, circumferential, filtering blebs. *Arch Ophthalmol.* Jun 2006;124(6):890–894.
2. Budenz DL, Hoffman K, Zacchei A. Glaucoma filtering bleb dysesthesia. *Am J Ophthalmol.* May 2001;131(5):626–630.
3. Palmberg P. Surgery for complications. In: Albert D, ed. *Ophthalmic Surgery: Principles and Techniques.* Vol 1. Malden, MA: Blackwell Science; 1999:476–491.
4. Lloyd M, Giegengack M, Morrison JC. Surgical reduction of dysesthetic blebs. *Arch Ophthalmol.* Dec 2008;126(12):1759–1764.
5. Jones E, Clarke J, Khaw PT. Recent advances in trabeculectomy technique. *Curr Opin Ophthalmol.* Apr 2005;16(2):107–113.
6. Wells AP, Cordeiro MF, Bunce C, Khaw PT. Cystic bleb formation and related complications in limbus- versus fornix-based conjunctival flaps in pediatric and young adult trabeculectomy with mitomycin C. *Ophthalmology.* Nov 2003;110(11):2192–2197.
7. Anis S, Ritch R, Shihadeh W, Liebmann J. Sutureless revision of overhanging filtering blebs. *Arch Ophthalmol.* Sept 2006;124(9):1317–1320.
8. Lanzl IM, Katz LJ, Shindler RL, Spaeth GL. Surgical management of the symptomatic overhanging filtering bleb. *J Glaucoma.* Aug 1999;8(4):247–249.
9. Morgan JE, Diamond JP, Cook SD. Remodelling the filtration bleb. *Br J Ophthalmol.* Aug 2002; 86(8):872–875.
10. Barton K. Bleb dysesthesia. *J Glaucoma.* Jun 2003;12(3):281–284.
11. Cordeiro MF, Constable PH, Alexander RA, Bhattacharya SS, Khaw PT. Effect of varying the mitomycin-C treatment area in glaucoma filtration surgery in the rabbit. *Invest Ophthalmol Vis Sci.* Jul 1997;38(8): 1639–1646.
12. Popovic V. Early hypotony after trabeculectomy. *Acta Ophthalmol Scand.* Jun 1995; 73(3):255–260.
13. Lynch MG, Brown RH. Treatment of excessive or overfiltering blebs. In: Spaeth GL, ed. *Ophthalmic Surgery: Principles and Practice.* 3rd ed. Philadelphia: Saunders; 2003:389–397.
14. Costa VP, Wilson RP, Moster MR, Schmidt CM, Gandham S. Hypotony maculopathy following the use of topical mitomycin C in glaucoma filtration surgery. *Ophthalmic Surg.* Jun 1993;24(6):389–394.
15. Stamper RL, McMenemy MG, Lieberman MF. Hypotonous maculopathy after trabeculectomy with subconjunctival 5-fluorouracil. *Am J Ophthalmol.* Nov 15 1992;114(5):544–553.
16. Zacharia PT, Deppermann SR, Schuman JS. Ocular hypotony after trabeculectomy with mitomycin C. *Am J Ophthalmol.* Sept 15 1993;116(3):314–326.
17. Scheie HG, Guehl JJ 3rd. Surgical management of overhanging blebs after filtering procedures. *Arch Ophthalmol.* Feb 1979;97(2):325–326.
18. Ulrich GG, Proia AD, Shields MB. Clinicopathologic features and surgical management of dissecting glaucoma filtering blebs. *Ophthalmic Surg Lasers.* Feb 1997;28(2):151–155.
19. Soong HK, Quigley HA. Dellen associated with filtering blebs. *Arch Ophthalmol.* Mar 1983;101(3):385–387.
20. Gagliese L. Pain and aging: the emergence of a new subfield of pain research. *J Pain.* Apr 2009;10(4):343–353.
21. Jin GJ, Crandall AS, Jones JJ. Phacotrabeculectomy: assessment of outcomes and surgical improvements. *J Cataract Refract Surg.* Jul 2007;33(7):1201–1208.
22. Siriwardena D, Khaw PT, King AJ, et al. Human antitransforming growth factor beta(2) monoclonal antibody—a new modulator of wound healing in trabeculectomy: a randomized placebo controlled clinical study. *Ophthalmology.* Mar 2002;109(3):427–431.
23. Onol M, Aktas Z, Hasanreisoglu B. Enhancement of the success rate in trabeculectomy: large-area mitomycin-C application. *Clin Experiment Ophthalmol.* May 2008;36(4):316–322.
24. Sanders R, MacEwen CJ, Haining WM. Trabeculectomy: effect of varying surgical site. *Eye (Lond).* 1993;7 (Pt 3):440–443.

25. La Borwit SE, Quigley HA, Jampel HD. Bleb reduction and bleb repair after trabeculectomy. *Ophthalmology.* Apr 2000;107(4):712–718.

26. Scott DR, Quigley HA. Medical management of a high bleb phase after trabeculectomies. *Ophthalmology.* Sept 1988;95(9):1169–1173.

27. Feldman RM, Tabet RR. Needle revision of filtering blebs. *J Glaucoma.* Oct-Nov 2008;17(7):594–600.

28. Grajewski A, Hodapp E, Huang A. Bubble dysesthesia. Poster presented at: American Glaucoma Society 5th Annual Meeting; February 2–4, 1995: Key West, FL.

29. Di Pascuale MA, Elizondo A, Gao YY, Raju VK, Tseng SC. Gigantic waves in the tear film generated by bubbles from a large glaucoma bleb. *Arch Ophthalmol.* Apr 2007;125(4):573–574.

30. Palmberg P, Zacchei AC. A new treatment for leaking or painful filtering blebs [ARVO abstract 2032]. *Invest Ophthalmol Vis Sci.* 1996;37(3):S444.

31. Feldman RM, Altaher G. Management of late-onset bleb leaks. *Curr Opin Ophthalmol.* Apr 2004;15(2):151–154.

32. Burnstein A, WuDunn D, Ishii Y, Jonescu-Cuypers C, Cantor LB. Autologous blood injection for late-onset filtering bleb leak. *Am J Ophthalmol.* Jul 2001;132(1):36–40.

33. Okada K, Tsukamoto H, Masumoto M, et al. Autologous blood injection for marked overfiltration early after trabeculectomy with mitomycin C. *Acta Ophthalmol Scand.* Jun 2001;79(3):305–308.

34. Hyung SM, Choi MY, Kang SW. Management of chronic hypotony following trabeculectomy with mitomycin C. *Korean J Ophthalmol.* Jun 1997;11(1):15–24.

35. Leen MM, Moster MR, Katz LJ, Terebuh AK, Schmidt CM, Spaeth GL. Management of overfiltering and leaking blebs with autologous blood injection. *Arch Ophthalmol.* Aug 1995;113(8):1050–1055.

36. Zaltas MM, Schuman JS. A serious complication of intrableb injection of autologous blood for the treatment of postfiltration hypotony. *Am J Ophthalmol.* Aug 15 1994;118(2):251–253.

37. Ayyala RS, Urban RC, Jr., Krishnamurthy MS, Mendelblatt DJ. Corneal blood staining following autologous blood injection for hypotony maculopathy. *Ophthalmic Surg Lasers.* Oct 1997;28(10):866–868.

38. Nuyts RM, Greve EL, Geijssen HC, Langerhorst CT. Treatment of hypotonous maculopathy after trabeculectomy with mitomycin C. *Am J Ophthalmol.* Sept 15 1994;118(3):322–331.

39. Gehring JR, Ciccarelli EC. Trichloracetic acid treatment of filtering blebs following cataract extraction. *Am J Ophthalmol.* Oct 1972;74(4):622–624.

40. Lynch MG. Surgical repair of leaking filtering blebs. *Ophthalmology.* Sept 2000;107(9):1687.

41. Cleasby GW, Fung WE, Webster RG, Jr. Cryosurgical closure of filtering blebs. *Arch Ophthalmol.* Mar 1972;87(3):319–323.

42. Douvas NG. Cystoid bleb cryotherapy. *Am J Ophthalmol.* Jul 1972;74(1):69–71.

43. El-Harazi SM, Fellman RL, Feldman RM, Dang YN, Chuang AZ. Bleb window cryopexy for the management of oversized, misplaced blebs. *J Glaucoma.* Feb 2001;10(1):47–50.

44. Tabet R, Feldman RM, Bell NP, Lee DA. "Bleb window"-pexy for the management of symptomatic, oversized blebs. *J Glaucoma.* Sept 2009;18(7):546–551.

45. Akova YA, Dursun D, Aydin P, Akbatur H, Duman S. Management of hypotony maculopathy and a large filtering bleb after trabeculectomy with mitomycin C: success with argon laser therapy. *Ophthalmic Surg Lasers.* Nov-Dec 2000;31(6):491–494.

46. Hennis HL, Stewart WC. Use of the argon laser to close filtering bleb leaks. *Graefes Arch Clin Exp Ophthalmol.* 1992;230(6):537–541.

47. Lynch MG, Roesch M, Brown RH. Remodeling filtering blebs with the neodymium:YAG laser. *Ophthalmology.* Oct 1996;103(10):1700–1705.

48. Iwach AG, Delgado ME, Adachi M, Makarewycz M, Wong P, Nguyen N. Filtering bleb modification with a THC:YAG (Holmium) laser. *Ophthalmic Surg Lasers.* May-Jun 2002;33(3):181–187.

49. Welcome BA, Skuta GL, Reynolds AC. Laser bleb reduction for bleb dissection with krypton green laser: technique and outcomes. *J Glaucoma.* Apr 2006;15(2):158–163.

50. Harizman N, Ben-Cnaan R, Goldenfeld M, Levkovitch-Verbin H, Melamed S. Donor scleral patch for treating hypotony due to leaking and/or overfiltering blebs. *J Glaucoma.* Dec 2005;14(6):492–496.

51. Schnyder CC, Shaarawy T, Ravinet E, Achache F, Uffer S, Mermoud A. Free conjunctival autologous graft for bleb repair and bleb reduction after trabeculectomy and nonpenetrating filtering surgery. *J Glaucoma.* Feb 2002;11(1):10–16.

52. Catoira Y, Wudunn D, Cantor LB. Revision of dysfunctional filtering blebs by conjunctival advancement with bleb preservation. *Am J Ophthalmol.* Nov 2000;130(5):574–579.

53. Ophir A, Pikkel J. Mini-trabeculectomy in eyes with high risk of scarring: midterm follow-up. *Am J Ophthalmol.* Jan 2001;131(1):13–18.

54. Thimmarayan SK, Rao VA, Gupta A. Mini-trabeculectomy in comparison to conventional trabeculectomy in primary open angle glaucoma. *Eur J Ophthalmol.* Sept-Oct 2006; 16(5):674–679.

55. Rahman R, Thaller VT. Bleb-limiting conjunctivoplasty for symptomatic circumferential trabeculectomy blebs. *J Glaucoma.* Jun 2003; 12(3):272–274.

19

BLEB-RELATED VISION LOSS

SHAI M. BAR-SELA

BLEB-RELATED VISION LOSS

Trabeculectomy is an effective procedure to control intraocular pressure (IOP) and to prevent progression of vision loss.[1] One of the risks associated with this procedure is oversized and exuberant blebs, which may result in reduction of visual acuity. Understanding the mechanisms and prognosis of this complication is important for evaluating and selecting the proper treatment.

CAUSES AND CONSEQUENCES OF PROGRESSION

Large blebs overhanging the cornea may cause visual acuity loss if they directly obstruct the visual axis, but they can also be problematic due to their effect on lid movements and resultant drying of the cornea.[2] Furthermore, the overhanging, "beer-belly" bleb can also induce corneal dryness as well as irregular astigmatism.

The trabeculectomy surgical technique itself may also affect the development of oversized blebs. Some authors believe that fornix-based conjunctival flaps result in more diffuse and less elevated blebs that are less likely to encroach on the limbus, compared to limbus-based conjunctival flaps.[3] Limbus-based conjunctival flaps are limited by scar formation at the conjunctival wound site, preventing posterior movement of aqueous and forcing bleb elevation toward the limbus. The use of antifibrotics, such as mitomycin-C and 5-fluorouracil, during filtering procedures may predispose to the development of larger ischemic blebs. Thin-walled ischemic blebs may continue to enlarge months to years postoperatively as the bleb wall constantly remodels.

MANAGEMENT

Laser Treatment

Various laser treatments can be used to contract oversized blebs. Fink et al used argon laser photocoagulation to shrink large blebs in 4 eyes; however 2 eyes developed leaks.[4] Sony et al treated 3 eyes with large blebs using frequency-doubled Nd:YAG photocoagulation after painting the area of the blebs with gentian violet to enhance the laser absorption. Several treatment sessions resulted in bleb shrinkage and remodeling.[5] Lynch et al applied a continuous wave multimode Nd:YAG laser in 4 eyes with symptomatic large blebs, 3 of which had undergone previous trabeculectomy with antifibrotic agents. Two eyes required retreatment, and one eye developed a bleb leak afterward.[6] These reports indicate that laser application success has been limited, and bleb leaks may occur.

Surgical Treatment

Oversized blebs can be divided into overhanging blebs, highly elevated blebs, and circumferential exuberant blebs. The particular surgical method should be selected based on the type and location of the bleb. More information about the management of each type is discussed in Chapter 18.

Overhanging Blebs. The overhanging portion of the bleb is generally a high elevated loose tissue that has been massaged over the cornea by the action of the eyelids. Using anterior segment optical coherence tomography, Kim et al demonstrated that the overhanging bleb has a coarse, multiloculated cystic structure.[7] The boundary of the loculations lies at the limbus. Supporting this finding, Ito et al used ultrasound biomicroscopy imaging to show that the overhanging part of the bleb is anatomically separated by a clear border of membrane from the conjunctival filtering part. Moreover, indocyanine green injected into the overhanging part of the bleb did not enter into the conjunctival part of the bleb or the anterior chamber, exemplifying that these 2 portions of the bleb are functionally separate.[8] Therefore, no significant leakage of aqueous

is expected from excision of the overhanging portion of the bleb since there is no exchange of aqueous between the section being removed and the main functional loculation.

Several surgical techniques have been described to treat overhanging blebs. Scheie et al described complete excision of the overhanging part of the bleb in 16 eyes that had undergone earlier trabeculectomy without application of antimetabolites. The procedure consists of blunt dissection of the overhanging part from the cornea, excision of the freed piece parallel to the limbus, and suturing of the cut edges of the conjunctival wound. The postoperative IOP remained at the preoperative level in all patients in the study, except for one who had late endophthalmitis.[2] Similar methodology was successfully applied by Lanzl et al in 4 eyes.[9]

However, filtration blebs after trabeculectomy with administration of antifibrotics are often extremely thin and cystic with friable conjunctiva, limiting the options of suturing the edges of the cut bleb due to the risk of perforations and leaks. Therefore, Anis et al described a sutureless surgery in 6 eyes, using an 18-mm diameter bandage contact lens to enable re-epithelialization of the cut edge of the bleb. The postoperative IOP was controlled in all eyes, but one eye developed persistent leak at the margin of the bleb, necessitating suturing and placement of cyanoacrylate glue.[10] We have found that in most cases simple observation will be adequate to allow leakage from the limbal incision to resolve, but when leakage is excessive at the time of the procedure, light cautery may be beneficial in sealing a leak, with the added benefit of potentially lowering the bleb and, making a smoother surface for improved tear coverage. No bandage lens is required. More recently, fibrin tissue glues, such as TISSEEL (Baxter, Deerfield, Illinois) and Evicel® (Ethicon, Inc., Somerville, New Jersey) have been used. Tissue glue stays in place for a few days, preventing leaks and allowing healing and epithelialization to occur.

In some cases an overhanging bleb may coexist with bleb-induced leakage or overfiltration. This combination of complications is more prevalent if antimetabolites were used during the trabeculectomy.[11-13] Consequently the surgical approach in these cases should include solutions for both problems: bleb dimension reduction for the overhanging part of the bleb and repair of the bleb's function to address the bleb-induced hypotony or leakage.[13] This may be as simple as re-covering the bleb with conjunctiva or may require addressing the hypotony from a melted scleral flap. These types of repairs are discussed in Chapter 21.

Highly Elevated Blebs. When a symptomatic elevated bleb does not coexist with bleb-induced leakage or overfiltration, the goal of bleb revision is to decrease the bleb's size while minimally affecting its function. A variety of nonincisional techniques have been reported, including use of an oversized soft contact lens,[14] Simmons shell,[15] and compression sutures.[16] La Borwit et al described such a technique for bleb reduction involving partial excision of large blebs. In this technique, the wound is covered with a conjunctival flap created posterior to the original and advanced to cover the filtration site. In cases where primary closure is impossible, a conjunctival autograft can be used. This conservative bleb reduction kept the postoperative IOP controlled, but was not effective in 45% of the cases in the study, necessitating further reduction of the bleb.[13]

When bleb leakage or overfiltration coexists with a high superior bleb, a more aggressive solution should be used, including excision of the ischemic portion of the bleb and closure of the wound with advancement of the posterior conjunctiva. If the defect cannot be closed primarily, a conjunctival autograft should be used.[17]

Circumferential Exuberant Blebs. The surgical approach for circumferential exuberant blebs is based on the segmentation of the bleb. Separating the circumferential oversized part of the bleb from the superior filtration site discontinues the flow to the circumferential part and causes the bleb to flatten.

Anis et al described a surgical method for bleb segmentation in 15 eyes. Their technique included incision of the blebs to segments at the 10:30 or 1:30 positions and suturing of the cut edges of the conjunctiva

and Tenon's capsule to the underlying sclera. Bleb reduction was successful in 14 patients, and only one patient had a transient bleb leak, which resolved spontaneously.[10]

In cases of ischemic, thin, and friable conjunctiva, suturing of the edges of the conjunctival wound may result in wound dehiscence or leak. Therefore, El-Harazi et al described a different method that does not involve conjunctival suturing called bleb window cryopexy. The procedure involves an incision of the bleb to create a 3 mm x 3 mm conjunctival window extending to bare sclera. Then light cryotherapy is applied to the sclera through the conjunctival window until the conjunctival edges begin to freeze. All patients in the study had a flattening of the bleb within 2 weeks and adequate IOP control, except for one patient who developed aqueous misdirection one week after the procedure.[18] An alternative version of this technique is to seal the conjunctival wounds with fibrin glue.[19] This glue enables a reliable wound closure with smoothly sealed edges, decreasing postoperative discomfort and allowing for early rehabilitation.

CORNEAL DRYING/DELLEN

One of the mechanisms of late vision loss after trabeculectomy is related to corneal drying in the area at the bleb-cornea interface, particularly if the bleb is elevated. It has been hypothesized that inadequate distribution of the tear film at the corneal border of the bleb during blinking is responsible.[20] Another explanation for bleb-induced corneal dryness is based on the finding that the return of aqueous production to normal levels after a period of postoperative decreased formation may cause bleb cavity expansion and elevation. In turn, the increased tension in the bleb wall decreases aqueous passage through the bleb wall into the tear film with resultant increase in IOP. As the IOP rises, the cycle continues, causing additional stretching of the bleb wall and further decrease in fluid conductivity.[21]

Corneal dryness, no matter the mechanism, may result in punctuate keratopathy or irregular astigmatism. Moreover, localized severe dryness may cause dellen formation in up to 9% of cases. Most dellen clear with lubrication therapy; however, corneal ulcers have been reported.[22] These ulcers typically resolve, leaving a vascularized scar with localized stromal thinning. These scars may result in permanent irregular astigmatism and resultant visual loss.

MANAGEMENT OF THE CORNEA

A variety of conservative measures can be used to treat symptomatic oversized blebs.[11] Topical lubrication, such as frequent use of artificial tear drops with or without ophthalmic ointment at bedtime, should be tried initially. In some cases insertion of punctual plugs may be required. In instances of intractable dellen, a bandage contact lens is an option.[11] Aqueous suppression may also be effective in reducing bleb size, which may improve wetting, particularly in the early postoperative period (but not early enough to allow bleb failure).[21] Generally, blebs will become smaller with medical treatment and resolution of the related symptoms. However, some patients continue suffering from bleb-related vision loss, and a surgical approach may be indicated.[13]

REFRACTIVE CONSIDERATIONS (ASTIGMATISM)

As mentioned previously, inadequate tear film distribution may lead to corneal drying and irregular astigmatism. Mechanical forces applied on the cornea by a large bleb may distort the corneal curvature compared with the preoperative state. Additionally, tight scleral flap sutures may induce astigmatism as well. Cautery used during surgery may also cause tissue contraction. Astigmatic corneal changes following trabeculectomy are typically with-the-rule[23,24] and can be classified into 3 categories: superior corneal steepening, superior corneal flattening, and a third group with complex, irregular patterns.[24] Astigmatism has been demonstrated to return to preoperative levels as soon as 12 weeks after surgery,[25] but can last longer than one year.[26]

If refractive changes persist and remain stable, spectacle correction may be used to improve visual acuity. Contact lenses should be used with caution depending on the size and shape of the bleb. Rigid gas permeable lenses might mechanically irritate and erode into the bleb at the limbus but can be fit tight to prevent rubbing against the bleb. The diameter of soft contact lenses is typically wider than that of the cornea, resulting in a poor fit if the bleb is elevated. Corneal refractive surgery with a procedure that does not require use of high pressure suction to create the flap can be considered. For more about refractive considerations, see Chapter 14.

FAILED FILTERING BLEB

The majority of this chapter has focused on visual dysfunction or loss from blebs that are too large. However, one must not forget that a nonfunctioning bleb with elevated IOP may also lead to late postoperative visual loss secondary to glaucomatous progression. Filtering surgery can fail with a flat bleb if the scleral flap scars closed or with a large encapsulated bleb if Tenon's layer becomes impermeable (see Chapter 15 and Chapter 18). In either situation, medical, laser, and incisional options can be utilized to lower the IOP and try to prevent further damage from glaucoma.

CONCLUSION

Trabeculectomy may result in an oversized bleb causing visual loss. This adverse effect is expected to be more common as a result of the widespread use of antimetabolites. Secondary to the development of an enlarged filtering bleb, corneal drying and/or astigmatism may cause transient or persistent visual dysfunction. Furthermore, an overhanging bleb may directly block the visual axis. If the bleb does not remodel with the tincture of time and conservative medical treatment, laser, or incisional surgical intervention may become necessary. The ultimate goal of these procedures is to restore vision to the preoperative state, while protecting from further glaucomatous damage.

COMMENTARY

LOUIS R. PASQUALE

Bleb-Related Vision Loss: Another mechanism to consider

An uncommon form of bleb-related vision loss is the low-lying bleb that is *not* hinged at the limbus, allowing it to slide down the cornea with a fairly low topographical profile. These blebs have an appearance somewhat similar to pterygia. These blebs do not necessarily cause ocular surface drying but, like pterygia, produce visual loss by obstructing the visual axis. The corneal portion of these blebs tends to be Seidel negative. This variant of bleb-related visual loss results from obliteration of corneal limbus stem cells that would normally serve as a barrier to prevent the constantly remodeling bleb from sliding down the cornea. The only real treatment for these blebs is surgical excision. Luckily the corneal portions of these blebs are almost invariably non-functional, and simple excision is often not accompanied by postoperative bleb leaks. There is always the risk of recurrence but the re-growth of these blebs is typically very slow.

These sliding blebs that are unanchored at the surgical limbus can be prevented from developing if one pays attention to how the surgical limbus is managed during the initial trabeculectomy. Exuberant coagulation of the surgical limbus during fornix-based flap trabeculectomy will destroy the corneal limbal stem cells and create a microenvironment that allows these types of blebs to develop. While the use of thermal coagulation is often needed during trabeculectomy surgery, overzealous use of this form of thermal ablation at the surgical limbus is to be avoided. Furthermore, if a trabeculectomy fails, I almost never revise the procedure at the same site. Reoperation at the same site can produce more damage to the corneal limbal stem cells, fostering this sort of unfavorable bleb formation. Rather than repeat surgery at the same site, consider a new site for trabeculectomy or tube shunt implantation.

Dr. Pasquale was supported by the Harvard Glaucoma Center of Excellence.

REFERENCES

1. The Advanced Glaucoma Intervention Study (AGIS): 4. Comparison of treatment outcomes within race. Seven-year results. *Ophthalmology.* Jul 1998;105(7):1146–1164.
2. Scheie HG, Guehl JJ 3rd. Surgical management of overhanging blebs after filtering procedures. *Arch Ophthalmol.* Feb 1979;97(2):325–326.
3. Wells AP, Cordeiro MF, Bunce C, Khaw PT. Cystic bleb formation and related complications in limbus- versus fornix-based conjunctival flaps in pediatric and young adult trabeculectomy with mitomycin C. *Ophthalmology.* Nov 2003; 110(11):2192–2197.
4. Fink AJ, Boys-Smith JW, Brear R. Management of large filtering blebs with the argon laser. *Am J Ophthalmol.* Jun 15 1986;101(6):695–699.
5. Sony P, Kumar H, Pushker N. Treatment of overhanging blebs with frequency-doubled Nd:YAG laser. *Ophthalmic Surg Lasers Imaging.* Sept-Oct 2004;35(5):429–432.
6. Lynch MG, Roesch M, Brown RH. Remodeling filtering blebs with the neodymium: YAG laser. *Ophthalmology.* Oct 1996;103(10): 1700–1705.
7. Kim WK, Seong GJ, Lee CS, Kim YG, Kim CY. Anterior segment optical coherence tomography imaging and histopathologic findings of an overhanging filtering bleb. *Eye (Lond).* Dec 2008;22(12):1520–1521.
8. Ito K, Miura K, Sugimoto K, Matsunaga K, Sasoh M, Uji Y. Use of indocyanine green during excision of an overhanging filtering bleb. *Jpn J Ophthalmol.* Jan-Feb 2007;51(1):57–59.
9. Lanzl IM, Katz LJ, Shindler RL, Spaeth GL. Surgical management of the symptomatic overhanging filtering bleb. *J Glaucoma.* Aug 1999;8(4):247–249.
10. Anis S, Ritch R, Shihadeh W, Liebmann J. Sutureless revision of overhanging filtering blebs. *Arch Ophthalmol.* Sept 2006;124(9): 1317–1320.
11. Allingham RR, Damji KF, Freedman S, Moroi SE, Shafranov G, Shields MB. Filtering Surgery. *Shield's Textbook of Glaucoma.* 5th ed. Philadelphia: Lippincott Williams & Wilkins; 2005: 568–609.
12. Greenfield DS, Budenz DL, Curtin VT. Late visual loss secondary to filtering bleb exuberance. *Arch Ophthalmol.* Jun 1996;114(6): 772–773.

13. La Borwit SE, Quigley HA, Jampel HD. Bleb reduction and bleb repair after trabeculectomy. *Ophthalmology*. Apr 2000;107(4):712–718.
14. Barton K. Bleb dysesthesia. *J Glaucoma*. Jun 2003;12(3):281–284.
15. Lynch MG, Brown RH. Treatment of excessive or overfiltering blebs. In: Spaeth GL, ed. *Ophthalmic Surgery: Principles and Practice*. 3rd ed. Philadelphia: Saunders; 2003:389–397.
16. Palmberg P, Zacchei AC. Compression sutures: a new treatment for leaking or painful filtering blebs [ARVO abstract]. *Invest Ophthalmol Vis Sci*. 1996;37:S444.
17. Harris LD, Yang G, Feldman RM, et al. Autologous conjunctival resurfacing of leaking filtering blebs. *Ophthalmology*. Sept 2000;107(9):1675–1680.
18. El-Harazi SM, Fellman RL, Feldman RM, Dang YN, Chuang AZ. Bleb window cryopexy for the management of oversized, misplaced blebs. *J Glaucoma*. Feb 2001;10(1):47–50.
19. Tabet R, Feldman RM, Bell NP, Lee DA. "Bleb window"-pexy for the management of symptomatic, oversized blebs. *J Glaucoma*. Sept 2009;18(7):546–551.
20. Anis S, Ritch R, Shihadeh W, Liebmann J. Surgical reduction of symptomatic, circumferential, filtering blebs. *Arch Ophthalmol*. Jun 2006;124(6):890–894.
21. Scott DR, Quigley HA. Medical management of a high bleb phase after trabeculectomies. *Ophthalmology*. Sept 1988;95(9):1169–1173.
22. Soong HK, Quigley HA. Dellen associated with filtering blebs. *Arch Ophthalmol*. Mar 1983;101(3):385–387.
23. Egrilmez S, Ates H, Nalcaci S, Andac K, Yagci A. Surgically induced corneal refractive change following glaucoma surgery: nonpenetrating trabecular surgeries versus trabeculectomy. *J Cataract Refract Surg*. Jun 2004;30(6):1232–1239.
24. Claridge KG, Galbraith JK, Karmel V, Bates AK. The effect of trabeculectomy on refraction, keratometry and corneal topography. *Eye (Lond)*. 1995;9(Pt 3):292–298.
25. Dietze PJ, Oram O, Kohnen T, Feldman RM, Koch DD, Gross RL. Visual function following trabeculectomy: effect on corneal topography and contrast sensitivity. *J Glaucoma*. Apr 1997;6(2):99–103.
26. Hayashi K, Hayashi H, Oshika T, Hayashi F. Fourier analysis of irregular astigmatism after trabeculectomy. *Ophthalmic Surg Lasers*. Mar-Apr 2000;31(2):94–99.

20

UVEITIS

MAHMOUD A. KHAIMI

UVEITIS

Delayed-onset postoperative inflammation can result from a diverse range of factors, such as blebitis, bleb-related endophthalmitis, underlying uveitis, mitomycin-C mediated inflammation, herpes infection, phaco-anaphylactic and phacogenic uveitis, intraocular lens (IOL) chafing of the iris, and sympathetic ophthalmia. Delayed postoperative uveitis is defined as inflammation occurring 6 weeks or later postoperatively and is a rare condition that may occur following a glaucoma filtering procedure. Currently, there are very few documented cases of this condition.[1] Even though it is rare, it is important to differentiate the infectious sources of delayed-onset postoperative uveitis after glaucoma filtering surgery from those that are noninfectious so that the appropriate treatment is administered.

LATE-ONSET POSTOPERATIVE UVEITIS: INFECTIOUS CASES (BLEBITIS AND BLEB-RELATED ENDOPHTHALMITIS)

Infectious cases of uveitis should be considered first. The most common form of late-onset postoperative uveitis after a filtering procedure is *blebitis*. Brown and colleagues were the first to use the term "blebitis" to describe a limited infection centered around a bleb with or without anterior chamber reaction and no vitreous involvement.[2] In contrast, on the other end of the spectrum, is *bleb-related endophthalmitis*, which is characterized by a more fulminant course with anterior chamber reaction and the presence of vitritis. Blebitis and bleb-related endophthalmitis typically manifest several months to years after the surgery.[3,4] Blebitis may often be a precursor to bleb-related endophthalmitis,[2,3] and early recognition of late-onset bleb-related infections should be taken seriously and promptly treated to avoid severe ocular and visual sequelae.

Clinical signs

Both forms of bleb-related infection can be differentiated by the extent of ocular inflammation. Patients with blebitis typically complain of redness, foreign body sensation, pain, photophobia, and conjunctival discharge. The conjunctiva around the bleb is also significantly injected. Additionally, the bleb itself usually has a whitish or chalky appearance with or without an epithelial defect. The anterior chamber may have variable degrees of reaction, and a hypopyon may be present in the anterior chamber as well as in the bleb itself.

Conversely, patients with bleb-related endophthalmitis typically present with a more fulminant course, which includes rapidly deteriorating vision, redness, pain, and diffuse conjunctival injection.[3–6] Vitritis, while absent in blebitis, is present in bleb-related endophthalmitis. The bleb is commonly opaque, and its contents are generally turbid in appearance. Additionally, the bleb may have an overlying epithelial defect, and fibrin and hypopyon are usually seen in the anterior chamber.[3–5] Seidel testing for leaks may be positive in both blebitis and bleb-related endophthalmitis.[4]

Treatment for blebitis

Classically, blebitis responds well to intense topical antibiotic treatment, and patients normally have complete recovery of their visual acuity and intraocular pressure.[2–5,7] A survey conducted by Reynolds and Skuta in 2001 among American Glaucoma Society (AGS) members found that management of blebitis was variable. The majority of specialists preferred to examine patients with symptoms of blebitis as soon as possible. Nearly half of the specialists surveyed always obtained conjunctival cultures at the onset of blebitis. Topical fluoroquinolones alone or in combination with one or 2 other antibiotics were the empirical treatment regimen by most physicians. A small percentage of specialists

used a combination of fortified topical agents (fortified aminoglycoside, vancomycin, or cephalosporin) for the treatment of isolated blebitis. Two-thirds of specialists surveyed preferred to use topical corticosteroids along with topical antibiotics. Surgical revision of a persistently leaking bleb was the treatment of choice among 77% of AGS members.[8,9]

Risk factors for bleb-related endophthalmitis

Antifibrotic agents such as mitomycin-C and 5-flurouracil have gained a valuable role as adjunctive antimetabolites in modern day trabeculectomy.[4] Subsequently, the appearance of thin-walled, cystic, avascular blebs has increased with the increased utilization of these antifibrotic agents.[10] Such blebs tend to leak more and are more vulnerable to exposure and trauma.[7] Numerous studies have shown that bleb leaks may lead to an increased risk of bleb-related infection.[7,11–15] Despite rising concern of increased risk of bleb-related endophthalmitis secondary to antifibrotic use,[16,17] reports by Mochizuki and Solomon have shown that the incidence of late bleb-related infection after trabeculectomy with antifibrotic use is similar to that after trabeculectomy without antifibrotic use.[11,18] Other established risk factors that have been associated with increased risk of bleb-related endophthalmitis include an inferiorly located bleb, conjunctivitis, blepharitis, and contact lens wear.[16,19–23]

Treatment for bleb-related endophthalmitis

Delayed-onset bleb-related endophthalmitis is caused by more virulent bacteria such as *Streptococcus*,[4,24–26] *Staphylococcus*,[24–27] and *Haemophilus influenzae*,[3–5,15,16,22,23,28] which necessitates early recognition and prompt and aggressive treatment.[23] Treatment of bleb-related endophthalmitis is similar to that of acute postoperative endophthalmitis in the anterior chamber. Vitreous cultures are obtained, and intravitreal and periocular antibiotics are administered.[21,29–31]

More detailed information on risk factors, clinical signs, prevention, and treatment for blebitis and bleb-related endophthalmitis is provided in Chapter 24.

LATE-ONSET POSTOPERATIVE UVEITIS: NONINFECTIOUS CAUSES (CAUSES OTHER THAN BACTERIAL OR FUNGAL BLEBITIS OR ENDOPHTHALMITIS)

It is imperative that the ophthalmologist first evaluate and rule out infectious causes of delayed-onset uveitis prior to considering non-infectious causes. Treatment with only immunosuppressive antiinflammatory medications (and no antibiotics) can exacerbate infections and worsen the patient's condition.

Underlying iridocyclitis

Patients with underlying iridocyclitis undergoing glaucoma filtering surgery may have prolonged and significant inflammation in the acute or delayed postoperative period. This entity should be considered in the differential diagnosis of patients with inflammation following glaucoma surgery.[32] Thorough investigation of past ocular history may give the ophthalmologist insight on previous preoperative episodes of uveitis, such as past history of red eye, pain, photophobia, and blurry vision. Workup, evaluation, and management would be similar to uveitis without previous filtering surgery in a glaucoma patient.

Mitomycin-C

Mitomycin-C has been associated with postoperative complications such as thin, avascular, leaky blebs[10] and hypotony maculopathy.[33] Mitomycin-C may also be implicated as one of the rare causes of late-onset postoperative uveitis after glaucoma filtering surgery, although currently there are no established scientific or clinical studies to substantiate such a hypothesis. Several anecdotal cases of delayed-onset uveitis in eyes that have undergone previous mitomycin-C filtering surgery have been reported. A study conducted by Nuyts and associates found that in one enucleated human eye that had previously undergone a mitomycin-C trabeculectomy, there was ciliary body epithelial disruption beneath the site of mitomycin-C application.[34] It was presumed that the ciliary body epithelial disruption resulted in aqueous hyposecretion and could have altered the blood-aqueous barrier, resulting in subsequent chronic low-grade uveitis. Thus, the adjunctive use of mitomycin-C with glaucoma filtering surgery could be an important risk factor for late-onset uveitis. Furthermore, mitomycin-C is a well-established cause of anterior chamber reaction upon entry into the eye.[35,36]

Herpes simplex and herpes zoster

Herpes simplex and herpes zoster are both known to cause chronic and recurrent iridocyclitis. After a primary infection, the herpes virus may lay dormant in the infected sensory ganglia and become reactivated[37] secondary to environmental stress factors. Patients with eyes that display delayed-onset postoperative uveitis following glaucoma filtering surgery should be carefully questioned about prior episodes of herpetic infection and examined for any key characteristic signs of herpetic involvement. The cornea should also be checked for the presence of dendritic epithelial keratitis, stromal keratitis, and neurotrophic keratopathy. Furthermore, in addition to anterior chamber reaction, the iris should be closely examined for signs of sector atrophy or patchy iris transillumination defects. If reactivation of a primary herpes infection is noted to be the cause of delayed-onset uveitis after a glaucoma filtering surgery, the treatment is typically in the form of topical steroids (if no epithelial involvement is present) to treat the anterior chamber reaction and possible long-term systemic antivirals.

Combined glaucoma and cataract surgery

Combined cataract extraction and glaucoma surgery is usually performed in patients with visually significant cataract and borderline or uncontrolled glaucoma status. When combining modern-day small incision cataract surgery with glaucoma filtering surgery, the specialist must consider phaco-anaphylactic uveitis, phacogenic uveitis, and IOL-mediated inflammation as causes of delayed-onset uveitis. Furthermore, a history of previous ocular surgery, greater technical difficulty of operation, and nonwhite race and brown iris pigmentation may set the stage for both early and late postoperative inflammation.[38]

Phaco-anaphylactic uveitis is a term used to describe a rare autoimmune inflammatory response to lens protein resulting from an abrogation of immune tolerance.[39–41] By definition, the lens capsule must be disrupted, and onset of inflammation has been reported to vary from one day to several decades after lens capsule violation.[40–43] Patients often present with ciliary injection, photophobia, and decreased vision. Clinical manifestations include varying degrees of ocular inflammation with anterior chamber and vitreal involvement, possible presence of hypopyon, granulomatous keratitic precipitates, and posterior synechiae. Inflammation of the choroid and retinal involvement are noted in the majority of cases.[41]

The inflammation associated with phaco-anaphylactic uveitis may fluctuate. Phaco-anaphylactic uveitis should be suspected after combined cataract and glaucoma surgical cases in which there is the presence of residual lens material, granulomatous inflammation, and a history of surgical or traumatic lens capsular rupture.[32] The definitive treatment includes removal of residual lens particles and the use of topical and systemic corticosteroids to control inflammation.

Phacogenic uveitis is a nongranulomatous variant of phaco-anaphylactic uveitis.[44] As with phaco-anaphylactic uveitis, phacogenic uveitis presents with inflammation secondary to lens protein following surgical or traumatic rupture of the lens capsule. Patients with phacogenic uveitis present similarly to those with phaco-anaphylactic uveitis, except for the fact that they rarely have keratitic precipitates. If keratitic precipitates are present, they are usually nongranulomatous.[44] Treatment is similar to phaco-anaphylactic uveitis with special attention given to

removing any remaining lens material. Ruling out infectious postoperative endophthalmitis is imperative, and intraocular antibiotics should be administered until a more definitive diagnosis is made.

Lower grade uveitis after combined phacoemulsification/trabeculectomy may also be infectious (i.e., *Propionibacterium acnes*) but is more commonly IOL-mediated. The inflammation generally occurs when the IOL is placed in the anterior chamber or sulcus after complicated lens extraction. Both anterior chamber- and sulcus-placed IOLs can cause chafing of the iris with consequential pigment release and breakdown of the blood-aqueous barrier. Therefore, eyes that have previously undergone a complicated surgical course during a combined glaucoma and cataract surgery in which an anterior chamber or sulcus lens was placed may be at long-term risk for delayed-onset inflammation. A few cells in the anterior chamber may be the presenting sign of chronic low-grade lens-induced uveitis, which must be differentiated from pigment release caused by iris chafing, although both pigment and white cells commonly coexist. These eyes should be carefully examined for iris transillumination or corectopia, indicating a mechanically induced source of inflammation. Ultrasound biomicroscopy is indicated where possible to demonstrate lens haptic rubbing against the iris and/or eroding through the ciliary body.[45] Inflammation in such eyes is initially treated with topical steroids, but definitive treatment includes repositioning or exchange of the IOL. If the cells in the anterior chamber appear totally unresponsive to topical corticosteroids, pigment release without inflammation should be considered, and in a filtered eye may not require intervention. Early differentiation is important in management and can usually be done by careful examination of the cells at the slit lamp.

Sympathetic ophthalmia

Sympathetic ophthalmia (SO) is a very rare cause of bilateral granulomatous panuveitis that can occur after trauma or ocular surgery to one eye. SO has rarely been documented as a complication following glaucoma filtering surgery, and in fact to date, there are only a few reported cases.[46,47] Most studies suggest that the condition of the eye undergoing the glaucoma surgical procedure is a more important predisposing factor than the actual type of glaucoma operation. Accordingly, case studies have shown that operating on a blind, painful eye or on a previously traumatized eye poses the greatest risk for SO.[46,48]

The previously injured or surgically operated eye is commonly referred to as the exciting eye and the fellow eye as the sympathizing eye. Symptoms of SO include an insidious onset of ciliary injection, pain, photophobia, and decreased vision in the sympathizing eye.[32] Clinically, most patients with SO present with low-grade persistent uveitis associated with mutton-fat keratitic precipitates, iris thickening, posterior synechiae, vitritis, disc edema, retinal vasculitis, and choroidal infiltration and thickening.[49,50] The exciting eye is typically blind, chronically inflamed, or phthisical.[51]

The mainstay of medical treatment of SO includes aggressive immunosuppression with the use of corticosteroids. Topical steroids and mydriatics are used to control anterior chamber inflammation, and systemic steroids are used for more severe and progressive cases. Other systemic immunosuppressive agents such as cyclosporine, cyclophosphamide, methotrexate, azathioprine, and chlorambucil have also been used in cases of corticosteroid intolerance and of nonresponders. For more information about SO, see Chapter 13.

Other rare causes of delayed-onset postoperative uveitis

Another possible cause of what appears to be late low-grade uveitis following filtering surgery is epithelial downgrowth (also referred to as epithelial ingrowth). The confusion occurs because this disorder is commonly accompanied by cells in the anterior chamber. These cells in the aqueous appear larger than normal because rather than being white blood cells, they are actually epithelial cells[52,53] floating freely. One other cause of anterior chamber cells nonresponsive to immunosuppression that should be considered is malignancy. Given that the age group in which most filters are performed is the same group in which many tumors occur, consideration should be directed towards malignancy, such as metastasis, lymphoma, and leukemia,. These tumors are sometimes responsive to topical corticosteroids but will recur on discontinuation, therefore recurrence should warrant further evaluation.

CONCLUSION

Recognizing the cause of intraocular inflammation in the late postoperative period following glaucoma filtering surgery is important because successful management is best accomplished by treating the underlying cause, whether infectious or noninfectious. Most noninfectious etiologies are uncommon, but if the clinician is familiar with the potential causes of inflammation, rapid diagnosis may be made and efficient treatment can be administered to ensure the best possible outcome.

Dr. Khaimi was supported by an Unrestricted Grant from Research to Prevent Blindness to the Dean McGee Eye Institute, University of Oklahoma College of Medicine.

COMMENTARY

PETER A. NETLAND

Dr. Khaimi has provided a comprehensive review of delayed-onset postoperative inflammation. Clinicians are frequently reminded of this while caring for patients, realizing that prompt recognition and treatment of these problems can avoid irreversible vision loss. Fortunately, these complications occur in a minority of patients. There is, however, a type of inflammation that occurs in the majority of patients, perhaps approaching 100% of patients treated with filtering surgery. This is the inflammation that occurs during the immediate postoperative period due to tissue trauma related to the surgical procedure itself.

The severity of the inflammatory response to surgery varies depending on the type of surgery and the type of glaucoma, as well as individual patient responses. Prolonged surgery with extensive tissue trauma in, for example, a patient with neovascular glaucoma or underlying uveitis may produce a more severe and prolonged postoperative inflammatory response. Managing this "routine" inflammation can lead to better bleb function and surgical outcomes after glaucoma surgery.[54] The mainstay of therapy for postoperative inflammation is topical corticosteroids.

After routine filtration surgery, a typical regimen is prednisolone acetate for 6 weeks, starting with 6 drops per day and decreasing the number of drops per day by one each week. Topical steroids may be used alone or in combination with nonsteroidal antiinflammatory drugs (NSAIDs), or even oral steroids when needed. Immunomodulatory drugs have been successfully used in combination with steroids to control postoperative inflammation in patients with uveitic glaucomas.[55] Antiangiogenesis drugs such as bevacizumab and panretinal photocoagulation may augment the effects of steroids in neovascular glaucoma because they produce a rapid clinical response, reducing neovascularization of the anterior segment and decreasing anterior segment inflammation.[54]

The response to steroid therapy is monitored, and therapy is intensified and prolonged as needed. For example, patients with silicone oil endotamponade may require prolonged postoperative treatment with steroids, averaging up to a year of topical steroid therapy, because of their propensity for inflammation.[56] If patients have evidence of generalized or focal inflammation around the bleb, steroid treatment is extended or intensified in an effort to avoid increased fibrosis and failure of the bleb. Treatment of focal inflammation around a bleb can be augmented with antifibrosis drugs, such as 5-fluourouracil given as a subconjunctival injection (5 mg in 0.1 mL) and repeated over several weeks as needed.

Topical corticosteroids provide excellent postoperative control of inflammation after filtering surgery and may be augmented with NSAIDs and antifibrosis drugs or immunomodulatory drugs in uveitic glaucoma, and with antivascular endothelial growth factor (anti-VEGF) drugs in neovascular glaucoma. Patients who have inflammatory conditions, such as neovascular glaucoma, uveitis, or silicone oil endotamponade, may require topical corticosteroids for a prolonged period of time. Attention to inflammation during the immediate postoperative period may influence outcomes after filtering surgery.

COMMENTARY
LEONARD K. SEIBOLD AND MALIK Y. KAHOOK

Inflammation during the immediate postoperative phase of aqueous filtration surgery is common and expected. It is the rare cases of delayed acute-onset or recurrent uveitis that are particularly worrisome as these are not expected findings and may herald serious infectious or inflammatory disorders. The challenge lies in determining the etiology. As Dr. Khaimi alludes to in this chapter, the primary goal is to delineate infectious from noninfectious causes. The appropriate treatment is dependent on the correct diagnosis. It is prudent to consider any late-onset inflammation as infectious until proven otherwise. To reiterate one of the chapter's key points, signs that should lead the treating physician to lean towards an infectious cause of inflammation include pain, dramatic decrease in vision, vitritis, and hypopyon, as well as fibrin within the bleb. When the diagnosis is in doubt, an anterior chamber paracentesis with culture is a quick, useful, and low-risk procedure to identify an offending agent. Gram stain results can be obtained quickly and guide initial antibiotic therapy. If suspicion is high, viral PCR can also be sent from the anterior chamber aspirate to identify other sources of persistent inflammation including cytomegalovirus (CMV) and herpes simplex virus (HSV). The aqueous may need to be diluted with balanced salt solution (BSS) or saline prior to sending off for PCR as the laboratory will often consider the volume of aspirate inadequate.

A key component of the workup of postoperative uveitis is a detailed preoperative history and examination. The surgeon should detail any prior ocular surgery as well as any prior uveitis. History of prior recurrent uveitis should alert the surgeon that intraocular surgery could exacerbate the condition. Concomitant cataract surgery with a glaucoma procedure may lead to persistent uveitis when complications occur with the cataract portion of the surgery. One cause of inflammation in eyes with IOLs relates to poorly positioned implants. Sutured IOLs, sulcus-fixated IOLs, poorly sized or placed anterior chamber IOLs can all result in significant inflammation due to contact with the iris. In any case, once infection has been ruled out, patients with exuberant inflammation after surgery should receive a higher frequency of topical steroids with a prolonged taper postoperatively as required to maintain a quiet eye. This will increase patient comfort and prevent bleb failure.

REFERENCES

1. Hamid M, Moubayed SP, Duval R, Fortin E, Lesk M, Li G. Recurrent anterior uveitis after trabeculectomy with mitomycin C. *Can J Ophthalmol*. Dec 2009;44(6):697–699.
2. Brown RH, Yang LH, Walker SD, Lynch MG, Martinez LA, Wilson LA. Treatment of bleb infection after glaucoma surgery. *Arch Ophthalmol*. Jan 1994;112(1):57–61.
3. Ciulla TA, Beck AD, Topping TM, Baker AS. Blebitis, early endophthalmitis, and late endophthalmitis after glaucoma-filtering surgery. *Ophthalmology*. Jun 1997;104(6):986–995.
4. Kangas TA, Greenfield DS, Flynn HW, Jr., Parrish RK 2nd, Palmberg P. Delayed-onset endophthalmitis associated with conjunctival filtering blebs. *Ophthalmology*. May 1997; 104(5):746–752.
5. Ayyala RS, Bellows AR, Thomas JV, Hutchinson BT. Bleb infections: clinically different courses of "blebitis" and endophthalmitis. *Ophthalmic Surg Lasers*. Jun 1997;28(6):452–460.
6. Poulsen EJ, Allingham RR. Characteristics and risk factors of infections after glaucoma filtering surgery. *J Glaucoma*. Dec 2000;9(6):438–443.
7. Wolner B, Liebmann JM, Sassani JW, Ritch R, Speaker M, Marmor M. Late bleb-related endophthalmitis after trabeculectomy with adjunctive 5-fluorouracil. *Ophthalmology*. Jul 1991;98(7):1053–1060.
8. Reynolds AC, Skuta GL, Monlux R, Johnson J. Management of blebitis by members of the American Glaucoma Society: a survey. *J Glaucoma*. Aug 2001;10(4):340–347.
9. Allingham RR, Damji K, Freedman S, Moroi SE, Shafranov G, Shields MB. Filtering surgery. *Shields' Textbook of Glaucoma*. 5th ed. Philadelphia: Lippincott Williams & Wilkins; 2005:568–609.
10. Kitazawa Y, Kawase K, Matsushita H, Minobe M. Trabeculectomy with mitomycin. A comparative study with fluorouracil. *Arch Ophthalmol*. Dec 1991;109(12):1693–1698.
11. Mochizuki K, Jikihara S, Ando Y, Hori N, Yamamoto T, Kitazawa Y. Incidence of delayed onset infection after trabeculectomy with adjunctive mitomycin C or 5-fluorouracil treatment. *Br J Ophthalmol*. Oct 1997;81(10): 877–883.
12. Gressel MG, Parrish RK 2nd, Folberg R. 5-fluorouracil and glaucoma filtering surgery: I. An animal model. *Ophthalmology*. Apr 1984;91(4):378–383.
13. Shields MB, Scroggs MW, Sloop CM, Simmons RB. Clinical and histopathologic observations concerning hypotony after trabeculectomy with adjunctive mitomycin C. *Am J Ophthalmol*. Dec 15 1993;116(6):673–683.
14. Soltau JB, Rothman RF, Budenz DL, et al. Risk factors for glaucoma filtering bleb infections. *Arch Ophthalmol*. Mar 2000;118(3): 338–342.
15. Waheed S, Ritterband DC, Greenfield DS, Liebmann JM, Seedor JA, Ritch R. New patterns of infecting organisms in late bleb-related endophthalmitis: a ten year review. *Eye (Lond)*. 1998;12(Pt 6):910–915.
16. Greenfield DS, Suner IJ, Miller MP, Kangas TA, Palmberg PF, Flynn HW, Jr. Endophthalmitis after filtering surgery with mitomycin. *Arch Ophthalmol*. Aug 1996;114(8):943–949.
17. Ticho U, Ophir A. Late complications after glaucoma filtering surgery with adjunctive

5-fluorouracil. *Am J Ophthalmol.* Apr 15 1993; 115(4):506–510.

18. Solomon A, Ticho U, Frucht-Pery J. Late-onset, bleb-associated endophthalmitis following glaucoma filtering surgery with or without antifibrotic agents. *J Ocul Pharmacol Ther.* Aug 1999;15(4):283–293.

19. Bellows AR, McCulley JP. Endophthalmitis in aphakic patients with unplanned filtering blebs wearing contact lenses. *Ophthalmology.* Aug 1981;88(8):839–843.

20. Higginbotham EJ, Stevens RK, Musch DC, et al. Bleb-related endophthalmitis after trabeculectomy with mitomycin C. *Ophthalmology.* Apr 1996;103(4):650–656.

21. Lehmann OJ, Bunce C, Matheson MM, et al. Risk factors for development of post-trabeculectomy endophthalmitis. *Br J Ophthalmol.* Dec 2000;84(12):1349–1353.

22. Mandelbaum S, Forster RK. Endophthalmitis associated with filtering blebs. *Int Ophthalmol Clin.* Summer 1987;27(2):107–111.

23. Mandelbaum S, Forster RK, Gelender H, Culbertson W. Late onset endophthalmitis associated with filtering blebs. *Ophthalmology.* Jul 1985;92(7):964–972.

24. Akova YA, Bulut S, Dabil H, Duman S. Late bleb-related endophthalmitis after trabeculectomy with mitomycin C. *Ophthalmic Surg Lasers.* Feb 1999;30(2):146–151.

25. Beck AD, Grossniklaus HE, Hubbard B, Saperstein D, Haupert CL, Margo CE. Pathologic findings in late endophthalmitis after glaucoma filtering surgery. *Ophthalmology.* Nov 2000;107(11):2111–2114.

26. Song A, Scott IU, Flynn HW, Jr., Budenz DL. Delayed-onset bleb-associated endophthalmitis: clinical features and visual acuity outcomes. *Ophthalmology.* May 2002;109(5):985–991.

27. Strmen P, Hlavackova K, Ferkova S, Vavrova K, Jakabovicova E, Vrastilova M. [Endophthalmitis after intraocular interventions]. *Klin Monbl Augenheilkd.* Oct 1997;211(4):245–249.

28. Kresloff MS, Castellarin AA, Zarbin MA. Endophthalmitis. *Surv Ophthalmol.* Nov-Dec 1998;43(3):193–224.

29. Kanski JJ. Treatment of late endophthalmitis associated with filtering blebs. *Arch Ophthalmol.* May 1974;91(5):339–343.

30. Olk RJ, Bohigian GM. The management of endophthalmitis: diagnostic and therapeutic guidelines including the use of vitrectomy. *Ophthalmic Surg.* Apr 1987;18(4):262–267.

31. Stern GA, Engel HM, Driebe WT, Jr. The treatment of postoperative endophthalmitis. Results of differing approaches to treatment. *Ophthalmology.* Jan 1989;96(1):62–67.

32. Carrasquillo AM, Goldstein DA. Postoperative uveitis. In: Tasman W, Jeager EA, eds. *Duane's Clinical Ophthalmology.* Vol 4. Philadelphia: Lippincott Williams & Wilkins; 2007. http://ovidsp.tx.ovid.com.ezproxyhost.library.tmc.edu/sp-2.3/ovidweb.cgi?&S=KCDHFPCIEGDDBGFCNCELBGGJGLJPAA00&Link+Set=S.sh.38%7c1%7csl_10. Accessed March 4, 2010.

33. Costa VP, Wilson RP, Moster MR, Schmidt CM, Gandham S. Hypotony maculopathy following the use of topical mitomycin C in glaucoma filtration surgery. *Ophthalmic Surg.* Jun 1993;24(6):389–394.

34. Nuyts RM, Felten PC, Pels E, et al. Histopathologic effects of mitomycin C after trabeculectomy in human glaucomatous eyes with persistent hypotony. *Am J Ophthalmol.* Aug 15 1994;118(2):225–237.

35. Derick RJ, Pasquale L, Quigley HA, Jampel H. Potential toxicity of mitomycin C. *Arch Ophthalmol.* Dec 1991;109(12):1635.

36. Morrow GL, Stein RM, Heathcote JG, Ikeda-Douglas JV, Feldman F. Ocular toxicity of mitomycin C and 5-fluorouracil in the rabbit. *Can J Ophthalmol.* Dec 1994;29(6):268–273.

37. Forrester JV, Dick AD, McMenamin PG, Roberts F. Microbiology and infection. *The Eye: Basic Sciences in Practice.* 3rd ed. Edinburgh: Saunders; 2008:435–463.

38. Corbett MC, Hingorani M, Boulton JE, Shilling JS. Factors predisposing to postoperative intraocular inflammation. *Eur J Ophthalmol.* Jan-Mar 1995;5(1):40–47.

39. Khalil MK, Lorenzetti DW. Lens-induced inflammations. *Can J Ophthalmol.* Apr 1986; 21(3):96–102.

40. Marak GE, Jr. Phacoanaphylactic endophthalmitis. *Surv Ophthalmol.* Mar-Apr 1992; 36(5):325–339.

41. Thach AB, Marak GE Jr., McLean IW, Green WR. Phacoanaphylactic endophthalmitis: a clinicopathologic review. *Int Ophthalmol.* Jul 1991;15(4):271–279.

42. Apple DJ, Mamalis N, Steinmetz RL, Loftfield K, Olson RJ, Notz RG. Phacoanaphylactic endophthalmitis following ECCE and IOL implantation. *J Am Intraocul Implant Soc.* Fall 1984;10(4):423–424.

43. McMahon MS, Weiss JS, Riedel KG, Albert DM. Clinically unsuspected phacoanaphylaxis after extracapsular cataract extraction with intraocular lens implantation. *Br J Ophthalmol.* Nov 1985;69(11):836–840.

44. Rao NA, See RF. Lens-induced uveitis and related intraocular inflammations. In: Tasman W, Jeager EA, eds. *Duane's Clinical Ophthalmology*. Vol 4. Philadelphia: Lippincott Williams & Wilkins; 2007. http://ovidsp.tx.ovid.com.ezproxyhost. library.tmc.edu/sp-2.3/ovidweb.cgi?&S=KCDHFP CIEGDDBGFCNCELBGGJGLJPAA00&Link+Set= S.sh.41%7c1%7csl_10. Accessed March 4, 2010.

45. Pavlin CJ, Harasiewicz K, Foster FS. Ultrasound biomicroscopic analysis of haptic position in late-onset, recurrent hyphema after posterior chamber lens implantation. *J Cataract Refract Surg.* Mar 1994;20(2):182–185.

46. Shammas HF, Zubyk NA, Stanfield TF. Sympathetic uveitis following glaucoma surgery. *Arch Ophthalmol.* Apr 1977;95(4):638–641.

47. Osamu I, Hiroshi K. A case of sympathetic ophthalmia following trabeculectomy. *J Eye.* 1999;16:521–524.

48. Scherer V, Schmidbauer J, Kasmann-Kellner B, Ruprecht KW. [Increased glare and distorted vision. Sympathetic ophthalmia after glaucoma surgery with uveal trauma]. *Ophthalmologe.* Dec 2000;97(12):896–897.

49. Goto H, Rao NA. Sympathetic ophthalmia and Vogt-Koyanagi-Harada syndrome. *Int Ophthalmol Clin.* Fall 1990;30(4):279–285.

50. Ramadan A, Nussenblatt RB. Visual prognosis and sympathetic ophthalmia. *Curr Opin Ophthalmol.* Jun 1996;7(3):39–45.

51. Gasch AT, Foster CS, Grosskreutz CL, Pasquale LR. Postoperative sympathetic ophthalmia. *Int Ophthalmol Clin.* Winter 2000;40(1):69–84.

52. Chiou AG, Kaufman SC, Kaz K, Beuerman RW, Kaufman HE. Characterization of epithelial downgrowth by confocal microscopy. *J Cataract Refract Surg.* Aug 1999;25(8):1172–1174.

53. Weiner MJ, Trentacoste J, Pon DM, Albert DM. Epithelial downgrowth: a 30-year clinico-pathological review. *Br J Ophthalmol.* Jan 1989; 73(1):6–11.

54. Netland PA. The Ahmed™ glaucoma valve in neovascular glaucoma (An AOS Thesis). *Transactions of the American Ophthalmological Society.* Dec 2009;107:325–342.

55. Da Mata A, Burk SE, Netland PA, Baltatzis S, Christen W, Foster CS. Management of uveitic glaucoma with Ahmed™ glaucoma valve implantation. *Ophthalmology.* Nov 1999; 106(11):2168–2172.

56. Ishida K, Ahmed, II, Netland PA. Ahmed™ glaucoma valve surgical outcomes in eyes with and without silicone oil endotamponade. *J Glaucoma.* Apr-May 2009;18(4):325–330.

21

LATE HYPOTONY WITHOUT LEAK

ANGELO P. TANNA

LATE HYPOTONY WITHOUT LEAK

Late ocular hypotony without a leak is a relatively common complication after trabeculectomy. In most eyes with a mature trabeculectomy, subconjunctival fibrosis is the rate-limiting factor in filtration; therefore, a reduction in resistance to filtration at the level of the scleral flap usually does not result in hypotony. However, in some eyes there is little subconjunctival fibrosis, and loss of resistance at the level of the scleral flap may result in excessive filtration and hypotony. The use of the antifibrotic agents, 5-flurouracil and mitomycin-C, results in reduced subconjunctival fibrosis and is one factor that increases the likelihood of postoperative hypotony due to the development of a very large and diffuse bleb surface area with the resultant possibility of overfiltration. Understanding how to prevent and manage this complication is important for surgeons who perform trabeculectomy.

RISK FACTORS

Myopia and young age are major risk factors for the development of hypotony maculopathy (see Chapter 22 for more information on hypotony maculopathy); however, some eyes tolerate very low intraocular pressures without adverse structural consequences. In eyes with late hypotony without a bleb leak and in the absence of hypotony maculopathy, choroidal detachment, optic disc edema, shallow anterior chamber, or corneal decompensation, patients can be closely monitored without intervention to reverse the hypotony.

DIFFERENTIAL DIAGNOSIS OF THE UNDERLYING PATHOLOGY CAUSING HYPOTONY

There are 4 basic mechanisms for hypotony: a bleb (or other wound) leak, overfiltration without an overt leak, excessive uveoscleral outflow by way of a cyclodialysis cleft or retinal tear, and aqueous hyposecretion (see Chapter 10 for more information about early hypotony).

Bleb leak

The presence of a bleb leak must be excluded by Seidel testing. Fluorescein solution (2%) may be easier to use and allow for better sensitivity for the detection of a leak than the use of a fluorescein-impregnated paper strip. If the anterior chamber is flat, the Seidel test may lead to a false negative result.

Overfiltration

Over time, scleral flap sutures lose tensile strength, and the scleral flap itself may become thin or even melt. In eyes with a mature trabeculectomy, subconjunctival fibrosis is often the rate limiting factor in filtration; therefore, a reduction in resistance to filtration at the level of the scleral flap usually does not result in hypotony. However, in some eyes there is little subconjunctival fibrosis, and loss of resistance at the level of the scleral flap may result in excessive filtration and hypotony.

The presence of a very diffuse, robust bleb in the setting of hypotony is the hallmark of overfiltration. Hypotony due to overfiltration can only occur if there is inadequate resistance at the level of the scleral flap *and* insufficient resistance at the level of the conjunctiva. In some cases overfiltration may result from insufficient tension of the scleral flap sutures. Occasionally, overfiltration can occur due to a defect in the scleral flap (e.g., due to melting of the scleral flap or a defect left behind at the location of an Axenfeld loop or from an unintentional full-thickness defect in the scleral flap near the site of the entry into the anterior chamber).

Cyclodialysis cleft

A cyclodialysis cleft, though very uncommon, should be suspected in the setting of hypotony in an eye with a flat or nearly flat bleb. It can occur as a result of surgical or subsequent trauma. Careful gonioscopy will usually disclose a cyclodialysis cleft when present; however, at times these are small or even

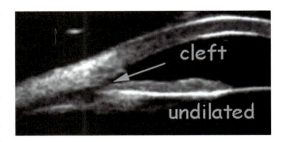

FIGURE 21.1 Ultrasound biomicroscopy image of a cyclodialysis cleft. Note the collection of fluid in the suprachoroidal space.

intermittently open making identification difficult. A cleft as small as 50 μm can be responsible for hypotony. Ultrasound biomicroscopy (UBM) is extremely valuable in the detection of a cyclodialysis cleft[1, 2] (Figure 21.1). Treatment with pilocarpine may open a cyclodialysis cleft, making gonioscopic detection easier in the office and also enhancing the surgeon's ability to treat the cleft with argon laser photocoagulation. Deepening the chamber with a viscoelastic agent may also be useful at the slit lamp to facilitate identification by gonioscopy or UBM.

Aqueous hyposecretion

As is the case for hypotony in the setting of a cyclodialysis cleft, the presence of a diminutive bleb suggests the possibility of aqueous hyposecretion. Even though IOP-lowering medications have been discontinued after surgery in the operated eye, aqueous hyposecretion may occur as a result of the use of a topical beta adrenergic antagonist in the fellow eye[3-6] or systemically. Similarly, the use of a systemic carbonic anhydrase inhibitor will also decrease aqueous production.[7, 8] Additionally, there is evidence that mitomycin-C may have direct toxicity on the ciliary epithelium, resulting in some degree of aqueous hyposecretion.[9]

Aqueous hyposecretion may also occur as a result of anterior uveitis of any etiology or anterior segment inflammation that occurs after intraocular surgery. So-called "ciliary body shutdown" is presumably the result of ciliary body inflammation and increased permeability of the blood-aqueous barrier. Increased uveoscleral outflow may further contribute to the resultant hypotony.[10-12] For further information on aqueous hyposecretion, see Chapters 34 and 39.

Ciliochoroidal effusion often results in a reduction in aqueous flow.[10] (For more on choroidal effusions, see Chapter 6.) This scenario is common in the setting of hypotony, but typically occurs as a result of initial hypotony of another etiology. Hypotony that ensues from overfiltration or hyposecretion due to inflammation may lead to serous ciliochoroidal detachment. The detachment then perpetuates the problem of aqueous hyposecretion,[10, 11, 13, 14] contributing to the persistence of hypotony. UBM is useful in the detection of ciliary body effusions. The presence of a cyclitic membrane that induces tractional ciliary body detachment can also be detected with UBM.[15] Differentiating the 2 mechanisms is crucial as treatment strategies are quite different.

PREVENTION

As is always the case, prevention of a complication is the best management. The judicious use of antifibrotic therapy is important as is the careful adjustment of scleral flap sutures to avoid overfiltration. While the use of releasable sutures or laser suture lysis may prevent early hypotony,[16-19] surgeons should avoid postoperative suture adjustment within the first week. Additionally, using a surgical technique that minimizes the risk of the inadvertent creation of a cyclodialysis cleft is of benefit. Rather than a sclerectomy, the entry into the anterior chamber should be anterior to Schwalbe's line. In creating the peripheral iridectomy, the iris should be grasped anteriorly and withdrawn gently. In theory, use of a flow-restricting device may also limit hypotony (see Chapter 29).

TREATMENT STRATEGIES

Overfiltration

Regardless of the mechanism of overfiltration, therapies aimed at increasing subconjunctival fibrosis may reverse hypotony. Various strategies for inducing subconjunctival inflammation and fibrosis are available, including diathermy, cryotherapy,[20, 21] electrocautery, laser photocoagulation,[22, 23] trichloroacetic acid,[24, 25] and subconjunctival autologous blood injection[26, 27] (see Chapter 18). These approaches are unreliable. However, repeat treatment may sometimes be successful when initial treatment is not adequate.[28, 29] See Chapters 10, 18, and 27 for more information. Additionally, a Simmons shell can be used as a temporizing measure while definitive therapy is planned.

Technique: Subconjunctival injection of autologous whole blood. The skin overlying an appropriate vein is prepared with 10% povidone-iodine solution. The ocular surface, eyelids, and periocular skin are prepared with 5% povidone-iodine solution. The slit-lamp microscope and solid eyelid speculum should be adjusted in advance. Venipuncture is performed, and approximately 0.5 mL of whole blood is drawn into a tuberculin syringe. This needle is then exchanged for a 27-gauge needle. The subconjunctival space is entered at least 8–10 mm from the region of the scleral flap. The blood is injected into the bleb such that it surrounds the bleb as extensively as possible. Sometimes a second subconjunctival injection site is utilized. Success of the procedure is poor when there is a bleb leak (whether focal or a diffuse "sweat"); however, a series of multiple injections over a period of a few weeks is often successful in triggering a fibrotic reaction and IOP elevation in the setting of overfiltration without a leak. Care must be taken to prevent the blood from reaching the anterior chamber. Viscoelastic may be useful but often results in IOP spikes.[30]

Technique: Simmons shell.[31, 32] The use of a Simmons shell typically results in substantial discomfort; however, the simultaneous use of a bandage contact lens often improves patient comfort. The Simmons shell forces apposition of the conjunctiva against the underlying sclera, limiting filtration during its use. This treatment may trigger subconjunctival fibrosis and reversal of hypotony; however, success is poor in eyes with late-onset hypotony.

An advantage of this technique is that it is effective in raising IOP while the shell is in place. As stated above, a Simmons shell may be used temporarily while further therapy is planned.

Resuturing or replacing the scleral flap

If the mechanism of overfiltration is inadequate suture tension of the scleral flap, resuturing the scleral flap will usually reverse hypotony. If the conjunctiva overlying the bleb is healthy and reasonably robust, transconjunctival suturing of the flap has been shown to be safe and effective.[33, 34]

Technique. 9–0 nylon on a VAS-100 needle (Ethicon, Inc., New Brunswick, New Jersey) should be used to tightly suture the scleral flap directly through the overlying conjunctiva with one or more interrupted sutures,[33, 34] as required to titrate flow, with the suture knots trimmed short. In cooperative patients this procedure can be performed at the slit lamp. This technique usually does not result in the development of a leak at the suture track; however, if a leak is present and persists for more than a few days, a 16 or 18 mm therapeutic soft contact lens can be used for a period of 1–2 weeks during which time the defect will usually heal. A topical fluoroquinolone antibiotic should be used during the time the contact lens is in place.

The sutures may be left in place indefinitely, as they are typically incorporated into the bleb. If a suture must be removed due to excessively elevated intraocular pressure, a leak may develop at the suture track. If this occurs, a large-diameter therapeutic soft contact lens should be used, as discussed above (Figures 21.2 and 21.3).

If the bleb is avascular and/or thin, transconjunctival suturing techniques will result in excessive damage to the conjunctival epithelium and stroma, and a persistent bleb leak may ensue. In such cases, the preferred option is to excise the avascular portion of the bleb and directly resuture the underlying scleral flap. The conjunctiva should then be closed by advancing the conjunctiva and suturing it to

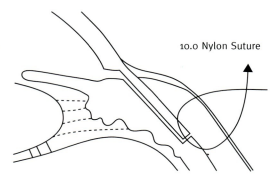

10.0 Nylon Suture

FIGURE 21.2 **Transconjunctival scleral flap resuturing** Nylon sutures (10.0) were applied through the conjunctiva into the scleral flap and the adjacent sclera and were knotted tightly over the conjunctiva.

From: Eha J, Hoffmann EM, Wahl J, Pfeiffer N. Flap suture— a simple technique for the revision of hypotony maculopathy following trabeculectomy with mitomycin C. *Graefes Arch Clin Exp Ophthalmol.* Jun 2008;246(6):869–874.

the limbus[35] or performing a free conjunctival autograft.[36] If the scleral flap is intact, but too friable to suture, the 2 best options are 1) the use of horizontal mattress compression sutures to secure the scleral flap (anchoring the sutures to healthy sclera surrounding the flap itself and compressing the flap onto the underlying scleral bed) or 2) the use of a replacement allograft such as dehydrated human donor pericardium or human donor sclera obtained from an eye bank or commercially prepackaged. If the scleral flap has melted or is otherwise compromised, a patch graft must be fashioned from replacement allograft tissue.

Cyclodialysis cleft

For information about treatment of cyclodialysis clefts, see Chapter 10.

Aqueous hyposecretion

Discontinue beta adrenergic antagonists administered systemically or in the fellow eye, if possible to do so safely. If spontaneous resolution does not occur prior to development of maculopathy or other complications,

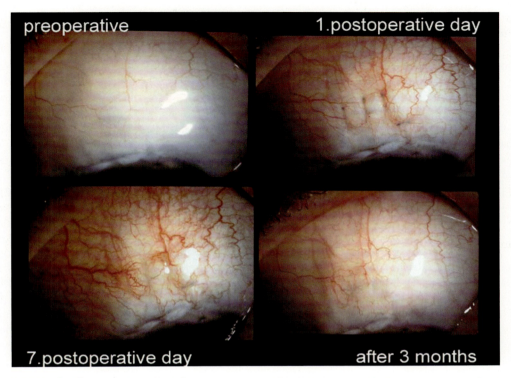

preoperative 1.postoperative day

7.postoperative day after 3 months

FIGURE 21.3 **Transconjunctival flap resuturing** Top left: large bleb following trabeculectomy with MMC before resuturing. Top right: 1st postoperative day after resuturing, backstitch-like. Bottom left: 7 days after surgery, the sutures are cutting through conjunctiva. Bottom right: after 3 months, sutures are buried under the conjunctiva. Same appearance after 3 and 6 months. Eha J, Hoffmann EM, Wahl J, Pfeiffer N. Flap suture—a simple technique for the revision of hypotony maculopathy following trabeculectomy with mitomycin C. *Graefes Arch Clin Exp Ophthalmol.* Jun 2008;246(6):869–874. Courtesy of Dr. Judith Eha.

any ciliochoroidal detachment should be addressed by drainage of suprachoroidal fluid (see Chapter 6). If superimposed overfiltration is also suspected, as is often the case, appropriate measures should be taken to reverse it. Eyes with tractional ciliary body detachment due to cyclitic membranes can be managed with vitrectomy and membrane peeling; however, the prognosis is poor. In eyes in which aqueous hyposecretion is suspected, a trial of topical, sub-Tenon's, intravitreal, or systemic corticosteroid therapy may be of benefit, particularly if there is active uveitis.

CONCLUSION

To properly manage hypotony, the surgeon must have a complete understanding of the mechanism(s) at play so that the appropriate treatment approach can be implemented. Late hypotony without a bleb leak is an increasingly common complication of trabeculectomy. As surgical techniques have evolved with the aim of minimizing subconjunctival fibrosis, the outcome has been more diffuse blebs and lower IOPs. Although this strategy seems to have reduced the risk of the development of thin, cystic blebs that are prone to develop leaks, it still has the increased risk of overfiltration. Other potential mechanisms, such as the presence of a cyclodialysis cleft or aqueous hyposecretion, demand different treatment strategies.

Dr. Tanna was supported by an Unrestricted Grant from Research to Prevent Blindness to Northwestern University.

COMMENTARY
L. JAY KATZ

The importance of identifying the mechanism of hypotony is crucial to the proper management of the cause. Dr. Tanna has clearly reviewed the 4 reasons for late hypotony after filtering surgery. Overfiltration hypotony associated with choroidal folds, maculopathy, and impaired vision has been reported in the years following the widespread use of antimetabolites such as 5-fluorouracil and mitomycin-C. High-risk patients have been identified, such as young white males, patients with myopia, or patients with no previous conjunctival surgery. Especially in these groups, measures to avoid overfiltration such as tighter scleral flaps, slow removal and cutting of scleral flap sutures, and judicious use (low concentration and shorter duration of application) of antimetabolites have been suggested. Intraoperative assessment of flow by irrigation through a paracentesis track is absolutely critical in assuring a tight sclera flap closure. When injecting fluid the eye should become firmer, at least transiently, and the flow at the flap should be slow with maintenance of a deep anterior chamber.

Although a number of conservative measures have been reported for overfiltration hypotony many, perhaps most, of these eyes end up needing a surgical revision. Additional scleral flap sutures and perhaps donor reinforcement tissue with a sliding or free conjunctival graft provide the best chance of successfully reversing the hypotony.

A cyclodialysis cleft may be difficult to detect on gonioscopy since the eye is soft. Injection of a viscoelastic into the anterior chamber firms the eye enough so that gonioscopy affords a better view to identify a cyclodialysis cleft, and carefully note the cleft location for surgical repair (suture cyclopexy) if conservative therapy (cycloplegia and argon laser application) fails.

COMMENTARY
MISHA F. SYED

Dr. Tanna discusses the complication of late hypotony without leakage after trabeculectomy. He describes the most common mechanisms for the development of late hypotony, including overfiltration, cyclodialysis cleft causing excessive uveoscleral outflow, and aqueous hyposecretion.

The structural causes of overfiltration within the bleb are explained very thoroughly, and it would be helpful to also mention potential ways to prevent the development of an overfiltering bleb. Prudent use of antimetabolites is mentioned in the chapter, but specifically there is not a mention of how best to place them on the sclera. After early placement of mitomycin-C and 5-fluorouracil directly over the area of intended scleral flap, and the resultant ischemic, thin, focal bleb formation, surgical technique can be adjusted to place antifibrotic agents posterior and adjacent to the scleral flap to facilitate creation of a diffuse, posteriorly positioned bleb. Also worth mentioning is the decrease in concentration of mitomycin-C used, as well as the duration of therapy intraoperatively. These adjustments in technique have decreased, although not eliminated, the incidence of an overfiltering bleb with or without a leak.

Risk factors for the development of hypotony and its resultant complications are also mentioned in this chapter. Specifically myopia and young age are described as characteristics that can predispose to hypotony, but it may be worth mentioning several other scenarios. Patients with thin sclera, whether from congenital or acquired causes, also may be at increased risk for hypotony after filtering surgery due to a thin scleral flap construction. Elderly patients could also become hypotonous from overfiltration if antimetabolites are used aggressively.

Overall, Dr. Tanna's contribution provides a very systematic overview of the mechanism of hypotony and discusses helpful treatment strategies for this challenging surgical complication.

Dr. Syed was supported by an Unrestricted Grant from Research to Prevent Blindness to the University of Texas Medical Branch.

REFERENCES

1. Gentile RC, Pavlin CJ, Liebmann JM, et al. Diagnosis of traumatic cyclodialysis by ultrasound biomicroscopy. *Ophthalmic Surg Lasers.* Feb 1996;27(2):97–105.

2. Hwang JM, Ahn K, Kim C, Park KA, Kee C. Ultrasonic biomicroscopic evaluation of cyclodialysis before and after direct cyclopexy. *Arch Ophthalmol.* Sept 2008;126(9):1222–1225.

3. Dunham CN, Spaide RF, Dunham G. The contralateral reduction of intraocular pressure by timolol. *Br J Ophthalmol.* Jan 1994;78(1):38–40.

4. Radius RL, Diamond GR, Pollack IP, Langham ME. Timolol. A new drug for management of chronic simple glaucoma. *Arch Ophthalmol.* Jun 1978;96(6):1003–1008.

5. Zimmerman TJ, Kass MA, Yablonski ME, Becker B. Timolol maleate: efficacy and safety. *Arch Ophthalmol.* Apr 1979;97(4):656–658.

6. Zimmerman TJ, Kaufman HE. Timolol. A beta-adrenergic blocking agent for the treatment of glaucoma. *Arch Ophthalmol.* Apr 1977; 95(4):601–604.

7. Kupfer C, Gaasterland D, Ross K. Studies of aqueous humor dynamics in man. V. Effects of acetazolamide and isoproterenol in young and old normal volunteers. *Invest Ophthalmol.* May 1976;15(5):349–355.

8. Larsson LI, Alm A. Aqueous humor flow in human eyes treated with dorzolamide and different doses of acetazolamide. *Arch Ophthalmol.* Jan 1998;116(1):19–24.

9. Mietz H. The toxicology of mitomycin C on the ciliary body. *Curr Opin Ophthalmol.* Apr 1996;7(2):72–79.

10. Liebmann JM, Sokol J, Ritch R. Management of chronic hypotony after glaucoma filtration surgery. *J Glaucoma.* Jun 1996;5(3):210–220.

11. Schubert HD. Postsurgical hypotony: relationship to fistulization, inflammation, chorioretinal lesions, and the vitreous. *Surv Ophthalmol.* Sept-Oct 1996;41(2):97–125.

12. Toris CB, Pederson JE. Aqueous humor dynamics in experimental iridocyclitis. *Invest Ophthalmol Vis Sci.* Mar 1987;28(3):477–481.

13. Chandler PA, Maumenee AE. A major cause of hypotony. *Am J Ophthalmol.* Nov 1961; 52:609–618.

14. Dellaporta A, Obear MF. Hyposecretion hypotony: experimental hypotony through detachment of the uvea. *Am J Ophthalmol.* Nov 1964;58:785–789.

15. Roters S, Engels BF, Szurman P, Krieglstein GK. Typical ultrasound biomicroscopic findings seen in ocular hypotony. *Ophthalmologica.* Mar-Apr 2002;216(2):90–95.

16. Kapetansky FM. Laser suture lysis after trabeculectomy. *J Glaucoma.* Aug 2003;12(4): 316–320.

17. Morinelli EN, Sidoti PA, Heuer DK, et al. Laser suture lysis after mitomycin C trabeculectomy. *Ophthalmology.* Feb 1996;103(2):306–314.

18. Geijssen HC, Greve EL. Prevention of hypotony after trabeculectomies with mitomycin. *Doc Ophthalmol.* 1993;85(1):45–49.

19. Savage JA, Condon GP, Lytle RA, Simmons RJ. Laser suture lysis after trabeculectomy. *Ophthalmology.* Dec 1988;95(12):1631–1638.

20. Cleasby GW, Fung WE, Webster RG Jr. Cryosurgical closure of filtering blebs. *Arch Ophthalmol.* Mar 1972;87(3):319–323.

21. Douvas NG. Cystoid bleb cryotherapy. *Am J Ophthalmol.* Jul 1972;74(1):69–71.

22. Lynch MG. Surgical repair of leaking filtering blebs. *Ophthalmology.* Sept 2000;107(9):1687.

23. Lynch MG, Roesch M, Brown RH. Remodeling filtering blebs with the neodymium:YAG laser. *Ophthalmology.* Oct 1996;103(10):1700–1705.

24. Barton K. Bleb dysesthesia. *J Glaucoma.* Jun 2003;12(3):281–284.

25. Gehring JR, Ciccarelli EC. Trichloracetic acid treatment of filtering blebs following cataract extraction. *Am J Ophthalmol.* Oct 1972;74(4): 622–624.

26. Burnstein A, WuDunn D, Ishii Y, Jonescu-Cuypers C, Cantor LB. Autologous blood injection for late-onset filtering bleb leak. *Am J Ophthalmol.* Jul 2001;132(1):36–40.

27. Choudhri SA, Herndon LW, Damji KF, Allingham RR, Shields MB. Efficacy of autologous blood injection for treating overfiltering or leaking blebs after glaucoma surgery. *Am J Ophthalmol.* Apr 1997;123(4):554–555.

28. Okada K, Tsukamoto H, Masumoto M, et al. Autologous blood injection for marked overfiltration early after trabeculectomy with mitomycin C. *Acta Ophthalmol Scand.* Jun 2001; 79(3):305–308.

29. Hyung SM, Choi MY, Kang SW. Management of chronic hypotony following trabeculectomy with mitomycin C. *Korean J Ophthalmol.* Jun 1997;11(1):15–24.

30. Nuyts RM, Greve EL, Geijssen HC, Langerhorst CT. Treatment of hypotonous maculopathy after trabeculectomy with mitomycin C. *Am J Ophthalmol.* Sept 15 1994;118(3):322–331.

31. Rajeev B, Thomas R. Corneal hazards in use of Simmons shell. *Aust NZ J Ophthalmol.* May 1991;19(2):145–148.

32. Simmons RJ, Kimbrough RL. Shell tamponade in filtering surgery for glaucoma. *Ophthalmic Surg.* Sept 1979;10(9):17–34.

33. Eha J, Hoffmann EM, Wahl J, Pfeiffer N. Flap suture—a simple technique for the revision of hypotony maculopathy following trabeculectomy with mitomycin C. *Graefes Arch Clin Exp Ophthalmol.* Jun 2008;246(6):869–874.

34. Shirato S, Maruyama K, Haneda M. Resuturing the scleral flap through conjunctiva for treatment of excess filtration. *Am J Ophthalmol.* Jan 2004;137(1):173–174.

35. Myers JS, Yang CB, Herndon LW, Allingham RR, Shields MB. Excisional bleb revision to correct overfiltration or leakage. *J Glaucoma.* Apr 2000;9(2):169–173.

36. Harris LD, Yang G, Feldman RM, et al. Autologous conjunctival resurfacing of leaking filtering blebs. *Ophthalmology.* Sept 2000; 107(9):1675–1680.

D. COMPLICATIONS COMMON TO THE EARLY AND LATE POSTOPERATIVE PERIOD

22

HYPOTONY MACULOPATHY

ROBERT L. STAMPER

HYPOTONY MACULOPATHY

Hypotony is often defined as intraocular pressure (IOP) less than 6 mm Hg. It has been reported to occur after glaucoma filtering surgery in up to 42% of cases and is usually associated with overfiltration or wound leaks.[1–4] Hypotony requiring revision, however, occurs in about 4% of filtering procedures.[5] Hypotony can follow any IOP-lowering procedure or even "simple" cataract surgery.[6,7] The advent of guarded filtering surgery has reduced the rate of hypotony significantly compared to full-thickness filtering surgery.[8] Unfortunately in the quest to increase success rates by using adjunctive antifibrotic agents, such as mitomycin-C (MMC) or 5-fluorouracil (5-FU), that prevent fibrotic wound healing, the incidence has increased again.[9] Higher doses of and longer exposure times to MMC are associated with a greater risk of hypotony.[10]

Most cases of hypotony are transient and self-limited to a few days or weeks after surgery. Transient hypotony does not seem to have any deleterious effect on long-term visual acuity.[11] However, persistent hypotony may result in structural changes that can become permanent. Hypotony maculopathy is one such condition manifesting from persistent hypotony that can result in permanent vision loss.

IDENTIFYING HYPOTONY MACULOPATHY

Hypotony maculopathy occurs in up to 10% of filtering operations with MMC or 5-FU[2,12–16] and in about 10% of eyes with chronic hypotony.[17] Maculopathy associated with hypotony was first described by Dellaporta.[18] Some years later, Gass, using fluorescein angiography, better characterized the condition.[19] In hypotony maculopathy, the sclera and choroid develop folds in the posterior pole, which can cause significant visual disturbances. The condition is recognized by characteristic striae or folds in the macular area that do not leak or stain with fluorescein. The posterior sclera appears partially collapsed, causing the folds.[20] The axial length of the eye may be shortened after both filtering and tube shunt surgery and more so in patients with hypotony.[21] The loss of vision is usually gradual after the hypotony has persisted for at least a month or more. Indocyanine green angiography has revealed some vascular abnormalities including vessel tortuosity and filling defects.[22]

ANTICIPATING AND PREVENTING HYPOTONY MACULOPATHY

Risk factors for hypotony maculopathy include youth, primary filtering procedure, and myopia.[15,23] Hypotony maculopathy is relatively rare in the black population, as demonstrated in African studies.[24,25] Hypotonous eyes with thin corneas may be less likely to develop hypotony maculopathy than those with thick corneas.[26] Additionally, the condition is likely to be bilateral if hypotony occurs in the second eye. Many cases are reversible both anatomically and functionally, even if present for many months (or even years), when hypotony is reversed.[15,27,28] However, the likelihood of complete functional reversal, may be dependent on the length of time the anatomic changes have persisted. If hypotony maculopathy persists for more than 6 months, the macular choroidal folds may become fixed and permanent, despite raising the IOP. Therefore, to manage maculopathy, manage the underlying hypotony as quickly as possible and aggressively before 6 months. Even if the folds become fixed, some improvement generally can occur with elevation of IOP.

The primary approach to dealing with hypotony maculopathy is prevention of hypotony. Use of the minimum concentration and duration of MMC or least amount of 5-FU is advocated. Similarly, application of the antifibrotic away from the sclerostomy site rather than over it may prevent some of the issues related to antifibrotics.[29–32] Suturing scleral flaps tightly and using sutures that can be modified later after some fibrosis has occurred (argon laser suture lysis or releasable sutures[33–36]) can be helpful. Careful surgical technique that prevents long-term wound leaks and late ischemic blebs should be undertaken.

MANAGEMENT OF HYPOTONY MACULOPATHY

The first approach for managing hypotony maculopathy is identifying the cause of the low IOP. Hypotony after filtration surgery may be caused by overfiltration (most common), leaking bleb, inadvertent cyclodialysis cleft, or persistent choroidal detachment (may be cause or effect). A leaking bleb is beyond the scope of this chapter (see Chapter 16); however, persistent bleb leaks in eyes treated with intraoperative MMC or 5-FU occasionally will respond to conservative measures such as large bandage contact lenses[37] and topical aminoglycoside treatment. Eventually, most will require surgical revision.

In the early postoperative period, it may not be easy to determine the cause of hypotony. (Chapter 10 addresses early postoperative hypotony in more detail.) Seidel testing is mandatory to rule out a leak. Leaks at the limbus and at suture sites are usually easily repaired in the office. Large filtering blebs, especially those that surround the limbus, almost always indicate overfiltration. Topical atropine should be utilized to facilitate closure of a cyclodialysis cleft, if present. By rotating the ciliary body and irido-zonular-lenticular apparatus posteriorly, atropine may also help to prevent peripheral anterior synechia.[38] Rapid tapering of steroid use is recommended to also permit some fibrosis at the filtering site. Pressure on the bleb site with an oversized bandage contact lens, torpedo pressure patch, or Simmons shell have their advocates, but compression sutures are a more definitive treatment for overfiltration in the early postoperative period. These sutures (7–0 or 8–0 polyglactin 910 [Vicryl™, Ethicon, Inc., Somerville, New Jersey]) are placed from the peripheral cornea to Tenon's capsule posterior to the bleb at each side of the bleb about 1 cm apart; they help to delimit the bleb and prevent fluid from tracking inferiorly.

Compression sutures can also be combined with irritation of the bleb to encourage fibrosis. The traditional irritants, such as cryoapplication, diathermy, or topical chemicals, are not effective if MMC or 5-FU have been used. Autologous blood injected into the bleb has been useful, although it may have to be repeated several times before results are seen.[39] One or 2 mL of blood is withdrawn from the antecubital vein using a 19-gauge needle. The needle is then switched to 25-gauge, 5/8 inch (1.5 cm), and about 0.5 mL of blood is injected into the bleb from a site about 1 cm temporal. These steps all must be done before the blood clots. Occasionally, some blood tracks into the anterior chamber, but it usually clears within 24 hours. IOP spikes are possible. The process can be repeated if there is little or no effect from the initial injection. Argon laser application to the bleb surface has been reported successful but has not gained widespread acceptance.[40]

Finally, if the more conservative approaches fail, surgical revision is indicated. The bleb is taken down, the scleral flap is resutured, and the bleb is resected and resutured. This approach is successful surprisingly frequently with reasonable IOP and improvement in vision in most patients.[41,42] Cohen et al has advocated near total closure of the scleral flap,

raising IOP to 25 mm Hg, in the early post-revision period as an effective method to rapidly reverse the maculopathy.[43] Later the sutures can be lysed with an argon laser or released to control the IOP (see above). Although in Cohen et al no patients suffered measurable additional glaucomatous damage,[43] that risk must be kept in mind, especially in those patients with advanced cupping. In our hands, such a risky approach has not been necessary. If IOP is restored to 10 mm Hg or more, with a little patience, the maculopathy slowly reverses, and vision usually recovers. Occasionally the scleral flap has melted and cannot be sutured down. In this case a tissue reinforcement graft of sclera, pericardium, or cornea may be used to replace the scleral flap.

CONCLUSION

Hypotony maculopathy can be frustrating for both the patient and the surgeon. The key to prevention is managing the low IOP before structural changes develop in the macula. Often conservative treatment is sufficient, but a subset of patients will require surgical intervention. Hopefully, successful treatment can be administered prior to irreversible structural changes.

COMMENTARY

JOHN S. COHEN

Hypotony maculopathy has become less common in recent years with improved trabeculectomy surgery techniques. The surgeon can minimize the risk with careful intraoperative scleral flap closure (to restrict aqueous filtration but permit flow with slight pressure at the flap edge) and postoperative timing of laser lysis and suture release.

When using antimetabolites, less rather than more concentration and duration of exposure is advisable, especially if the surgeon's experience is limited. Antimetabolite application should extend beyond the site of surgery in the areas that bleb formation is desired (i.e., posterior and lateral). Filtering surgery in younger patients, and especially if they are myopic, has a higher risk of hypotony maculopathy. 5-Fluorouracil is often used instead of mitomycin-C to decrease this risk.

When closing the scleral flap, I prefer 5 releasable sutures (or conventional sutures if preferred) in a triangular scleral flap (Figure 22.1). Use of multiple sutures permits the surgeon to incrementally titrate increases in aqueous filtration postoperatively as healing progresses and risk of overfiltration decreases.[44–46]

If overfiltration and hypotony maculopathy do occur, conservative measures are safe and psychologically helpful for the patient (and surgeon), but neither the patient nor surgeon should be discouraged if they do not work. In my experience, aggressive intervention is usually needed.

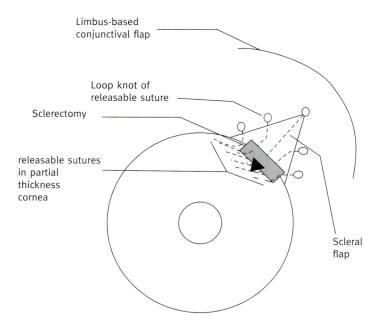

Limbus-based
conjunctival flap

Loop knot of
releasable suture

Sclerectomy

releasable sutures
in partial
thickness
cornea

Scleral
flap

FIGURE 22.1   Superonasal, triangular, limbus-based scleral flap with 5 releasable sutures under limbus-based conjunctival flap.

As the postoperative course progresses and if the IOP is borderline, the surgeon should consider that addition of glaucoma medications is often better and safer than aggressively striving for low IOP without medications. The best management of hypotony maculopathy is prevention, which brings to mind a quote of unknown origin that I first heard from Alan Kolker, MD: "Good judgment comes from experience, but experience comes from bad judgment." Hopefully we can minimize "bad judgment."

COMMENTARY
JEFFREY S. SCHULTZ

Hypotony maculopathy is the bane of the glaucoma surgeon's existence: it's the surgery that seems to be working all too well. Not all eyes with hypotony are destined to develop maculopathy. As Dr. Stamper points out, those at greatest risk to develop maculopathy are young myopes with concurrent antimetabolite use during filtering surgery. In eyes with maculopathy, the elastic sclera shrinks as the pressure is lowered, leading the relatively inelastic retina to develop folds in order to accommodate loss of surface area of the globe. In order to reverse these changes, the eye needs to be pressurized to a significantly higher level to restretch the sclera and overcome its elastic resistance as in blowing up a balloon.

There are many treatments reported by Dr. Stamper, and this suggests that nothing works perfectly. Although prevention is the mainstay, even with tight scleral flaps and minimal antimetabolite use, as we carefully lyse or remove flap sutures to improve outflow in a poorly functioning trabeculectomy, some eyes may go from a pressure of 40 mm Hg to a pressure of 2 mm Hg with the cutting of just one suture. In the absence of a wound leak, hypotony in the early postoperative period is typically related to a scleral flap issue, as the conjunctiva offers little resistance to flow. While attempts to either decrease the surface area of the bleb or increase its resistance may be helpful in some eyes, more definitive treatment involves resuturing and tightening the scleral flap.

Late hypotony in an eye with a previously functional filter often represents a breakdown of the bleb, with increased flow through a small cystic area of bleb typically surrounded by peripheral scar tissue. These eyes typically require surgical revision with the inherent risk of loss of pressure control. Some late hypotony occurs with diffuse enlargement of the bleb; this may be related to degradation of the scleral flap or flap sutures. These eyes may respond quite well to scleral flap tightening sutures through the intact conjunctiva, as these blebs rarely leak after suture placement.

REFERENCES

1. Gedde SJ, Schiffman JC, Feuer WJ, Herndon LW, Brandt JD, Budenz DL. Three-year follow-up of the Tube versus Trabeculectomy study. *Am J Ophthalmol*. Nov 2009;148(5):670–684.

2. Bindlish R, Condon GP, Schlosser JD, D'Antonio J, Lauer KB, Lehrer R. Efficacy and safety of mitomycin-C in primary trabeculectomy: five-year follow-up. *Ophthalmology*. Jul 2002;109(7):1336–1341; discussion 1341–1332.

3. Shigeeda T, Tomidokoro A, Chen YN, Shirato S, Araie M. Long-term follow-up of initial trabeculectomy with mitomycin C for primary open-angle glaucoma in Japanese patients. *J Glaucoma*. Jun 2006;15(3):195–199.

4. Ticho U, Ophir A. Late complications after glaucoma filtering surgery with adjunctive 5-fluorouracil. *Am J Ophthalmol*. Apr 15 1993;115(4):506–510.

5. Scott IU, Greenfield DS, Schiffman J, et al. Outcomes of primary trabeculectomy with the use of adjunctive mitomycin. *Arch Ophthalmol*. Mar 1998;116(3):286–291.

6. Morinelli EN, Sidoti PA, Heuer DK, et al. Laser suture lysis after mitomycin C trabeculectomy. *Ophthalmology*. Feb 1996;103(2):306–314.

7. Schubert HD. Postsurgical hypotony: relationship to fistulization, inflammation, chorioretinal lesions, and the vitreous. *Surv Ophthalmol*. Sept-Oct 1996;41(2):97–125.

8. Blondeau P, Phelps CD. Trabeculectomy vs thermosclerostomy. A randomized prospective clinical trial. *Arch Ophthalmol*. May 1981;99(5):810–816.

9. Zacharia PT, Deppermann SR, Schuman JS. Ocular hypotony after trabeculectomy with mitomycin C. *Am J Ophthalmol*. Sept 15 1993;116(3):314–326.

10. Sanders SP, Cantor LB, Dobler AA, Hoop JS. Mitomycin C in higher risk trabeculectomy: a prospective comparison of 0.2- to 0.4-mg/cc doses. *J Glaucoma*. Jun 1999;8(3):193–198.

11. Schwenn O, Kersten I, Dick HB, Muller H, Pfeiffer N. Effects of early postfiltration ocular hypotony on visual acuity, long-term intraocular pressure control, and posterior segment morphology. *J Glaucoma*. Apr 2001;10(2):85–88.

12. Cheung JC, Wright MM, Murali S, Pederson JE. Intermediate-term outcome of variable dose mitomycin C filtering surgery. *Ophthalmology*. Jan 1997;104(1):143–149.

13. Costa VP, Wilson RP, Moster MR, Schmidt CM, Gandham S. Hypotony maculopathy following the use of topical mitomycin C in glaucoma filtration surgery. *Ophthalmic Surg*. Jun 1993;24(6):389–394.

14. Shields MB, Scroggs MW, Sloop CM, Simmons RB. Clinical and histopathologic observations concerning hypotony after trabeculectomy with adjunctive mitomycin C. *Am J Ophthalmol*. Dec 15 1993;116(6):673–683.

15. Suner IJ, Greenfield DS, Miller MP, Nicolela MT, Palmberg PF. Hypotony maculopathy after filtering surgery with mitomycin C. Incidence and treatment. *Ophthalmology*. Feb 1997;104(2):207–214; discussion 214–205.

16. Whiteside-Michel J, Liebmann JM, Ritch R. Initial 5-fluorouracil trabeculectomy in young patients. *Ophthalmology*. Jan 1992;99(1):7–13.

17. Costa VP, Smith M, Spaeth GL, Gandham S, Markovitz B. Loss of visual acuity after trabeculectomy. *Ophthalmology*. May 1993;100(5):599–612.

18. Dellaporta A. Fundus changes in postoperative hypotony. *Am J Ophthalmol*. Dec 1955;40(6):781–785.

19. Gass JDM. Hypotony maculopathy. In: Bellows JG, ed. *Contemporary Ophthalmology: Honoring Sir Steward Duke-Elder*. Baltimore: The Willams & Wilkins Company; 1972:343–366.

20. Loewenstein A, McKinnon S, DiBernardo C. Echographic diagnosis of scleral fold in hypotony. *Am J Ophthalmol*. Aug 1997;124(2):260–261.

21. Francis BA, Wang M, Lei H, et al. Changes in axial length following trabeculectomy and glaucoma drainage device surgery. *Br J Ophthalmol*. Jan 2005;89(1):17–20.

22. Masaoka N, Sawada K, Komatsu T, Fukushima A, Ueno H. Indocyanine green angiographic findings in 3 patients with traumatic hypotony

maculopathy. *Jpn J Ophthalmol.* May-Jun 2000;44(3):283–289.

23. Stamper RL, McMenemy MG, Lieberman MF. Hypotonous maculopathy after trabeculectomy with subconjunctival 5-fluorouracil. *Am J Ophthalmol.* Nov 15 1992;114(5):544–553.

24. Quigley HA, Buhrmann RR, West SK, Isseme I, Scudder M, Oliva MS. Long term results of glaucoma surgery among participants in an east African population survey. *Br J Ophthalmol.* Aug 2000;84(8):860–864.

25. Singh K, Byrd S, Egbert PR, Budenz D. Risk of hypotony after primary trabeculectomy with antifibrotic agents in a black west African population. *J Glaucoma.* Apr 1998;7(2):82–85.

26. Nicolela MT, Carrillo MM, Yan DB, Rafuse PE. Relationship between central corneal thickness and hypotony maculopathy after trabeculectomy. *Ophthalmology.* Jul 2007;114(7):1266–1271.

27. Delgado MF, Daniels S, Pascal S, Dickens CJ. Hypotony maculopathy: improvement of visual acuity after 7 years. *Am J Ophthalmol.* Dec 2001; 132(6):931–933.

28. Oyakhire JO, Moroi SE. Clinical and anatomical reversal of long-term hypotony maculopathy. *Am J Ophthalmol.* May 2004;137(5):953–955.

29. Derick RJ, Pasquale L, Quigley HA, Jampel H. Potential toxicity of mitomycin C. *Arch Ophthalmol.* Dec 1991;109(12):1635.

30. Khaw PT, Baez KA, Sherwood MB, Hitchings RA, Miller MH, Rice NS. Dangers of direct injection of antimetabolites into filtration blebs. *Eye (Lond).* 1993;7(Pt 3):481–482.

31. Mazey BJ, Siegel MJ, Siegel LI, Dunn SP. Corneal endothelial toxic effect secondary to fluorouracil needle bleb revision. *Arch Ophthalmol.* Nov 1994;112(11):1411.

32. Nuyts RM, Van Diemen HA, Greve EL. Occlusion of the retinal vasculature after trabeculectomy with mitomycin C. *Int Ophthalmol.* 1994; 18(3):167–170.

33. de Barros DS, Gheith ME, Siam GA, Katz LJ. Releasable suture technique. *J Glaucoma.* Aug 2008;17(5):414–421.

34. Raina UK, Tuli D. Trabeculectomy with releasable sutures: a prospective, randomized pilot study. *Arch Ophthalmol.* Oct 1998;116(10): 1288–1293.

35. Chopra H, Goldenfeld M, Krupin T, Rosenberg LF. Early postoperative titration of bleb function: argon laser suture lysis and removable sutures in trabeculectomy. *J Glaucoma.* Apr 1992;1(1):54–57.

36. Ralli M, Nouri-Mahdavi K, Caprioli J. Outcomes of laser suture lysis after initial trabeculectomy with adjunctive mitomycin C. *J Glaucoma.* Feb 2006;15(1):60–67.

37. Shoham A, Tessler Z, Finkelman Y, Lifshitz T. Large soft contact lenses in the management of leaking blebs. *CLAO J.* Jan 2000;26(1): 37–39.

38. Burgansky-Eliash Z, Ishikawa H, Schuman JS. Hypotonous malignant glaucoma: aqueous misdirection with low intraocular pressure. *Ophthalmic Surg Lasers Imaging.* Mar-Apr 2008;39(2):155–159.

39. Okada K, Tsukamoto H, Masumoto M, et al. Autologous blood injection for marked overfiltration early after trabeculectomy with mitomycin C. *Acta Ophthalmol Scand.* Jun 2001; 79(3):305–308.

40. Akova YA, Dursun D, Aydin P, Akbatur H, Duman S. Management of hypotony maculopathy and a large filtering bleb after trabeculectomy with mitomycin C: success with argon laser therapy. *Ophthalmic Surg Lasers.* Nov-Dec 2000;31(6):491–494.

41. Bashford KP, Shafranov G, Shields MB. Bleb revision for hypotony maculopathy after trabeculectomy. *J Glaucoma.* Jun 2004;13(3): 256–260.

42. Tannenbaum DP, Hoffman D, Greaney MJ, Caprioli J. Outcomes of bleb excision and conjunctival advancement for leaking or hypotonous eyes after glaucoma filtering surgery. *Br J Ophthalmol.* Jan 2004;88(1):99–103.

43. Cohen SM, Flynn HW Jr., Palmberg PF, Gass JD, Grajewski AL, Parrish RK 2nd. Treatment of hypotony maculopathy after trabeculectomy. *Ophthalmic Surg Lasers.* Sept–Oct 1995;26(5):435–441.

44. Cohen JS, Osher RH. Releasable sclera flap sutures. In: Krupin T, Wax MB, eds. *Ophthalmology Clinics of North America: New Techniques in Glaucoma Surgery.* Vol 1. Philadelphia: W.B. Saunders; 1988.

45. Kolker AE, Kass MA, Rait JL. Trabeculectomy with releasable sutures. *Arch Ophthalmol.* Jan 1994;112(1):62–66.

46. Cohen JS, Khatana AK, Osher RH. Combined cataract implant and filtering surgery. In: Steinert RF, ed. *Cataract Surgery: Technique, Complications, Management.* 2nd ed. Philadelphia: Saunders; 2004:223–246.

23

HYPHEMA

PETER T. WOLLAN

HYPHEMA

One of the most common complications of filtering surgery is postoperative anterior chamber bleeding, or hyphema. Rates of postoperative hyphema in the literature vary, but have been reported to be up to 53%.[1-5] However, recent data from the Tube Versus Trabeculectomy Study found that postoperative hyphema occurred in only 8% of eyes (8 of 105 eyes),[6] possibly a sign of improving surgical technique.

The severity of hyphema after trabeculectomy varies greatly. Bleeding in the anterior chamber may be so mild that visual acuity and surgical outcome are unaffected. On the other hand, a total hyphema may obstruct the visual axis and potentially result in fibrosis and failure of the filtering procedure. Furthermore, some patients with glaucoma who require surgical intervention also have visual impairment or blindness in the fellow eye. Loss of vision from hyphema in the operated eye, even if only temporary, can be functionally, and possibly psychologically, debilitating to the patient.

REDUCING RISK OF HYPHEMA

The first step in reducing the risk for hyphema is obtaining a good medical history. Does the patient have any bleeding disorders, such as hemophilia or thrombocytopenia? Is the patient taking any medications that interfere with clotting or platelet aggregation, such as aspirin, clopidogrel, and/or warfarin? The use of antiplatelet and anticoagulation therapy is associated with a higher incidence of hyphemas.[7]

Platelets stop bleeding by plugging the hole in the broken vessel wall. Alternatively, antiplatelet medications inhibit platelet aggregation and therefore prolong bleeding time. Aspirin permanently alters developing platelets, and therefore its antiplatelet effect lasts until the complete cohort of affected platelets is turned over, approximately 2 weeks. Nonsteroidal antiinflammatory drugs (NSAIDs) inhibit platelet aggregation in a manner similar to aspirin, but the effect is to existing circulating platelets only and wears off in 2–3 days.[8] Ticlopidine (i.e., Ticlid; Roche Laboratories, Inc., Nutley, New Jersey) and clopidogrel (i.e., Plavix; Bristol-Myers Squibb/Sanofi Pharmaceuticals Partnership, Bridgewater, New Jersey) also affect platelet aggregation by binding to the $P2Y_{12}$, resulting in irreversible platelet inhibition. The effects of clopidogrel wear off approximately one week after treatment is terminated, while ticlopidine's effects take up to 13 days to wear off, depending on the dosage.[9] Various herbal medicines have been anecdotally implicated as having antiplatelet properties, but a recent *in vivo* study using aspirin as a control showed that platelet function was not affected by ginkgo biloba, ginseng, garlic, St. John's wort, or saw palmetto.[10]

Warfarin is an anticoagulant medication that disrupts the production of clotting factors.[11] The functional status of the coagulation cascade is grossly measured by the International Normalized Ratio (INR). If the preoperative INR is elevated above normal, intraoperative bleeding will be more difficult to control. Certain vitamins and herbal supplements are known or suspected to impair clotting. Vitamin E inhibits coagulation by interacting with vitamin K, which is required for regulation of the clotting cascade and production of clotting factors.[12] Ginkgo biloba is suspected to potentiate the anticoagulant effects of warfarin.[13]

There are no standard guidelines regarding the use of these medications prior to trabeculectomy. Prior to stopping antiplatelet or anticoagulation therapy, it is important to consult with the prescribing physician because discontinuation may be too risky due to the increased risk of stroke or myocardial infarction.[7] If anticoagulant medications cannot be safely discontinued, it may be prudent to assure that the INR is at least in the target range, but not higher than the patient's clinical situation requires. Another approach is to switch the patient temporarily to a low-molecular-weight heparin product, but this should be done under the supervision of the physician who is monitoring the anticoagulation. Furthermore, significant blood pressure elevation should be controlled preoperatively and intraoperatively to lower risk of bleeding, as well as cardiac and cerebral vascular events.

INTRAOPERATIVE HYPHEMA

To reduce the occurrence of hyphema intraoperatively, consider the bleeding source. Iris vessels may be severed when creating the iridectomy. These tend to have limited bleeding potential. Ciliary processes may also present under the iris when performing iridectomy and if cut often result in pronounced bleeding that is difficult to control. This scenario is more likely when the sclerostomy is posterior and also in severely hyperopic eyes. Bleeding from the ciliary body can be difficult to control and may result not only in hyphema but also vitreous hemorrhage. Finally, the scleral vasculature can be a source of bleeding. In addition to hyphema, bleeding from these vessels may externally seal the sclerostomy closed, compromising the success of the procedure. If intraocular bleeding occurs intraoperatively, 23-gauge "needle tip" cautery may be used to stop the hemorrhage. Tamponade of leaking vessels may also be achieved by raising the intraocular pressure (IOP) through tightly suturing the sclerostomy or by inflating the anterior chamber with an ophthalmic viscoelastic device. Intraoperative management of hemorrhage and hyphema is discussed in more detail in Chapter 5.

MANAGING/PREVENTING POSTOPERATIVE HYPHEMA

The first step in preventing postoperative hyphema is careful control of intraocular bleeding. Occasionally, hyphema is noted on the first postoperative day despite there being none at the completion of the surgical case. One explanation for this scenario is that the IOP was so low that a Valsalva maneuver by the patient raised the IOP enough to reopen a cauterized vessel. Similarly, IOP lowering achieved by removal of releasable sutures or laser suture lysis can place the patient at risk for hemorrhage by acutely stretching blood vessels with a change in IOP. Hyphema may also occur later in the postoperative period following needle revision of inadequately functioning blebs.[14,15] Instructing the patient to avoid heavy lifting, bending, and straining may prevent hyphema (as well as the more serious suprachoroidal hemorrhage). A "pseudo-hyphema" can also result from autologous blood injection of an overfiltering bleb if the blood passes through the sclerostomy into the anterior chamber.

If a hyphema occurs at any time in the postoperative period, action should be taken to limit adverse consequences. Restriction of the patient's activity with bed rest and head elevation may hasten the recovery of visual acuity and prevent rebleeding. An eye shield should be worn throughout the day and night to protect from inadvertent ocular trauma. Aspirin and NSAIDs should be avoided. Most hyphemas are small and transient and can therefore just be observed with the routine postoperative regimen.

Larger or total hyphemas might require increased dosing of topical steroids to limit the fibrinous reaction in the anterior chamber. Topical cycloplegic agents can be useful to minimize the patient's discomfort. If the IOP becomes elevated because flow through the sclerostomy is obstructed by a blood clot, topical and/or oral glaucoma medications should be used. In patients with sickle cell disease or trait, systemic carbonic anhydrase inhibitors should be avoided since they lower the pH of the aqueous and therefore may cause red blood cells to sickle,[16] making it more difficult to pass through the already dysfunctional trabecular meshwork. No research in the literature suggests that topical carbonic anhydrase inhibitors also produce the same effect; nonetheless, to err on the side of caution, they should be avoided in those with sickle cell disease, at least until a conclusive answer is reached. If medications are insufficient to control IOP, a surgical washout of the anterior chamber may become necessary. This action is usually unnecessary, because once the clot hemolyzes, the trabeculectomy is typically able to clear the hyphema. Tissue plasminogen activator may also be useful in clearing an extensive hyphema but risk of rebleeding is high.[17–19] (See Chapter 5 for further discussion.)

CONCLUSION

Although postoperative hyphema following trabeculectomy is usually transient and self-limited, it can induce anxiety for both the patient and the surgeon. Careful preoperative assessment of bleeding risk, meticulous control of intraoperative hemorrhage, and supportive (yet aggressive, if necessary) postoperative care are the keys to successfully managing this bothersome complication.

COMMENTARY

DAVID A. LEE

Dr. Peter Wollan thoroughly covered commonly used medications that can increase the risk of hyphema in patients undergoing glaucoma surgery. However, if a large hyphema has occurred and there is a significant risk of rebleeding with severe ocular damage, then aminocaproic acid (50 mg/kg), an antifibrinolytic, may be administered topically[20] or systemically to prevent rebleeding. Aminocaproic acid has its own risks of side effects, including deep venous thrombosis, nausea, and vomiting.

Certain types of glaucoma have increased risks of spontaneous or postoperative bleeding. These types of glaucoma include neovascular glaucoma, usually from ocular ischemia due to proliferative diabetic retinopathy or retinal vein occlusion; uveitic glaucoma, especially in actively inflamed eyes with a disrupted blood-ocular barrier; and traumatic glaucoma with vascularized scar tissue. Eyes that have had previous extensive intraocular surgery, usually to treat glaucoma or repair retinal detachment, may be at greater risk of bleeding during or after glaucoma surgery due to residual scar tissue. Reducing the risk of hyphema in eyes with ischemic disease includes strategies such as panretinal laser photocoagulation and injections of anti-VEGF (vascular endothelial growth factor) agents, such as ranibizumab (Lucentis®; Genentech, Inc., South San Francisco, California) or bevacizumab (Avastin®; Genentech, Inc.), which can also improve the success rate of subsequent glaucoma surgery.[21] Active inflammation should be aggressively treated with topical, subconjunctival, and even intraocular injections of steroids prior to and after glaucoma surgery to avoid hyphema and improve surgical success. Whenever possible, areas of significant ocular scar tissue should be avoided when deciding on the location to perform glaucoma surgery to reduce technical difficulties and improve success. A simple but effective procedure to check conjunctival mobility uses a cotton swab to identify areas of scarring, and locations that should be avoided.

Obviously, avoiding hyphema with its potential risk of corneal blood staining and failure of the glaucoma surgery is much preferred over treatment after it occurs. Meticulous surgical technique is essential, including delicate handling of the conjunctiva with nontoothed (Chandler-Gills) forceps, topical application of epinephrine 1% to produce vasoconstriction and hemostasis, and judicious use of wet field cautery to avoid charring. A simple technique that aids in the conjunctival dissection, hemostasis, and local anesthesia is a subconjunctival injection of 2% lidocaine and epinephrine with a 30-gauge needle at the beginning of the case before the conjunctiva is incised.

Dr. Lee was supported by a Challenge Grant from Research to Prevent Blindness to The University of Texas Medical School at Houston and the Hermann Eye Fund.

REFERENCES

1. Alemu B. Trabeculectomy: complications and success in IOP control. *Ethiop Med J.* Jan 1997; 35(1):1–11.

2. Edmunds B, Thompson JR, Salmon JF, Wormald RP. The National Survey of Trabeculectomy. III. Early and late complications. *Eye.* May 2002; 16(3):297–303.

3. Jampel HD, Musch DC, Gillespie BW, Lichter PR, Wright MM, Guire KE. Perioperative complications of trabeculectomy in the Collaborative Initial Glaucoma Treatment Study (CIGTS). *Am J Ophthalmol.* Jul 2005;140(1):16–22.

4. Konstas AG, Jay JL. Modification of trabeculectomy to avoid postoperative hyphaema. The 'guarded anterior fistula' operation. *Br J Ophthalmol.* Jun 1992;76(6):353–357.

5. Matsuda T, Tanihara H, Hangai M, Chihara E, Honda Y. Surgical results and complications of trabeculectomy with intraoperative application of mitomycin C. *Jpn J Ophthalmol.* 1996; 40(4):526–532.

6. Gedde SJ, Herndon LW, Brandt JD, Budenz DL, Feuer WJ, Schiffman JC. Surgical complications in the Tube Versus Trabeculectomy Study during the first year of follow-up. *Am J Ophthalmol.* Jan 2007;143(1):23–31.

7. Cobb CJ, Chakrabarti S, Chadha V, Sanders R. The effect of aspirin and warfarin therapy in trabeculectomy. *Eye.* May 2007;21(5):598–603.

8. Schafer AI. Effects of nonsteroidal antiinflammatory drugs on platelet function and systemic hemostasis. *J Clin Pharmacol.* Mar 1995;35(3):209–219.

9. Wallentin L. P2Y(12) inhibitors: differences in properties and mechanisms of action and potential consequences for clinical use. *Eur Heart J.* Aug 2009;30(16):1964–1977.

10. Beckert BW, Concannon MJ, Henry SL, Smith DS, Puckett CL. The effect of herbal medicines on platelet function: an in vivo experiment and review of the literature. *Plast Reconstr Surg.* Dec 2007;120(7):2044–2050.

11. Hill CE, Duncan A. Overview of pharmacogenetics in anticoagulation therapy. *Clin Lab Med.* Dec 2008;28(4):513–524.

12. Traber MG. Vitamin E and K interactions—a 50-year-old problem. *Nutr Rev.* Nov 2008;66(11):624–629.

13. Izzo AA, Ernst E. Interactions between herbal medicines and prescribed drugs: a systematic review. *Drugs.* 2001;61(15):2163–2175.

14. Mardelli PG, Lederer CM Jr., Murray PL, Pastor SA, Hassanein KM. Slit-lamp needle revision of failed filtering blebs using mitomycin C. *Ophthalmology.* Nov 1996;103(11):1946–1955.

15. Chang SH, Hou CH. Needling revision with subconjunctival 5-fluorouracil in failing filtering blebs. *Chang Gung Med J.* Feb 2002;25(2): 97–103.

16. Walton W, Von Hagen S, Grigorian R, Zarbin M. Management of traumatic hyphema. *Surv Ophthalmol.* Jul–Aug 2002;47(4):297–334.

17. Williams DF, Han DP, Abrams GW. Rebleeding in experimental traumatic hyphema treated with intraocular tissue plasminogen activator. *Arch Ophthalmol.* Feb 1990;108(2):264–266.

18. Kim MH, Koo TH, Sah WJ, Chung SM. Treatment of total hyphema with relatively low-dose tissue plasminogen activator. *Ophthalmic Surg Lasers.* Sept 1998;29(9):762–766.

19. Starck T, Hopp L, Held KS, Marouf LM, Yee RW. Low-dose intraocular tissue plasminogen activator treatment for traumatic total hyphema, postcataract, and penetrating keratoplasty fibrinous membranes. *J Cataract Refract Surg.* Mar 1995;21(2):219–224.

20. Crouch ER Jr., Williams PB, Gray MK, Crouch ER, Chames M. Topical aminocaproic acid in the treatment of traumatic hyphema. *Arch Ophthalmol.* Sept 1997;115(9):1106–1112.

21. Duch S, Buchacra O, Milla E, Andreu D, Tellez J. Intracameral bevacizumab (Avastin®) for neovascular glaucoma: a pilot study in 6 patients. *JGlaucoma.* Feb 2009;18(2): 140–143.

24

ENDOPHTHALMITIS

JOHN T. LIND AND STEVEN J. GEDDE

ENDOPHTHALMITIS

Bleb-related endophthalmitis is one of the most visually devastating complications of glaucoma filtering surgery. Endophthalmitis associated with a functioning filtering bleb may develop months or years postoperatively. Early postoperative endophthalmitis occurs within 6 weeks following the surgery, and late endophthalmitis occurs after this 6-week window. Early detection and rapid institution of appropriate treatment is important in optimizing outcomes and preserving vision.

DEFINITIONS

Blebitis is defined as an infection localized to the bleb and surrounding tissues, including the anterior chamber. Blebitis lacks vitreous involvement. Ocular signs of blebitis may include hyperemia around the bleb site, focal infiltrate in the bleb, bleb purulence, and anterior chamber reaction. Bleb-related endophthalmitis encompasses the findings of blebitis with concurrent vitreous inflammation. The presence of vitreous inflammation differentiates bleb-related endophthalmitis from blebitis (Figure 24.1).

DEMOGRAPHICS AND RISK FACTORS FOR THE DEVELOPMENT OF BLEBITIS AND ENDOPHTHALMITIS

Bleb leaks

Risk factors for bleb-related infections are listed in Table 24.1. Bleb morphology and the presence of a bleb leak affect the risk of blebitis or endophthalmitis. Bleb leaks have been identified as the single most important risk factor for the development of bleb-related infections. In a case-control study by Soltau

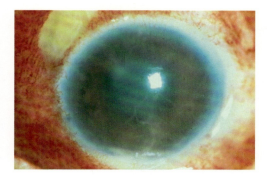

FIGURE 24.1   Bleb-Related Endophthalmitis

et al, Seidel-positive bleb leaks increased the risk of bleb infection nearly 26-fold.[1] A multicenter study also found that a bleb leak is a major risk factor for blebitis and endophthalmitis.[2] In a review of 20 endophthalmitis cases, 55% of the patients (11 patients) had a Seidel-positive leak following filtering surgery, and three-quarters (15 patients) were noted to have a thin or avascular bleb. Recurrent bleb leaks were observed in over a third of the patients.[3] Song et al found that bleb leaks occurred in 27% of eyes (13 of 49 eyes) with delayed-onset bleb-related endophthalmitis.[4] It is recommended that the clinician routinely monitor patients for bleb leaks and make appropriate interventions to resolve the leak once it is identified.

Table 24.1.   Risk Factors for the Development of Blebitis and Bleb-Related Endophthalmitis

- Blepharitis
- Contact Lens Wear
- Inferior Bleb Location
- Full-Thickness Procedure
- Adjunctive Use of an Antifibrotic Agent
- Conjunctivitis
- Nasolacrimal Duct Obstruction
- Bleb Leak
- Cystic, Thin-Walled Bleb Morphology
- Prophylactic Antibiotic Use

Antifibrotic usage

The advent of antifibrotic agents has improved the success rate of traditional filtering surgery but has also increased the incidence of bleb-related infections.[5–8] Greenfield et al demonstrated that mitomycin-C (MMC) increases the risk of bleb leak.[9] This increased infection rate is presumably related to alterations in bleb morphology, including an increase in permeability or avascularity and a decrease in bleb thickness.

Clinical studies have reported differing rates of blebitis and bleb-related infections associated with antifibrotic usage. DeBry et al estimated the incidence of a bleb leak or infection after trabeculectomy with MMC to be as high as 23% over a 5-year period.[10] Bindlish et al reported that blebitis and endophthalmitis occurred in 5.7% (7 of 124 eyes) and 0.8% (1 of 123 eyes) of eyes, respectively.[11] However, Mochizuki et al found the incidence of bleb-related infection was 1.1% in patients receiving a trabeculectomy with MMC (7 of 662 procedures) and 1.3% in patients who underwent a trabeculectomy with 5-fluorouracil (3 of 228 procedures).[12] Surgeons have titrated the exposure and concentration of MMC in an attempt to optimize surgical success while minimizing bleb-related complications. A patient's past ocular surgery and expected healing response can help guide MMC dosing during a filtering operation.

Thin conjunctiva

In a histopathologic study, Matsuo et al demonstrated that blebs with recurrent blebitis have extraordinarily thin conjunctiva.[13] In some cases the conjunctival specimens displayed a 1–2 layer thick epithelium. Loss of goblet cells was identified as an exacerbating factor for possible infection. It has been postulated that the mucin-producing goblet cells produce both physical and biologic barriers to infection, and the lack of these cells could predispose the bleb to leakage and infection.[13] The lack of host inflammatory reaction and available blood supply of tissue treated with an adjunctive antifibrotic agent could also contribute to an increased rate of infection and decreased host responses to bacterial infections.[14]

Bleb location

An inferior location to the bleb has also been identified as a modifiable risk factor for bleb-related infections. A study by Wolner et al reported that an inferior filter carries a 4 times greater relative risk of bleb-related endophthalmitis.[15] Greenfield et al found the incidence of endophthalmitis was 1.3% and 7.8% in superior and inferior trabeculectomy procedures with MMC, respectively.[16] Higginbotham et al reported that endophthalmitis developed in 1.1% of eyes with superior blebs (2 of 179 eyes) compared to 8% of patients with inferior blebs (4 of 50 eyes).[17]

Postoperative antibiotics

Jampel et al noted that continuous and episodic use of postoperative antibiotics was an independent risk factor for the development of late-onset infection after traditional filtering surgery.[2] It has been postulated that chronic antibiotic use can select out more virulent organisms. If a bleb infection develops in this setting, it is more serious and refractory to treatment.

ORGANISMS CAUSING BLEBITIS AND ENDOPHTHALMITIS

The normal flora of the ocular adenexa is likely responsible for the majority of blebitis and early endophthalmitis cases. Gram-positive specimens are most commonly isolated from positive cultures of bleb-related infections. In a series of 10 patients with blebitis, conjunctival swabs grew *Staphylococcus epidermidis* in 4 patients, *Staphylococcus aureus* in 3 patients, a combination of *S. epidermidis* and *S. aureus* in 1 patient, and a combination of *Serratia marescens* and *S. epidermidis* in 1 patient.[18] *S. epidermidis* was identified as the causative organism by vitreous culture in two-thirds of the early bleb-related endophthalmitis cases (4 of 6 patients), while the same organism caused only 4% (1 of 27 cases) of the late endophthalmitis cases.[18] It is postulated that

S. epidermidis, being part of the normal flora of the ocular surface, causes infection by direct inoculation at the time of surgery.

Table 24.2 shows the causative agent in several studies of late-occurring bleb-related endophthalmitis.[4,19,20,36] Once again, gram-positive organisms, such as staphylococci and streptococci, are the predominant infectious agents in culture-proven endophthalmitis. However, when selecting antibiotic therapy, it is important to consider gram-negative pathogens as well as methicillin-resistant *S. aureus* in some patient populations.[21]

CLINICAL DIAGNOSIS OF BLEBITIS AND ENDOPHTHALMITIS

Patients with bleb-related infections may present days to many years following surgery with complaints of ocular redness, pain, light sensitivity, diminished vision, and/or foreign body sensation. Education of patients who have undergone successful trabeculectomy with the pneumonic RSVP (**R**edness, light **S**ensitivity, decreased **V**ision, and **P**ain) can help to promote timely diagnosis and treatment of bleb infections. Prompt recognition, evaluation, and treatment of these patients are of paramount importance for saving vision, preventing fulminant endophthalmitis, and possibly even preserving bleb function.

Several clinical findings should heighten the clinician's suspicion of blebitis. The eye may be injected with prominent hyperemia surrounding the bleb (Figure 24.2). A Seidel-positive leak (Figure 24.3) may be present with possible purulent material being expressed from the defect in the bleb. The eye may be hypotonous secondary to aqueous leakage or intraocular inflammation, causing decreased aqueous production. Conversely, the intraocular pressure may be elevated secondary to bleb failure related to the intraocular inflammation plugging the sclerostomy or frank bleb scarring. The amount of cell and flare in the anterior chamber is variable. A hypopyon may be present, and gonioscopic examination can be used to look for a small, layered hypopyon, which might not be easily detected by slit-lamp biomicroscopy.

Table 24.2. Causative Agents of Culture Positive Cases of Bleb-Related Endophthalmitis, % (no. cases)

STUDY	STREPTOCOCCUS	STAPHLOCOCCUS	MORAXELLA	ENTEROCOCCI	SERRATIA	HEMOPHILUS	ENTEROBACTER	PSEUDOMONAS	OTHER	NOTES
Song, 2001, 39 cases[4]	41 (16)	28 (11)	15 (6)	23 (9)	8 (3)	3 (1)	3 (1)	—	3 (1)	Several cases positive for *Staph and Strep* species
Busbee, 1996–2001, 27 cases[36]	52 (14)	22 (6)	7 (2)	4 (1)	—	4 (1)	—	4 (1)	7 (2)	One case positive for *Candida albicans*
Waheed, 1998, 42 cases[20]	19 (8)	59 (25)	5 (2)	—	2 (1)	5 (2)	—	—	10 (4)	
Kangas, 1997, 31 cases[19]	47 (15)	23 (7)	6 (2)	6 (2)	—	16 (5)	—	—	3 (1)	One case positive for *Staph and Strep* species
Busbee, 1989–1995, 17 cases[36]	24 (4)	29 (5)	6 (1)	18 (3)	12 (2)	6 (1)	—	12 (2)	—	One case positive for *Staph and Strep* species

* culture not positive

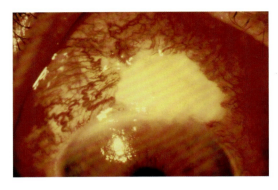

FIGURE 24.2   Blebitis

All patients with intraocular inflammation following trabeculectomy should be dilated to examine for posterior segment inflammation. If the posterior segment examination is obscured by fibrin or a dense cataract, B-scan ultrasonography should be performed to examine the vitreous cavity for inflammatory debris. It is frequently useful to compare the ultrasound findings between the unaffected and affected eye.

PREVENTION/TREATMENT OF BLEBITIS AND BLEB-RELATED ENDOPHTHALMITIS

Prevention involves anticipating which patients are at risk for developing these complications and providing medical and/or surgical correction to lower the eye's risk. As previously discussed, bleb leaks are one of the major risk factors for developing infection. By routinely checking for leaks, the clinician

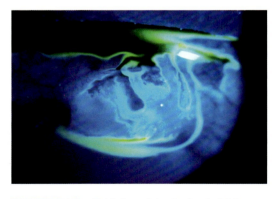

FIGURE 24.3   Seidel-positive leak of a bleb

can address this complication and prevent it from progressing to a vision-threatening infection. Bleb revisions,[22,23] bandage contact lenses,[24–26] pressure patching,[22] compression sutures,[27] autologous blood injection,[28,29] tissue glue,[24,30,31] aqueous suppressants,[32] laser surgery,[33,34] cryotherapy, and bleb needling[29] have been used to treat bleb leaks. Burnstein et al demonstrated that surgical treatment of bleb leaks with conjunctival advancement greatly reduced recurrence of bleb leaks and rates of blebitis and endophthalmitis compared with nonsurgical interventions.[22]

The utility of culturing the conjunctival surface in the setting of a bleb infection has not been proven. Studies have demonstrated that the cultures from the ocular surface and those obtained from anterior chamber and vitreous taps have shown poor correlation.[18] Reynolds et al surveyed members of the American Glaucoma Society (AGS) in 1999 to evaluate practice patterns for the evaluation and treatment of blebitis (204 respondents).[35] Thirty-four percent of glaucoma specialists (69 respondents) indicated that they "almost never or never" obtain cultures compared to 28% (57 respondents) who responded that they "always or almost always" obtain cultures.[35] In contrast, vitreous cultures should always be obtained when confronted with bleb-related endophthalmitis. Vitreous cultures are positive in greater than 50% of samples taken.[18,36] Anterior chamber aqueous cultures generally correlate with vitreous cultures from the posterior segment. In one series of 18 patients in which both anterior chamber and vitreous samples were taken, 16 either grew the same infectious organism in both the anterior chamber and vitreous cultures or revealed no growth in either culture. The 2 patients in whom cultures did not correlate revealed no growth in the aqueous sample, while the vitreous sample showed organism growth.[18]

Practice patterns differ for the treatment of blebitis, as indicated by a survey of AGS members.[35] Thirty-one percent of respondents (63 respondents of 204 total) advise their patients to keep topical antibiotics at home in case they develop symptoms of blebitis. Fifty-one percent of respondents (104 respondents) start only topical fluoroquinolones at the onset of blebitis. Oral and intravenous antibiotics were "almost never or never" used by 80% (163 respondents) and 92% (188 respondents) of respondents, respectively. Subconjunctival injection of antibiotics at the onset of isolated blebitis was used by 12% (24 respondents) of AGS members who responded to this survey.[35]

The role of corticosteroids was also explored in the same AGS survey. Sixty-two percent of the respondents (126 respondents) used steroids at some point in the treatment of blebitis. Only 2% (4 respondents) used them at the onset of treatment, while 54% (110 respondents) used them "once improvement of blebitis is noted."[35] If steroids are used initially, it may be unclear whether clinical improvement is a result of appropriate antibiotic therapy or suppression of inflammation by the steroid.

The antibiotic regimen should be tailored to the suspected infectious organisms and should be altered based upon the patient's response to treatment. Prasad and Latina advocate fortified antibiotics of either vancomycin (25 to 50 mg/ml) or cephazolin (50 mg/ml) with tobramycin (14 mg/ml) alternating every half hour for the first 1–2 days. An alternative regimen involves use of a fourth generation fluoroquinolone (gatifloxacin, 0.3% or moxifloxicin, 0.5%) every hour. A loading dose of either regimen of 4 drops separated by 5 minutes is also advocated by the authors.[37]

Due to the emergence of methacillin-resistant *Staphlococcus aureus* (MRSA) infections and other resistant pathogens, antibiotic regimens have to be carefully considered. Blomquist noted that MRSA has been found to cause bleb-related infections, and this organism has considerable resistance to conventional antibiotics used to treat infections. Fluoroquinolones were frequently found to be used inappropriately in ophthalmic infections and have indeterminate or resistant sensitivities when tested.[21] Therefore, we advocate use of fortified antibiotics for the treatment of all bleb-related infections if available, and we reserve use of fluoroquinolones for cases where fortified antibiotics are not available.

Bleb-related endophthalmitis requires more intensive treatment than blebitis. In addition to topical fortified antibiotics, bleb-related endophthalmitis requires removal of a vitreous sample for culture and injection of intravitreal antibiotics with possible adjunctive steroids. Vancomycin (1 mg/0.1 mL) in combination with ceftazidime (2.25 mg/0.1 mL), amikacin (0.4 mg/0.1 mL), or gentamycin (0.1 mg/0.1 mL) has been advocated.[37] The role of adjunctive, concurrent steroid injection for endophthalmitis remains controversial. A retrospective, nonrandomized, comparative trial of endophthalmitis after cataract surgery showed that adjunctive intravitreal steroid injection reduced the chance of improvement of 3 lines of visual acuity. Final mean visual acuity was also worse in the steroid group compared with the group that did not receive intravitreal steroid.[38]

No multicenter, prospective, randomized clinical trials have evaluated the outcomes of vitrectomy versus a vitreous tap with injection of intravitreal antibiotics for bleb-related endophthalmitis. The Endophthalmitis Vitrectomy Study (EVS) elucidated criteria for the necessity of vitrectomy in patients who developed endophthalmitis after cataract extraction or secondary intraocular lens implantation.[39] The results of EVS cannot be extrapolated to bleb-related endophthalmitis, because the forms of endophthalmitis have different causative organisms and different time courses for the onset of infection following surgery. Busbee et al reported that patients who received vitrectomy for bleb-related endophthalmitis had better visual outcomes when compared with patients who underwent a vitreous tap with injection of intravitreal antibiotics. In patients who received vitrectomy (18 patients total), 30% had visual acuity better than 20/50, and 60% achieved 20/400 or better vision. In contrast, no patients who had only a tap and injection (20 patients total) obtained 20/50 or better visual acuity, and only 25% had vision at the level of 20/400 or better. However, it is noteworthy, that the presenting range of visual acuity was worse in the tap and injection group, but the median presenting acuity was the same.[36] However, Song et al reported different results. In this series, 15% of the tap and injection group (4 of 26 eyes) achieved vision of better than 20/50, and 69% of patients had vision at 20/400 or better (18 of 26 eyes). In the vitrectomy group, 5% had vision better than 20/50 (1 of 22 eyes) and 36% had vision of 20/400 or better (8 of 22 eyes).[4] The role of vitrectomy is left to the judgment of the treating ophthalmologist, but there is potential benefit in offering surgery that debulks the infectious organisms and removes toxic byproducts of the bacteria and host response.

OUTCOMES OF BLEBITIS AND BLEB-RELATED ENDOPHTHALMITIS

Clinical outcomes differ for those patients who present with blebitis as opposed to bleb-related endophthalmitis. In a series of 8 patients with blebitis after trabeculectomy with MMC, Ayyala et al reported 100% success of treatment in returning the patients to preinfection levels of visual acuity and intraocular pressure.[40] In contrast, bleb-associated endophthalmitis can have devastating visual consequences. Busbee et al noted that the incidence of No Light Perception at 12 months following treatment was 35% (24 of 68 patients). In patients

who were culture positive, the mean visual acuity was worse (Hand Motion) when compared to culture negative patients who had a mean visual acuity of 20/100.[36] Song et al reported that 22% of eyes with bleb-related endophthalmitis had enucleation or evisceration (11 of 49 eyes). These eyes had Light Perception or No Light Perception vision. Patients infected with *Streptococcus* were more likely to require an enucleation or evisceration.[4]

CONCLUSION

Blebitis and bleb-related endophthalmitis are 2 conditions that can lead to potentially serious and devastating complications. Patients exhibiting signs of either condition need to be carefully managed to avoid loss of bleb function, vision, and even the eye.

Dr. Gedde was supported by National Eye Institute grant P30EY014801, Department of Defense Grant W81XWH-09–1-0675, and an Unrestricted Grant from Research to Prevent Blindness to the Bascom Palmer Eye Institute, Miller School of Medicine, University of Miami.

COMMENTARY
SILVIA D. ORENGO-NANIA

Ocular infection following glaucoma surgery may be the worst possible outcome of a surgery done to prevent vision loss. As with glaucoma, which requires vigilant follow-up because there is no cure, there is no time after surgery that one should not be vigilant watching for and preventing infection. It is critical that the physician educate the patient regarding this perpetual risk and remind the patient of it periodically. During the informed consent process and postoperatively, patients should be told that they should call immediately if they develop excessive tearing, discomfort, redness, and blurred vision at any time in their lives.

A routine examination in patients at risk for bleb leaks, which includes thin blebs, eye rubbers, or chronic blepharitis, should be evaluated for bleb leaks. This evaluation should include Seidel testing and also be performed in any patient without complaints whose intraocular pressure is lower than usual or who has a history of trauma to the face. It is also important to remember when checking for leaks in patients who are hypotonous that just painting the bleb with flourescein is not enough and that mild pressure should be applied to the eye through the eyelid to expose an occult leak.

As mentioned, early and broad coverage treatment is the key to a favorable outcome. If fortified antibiotics are difficult to obtain, flurouquinolones should be started immediately. If the patient is monocular and has no reliable way of getting the drops in, hospitalization is indicated to ensure proper administration of frequent eye drops.

COMMENTARY

LOUIS R. PASQUALE

Diagnosing Blebitis: Making a definitive diagnosis of blebitis can be challenging, but it is critically important because an early diagnosis can prevent bleb-related endophthalmitis. When the bleb is frankly yellow, as shown in Figure 24.2, it is not difficult to make a diagnosis of blebitis. However, early on in the course, a patient with blebitis can have an infiltrate or abscess in the filtration bleb that has a cloudy grey appearance, making it difficult to distinguish from the normal porcelain appearance of the bleb. In contrast, when such an infiltrate is present in the transparent cornea, it is easy to spot. The authors point out several examination features consistent with blebitis, but I would like to add another simple diagnostic maneuver. It is natural to gravitate to a slit-lamp exam when making an assessment of blebitis; however, the slit beam will blanch out the conjunctival features, making it even more difficult to tell whether an early infiltrate or abscess is present. I recommend lifting the lid and inspecting the bleb with normal room light. This maneuver, also recommended for the assessment of scleritis, can be helpful and allow the examiner to feel confident that a patient has early blebitis.

Treating bleb leaks: The authors correctly point out that bleb leaks should always be sought out and addressed because they represent an important risk factor for subsequent bleb-related infections. Painting the bleb with a moistened fluorescein strip represents an effective way to definitively identify bleb leaks, particularly ones that are subtle. They also point out that surgical revision with advancement of healthy conjunctiva represents the most effective way to address bleb leaks. At times, patients are not amenable to returning to the operating room for bleb repair once conservative treatments fail. In these instances, it is important to give patients "blebitis precautions" and to document that these instructions were discussed. Specifically the patient should be instructed to seek immediate assistance if the operative eye were to develop redness or pain with or without light sensitivity or change in vision. Whether these patients should be given an emergency prescription for antibiotics is a matter for debate; I agree that prophylactic daily antibiotic therapy should be avoided.

Dr. Pasquale was supported by the Harvard Glaucoma Center for Excellence.

REFERENCES

1. Soltau JB, Rothman RF, Budenz DL, et al. Risk factors for glaucoma filtering bleb infections. *Arch Ophthalmol.* Mar 2000;118(3):338–342.
2. Jampel HD, Quigley HA, Kerrigan-Baumrind LA, Melia BM, Friedman D, Barron Y. Risk factors for late-onset infection following glaucoma filtration surgery. *Arch Ophthalmol.* Jul 2001;119(7):1001–1008.
3. Poulsen EJ, Allingham RR. Characteristics and risk factors of infections after glaucoma filtering surgery. *J Glaucoma.* Dec 2000;9(6):438–443.
4. Song A, Scott IU, Flynn HW Jr., Budenz DL. Delayed-onset bleb-associated endophthalmitis: clinical features and visual acuity outcomes. *Ophthalmology.* May 2002;109(5):985–991.
5. Five-year follow-up of the Fluorouracil Filtering Surgery Study. The Fluorouracil Filtering Surgery Study Group. *Am J Ophthalmol.* Apr 1996;121(4):349–366.
6. Cheung JC, Wright MM, Murali S, Pederson JE. Intermediate-term outcome of variable dose mitomycin C filtering surgery. *Ophthalmology.* Jan 1997;104(1):143–149.
7. Khaw PT. Advances in glaucoma surgery: evolution of antimetabolite adjunctive therapy. *J Glaucoma.* Oct 2001;10(5)(suppl 1):S81–S84.
8. Loon SC, Chew PT. A major review of antimetabolites in glaucoma therapy. *Ophthalmologica.* 1999;213(4):234–245.
9. Greenfield DS, Liebmann JM, Jee J, Ritch R. Late-onset bleb leaks after glaucoma filtering surgery. *Arch Ophthalmol.* Apr 1998;116(4):443–447.
10. DeBry PW, Perkins TW, Heatley G, Kaufman P, Brumback LC. Incidence of late-onset bleb-related complications following trabeculectomy with mitomycin. *Arch Ophthalmol.* Mar 2002;120(3):297–300.
11. Bindlish R, Condon GP, Schlosser JD, D'Antonio J, Lauer KB, Lehrer R. Efficacy and safety

of mitomycin-C in primary trabeculectomy: five-year follow-up. *Ophthalmology*. Jul 2002;109(7):1336–1341; discussion 1341–1332.

12. Mochizuki K, Jikihara S, Ando Y, Hori N, Yamamoto T, Kitazawa Y. Incidence of delayed onset infection after trabeculectomy with adjunctive mitomycin C or 5-fluorouracil treatment. *Br J Ophthalmol*. Oct 1997;81(10):877–883.

13. Matsuo H, Tomita G, Araie M, et al. Histopathological findings in filtering blebs with recurrent blebitis. *Br J Ophthalmol*. Jul 2002;86(7):827.

14. Belyea DA, Dan JA, Stamper RL, Lieberman MF, Spencer WH. Late onset of sequential multifocal bleb leaks after glaucoma filtration surgery with 5-fluorouracil and mitomycin C. *Am J Ophthalmol*. Jul 1997;124(1):40–45.

15. Wolner B, Liebmann JM, Sassani JW, Ritch R, Speaker M, Marmor M. Late bleb-related endophthalmitis after trabeculectomy with adjunctive 5-fluorouracil. *Ophthalmology*. Jul 1991;98(7):1053–1060.

16. Greenfield DS, Suner IJ, Miller MP, Kangas TA, Palmberg PF, Flynn HW Jr. Endophthalmitis after filtering surgery with mitomycin. *Arch Ophthalmol*. Aug 1996;114(8):943–949.

17. Higginbotham EJ, Stevens RK, Musch DC, et al. Bleb-related endophthalmitis after trabeculectomy with mitomycin C. *Ophthalmology*. Apr 1996;103(4):650–656.

18. Ciulla TA, Beck AD, Topping TM, Baker AS. Blebitis, early endophthalmitis, and late endophthalmitis after glaucoma-filtering surgery. *Ophthalmology*. Jun 1997;104(6):986–995.

19. Kangas TA, Greenfield DS, Flynn HW Jr., Parrish RK 2nd, Palmberg P. Delayed-onset endophthalmitis associated with conjunctival filtering blebs. *Ophthalmology*. May 1997;104(5):746–752.

20. Waheed S, Ritterband DC, Greenfield DS, Liebmann JM, Seedor JA, Ritch R. New patterns of infecting organisms in late bleb-related endophthalmitis: a ten year review. *Eye (Lond)*. 1998;12(Pt 6):910–915.

21. Blomquist PH. Methicillin-resistant Staphylococcus aureus infections of the eye and orbit (an American Ophthalmological Society thesis). *Trans Am Ophthalmol Soc*. 2006;104:322–345.

22. Burnstein AL, WuDunn D, Knotts SL, Catoira Y, Cantor LB. Conjunctival advancement versus nonincisional treatment for late-onset glaucoma filtering bleb leaks. *Ophthalmology*. Jan 2002;109(1):71–75.

23. Harris LD, Yang G, Feldman RM, et al. Autologous conjunctival resurfacing of leaking filtering blebs. *Ophthalmology*. Sept 2000;107(9):1675–1680.

24. Petursson GJ, Fraunfelder FT. Repair of an inadvertent buttonhole or leaking filtering bleb. *Arch Ophthalmol*. May 1979;97(5):926–927.

25. Blok MD, Kok JH, van Mil C, Greve EL, Kijlstra A. Use of the Megasoft Bandage Lens for treatment of complications after trabeculectomy. *Am J Ophthalmol*. Sept 15 1990;110(3):264–268.

26. Budenz DL, Chen PP, Weaver YK. Conjunctival advancement for late-onset filtering bleb leaks: indications and outcomes. *Arch Ophthalmol*. Aug 1999;117(8):1014–1019.

27. Palmberg P, Zacchei AC. Compression sutures: a new treatment for leaking or painful filtering blebs [ARVO abstract 2032]. *Invest Ophthalmol Vis Sci*. 1996;37(3):S444.

28. Choudhri SA, Herndon LW, Damji KF, Allingham RR, Shields MB. Efficacy of autologous blood injection for treating overfiltering or leaking blebs after glaucoma surgery. *Am J Ophthalmol*. Apr 1997;123(4):554–555.

29. Leen MM, Moster MR, Katz LJ, Terebuh AK, Schmidt CM, Spaeth GL. Management of overfiltering and leaking blebs with autologous blood injection. *Arch Ophthalmol*. Aug 1995;113(8):1050–1055.

30. Awan KJ, Spaeth PG. Use of isobutyl-2-cyanoacrylate tissue adhesive in the repair of conjunctival fistula in filtering procedures for glaucoma. *Ann Ophthalmol*. Aug 1974;6(8):851–853.

31. Zalta AH, Wieder RH. Closure of leaking filtering blebs with cyanoacrylate tissue adhesive. *Br J Ophthalmol*. Mar 1991;75(3):170–173.

32. Shields MB, Scroggs MW, Sloop CM, Simmons RB. Clinical and histopathologic observations concerning hypotony after trabeculectomy with adjunctive mitomycin C. *Am J Ophthalmol*. Dec 15 1993;116(6):673–683.

33. Geyer O. Management of large, leaking, and inadvertent filtering blebs with the neodymium:YAG laser. *Ophthalmology*. Jun 1998;105(6):983–987.

34. Lynch MG, Roesch M, Brown RH. Remodeling filtering blebs with the neodymium:YAG laser. *Ophthalmology*. Oct 1996;103(10):1700–1705.

35. Reynolds AC, Skuta GL, Monlux R, Johnson J. Management of blebitis by members of the American Glaucoma Society: a survey. *J Glaucoma*. Aug 2001;10(4):340–347.

36. Busbee BG, Recchia FM, Kaiser R, Nagra P, Rosenblatt B, Pearlman RB. Bleb-associated endophthalmitis: clinical characteristics and visual outcomes. *Ophthalmology*. Aug 2004;111(8):1495–1503; discussion 1503.

37. Ceballos EM, Gedde SJ. Bleb infections after glaucoma filtering surgery. *Comprehensive Ophthalmology Update*. 2000;1(5):287–292.

38. Shah GK, Stein JD, Sharma S, et al. Visual outcomes following the use of intravitreal steroids in the treatment of postoperative endophthalmitis. *Ophthalmology*. Mar 2000;107(3):486–489.

39. Wisniewski SR, Capone A, Kelsey SF, Groer-Fitzgerald S, Lambert HM, Doft BH. Characteristics after cataract extraction or secondary lens implantation among patients screened for the Endophthalmitis Vitrectomy Study. *Ophthalmology*. Jul 2000;107(7):1274–1282.

40. Ayyala RS, Bellows AR, Thomas JV, Hutchinson BT. Bleb infections: clinically different courses of "blebitis" and endophthalmitis. *Ophthalmic Surg Lasers*. Jun 1997;28(6):452–460.

25

PTOSIS

MARC R. CRIDEN

PTOSIS

Ptosis of the upper eyelids is a well-known complication of most forms of ocular surgery. The incidence of ptosis following glaucoma surgery is reported to range from 6 to 12%.[1, 2] The etiology has not been entirely established; however, it is believed to be multifactorial, and several contributing factors have been identified. Identification of the etiology is important since this will often dictate the management. The ptosis may be transient, resolving within days, or persistent. The management of acquired ptosis following glaucoma surgery is critical since surgical over correction can expose a filtering bleb and lead to serious complications, including endophthalmitis.

ETIOLOGY AND PREVENTION

Transient ptosis following surgery is more common than persistent ptosis and may recover within 12 to 72 hours. It may be caused by anesthetic, lid edema, or hematoma formation in the eyelid or muscle. A retrobulbar or peribulbar block with lidocaine may affect the levator muscle. Similarly, direct infiltration of the eyelid will block the distal fibers of the oculomotor nerve.

The primary factors postulated to cause ptosis include muscle or nerve damage from local block,[3] a superior rectus bridle suture or corneal traction suture,[4] general anesthesia, eyelid edema, traction applied by the speculum, and levator aponeurosis dehiscence.[5]

The lid speculum has been identified as a cause of ptosis regardless of the type of ocular surgery. Superior forces are placed on the upper eyelid while a superior bridle suture or corneal traction suture directs forces downward. These opposing forces may cause a stretching or frank dehiscence of the levator aponeurosis. One study specifically looked at the role of the bridle suture and did not find a significant contribution to ptosis development versus those cases that did not use a bridle suture. Rather, lid edema, neuromuscular block, and the lid speculum itself were identified as causative factors.[6]

It has been suggested that prolonged eyelid edema leads to disinsertion of the levator aponeurosis in susceptible populations, such as the elderly.[5] This has not been borne out in other studies;[3] however, some of the same factors that cause prolonged edema may also cause persistent ptosis, specifically inflammation.[7] Common inflammatory triggers include size of conjunctival incision, exposed sutures, hematoma formation, and medicamentosa. The edema typically resolves after removing the offending agent or treating the inflammation.

Glaucoma surgeries often involve incisions near the superior conjunctival fornix. Closure of the conjunctival wound of a limbus-based trabeculectomy may result in tethering of the conjunctiva and tractional ptosis with possible restrictive strabismus. Revision of filtering blebs with excision of thin, ischemic conjunctiva and advancement of healthier conjunctiva shortens the distance between the limbus and the fornix and may directly cause tractional ptosis. To prevent this, a relaxing incision in the fornix may be made when advancing conjunctiva. A similar technique may be useful to treat the traction.

ANESTHESIA

Retrobulbar with or without orbicularis blocks are the preferred choice of anesthesia for glaucoma surgery and are considered very safe, effective, and transient. Bupivicaine (0.5% – 0.75%) and lidocaine (1% – 2%) without epinephrine are the most commonly used. Recently, hyaluronidase has become more commercially available. This supplement to local anesthesia blocks improves the tissue spread of the anesthetic by breaking down connective tissue ground substance and increasing diffusion, thus requiring less anesthetic. Although this may aid anesthesia efficacy, it may also add to eyelid akinesia and ptosis.

Bupivicaine has a duration of action of approximately 6 hours, with lidocaine lasting 30 minutes. If the ptosis lasts significantly longer than the expected duration of action, then the toxic effects of these agents must be considered.[8] Recovery from the myotoxic effects is known to occur but is often slow and may require several months.

Subconjunctival anesthesia using mepivacaine 2% and bupivacaine 0.75% has been shown to be an effective alternative to peribulbar blocks and thus decrease the complication risk of hemorrhage and toxic effects.[9]

MANAGEMENT

Any of these factors that contribute to transient ptosis may also lead to permanent ptosis even if some resolution has occurred. If it has been determined that the ptosis is not transient and requires correction, then several options are available. No clear consensus exists for how long to wait before declaring postoperative ptosis irreversible. Three months is the typical duration for observation; however, intervention may be delayed if improvement has not reached a stable plateau.

The ptosis evaluation consists of determining the cause as specifically as possible (involutional, neurogenic, myogenic, mechanical), measuring the marginal reflex distance 1 (MRD1), lid crease position, and levator excursion. These will help in determining the most appropriate surgical technique. It is also imperative to evaluate the size and position of the filtering bleb. Overcorrecting the lid height and exposing the filtering bleb will place it at high risk for breakdown with leakage and possible endophthalmitis. The surgical goal of raising the lid is to maximize the visual field while still providing adequate coverage of the filtering bleb. Patients should be made aware that a successful surgical outcome might still result in slight lid height asymmetry.

Both external and internal approaches for surgical repair are acceptable. An external approach directly addresses the aponeurotic dehiscence and corrects it by advancement. This technique works for both mild and severe cases of ptosis. The posterior transconjunctival approach is accomplished by a conjunctival-Mullerectomy (Putterman procedure). This approach is also very safe, reproducible, and rarely results in overcorrection. It is best suited for ptosis of 2 mm or less.[10]

CONCLUSION

Ptosis is an inherent risk of any intraocular surgical procedure, and this possibility should always be included as part of any preoperative discussion. Fortunately, most cases of postoperative ptosis are transient. With careful planning regarding anesthesia and instrumentation, the risk can be minimized. Attention to lid speculum tension, surgical duration, and postoperative inflammation can also minimize the rate and severity of post-trabeculectomy ptosis. It is reasonable to exercise initial conservative management with observation prior to pursuing surgical repair. Surgical repair should respect the presence of a filtering bleb to maintain its integrity.

COMMENTARY

ROBERT J. NOECKER

Dr. Criden discusses many of the factors that can lead to the recognized complication of ptosis following glaucoma surgery. Although some of these issues may be inherent in the surgery, some of the risks may be mitigated by changes in technique.

As a general rule, the less tension that is placed on the eyelid, the less chance for eyelid tissue attenuation, which is where the choice of speculum becomes important. While exposure is of paramount importance in glaucoma surgery, the amount of tension on eyelid structure should be minimized. Use of a flexible speculum, such as a Barraquer speculum, may be less traumatic to the levator than a fixed speculum. If the fixed speculum is used, then the minimum amount of acceptable opening should be used.

Peribulbar and retrobulbar blocks can cause eyelid tissue stretching. Use of lidocaine gel preoperatively and subconjunctival lidocaine intraoperatively can help to eliminate or reduce the need for anesthesia given via the peribulbar or retrobulbar route. I have found that administering subconjunctival lidocaine with mitomycin-C at the beginning of the case provides more than adequate anesthesia for a trabeculectomy.

Antiinflammatory therapy to minimize postoperative tissue swelling is also paramount in preventing ptosis. Intravenous administration of dexamethasone intraoperatively can help improve comfort and decrease edema. Intracameral dexamethasone and sub-Tenon's triamcinolone during surgery can create a very quiet postoperative environment with minimal periocular swelling.

Lastly, avoiding scarring and trauma in the superior fornices can help to limit edema. Clear corneal traction sutures avoid the tension on the superior rectus that muscle traction sutures place. Consideration should be given to avoiding posterior conjunctival incisions in patients who are at risk for ptosis. Fornix-based conjunctival incisions may reduce that risk. When preventative approaches are undertaken, the incidence of ptosis can be minimized with modern glaucoma surgical techniques. These technique changes to reduce ptosis should be balanced against the reason why an alternative technique is used and possible effects on surgical success.

REFERENCES

1. Jampel H, Musch D, Gillepsie B, Lichter P, Wright M, Guire K. Perioperative complications of trabeculectomy in the Collaborative Initial Glaucoma Treatment Study (CIGITS). *Am JOphthalmol.* 2005;140(1):16–22.

2. Song M, Shin D, Spoor T. Incidence of ptosis following trabeculectomy: A comparative study. *Korean JOphthalmol.* 1996;10:97–103.

3. Kaplan L, Jaffe N, Clayman H. Ptosis and cataract surgery. A multivariant computer analysis and retrospective study. *Ophthalmology.* 1985;92:237–242.

4. Alpar J. Acquired ptosis following cataract and glaucoma surgery. *Glaucoma*. 1982;4:66–68.
5. Paris G, Quickert M. Disinsertion of the levator aponeurosis superioris muscle after cataract surgery. *Am JOphthalmol*. 1976;81:337.
6. Patel JI, Blount M, Jones C. Surgical blepharoptosis—the bridle suture factor? *Eye (Lond)*. Sept 2002;16(5):535–537.
7. Feibel R, Custer P, Gordon M. Postcataract ptosis: A randomized, double-masked comparison of peribulbar and retrobulbar anesthesia. *Ophthalmology*. 1993;100: 660–665.
8. Ropo A, Ruusuvaara P, Paloheimo M, Maunuksela EL, Nikki P. Periocular anaesthesia: technique, effectiveness and complications with special reference to postoperative ptosis. *Acta Ophthalmol (Copenh)*. Dec 1990;68(6):728–732.
9. Azuara-Blanco A, Moster M, Marr B. Subjunctival versus peribular anesthesia in trabeculectomy: a prospective randomized study. *Ophthalmic Surg Lasers*. 1997;28:896.
10. Michels K, Vagefi M, Zwick O, Torres J, Seiff S, Dailey R. Muller muscle-conjunctiva resection to correct ptosis in high-risk patients. *Ophthalmic Plast Reconstruct Surg*. 2007;23(5):363–366.

E. COMPLICATIONS OF ANTIFIBROTIC AGENTS

26

CORNEAL COMPLICATIONS

CLARK L. SPRINGS

CORNEAL COMPLICATIONS

The desired effects of antifibrotic agents 5-fluorouracil (5-FU) and mitomycin-C (MMC) in glaucoma filtration surgery result from their ability to limit postoperative scarring by inhibiting vascular proliferation and fibroblastic transformation. However, these same mechanisms of action can have deleterious effects on surrounding normal tissues such as the cornea. Knowing how to use these agents is important in preventing antifibrotic-related complications.

MECHANISM OF ACTION OF 5-FLUOROURACIL AND MITOMYCIN-C

5-FU is an inhibitor of DNA synthesis, specifically thymidylate synthetase, and blocks thymidine from being incorporated into DNA. In addition to affecting DNA synthesis, 5-FU also may be incorporated into RNA, interfering with RNA synthesis and therefore protein synthesis. Thus, it is more toxic to actively proliferating cells.[1, 2] In glaucoma filtration surgery, 5-FU is generally administered intraoperatively (50 mg/mL for 5 minutes). 5-FU can also be administered as a subconjunctival injection postoperatively with a dosage of 5.0–7.5 mg in 0.1–0.15 mL solution directly from the 50 mg/mL bottle. A series of injections may be given over several weeks and titrated based on clinical response. In addition to glaucoma filtration surgery, 5-FU has also been used for other ophthalmic applications such as pterygium surgery, lacrimal surgery, and during vitrectomy to prevent proliferative vitreoretinopathy.[1]

MMC is an alkylating agent that crosslinks DNA.[3] It requires enzymatic activation via cytochrome p450 prior to exerting its inhibitory effects on DNA synthesis. MMC activity is independent of cell cycle and affects both actively replicating and nonreplicating cells.[4] However, variations in enzymatic activity among individuals may contribute to the differences in efficacy, as well as toxicity of MMC.[5] In glaucoma filtration surgery, MMC is typically administered as a single intraoperative application. It is applied after dissection of the conjunctival flap and prior to the formation of the scleral flap. Most surgeons use a dose of 0.1–0.5 mg/mL with an exposure time of 1–5 minutes depending upon the clinical indication. MMC use has also been well established for refractive surgery to prevent corneal haze after photorefractive keratectomy in patients at high risk of developing corneal haze, pterygium surgery, and corneal intraepithelial neoplasia.[3] For more information on 5-FU and MMC in glaucoma surgery, see Chapter 3.

DELAYED CORNEAL EPITHELIOPATHY AND LIMBAL STEM CELL DEFICIENCY

The most frequently observed complication of 5-FU is corneal epithelial toxicity, occurring in 50%–100% of eyes undergoing more than one injection per week.[6] Its effects are dose dependent and more common with total doses of more than 100 mg.[7] Epithelial toxicity can range from mild epitheliopathy, frank corneal epithelial defects, whorl-like epitheliopathy (indicating partial limbal stem cell deficiency) to complete limbal stem cell deficiency (Figure 26.1). Epithelial defects typically resolve in 1–2 weeks after cessation of 5-FU, but can persist for up to 4 weeks.[8, 9] However, more severe complications can develop, such as bacterial keratitis, corneal melting, and perforation.[6] It is important to note that epithelial complications are uncommon with a single *intraoperative* application of 5-FU.[2]

5-FU is a cell-cycle-specific antimetabolite and preferentially affects the rapidly proliferating cells of the corneal epithelium. It, therefore, affects the more mitotically active basal layers of the corneal epithelium. Limbal stem cells are more resistant to the effects of 5-FU due to a slower cell cycle than basal epithelial cells. However, glaucoma patients may be more susceptible to limbal stem cell toxicity due to a shortened limbal stem cell cycle because of more rapid regeneration due to epithelial stressors, such as ocular surface disease and medicamentosa, from topical glaucoma

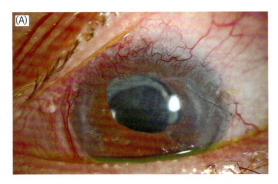

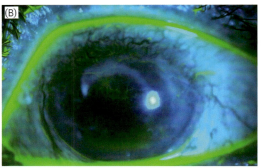

FIGURE 26.1 Corneal opacification and neovascularization secondary to limbal stem cell deficiency (A) and its fluorescein staining pattern (B).

therapy.[10] A case of limbal stem cell deficiency requiring limbal stem cell transplantation was reported by Manche et al in a patient receiving both intraoperative MMC and postoperative 5-FU.[11] Traverso et al described a technique to reduce reflux of 5-FU into the tear film by applying a swab to the injection site immediately after injection, which resulted in a significant reduction in epithelial complications.[12]

Corneal epithelial complications are rare following one-time intraoperative application of MMC. In refractive surgery where MMC is applied to bare corneal stroma on a cellulose corneal light shield at 0.2–0.4 mg/mL for up to 2 minutes, epithelialization occurs at the same rate as in virgin eyes.[13] If MMC drops are administered, epithelial complications and tear film disturbance are common, but typically resolve after cessation of therapy.[14, 15] Severe sight-threatening complications have been reported following usage of MMC drops, often in the presence of a corneal or conjunctival epithelial defect. Dudney and coauthors reported a case of limbal stem cell deficiency in a patient with corneal epithelial neoplasia who received 5, 1-week courses of 0.4 mg/mL MMC.[16] Rubinfeld and coauthors reported a series of 10 patients who developed severe complications such as corneal edema, scleral and corneal melting, corneal perforation, iritis, and secondary glaucoma after receiving 0.2 mg/mL MMC drops following pterygium surgery with no autograft for 3–28 days.[17] Since this report, the use of MMC drops after pterygium surgery has fallen out of favor.

INDUCED ASTIGMATISM

Trabeculectomy has a significant effect on corneal curvature. Dietze et al found mean central corneal astigmatism to increase by 1.4 D after trabeculectomy, but by 12 weeks it returned to within 1 D of preoperative levels in 12 of 13 patients.[18] Cunliffe and coauthors found an induction of with-the-rule (WTR) astigmatism following trabeculectomy without MMC that returned to preoperative levels by 2 months.[19] Claridge and coauthors found the induced WTR astigmatism following trabeculectomy was 2.63 D at 1 month, which stabilized but persisted at 3 months at 1.24 D.[20] Reasons proposed for the induction of WTR astigmatism are from tight scleral flap sutures and a reduction in internal corneal radius by the creation of the internal sclerostomy.

There is no significant association between 5-FU use in trabeculectomy and corneal astigmatism. However, trabeculectomy with MMC has been associated with less WTR astigmatism than non-MMC trabeculectomy, presumably due to its inhibitory effect on wound healing.[21] Hong and coauthors found induced WTR astigmatism following trabeculectomy without MMC was 2.63 D one month postoperatively and 1.42 D 12 months postoperatively. In trabeculectomy with MMC, the induced WTR astigmatism was significantly less at 1.01 and –0.34 D at one and 12 months postoperatively, respectively. Kook and coauthors found similar results with regard to induced astigmatism and MMC trabeculectomy; additionally, they found that these changes were similar regardless of the preoperative status of the cornea, whether WTR or against-the-rule.[22]

CORNEAL ENDOTHELIAL TOXICITY

The contributory role of antimetabolites in corneal endothelial cell loss is difficult to ascertain due to multiple confounding factors. Glaucoma patients tend to have a lower endothelial cell count than controls. Further, endothelial cell count is inversely proportional to intraocular pressure and the number of topical glaucoma medications used.[23] Additional perioperative conditions may exist that can contribute to an accelerated rate of endothelial cell loss in glaucoma patients undergoing filtration surgery, such as postoperative hypotony with flat anterior chamber, postoperative inflammation, laser iridotomy, and topical medications.

Regardless, in a laboratory model, Nuyts and coauthors found that MMC and 5-FU are toxic to the endothelium when applied at a higher concentration and duration than used in clinical practice. Interestingly, however, the authors concluded that at concentrations and durations used in clinical practice, toxicity would not be expected, unless there were unusual circumstances allowing for access of the antimetabolite into the anterior chamber.[24] Chang and coauthors demonstrated a dose-dependent increase in endothelial apoptosis, corneal thickness, and subsequent loss of corneal clarity in rabbit eyes after a single application of MMC.[25]

Clinically, a 15% decrease in endothelial cell density was reported at 1 year following 5-FU injections.[9] Similarly, MMC-assisted trabeculectomy has been associated with a 10%–11% greater endothelial cell loss in comparison to a control group with no antifibrotic use.[26] Fukuchi and colleagues reported 2 patients with moderate corneal guttata who developed severe endothelial damage after trabeculectomy with MMC. However, in both patients, a flat or shallow anterior chamber was present postoperatively, which is a known risk factor for endothelial cell loss.[27, 28] Mohammadpour and coauthors reported a case of inferior corneal decompensation following MMC trabeculectomy in a patient with uveitic glaucoma. The authors speculate that the inferior cornea was exposed to MMC for a prolonged period due to trapped MMC in the lower conjunctival fornix while the eye was infraducted during surgery.[29]

In refractive surgery, MMC is usually applied to bare corneal stroma following excimer laser ablation in similar concentrations and durations as in glaucoma filtration surgery. Because the corneal epithelial barrier is bypassed, this method of MMC application leads to a higher anterior chamber concentration than would be expected in glaucoma filtration surgery.[30] However, to date no reports of corneal edema have been reported following intraoperative MMC application in refractive surgery. One case of permanent corneal edema was reported following MMC use in phototherapeutic keratectomy with only postoperative drop use (14 postoperative drops of 0.2 mg/mL MMC); there was not a single intraoperative application.[31] No significant endothelial cell loss or change in endothelial cell morphology was seen at 18 months following application of 0.2 mg/mL MMC for 12 seconds following photorefractive keratectomy to the corneal stroma.[32] However, Chayet and coauthors reported a 9% rate of endothelial cell loss in photorefractive keratectomy following a 30-second intraoperative application of 0.2 mg/mL MMC.[33] In pterygium surgery, Avisar and coauthors found a 21% reduction of endothelial cell loss following a single 5 minute application of 0.2 mg/mL MMC.[34]

CONCLUSION

Corneal complications following the judicious use of antifibrotic agents in glaucoma filtration surgery are generally mild, epithelial-related, and often self-limited without the need for significant intervention. More severe and long-term complications such as limbal stem cell deficiency and corneal decompensation are possible but are fortunately rare.

DR. Springs was supported by an Unrestricted Grant from Research to Prevent Blindness to the Glick Eye Institute, Indiana University School of Medicine.

COMMENTARY
TONY REALINI

Although there can be no question that the application of antifibrotic agents in glaucoma surgery has improved surgical success rates, such benefits do not come without cost. Corneal complications following antifibrotic exposure—particularly 5-FU—are common and can be dose-limiting and thus can impact surgical success. Fortunately, the vast majority of complications are self-limiting and resolve in short order; vision-threatening corneal complications of these agents are rare.

From a clinical standpoint, management of corneal complications of antifibrotic therapy should be aimed at prevention. Several perioperative steps can be taken to reduce the occurrence of these issues. First, choose the correct agent for the patient. Patients with concomitant ocular surface disease may be better suited to MMC therapy over 5-FU therapy, as the corneal epithelium side effect profile of MMC is more favorable. Second, minimize exposure to the smallest dose necessary. There are as many combinations of MMC concentration and exposure time as there are glaucoma surgeons, but it is worth considering that we have minimal data supporting the use of more versus less drug for a given patient. Some surgeons utilize antifibrotic therapy uniformly in all cases, but there are certainly some patients who do not require it for surgical success, so there may be some overuse of these agents. Third, irrigate, irrigate, irrigate! After exposure, copiously irrigate the ocular surface—both the scleral bed and the cornea—with at least 50 mL of balanced salt solution to terminate tissue exposure. When subconjunctival 5-FU is used postoperatively, the injection site can be sealed with a cotton applicator to minimize egress of 5-FU to the ocular surface. Fourth, a clinical pearl: if you use a sponge-based corneal protector and leave it in place during antifibrotic exposure, replace it after irrigation because it has undoubtedly absorbed some of the drug and if not replaced will act as a slow-release reservoir on the cornea for the remainder of the case.

Antifibrotic agents represent perhaps the single most important improvement to Cairns' trabeculectomy procedure in the more than 40 years since its original description. Used judiciously, they can offer maximal benefit with minimal risk.

REFERENCES

1. Abraham LM, Selva D, Casson R, Leibovitch I. The clinical applications of fluorouracil in ophthalmic practice. *Drugs.* 2007;67(2):237–255.
2. Lama PJ, Fechtner RD. Antifibrotics and wound healing in glaucoma surgery. *Surv Ophthalmol.* May-Jun 2003;48(3):314–346.
3. Abraham LM, Selva D, Casson R, Leibovitch I. Mitomycin: clinical applications in ophthalmic practice. *Drugs.* 2006;66(3):321–340.
4. Smith S, D'Amore PA, Dreyer EB. Comparative toxicity of mitomycin C and 5-fluorouracil in vitro. *Am J Ophthalmol.* Sept 15 1994;118(3):332–337.
5. Cummings J, Spanswick VJ, Tomasz M, Smyth JF. Enzymology of mitomycin C metabolic activation in tumour tissue: implications for enzyme-directed bioreductive drug development. *Biochem Pharmacol.* Aug 15 1998;56(4):405–414.
6. Lee DA, Hersh P, Kersten D, Melamed S. Complications of subconjunctival 5-fluorouracil following glaucoma filtering surgery. *Ophthalmic Surg.* Mar 1987;18(3):187–190.
7. Shapiro MS, Thoft RA, Friend J, Parrish RK, Gressel MG. 5-Fluorouracil toxicity to the ocular surface epithelium. *Invest Ophthalmol Vis Sci.* Apr 1985;26(4):580–583.
8. Fluorouracil Filtering Surgery Study one-year follow-up. The Fluorouracil Filtering Surgery Study Group. *Am J Ophthalmol.* Dec 15 1989;108(6):625–635.
9. Knapp A, Heuer DK, Stern GA, Driebe WT Jr. Serious corneal complications of glaucoma filtering surgery with postoperative 5-fluorouracil. *Am J Ophthalmol.* Feb 15 1987;103(2):183–187.
10. Tseng SC, Zhang SH. Limbal epithelium is more resistant to 5-fluorouracil toxicity than corneal epithelium. *Cornea.* Jul 1995;14(4):394–401.
11. Manche EE, Afshari MA, Singh K. Delayed corneal epitheliopathy after antimetabolite-augmented trabeculectomy. *J Glaucoma.* Aug 1998;7(4):237–239.
12. Traverso CE, Facino M, Murialdo U, Corazza M, Gandolfo E, Calabria G. Decreased corneal complications after no-reflux, low-dose 5 fluorouracil subconjunctival injection following trabeculectomy. *Int Ophthalmol.* 1994;18(4):247–250.
13. Lacayo GO, 3rd, Majmudar PA. How and when to use mitomycin-C in refractive surgery. *Curr Opin Ophthalmol.* Aug 2005;16(4):256–259.
14. Frucht-Pery J, Sugar J, Baum J, et al. Mitomycin C treatment for conjunctival-corneal intraepithelial neoplasia: a multicenter experience. *Ophthalmology.* Dec 1997;104(12):2085–2093.
15. Dogru M, Erturk H, Shimazaki J, Tsubota K, Gul M. Tear function and ocular surface changes with topical mitomycin (MMC) treatment for primary corneal intraepithelial neoplasia. *Cornea.* Oct 2003;22(7):627–639.
16. Dudney BW, Malecha MA. Limbal stem cell deficiency following topical mitomycin C treatment of conjunctival-corneal intraepithelial neoplasia. *Am J Ophthalmol.* May 2004;137(5):950–951.
17. Rubinfeld RS, Pfister RR, Stein RM, et al. Serious complications of topical mitomycin-C after pterygium surgery. *Ophthalmology.* Nov 1992;99(11):1647–1654.
18. Dietze PJ, Oram O, Kohnen T, Feldman RM, Koch DD, Gross RL. Visual function following trabeculectomy: effect on corneal topography and contrast sensitivity. *J Glaucoma.* Apr 1997;6(2):99–103.
19. Cunliffe IA, Dapling RB, West J, Longstaff S. A prospective study examining the changes in factors that affect visual acuity following trabeculectomy. *Eye.* 1992;6(Pt 6):618–622.
20. Claridge KG, Galbraith JK, Karmel V, Bates AK. The effect of trabeculectomy on refraction, keratometry and corneal topography. *Eye.* 1995;9(Pt 3):292–298.
21. Hong YJ, Choe CM, Lee YG, Chung HS, Kim HK. The effect of mitomycin-C on postoperative corneal astigmatism in trabeculectomy and a triple procedure. *Ophthalmic Surg Lasers.* Jun 1998;29(6):484–489.
22. Kook MS, Kim HB, Lee SU. Short-term effect of mitomycin-C augmented trabeculectomy on

axial length and corneal astigmatism. *J Cataract Refract Surg.* Apr 2001;27(4):518–523.

23. Gagnon MM, Boisjoly HM, Brunette I, Charest M, Amyot M. Corneal endothelial cell density in glaucoma. *Cornea.* May 1997;16(3):314–318.

24. Nuyts RM, Pels E, Greve EL. The effects of 5-fluorouracil and mitomycin C on the corneal endothelium. *Curr Eye Res.* Jun 1992;11(6):565–570.

25. Chang SW. Early corneal edema following topical application of mitomycin-C. *J Cataract Refract Surg.* Aug 2004;30(8):1742–1750.

26. Sihota R, Sharma T, Agarwal HC. Intraoperative mitomycin C and the corneal endothelium. *Acta Ophthalmol Scand.* Feb 1998;76(1):80–82.

27. Fiore PM, Richter CU, Arzeno G, et al. The effect of anterior chamber depth on endothelial cell count after filtration surgery. *Arch Ophthalmol.* Nov 1989;107(11):1609–1611.

28. Smith DL, Skuta GL, Lindenmuth KA, Musch DC, Bergstrom TJ. The effect of glaucoma filtering surgery on corneal endothelial cell density. *Ophthalmic Surg.* May 1991;22(5):251–255.

29. Mohammadpour M, Jabbarvand M, Javadi MA. Focal corneal decompensation after filtering surgery with mitomycin C. *Cornea.* Dec 2007;26(10):1285–1287.

30. Song JS, Kim JH, Yang M, Sul D, Kim HM. Mitomycin-C concentration in cornea and aqueous humor and apoptosis in the stroma after topical mitomycin-C application: effects of mitomycin-C application time and concentration. *Cornea.* May 2007;26(4):461–467.

31. Pfister RR. Permanent corneal edema resulting from the treatment of PTK corneal haze with mitomycin: a case report. *Cornea.* Oct 2004;23(7):744–747.

32. Goldsberry DH, Epstein RJ, Majmudar PA, et al. Effect of mitomycin C on the corneal endothelium when used for corneal subepithelial haze prophylaxis following photorefractive keratectomy. *J Refract Surg.* Sept 2007;23(7):724–727.

33. Morales AJ, Zadok D, Mora-Retana R, Martinez-Gama E, Robledo NE, Chayet AS. Intraoperative mitomycin and corneal endothelium after photorefractive keratectomy. *Am J Ophthalmol.* Sept 2006;142(3):400–404.

34. Avisar R, Avisar I, Bahar I, Weinberger D. Effect of mitomycin C in pterygium surgery on corneal endothelium. *Cornea.* Jun 2008;27(5):559–561.

27

NONCORNEAL COMPLICATIONS

ANURAG SHRIVASTAVA AND KULDEV SINGH

NONCORNEAL COMPLICATIONS

Most glaucoma specialists advocate the use of 5-fluorouracil (5-FU) and mitomycin-C (MMC) in various concentrations during the intra-operative and postoperative periods to help inhibit postoperative scarring, the primary cause of filtration surgery failure. Although the increased use of antifibrotic agents as adjunctive therapy to guarded filtration surgery has improved the likelihood of operative success,[1–5] there are many additional complications associated with this class of medications.[3,6–10] It is the nature of filtration surgery as it is performed today that successful drainage of aqueous comes with a price. Any adjunct that improves the intraocular pressure (IOP)-lowering success of surgery must be assessed in light of this increased risk.

LEAKING BLEB

A leaking bleb is one of the most common complications seen after trabeculectomy and may occur at any point postoperatively. This complication has been reported with an incidence ranging between 17% and 42% according to one review.[11] More recent estimates have been somewhat lower, at between 8% and 14.6%.[8,12] The longer the postoperative follow-up, the greater the cumulative likelihood of bleb leakage. It is imperative that the bleb be checked periodically for leaks, primarily through examination and standard Seidel testing.[13,14] Use of antifibrotic therapy is associated with increased formation of thin-walled cystic blebs, which are more likely to result in both short-term and long-term complications.[11,15,16] The timing of a bleb leak will dictate management. Many early postoperative bleb leaks resolve without intervention but can significantly decrease the likelihood of trabeculectomy success.[17]

Early postoperative bleb leaks are often attributed to surgical technique and can generally be avoided by use of appropriate blunt instruments and careful attention to surgical detail. The simple use of nontoothed forceps when handling the conjunctiva can prevent small buttonhole conjunctival tears, which often result in early postoperative bleb leaks. However, even with careful manipulation, friable conjunctival tissue can be prone to small tears.[18] While some have advocated the use of light cautery, or even tissue adhesives[19] to close bleb leaks, the use of such techniques has diminished in the antifibrotic era. Intraoperative suturing of buttonholes is definitive. Depending on location of the buttonhole and the location of the conjunctival incision, buttonholes may be incorporated into the incisions or may be closed with a purse string suture of 9–0 to 11–0. (For more details, see Chapter 4.) Limbus-based flaps are less likely to be associated with early postoperative wound leakage than fornix-based flaps,[20–22] regardless of the suture material or technique. However, it should be noted that in general, early postoperative wound leakage is rarely a problem, regardless of incision location, if the procedure is performed with care. Although, even with appropriate surgical technique, slow bleb leaks and buttonholes may go undetected and may need to be assessed and managed postoperatively. Such bleb leaks are underdiagnosed when physicians do not routinely perform Seidel testing in the postoperative period.

Minor bleb leaks in the early postoperative period can be treated conservatively as they often resolve spontaneously without intervention, although they are a risk factor for surgical failure.[17] Techniques that have been described to treat such leaks (other than simple observation) include placement of a large diameter bandage contact lens,[19,23,24] symblepharon rings,[25] cyanoacrylate glue,[26, 27] Simmons shell,[28,29] pressure patching,[30] and aqueous suppression.[31] In the absence of irido-corneal or lenticulo-corneal touch, conservative therapy with cycloplegics, with or without aqueous suppression, in conjunction with topical antibiotic coverage may be adequate. Small buttonholes that evaded careful intraoperative inspection generally prove to be self-limited, although patients with early postoperative hypotony must be examined frequently in the postoperative period to monitor for choroidal effusion/hemorrhage, infection, and corneal decompensation (see Chapter 10).

Late bleb leakage is most often associated with thin-walled cystic blebs, which more commonly develop after treatment with antifibrotic agents, particularly MMC.[11,15,16] Along with the previously described conservative techniques, autologous blood injections,[32–36] needle revision[37,38] with or without antifibrotics, and continuous wave Nd:YAG laser application[39,40] have been shown to be associated with variable success. Burnstein et al reported a retrospective series of 51 eyes comparing long-term outcomes of late bleb leak management using conservative therapies (aqueous suppression, bandage contact lenses, cyanoacrylate glue, autologous blood injections) and surgical revision (conjunctival advancement with preservation of the preexisting bleb). In this series, the surgical revision group had a Kaplan-Meier cumulative probability of success twice that of the conservatively treated group (0.42 versus 0.8, respectively, at 2 years), with the surgical group being associated with a dramatically lower incidence of infection (0 of 34 eyes) than the nonincisional group (6 of 37 eyes).[30] Budenz et al reported similar results in a retrospective review demonstrating success with conjunctival advancement in 22 of 24 eyes with late bleb leaks.[24] Azusa recently described a case series of 6 patients with intractable late-onset bleb leaks that were all successfully repaired utilizing amniotic patch grafts instead of conjunctival advancement.[41] However, Budenz and Rauscher have described a similar series where amniotic grafting had a significant failure rate approaching 50%.[42,43] We prefer surgical revision of late bleb leaks in thin-walled cystic blebs with chronic hypotony, sometimes by resecting a portion or all of the affected conjunctiva and replacing it with an advancement, rotational, or free conjunctival graft.[44] Further study into the best

OVERFILTRATION

While overfiltration following trabeculectomy is less frequent than following full-thickness procedures,[45, 46] the almost universal use of antimetabolites has led to an increased risk of exuberant filtration and hypotony.[47] Overfiltration in partial-thickness procedures may also be related to surgical technique, specifically loose suturing of the scleral flap or premature suture lysis. The techniques available to help reduce the likelihood of overfiltration overlap with those used to avoid late bleb leaks and thin cystic blebs. The goal is to avoid overfiltration by optimizing resistance to outflow via the fistula.

Intraoperatively, we prefer the use of at least 2, 10–0 nylon sutures on the nasal and temporal sides of a semicircular, rectangular, or triangular scleral flap with moderate tension utilizing slip knots. Flow through the sclerostomy is further checked at the flap with multiple dry surgical spear sponges, and additional sutures are placed if aqueous egress is determined to be excessive. While antifibrotic drugs may not directly contribute to overfiltration in most cases, these agents prevent healing that would limit excessive flow. One should aim for significant flap resistance, little early postoperative flow, and moderately higher IOP in the early postoperative period when antifibrotics are used. Great care should be taken to avoid inadvertently cutting or puncturing the scleral flap, particularly when using antifibrotics. If this scenario occurs, the risk of postoperative overfiltration is high. Suture closure or even a patch graft to limit outflow may be required to achieve adequately low flow. While persistent overfiltration is the primary reason for hypotony following antimetabolite-augmented trabeculectomy, direct MMC toxicity to the ciliary body may decrease aqueous humor production, thereby further contributing to the hypotony.[48]

In the postoperative period, laser remodeling,[39,40] bandage contact lens,[23,24] autologous blood injections,[32–36] compression suturing,[49,50] Simmons shell,[28,29] gas/viscoelastic injection,[51] and surgical revision (see below) have all been advocated for overfiltration with variable results. Choice of surgical technique should be based on the cause of overfiltration. In some cases hypotony is caused by a low-resistance, thin-walled bleb and in others by a sclerostomy that is too wide open. Recent reviews of bleb revision show excellent results. One study demonstrated a 77.1% success rate (IOP between 8 and 21 mm Hg without medication) after revision.[52] In addition, a review by Cohen et al of 9 hypotonous eyes demonstrated a 66% reversal of visual acuity loss (6 of 9 eyes) from hypotony maculopathy following resuturing of the scleral flap.[53] A larger review of 27 hypotonous eyes and 13 eyes with bleb leaks that underwent surgical revision by conjunctival advancement, with or without resuturing of the scleral flap or placement of a graft, demonstrated an 83% (33 of 40 eyes) qualified success rate (resolution of hypotony or leak with IOP 6–21 mmHg without further glaucoma surgery, with or without medications).[54] When conservative therapy with cycloplegics, cessation of topical steroid use, and bandage contact lens use are unsuccessful, we advocate surgical revision of the bleb with resuturing of the scleral flap, thereby decreasing the egress of aqueous humor via the sclerostomy. See Chapter 10 and 21 for more information on overfiltration.

BLEB-RELATED INFECTIONS

One of the most devastating consequences following any intraocular surgery is postoperative infection, and in the context of guarded filtration surgery, the spectrum ranges from simple blebitis to panophthalmitis. The incidence of blebitis has been reported as high as 5.7%,[8,12,55,56] with the incidence of bleb-related endophthalmitis being significantly lower, ranging from 0.3%–1.5%.[55,57–60] Given the average endophthalmitis rate of 0.093% for all types of intraocular surgery,[61] it is clear that guarded filtration surgery is associated with a substantial lifelong risk of this complication. The question of how much additional risk is created with the use of antimetabolites remains unanswered.

Late bleb leakage has been repeatedly demonstrated as a risk factor for infection, with one study finding a 26-fold increased rate when compared to Seidel negative controls.[9] Furthermore, thin-walled cystic blebs are often implicated in these situations, as barriers to resistance are compromised in such circumstances,[31,62] allowing causative organisms access to the subconjunctival space and, ultimately, the intraocular space, via the sclerostomy. In a case-control series by Lehmann et al, adjunctive antimetabolite use with trabeculectomy significantly decreased the mean postoperative duration prior to infection and further demonstrated a trend towards increased overall risk of this complication.[58] A retrospective review by Poulsen et al demonstrated that only 3 out of 20 eyes presenting with ocular infection in their series had simple blebitis without intraocular signs of infection. The remaining 17 presented with endophthalmitis, with 75% of all eyes noted to have thin and/or avascular blebs and more than half demonstrating bleb leaks.[63] As with all cases of intraocular infection, prompt diagnosis and aggressive treatment are critical in optimizing patient outcomes.

The most common pathogens cultured in cases of bleb-related endophthalmitis have evolved in the antifibrotic era, and, furthermore, different organisms are cultured at different times during the postoperative period. Early bleb infections are generally considered less virulent and are associated most commonly with *Staphylococcus epidermidis* and normal conjunctival flora.[64–66]

Bleb-related endophthalmitis in the early postoperative period is commonly associated with *Propionibacterium acnes* or coagulase-negative *Staphylococcus* species, whereas later infections are usually caused by *Streptococcus* species and *Haemophilus influenzae*.[10,67]

For prevention of infection, as with all intraocular surgery, sterile intraoperative technique is essential, as is repair of late leaking blebs. Ultimately, using less antifibrotic agent may reduce the risk significantly. For further information, see Chapter 24.

CONCLUSION

Any technique that allows for greater bleb preservation and lower IOP following trabeculectomy is bound to be associated with greater risk of complications. Eyes without blebs do not develop bleb leaks, are not prone to overfiltration, and rarely develop intraocular infections. Thus, much of the increased risk associated with the use of antifibrotic drugs can be attributed to the surgical procedure, trabeculectomy, rather than the use of agents that improve the likelihood of success. Nevertheless, there are some characteristic complications associated with antifibrotic use that must be considered, particularly the ischemic necrosis of the conjunctiva, which predisposes to many long-term problems.

Dr. Shrivastava was supported by an Unrestricted Grant from Research to Prevent Blindness to the Albert Einstein College of Medicine.

COMMENTARY

JASON A. GOLDSMITH

There exists a widely held belief that the use of antimetabolite agents in trabeculectomy surgery has led to an increased incidence of postoperative complications. This opinion, however, may be in error. There may not be a direct causal relationship between antimetabolite use and the formation of dysmorphic, dysfunctional, and dysesthetic blebs. There may, in fact, be a confounding variable, namely limitation of posterior aqueous flow secondary to the establishment of a semicircular band of scar tissue, and this scar tissue may result from improper application of antimetabolite agents. The observed relationship between antimetabolite use and increased complication rate is likely more complex, and includes the paradoxical conclusion that when properly used in a diffuse administration, antimetabolite therapy is one key component to high-quality blebs with a low risk for complications.

Dr. Goldsmith was supported by an Unrestricted Grant from Research to Prevent Blindness to the University of Utah.

COMMENTARY
ALBERT S. KHOURI

The use of antifibrotic agents during filtering surgery is generally standard practice. It is under unusual circumstances that a glaucoma surgeon opts against the use of MMC or 5-FU. The improved success of trabeculectomy with antifibrotics comes at a price of increased risk of complications. Large avascular blebs are an unfortunate occurrence when too much of a good thing is used. Such bleb morphology inflicts a lifelong risk of leak and bleb-related endophthalmitis. Symptomatic dysesthesia is also more likely to occur with large overhanging or circumferential blebs.

Delayed bleb leaks can occur years after surgery and may remain undetected until patients present with blebitis or endophthalmitis. I routinely "paint" blebs with a wet fluorescein strip, which simplifies identification of leaks. Early leaks are usually not as difficult to detect, as they predictably occur at the incision or at a conjunctival button hole. Early leaks, however, can be as challenging to manage. In the early postoperative period, a leaking bleb will delay suture lysis, leading to a low or flat bleb with a higher likelihood of failure even after the leak stops. Aqueous suppression is sometimes used to "slow down" a leak. This, however, will also affect aqueous flow through the sclerostomy site and may inadvertently influence filtration and bleb survival. I prefer to surgically revise a leaking bleb within days if conservative measures fail.

Overfiltration and hypotony are more common with antifibrotic use. The best time to manage this complication is intraoperatively with judicious tightening of scleral flap sutures. I routinely place 4 sutures in a rectangular flap and occasionally add a fifth (or more as needed) until outflow resistance is optimized. In experienced hands it probably makes no difference, but I find titrating tension on a slip knot easier to gauge than the often used 3–1-1 throw knot. Avoiding suture lysis within the first 5–7 days is critical as the chances of hypotony are substantial with early suture release. Even when everything is done right, unfortunately some eyes still end up with hypotony. Extra caution must be exercised when using adjunctive antifibrotics in young myopic eyes as these eyes are more at risk for hypotony maculopathy.

Perhaps most serious is the lifelong increased risk of bleb-related endophthalmitis. Eyes with recurrent limited leaks may have been treated repeatedly with topical antibiotics, and are likely to harbor more resistant bacterial strains. Recommendations of the Endophthalmitis Vitrectomy Study were based on cataract patients within 6 weeks of surgery. Those, albeit helpful, do not directly apply to bleb-related endophthalmitis, which tends to be aggressive and progress rapidly within hours or days. Early intervention in consult with a retina specialist is necessary to avoid catastrophic consequences.

REFERENCES

1. Five-year follow-up of the Fluorouracil Filtering Surgery Study. The Fluorouracil Filtering Surgery Study Group. *Am J Ophthalmol.* Apr 1996;121(4):349–366.
2. Cheung JC, Wright MM, Murali S, Pederson JE. Intermediate-term outcome of variable dose mitomycin C filtering surgery. *Ophthalmology.* Jan 1997;104(1):143–149.
3. Greenfield DS, Liebmann JM, Jee J, Ritch R. Late-onset bleb leaks after glaucoma filtering surgery. *Arch Ophthalmol.* Apr 1998;116(4):443–447.
4. Katz GJ, Higginbotham EJ, Lichter PR, et al. Mitomycin C versus 5-fluorouracil in high-risk glaucoma filtering surgery. Extended follow-up. *Ophthalmology.* Sept 1995;102(9): 1263–1269.
5. Skuta GL, Beeson CC, Higginbotham EJ, et al. Intraoperative mitomycin versus postoperative 5-fluorouracil in high-risk glaucoma filtering surgery. *Ophthalmology.* Mar 1992;99(3):438–444.
6. Asrani SG, Wilensky JT. Management of bleb leaks after glaucoma filtering surgery. Use of autologous fibrin tissue glue as an alternative. *Ophthalmology.* Feb 1996;103(2):294–298.

7. Belyea DA, Dan JA, Stamper RL, Lieberman MF, Spencer WH. Late onset of sequential multifocal bleb leaks after glaucoma filtration surgery with 5-fluorouracil and mitomycin C. *Am J Ophthalmol.* Jul 1997;124(1):40–45.

8. DeBry PW, Perkins TW, Heatley G, Kaufman P, Brumback LC. Incidence of late-onset bleb-related complications following trabeculectomy with mitomycin. *Arch Ophthalmol.* Mar 2002; 120(3):297–300.

9. Soltau JB, Rothman RF, Budenz DL, et al. Risk factors for glaucoma filtering bleb infections. *Arch Ophthalmol.* Mar 2000;118(3):338–342.

10. Song A, Scott IU, Flynn HW Jr., Budenz DL. Delayed-onset bleb-associated endophthalmitis: clinical features and visual acuity outcomes. *Ophthalmology.* May 2002;109(5):985–991.

11. Loon SC, Chew PT. A major review of antimetabolites in glaucoma therapy. *Ophthalmologica.* 1999; 213(4):234–245.

12. Bindlish R, Condon GP, Schlosser JD, D'Antonio J, Lauer KB, Lehrer R. Efficacy and safety of mitomycin-C in primary trabeculectomy: five-year follow-up. *Ophthalmology.* Jul 2002;109(7): 1336–1341; discussion 1341–1332.

13. Cain W Jr., Sinskey RM. Detection of anterior chamber leakage with Seidel's test. *Arch Ophthalmol.* Nov 1981;99(11):2013.

14. Azuara-Blanco A, Katz LJ. Prevention and management of complications of glaucoma surgery. In: Tasman W, Jeager EA, eds. *Duane's Clinical Ophthalmology.* Vol 6. Philadelphia: Lippincott Williams & Wilkins; 2007. http://ovidsp.tx.ovid.com.ezproxyhost.library.tmc.edu/sp-2.3/ovidweb.cgi?&S=KCDHFPCIEGDDBGFCNCELBGGJGLJPAA00&Link+Set=S.sh.17%7c1%7csl_10. Accessed March 15, 2010.

15. Khaw PT. Advances in glaucoma surgery: evolution of antimetabolite adjunctive therapy. *J Glaucoma.* Oct 2001;10(5)(suppl 1): S81–S84.

16. Khaw PT, Clarke J. Antifibrotic agents in glaucoma surgery. In: Yanoff M, Duker JS, eds. *Ophthalmology.* 3rd ed. Philadelphia, PA: Mosby; 2008. http://www.mdconsult.com.ezproxyhost.library.tmc.edu/das/book/body/189231676–3/968258247/1869/552.html#4-u1.0-B978–0-323–04332–8..00211–0_4734. Accessed March 15, 2010.

17. Parrish RK, 2nd, Schiffman JC, Feuer WJ, Heuer DK. Prognosis and risk factors for early postoperative wound leaks after trabeculectomy with and without 5-fluorouracil. *Am J Ophthalmol.* Nov 2001;132(5):633–640.

18. Brown SV. Management of a partial-thickness scleral-flap buttonhole during trabeculectomy. *Ophthalmic Surg.* Nov-Dec 1994;25(10):732–733.

19. Petursson GJ, Fraunfelder FT. Repair of an inadvertent buttonhole or leaking filtering bleb. *Arch Ophthalmol.* May 1979;97(5):926–927.

20. Batterbury M, Wishart PK. Is high initial aqueous outflow of benefit in trabeculectomy? *Eye (Lond).* 1993;7 (Pt 1):109–112.

21. Kohl DA, Walton DS. Limbus-based versus fornix-based conjunctival flaps in trabeculectomy: 2005 update. *Int Ophthalmol Clin.* Fall 2005;45(4):107–113.

22. Shuster JN, Krupin T, Kolker AE, Becker B. Limbus- v fornix-based conjunctival flap in trabeculectomy. A long-term randomized study. *Arch Ophthalmol.* Mar 1984;102(3):361–362.

23. Blok MD, Kok JH, van Mil C, Greve EL, Kijlstra A. Use of the Megasoft Bandage Lens for treatment of complications after trabeculectomy. *Am J Ophthalmol.* Sept 15 1990;110(3):264–268.

24. Budenz DL, Chen PP, Weaver YK. Conjunctival advancement for late-onset filtering bleb leaks: indications and outcomes. *Arch Ophthalmol.* Aug 1999;117(8):1014–1019.

25. Hill RA, Aminlari A, Sassani JW, Michalski M. Use of a symblepharon ring for treatment of over-filtration and leaking blebs after glaucoma filtration surgery. *Ophthalmic Surg.* Oct 1990;21(10):707–710.

26. Awan KJ, Spaeth PG. Use of isobutyl-2-cyanoacrylate tissue adhesive in the repair of conjunctival fistula in filtering procedures for glaucoma. *Ann Ophthalmol.* Aug 1974;6(8):851–853.

27. Zalta AH, Wieder RH. Closure of leaking filtering blebs with cyanoacrylate tissue adhesive. *Br J Ophthalmol.* Mar 1991;75(3):170–173.

28. Rajeev B, Thomas R. Corneal hazards in use of Simmons shell. *Aust NZ J Ophthalmol.* May 1991;19(2):145–148.

29. Simmons RJ, Kimbrough RL. Shell tamponade in filtering surgery for glaucoma. *Ophthalmic Surg.* Sept 1979;10(9):17–34.

30. Burnstein AL, WuDunn D, Knotts SL, Catoira Y, Cantor LB. Conjunctival advancement versus nonincisional treatment for late-onset glaucoma filtering bleb leaks. *Ophthalmology.* Jan 2002;109(1):71–75.

31. Shields MB, Scroggs MW, Sloop CM, Simmons RB. Clinical and histopathologic observations concerning hypotony after trabeculectomy with adjunctive mitomycin C. *Am J Ophthalmol.* Dec 15 1993;116(6):673–683.

32. Azuara-Blanco A, Katz LJ. Dysfunctional filtering blebs. *Surv Ophthalmol.* Sept–Oct 1998;43(2):93–126.

33. Choudhri SA, Herndon LW, Damji KF, Allingham RR, Shields MB. Efficacy of autologous blood injection for treating overfiltering or leaking blebs after glaucoma surgery. *Am J Ophthalmol.* Apr 1997;123(4):554–555.

34. Leen MM, Moster MR, Katz LJ, Terebuh AK, Schmidt CM, Spaeth GL. Management of overfiltering and leaking blebs with autologous blood injection. *Arch Ophthalmol.* Aug 1995;113(8):1050–1055.

35. Smith MF, Magauran RG, 3rd, Betchkal J, Doyle JW. Treatment of postfiltration bleb leaks with autologous blood. *Ophthalmology.* Jun 1995;102(6):868–871.

36. Wise JB. Treatment of chronic postfiltration hypotony by intrableb injection of autologous blood. *Arch Ophthalmol.* Jun 1993;111(6):827–830.

37. Fine LC, Chen TC, Grosskreutz CL, Pasquale LR. Management and prevention of thin, cystic blebs. *Int Ophthalmol Clin.* Winter 2004;44(1):29–42.

38. Solish AM. Treatment of leaking filtering blebs using needle expansion and adjunctive metabolites: Clinical experimental evidence for an alternative theory of leaking filtration blebs. Poster presented at: American Glaucoma Society 12th Annual Meeting; March 2002; San Juan, Puerto Rico.

39. Geyer O. Management of large, leaking, and inadvertent filtering blebs with the neodymium:YAG laser. *Ophthalmology.* Jun 1998;105(6):983–987.

40. Lynch MG, Roesch M, Brown RH. Remodeling filtering blebs with the neodymium:YAG laser. *Ophthalmology.* Oct 1996;103(10):1700–1705.

41. Nagai-Kusuhara A, Nakamura M, Fujioka M, Negi A. Long-term results of amniotic membrane transplantation-assisted bleb revision for leaking blebs. *Graefes Arch Clin Exp Ophthalmol.* Apr 2008;246(4):567–571.

42. Budenz DL, Barton K, Tseng SC. Amniotic membrane transplantation for repair of leaking glaucoma filtering blebs. *Am J Ophthalmol.* Nov 2000;130(5):580–588.

43. Rauscher FM, Barton K, Budenz DL, Feuer WJ, Tseng SC. Long-term outcomes of amniotic membrane transplantation for repair of leaking glaucoma filtering blebs. *Am J Ophthalmol.* Jun 2007;143(6):1052–1054.

44. Harris LD, Yang G, Feldman RM, et al. Autologous conjunctival resurfacing of leaking filtering blebs. *Ophthalmology.* Sept 2000;107(9):1675–1680.

45. Shields MB. Trabeculectomy vs full-thickness filtering operation for control of glaucoma. *Ophthalmic Surg.* Aug 1980;11(8):498–505.

46. Watkins PH Jr., Brubaker RF. Comparison of partial-thickness and full-thickness filtration procedures in open-angle glaucoma. *Am J Ophthalmol.* Dec 1978;86(6):756–761.

47. Rahman A, Mendonca M, Simmons RB, Simmons RJ. Hypotony after glaucoma filtration surgery. *Int Ophthalmol Clin.* Winter 2000;40(1):127–136.

48. Mietz H. The toxicology of mitomycin C on the ciliary body. *Curr Opin Ophthalmol.* Apr 1996;7(2):72–79.

49. Palmberg P, Zacchei AC. Compression sutures: a new treatment for leaking or painful filtering blebs [ARVO abstract 2032]. *Invest Ophthalmol Vis Sci.* 1996;37(3):S444.

50. Quaranta L, Pizzolante T. Endophthalmitis after compression sutures for enlarged conjunctival filtration bleb following trabeculectomy. *Ophthalmic Surg Lasers Imaging.* Jul-Aug 2009;40(4):432–433.

51. Kurtz S, Leibovitch I. Combined perfluoro-propane gas and viscoelastic material injection for anterior chamber reformation following trabeculectomy. *Br J Ophthalmol.* Nov 2002;86(11):1225–1227.

52. Dintelmann T, Lieb WE, Grehn F. [Filtering bleb revision. Techniques and outcome]. *Ophthalmologe.* Dec 2002;99(12):917–921.

53. Cohen SM, Flynn HW Jr., Palmberg PF, Gass JD, Grajewski AL, Parrish RK 2nd. Treatment of hypotony maculopathy after trabeculectomy. *Ophthalmic Surg Lasers.* Sept-Oct 1995;26(5):435–441.

54. Tannenbaum DP, Hoffman D, Greaney MJ, Caprioli J. Outcomes of bleb excision and conjunctival advancement for leaking or hypotonous eyes after glaucoma filtering surgery. *Br J Ophthalmol.* Jan 2004;88(1):99–103.

55. Mac I, Soltau JB. Glaucoma-filtering bleb infections. *Curr Opin Ophthalmol.* Apr 2003;14(2):91–94.

56. Parrish R, Minckler D. "Late endophthalmitis"—filtering surgery time bomb? *Ophthalmology.* Aug 1996;103(8):1167–1168.

57. Katz LJ, Cantor LB, Spaeth GL. Complications of surgery in glaucoma. Early and late bacterial endophthalmitis following glaucoma filtering surgery. *Ophthalmology.* Jul 1985;92(7):959–963.

58. Lehmann OJ, Bunce C, Matheson MM, et al. Risk factors for development of post-trabeculectomy endophthalmitis. *Br J Ophthalmol.* Dec 2000;84(12):1349–1353.

59. Mochizuki K, Jikihara S, Ando Y, Hori N, Yamamoto T, Kitazawa Y. Incidence of delayed onset infection after trabeculectomy with adjunctive mitomycin C or 5-fluorouracil treatment. *Br J Ophthalmol.* Oct 1997;81(10):877–883.

60. Wilson P. Trabeculectomy: long-term follow-up. *Br J Ophthalmol.* Aug 1977;61(8):535–538.

61. Aaberg TM, Jr., Flynn HW, Jr., Schiffman J, Newton J. Nosocomial acute-onset postoperative endophthalmitis survey. A 10-year review of incidence and outcomes. *Ophthalmology.* Jun 1998;105(6):1004–1010.

62. Nuyts RM, Felten PC, Pels E, et al. Histopathologic effects of mitomycin C after trabeculectomy in human glaucomatous eyes with persistent hypotony. *Am J Ophthalmol.* Aug 15 1994;118(2):225–237.

63. Poulsen EJ, Allingham RR. Characteristics and risk factors of infections after glaucoma filtering surgery. *J Glaucoma.* Dec 2000;9(6):438–443.

64. Ciulla TA, Beck AD, Topping TM, Baker AS. Blebitis, early endophthalmitis, and late endophthalmitis after glaucoma-filtering surgery. *Ophthalmology.* Jun 1997;104(6):986–995.

65. Olson JC, Flynn HW Jr., Forster RK, Culbertson WW. Results in the treatment of postoperative endophthalmitis. *Ophthalmology.* Jun 1983;90(6):692–699.

66. Puliafito CA, Baker AS, Haaf J, Foster CS. Infectious endophthalmitis. Review of 36 cases. *Ophthalmology.* Aug 1982;89(8):921–929.

67. Waheed S, Ritterband DC, Greenfield DS, Liebmann JM, Seedor JA, Ritch R. New patterns of infecting organisms in late bleb-related endophthalmitis: a ten year review. *Eye.* 1998;12 (Pt 6):910–915.

F. REVISION OF FILTERING SURGERY

28

NEEDLING AND REVISION COMPLICATIONS

ALFRED M. SOLISH

NEEDLING AND REVISION COMPLICATIONS

Needle revision refers to a surgical procedure in which a fine gauge needle or needle-knife is used to incise scar tissue in the vicinity of a filtration opening. Initially described for temporary relief of elevated intraocular pressure (IOP) in the case of encapsulated filtering blebs,[1] needle revision has been used to establish flow in the setting of a nonexistent bleb, enhance aqueous flow when a bleb is present, and to alter tectonic features of a filtration bleb.[2] Among the many advantages of needle revision are rapidity, low cost (especially when performed in the office), minimal preparation, and rapid recovery. Compared to full surgical revision, needle revision involves relatively little disruption of tissue, resulting in minimal inflammation.

Needle revision can be used to rearrange bleb architecture to decrease bleb height, a bleb morphology that is associated with corneal dellen and dysesthesia (see Chapters 18 and 19). Flow can be redirected using needle revision to reduce flow through bleb leaks,[3] which may result in closure and/or prevent reformation of "overhanging" blebs. Although incision of relatively thin scar tissue with a needle establishes fluid flow, scar reformation is likely to occur without some sort of inhibition of scar formation. The introduction of antifibrotics, such as 5-fluorouracil (5-FU)[4] and mitomycin-C (MMC),[5] and antiangiogenics, such as bevacizumab,[6] have enhanced our ability to prevent reformation of scar tissue.

Needle revision is a useful procedure that can revise bleb architecture and redirect fluid flow with little inflammation. Understanding complications associated with this procedure is important for an ultimately successful glaucoma procedure.

SETTING OF NEEDLE REVISION AND ANESTHESIA TECHNIQUE

Needle revision can be performed in a variety of settings: the operating room, complete with the operating microscope, full preparation, and draping; the office minor procedure room using the operating microscope; or even at the slit lamp in the examination lane. Procedure time, cost, and equipment preference and availability are among other factors that may influence the choice of venue. Anesthesia methods also vary. Topical anesthesia, subconjunctival block, and retrobulbar injection can all be used. Generally, topical anesthesia with viscous lidocaine is adequate in most patients.

USE OF ANTIMETABOLITES IN NEEDLE REVISION

To prevent complications, the needling technique should differ depending on which antimetabolite is being used. MMC is absorbed into surrounding tissue in 15–20 minutes, so a delay between injection of antimetabolite and needle revision is advisable. 5-FU may safely be injected subconjunctivally in the presence of a functioning sclerostomy. However, intracameral 5-FU has been observed to cause profound cataract.[7] It may be prudent to avoid injection directly into a newly functioning bleb,[8] but injection into the subconjunctival space next to or away from the bleb appears safe.

COMPLICATIONS

Since there are a wide range of venues, techniques, and anesthesia usage, complications will vary somewhat based on the surgeon's choices. Complications will also vary based on the selection and use of antiscarring medications.

Expected complications

Since a very thin instrument (typically a 25- to 30-gauge needle or knife of a similar size) is used to incise scar tissue, very little tissue is usually cut at any one time. Therefore, multiple needling procedures may be needed to maintain flow.[3] Even in one sitting, multiple entries may be required to initiate adequate flow. Each needle entry through the conjunctiva results in a small conjunctival opening; most surgeons do not suture the entry site. Since antiscarring medications are used, the entry site may leak for up to 2 weeks,

particularly when larger bore needles (25- or 23-gauge) are used. The use of bevacizumab may also be associated with prolongation of leakage through the needle entry site.

Conjunctival leaks at the entry site generally seal without intervention. Low-grade inflammation may result if a suture is used, at least until the suture is removed or dissolves. It is not known whether the use of suture or the type of suture material has an impact on success rate. Other surgeons use cautery to seal the needle hole at the entry site. Sealing the needle hole is not believed to affect outcome since the entry site is typically more than a centimeter away from the main loculation of the bleb.

Hyphema and subconjunctival hemorrhage are common since scar tissue is generally well vascularized. Though the tiny needle opening has many advantages, the tiny opening prohibits surgical hemostasis, or cautery. Even when the patient is being treated with anticoagulation therapy, bleeding will cease in a very short time. Although suprachoroidal hemorrhage is a risk, it is extremely rare. It is not uncommon for the patient to notice blood-tinged tears postoperatively. Reassurance is indicated as this is an expected phenomenon.

As in other forms of filtration surgery, hyphema may persist for a more prolonged period. An explanation for this phenomenon may be decreased aqueous inflow. As prolonged hyphema will affect visual acuity, a 27- or 30-gauge needle may be used to perform a paracentesis and washout at the 6-o'clock position. Topical antibiotics should be used postoperatively as well as when performing this procedure.

The anterior chamber may shallow since, in effect, needle revision may be a "full-thickness" procedure. However, this complication occurs infrequently, probably because the needle opening is very small. When the chamber shallows, cycloplegics are usually effective. Reformation with a viscoelastic may be required. See Chapter 11 for more information on management of a shallow anterior chamber.

Surgical complications not unique to needle revision

By far, the most frequent complication of any glaucoma surgical procedure is failure to achieve the desired result. When used to control IOP, needle revision success rates are estimated to range from 27% to 90%, depending on the morphology of the bleb, technique, number of needling procedures, and time since original filtering surgery.[2,9-13] Infection is rare, as in other intraocular procedures (see Chapter 24). Due to the rarity of infection, it is difficult to quantify or compare needle revision to other surgical procedures. Preoperative as well as postoperative treatment with topical antibiotics is recommended. Lastly, as in filtration surgery with 5-FU, corneal epitheliopathy may occur following needle revision with 5-FU, particularly when multiple antimetabolite injections are required.[14]

Surgical complications unique to needle revision

Large conjunctival tears may result from sudden patient movement or particularly tough scar tissue. Needle revision often includes not only punctures of the scar tissue, but also movement of the needle through an arc so as to linearly cut scar tissue. During these rotational movements, the scar tissue may give way, resulting in a sudden movement. This movement may in turn result in a conjunctival tear or perforation. On rare occasions, these tears may need to be sutured. A purse-string suture is recommended where technically feasible. Small perforations of the conjunctiva occur more frequently and usually close spontaneously without additional therapy.

A rare complication of needle revision is vitreous prolapse to the conjunctival surface. On occasion, vitreous filling the anterior chamber may not be evident, and needle revision may permit the vitreous to prolapse through the conjunctival needle wound via the sclerostomy. A return to the operating room for anterior vitrectomy may be required. All cases that I am aware of have occurred in the setting of corneal transplantation. One case did not require an anterior vitrectomy. The wound closed spontaneously, and the IOP remained low. See Chapter 7 for more information about vitreous prolapse.

Subconjunctival injection of antimetabolite, particularly MMC, may result in a unique clinical picture similar to endophthalmitis.

The eyelid becomes swollen and tender, and the patient may be unable to open the eye (Figure 28.1A). This reaction is limited to the eyelid and is not an infectious process. When the lid is opened, the conjunctiva is white and quiet, and the anterior chamber is without significant flare and cell (Figure 28.1B). Conservative management is indicated, using cool compresses and topical steroids. The condition resolves spontaneously. This complication is idiosyncratic and not associated with MMC concentration or the injection site. It seems to occur most frequently when MMC is used immediately prior to the needle revision and a 5-FU injection is used immediately following the procedure. Therefore, that particular combination is not recommended for concomitant treatment. Success may be achieved when 5-FU injections are used after a delay of several days.

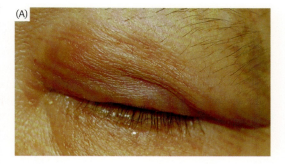

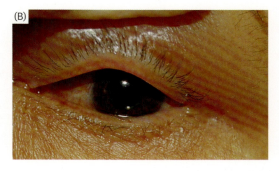

FIGURE 28.1 Mitomycin-C reaction following bleb needling. The eyelid may become swollen and tender with subconjunctival injection of MMC. The eye may appear "hot" or infected (A), but when the eyelid is lifted, the eye is shown to be quiet and the reaction mostly limited to the eyelid (B).

Cataract surgery has been shown to significantly affect the functioning of a bleb that has been successfully needled. In one study, nearly 25% of the blebs failed following cataract surgery.[15] When contemplating cataract surgery, the necessity for a repeat needle revision should be expected.

CONCLUSION

Needle revision can resuscitate failed glaucoma filtering blebs in a cost-effective manner. Although not free of complications, needle bleb revision may prevent the need to perform more extensive revision, another filtering procedure, or implantation of a tube shunt. Every glaucoma surgeon should be familiar with the techniques and potential pitfalls of needle bleb revision, and this procedure should be considered in the management algorithm of poorly functioning filtering blebs.

COMMENTARY
PETER T. CHANG

Successful needle revision can result in a long-term pressure reduction in eyes with a failed or failing bleb following trabeculectomy. Needle revision may be performed in the early or late postoperative period, although some authors have reported revision within 4 months of surgery to be highly correlated with successful outcome.[12] For the cases in which the bleb height is very low or flat, the risk of inadvertent conjunctival buttonhole or tear may be reduced by hydrodissection or viscodissection prior to the actual needling. This may be accomplished by having the needle attached to a syringe filled with balanced salt solution or ophthalmic viscoelastic device and injected subconjunctivally as the needle makes the initial entry through the conjunctiva. Lidocaine may also be used to provide further local anesthesia.

Eyes requiring multiple needle revisions have been reported to have lower long-term IOP control than those requiring one revision.[16] Repeated attempts after failed revisions may be inappropriate considering the lower probability of success.

COMMENTARY
RICHARD K. PARRISH, II

The authors describe the obvious simplicity of immediately increasing the rate of aqueous outflow by perforating a thick husk-like layer of fibrovascular tissue at the filtering site with a needle. The success of this technique likely depends on several factors: the activity of inflammation associated with wound healing at the filtering site; the use of antiscarring agents, such as 5-FU or MMC at the time of the filtering surgery; or the bleb morphology, such as flat blebs that are associated with tightly adherent scleral flaps to the underlying tissue or highly elevated blebs that are associated with a tensely engorged vasculature.

Scleral flaps that remain fixed to the underlying tissue after laser suture in the early postoperative period can be pried open and the tip of the needle advanced safely into the anterior chamber to promote aqueous drainage. Multiple small perforations or linear cuts into the lateral wall of thickened blebs, erroneously referred to as "encapsulated blebs" in the absence of any capsular architecture, may also rapidly lower tissue resistance to drainage. However, being able to predict the long-term outcome is difficult and is reflected in reported success rates that vary from 27% to 90% in the early postoperative period. No high-quality, long-term, evidence-based medical data compellingly supports this practice, and yet this procedure is uniformly practiced on the basis of a perceived very low risk and reasonably high benefit. Risk ratio for failure in a small (49 eyes of 43 patients) retrospective, nonrandomized comparative case series was 3.781 (P=0.047) for fornix-based trabeculectomies compared with limbus-based trabeculectomies.[17] Gender, race, type of glaucoma, previous surgery, antimetabolite used for the initial trabeculectomy, and lens status were not predictive of success in that study. In another small retrospective comparative observational case series (65 patients received 5-FU and 43 received MMC.) the overall survival rate was 49.5% and the mean time to failure was 7.7 months.[18]

In view of the high safety profile and minimally invasive nature of the intervention, bleb needling will likely continue, even in the absence of better information.

Dr. Parrish was supported by National Eye Institute grant P30EY014801, Department of Defense grant W81XWH-09-1-0675, and an Unrestricted Grant from Research to Prevent Blindness to Bascom Palmer Eye Institute, Miller School of Medicine, University of Miami.

REFERENCES

1. Pederson JE, Smith SG. Surgical management of encapsulated filtering blebs. *Ophthalmology.* Jul 1985;92(7):955–958.
2. Feldman RM, Tabet RR. Needle revision of filtering blebs. *J Glaucoma.* Oct-Nov 2008;17(7):594–600.
3. Solish AM, Solish SP. Treatment of leaking filtration blebs using mitomycin-C. *J Glaucoma.* Feb 1999;8(1):S20.
4. Solish A. Re-opening failed filtration fistulae using bleb needling and 5-fluorouracil [ARVO abstract]. *Invest Ophthalmol Vis Sci.* Mar 1989;30(3):416.
5. Mardelli PG, Lederer CM Jr., Murray PL, Pastor SA, Hassanein KM. Slit-lamp needle revision of failed filtering blebs using mitomycin C. *Ophthalmology.* Nov 1996;103(11):1946–1955.
6. Kahook MY, Schuman JS, Noecker RJ. Needle bleb revision of encapsulated filtering bleb with bevacizumab. *Ophthalmic Surg Lasers Imaging.* Mar-Apr 2006;37(2):148–150.
7. Libre PE. Transient, profound cataract associated with intracameral 5-fluorouracil. *Am J Ophthalmol.* Jan 2003;135(1):101–102.
8. Mazey BJ, Siegel MJ, Siegel LI, Dunn SP. Corneal endothelial toxic effect secondary to fluorouracil needle bleb revision. *Arch Ophthalmol.* Nov 1994;112(11):1411.
9. Shin DH, Juzych MS, Khatana AK, Swendris RP, Parrow KA. Needling revision of failed filtering blebs with adjunctive 5-fluorouracil. *Ophthalmic Surg.* Apr 1993;24(4):242–248.
10. Shetty RK, Wartluft L, Moster MR. Slit-lamp needle revision of failed filtering blebs using high-dose mitomycin C. *J Glaucoma.* Feb 2005;14(1):52–56.
11. Hung JW, Bellows AR. Bleb revision. In: Chen TC, ed. *Surgical Techniques in Ophthalmology: Glaucoma Surgery.* Philadelphia: Saunders; 2008.
12. Gutierrez-Ortiz C, Cabarga C, Teus MA. Prospective evaluation of preoperative factors associated with successful mitomycin C needling of failed filtration blebs. *J Glaucoma.* Apr 2006;15(2):98–102.
13. Iwach AG, Delgado MF, Novack GD, Nguyen N, Wong PC. Transconjunctival mitomycin-C in needle revisions of failing filtering blebs. *Ophthalmology.* Apr 2003;110(4):734–742.
14. Durak I, Ozbek Z, Yaman A, Soylev M, Cingil G. The role of needle revision and 5-fluorouracil application over the filtration site in the management of bleb failure after trabeculectomy: a prospective study. *Doc Ophthalmol.* Mar 2003;106(2):189–193.
15. Rotchford AP, King AJ. Cataract surgery after needling revision of trabeculectomy blebs. *J Glaucoma.* Sept 2007;16(6):562–566.
16. Greenfield DS, Miller MP, Suner IJ, Palmberg PF. Needle elevation of the scleral flap for failing filtration blebs after trabeculectomy with mitomycin C. *Am J Ophthalmol.* Aug 1996;122(2):195–204.
17. Hawkins AS, Flanagan JK, Brown SV. Predictors for success of needle revision of failing filtration blebs. *Ophthalmology.* Apr 2002;109(4):781–785.
18. Palejwala N, Ichhpujani P, Fakhraie G, Myers JS, Moster MR, Katz LJ. Single needle revision of failing filtration blebs: a retrospective comparative case series with 5-fluorouracil and mitomycin C. *Eur J Ophthalmol.* Nov-Dec 2010;20(6): 1026–1034.

G. COMPLICATIONS SPECIFIC TO EX-PRESS™ SHUNTS

29

COMPLICATIONS SPECIFIC TO EX-PRESS™ SHUNTS

STEVEN R. SARKISIAN, JR.

COMPLICATIONS SPECIFIC TO EX-PRESS™ SHUNTS

The EX-PRESS™ Glaucoma Filtration Device (Alcon Laboratories, Inc., Fort Worth, Texas) has been commercially available in the United States since 2002 and was originally developed by Optonol, Inc. (Kansas City, Kansas) for implantation directly under the conjunctiva for an indication of control of intraocular pressure (IOP). It is a nonvalved, stainless steel device almost 3 mm long with an external diameter of approximately 400 microns and a 50 or 200 micron lumen, depending on the model. It has an external disc at one end and a spur-like extension on the other to prevent extrusion.

The EX-PRESS™ shunt is one option for controlling IOP available to today's glaucoma surgeon. The challenges and complications involved with EX-PRESS™ shunts are addressed below, as well as how to manage and prevent such scenarios.

IMPLANTATION OF AN EX-PRESS™ SHUNT

The original unguarded technique of implantation under the conjunctiva resulted in numerous complications, including hypotony, extrusion, and, most commonly, erosion of the implant.[1-11] Typically, there was a period of hypotony followed by failure and erosion of the implant. Endophthalmitis has also been associated with an exposed implant.[6]

To avoid complications associated with subconjunctival implantation, Dahan and Carmichael proposed implanting the device under a scleral flap.[12] This technique has greatly reduced erosions, and EX-PRESS™ shunts have been reported to have a lower rate of hypotony than trabeculectomy (15.8% with EX-PRESS™ shunt versus 22.5% in trabeculectomy).[13] Since 2003, the manufacturer has recommended all users only implant the device under a scleral flap.

WHAT TO DO WHEN AN EX-PRESS™ SHUNT FAILS

Like all filtration surgery, failure is most commonly from episcleral and subconjunctival fibrosis.[14] As with traditional filtration surgery, intraoperative adjunctive antimetabolites, such as mitomycin-C, may be used to limit the degree of postoperative scarring. However, should failure due to fibrosis occur, there are several options. The first is to add topical medications or perform laser trabeculoplasty. The second is to perform bleb revision or needling with an antifibrotic agent. Finally, as in a failed trabeculectomy, the surgeon may abandon the EX-PRESS™ shunt and perform a second unrelated procedure.

Typically, the failed EX-PRESS™ shunt does not need to be removed when performing additional glaucoma surgery if the implant is well covered and in good position. Removing it may require a large wound. Therefore, the site of implantation and scleral flap should be avoided to prevent inadvertent exposure. If overfiltration occurs due to hypotony from a poor flap or after lysis of a flap suture, the treatment would be exactly as for hypotony from a trabeculectomy without the device (see Chapter 10).

SHUNT OCCLUSION

The EX-PRESS™ shunt is designed not only with a port at the tip of the device, but also with holes on the sides (Figure 29.1). Therefore, if the tip becomes occluded by fibrin, blood, or iris tissue, there may still be flow through the device. In a review of patients with EX-PRESS™ shunts, the most common device-related complication was shunt occlusion (6 of 345 total cases), which can be relieved by Nd:YAG laser photolysis at the tip of the implant, even if the blockage is not visible.[15] There were also several implants in which the tip was touching the iris (Figure 29.2); none were occluded by the iris nor was there any decrease in vision, inflammation, or macular edema, and intervention was not required.

MIGRATION OF THE EX-PRESS™ SHUNT

To prevent dislocation or migration of an EX-PRESS™ shunt into the anterior chamber or the subconjunctival space, great care must be taken to make certain that the correct needle is used for the preincision site, the flap is well constructed, and the implant is resting

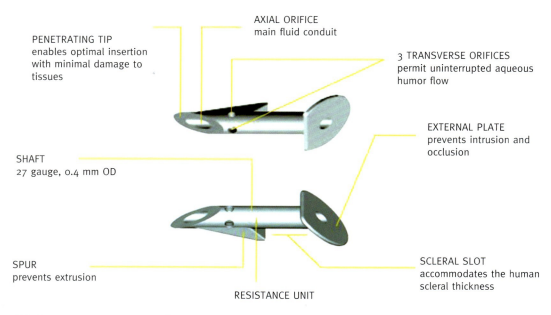

AXIAL ORIFICE
main fluid conduit

PENETRATING TIP
enables optimal insertion with minimal damage to tissues

3 TRANSVERSE ORIFICES
permit uninterrupted aqueous humor flow

EXTERNAL PLATE
prevents intrusion and occlusion

SHAFT
27 gauge, 0.4 mm OD

SPUR
prevents extrusion

SCLERAL SLOT
accommodates the human scleral thickness

RESISTANCE UNIT

FIGURE 29.1   EX-PRESS™ Glaucoma Filtration Device, model R-50

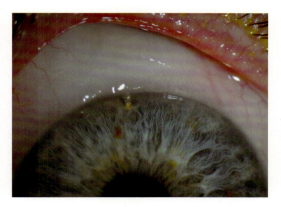

FIGURE 29.2 Tip of EX-PRESS™ shunt in contact with iris. If outflow through the device becomes obstructed, Nd:YAG laser photolysis may be used to reestablish flow. In this case, the evidence of an ischemic conjunctival bleb suggests that the device is patent.

flush with the scleral bed immediately following insertion. If the flap is too thin or not completely covering the EX-PRESS™ shunt, or if the plate does not sit flush with the sclera, there is an increased risk of exposure.

The original version of the EX-PRESS™ shunt, model R-50 (Figure 29.1), was designed for subconjunctival implantation and requires a 27-gauge needle for preinsertion track formation. Although the R-50 works well under a scleral flap, the newer P series shunts were designed specifically for implantation under a flap. They require a 25-gauge needle track because they have a slightly squared off shape. The subtle square shape prevents rotation and malposition once the implant is in place; however, it is difficult to insert through a 27-gauge needle tract. The P series shunts are also shorter than the R-50.

Using the correct needle size for implanting an EX-PRESS™ shunt is underscored by a report of an EX-PRESS™ shunt migrating into the anterior chamber. Using too large a needle, for example, using a 25-gauge needle for insertion of an R-50 model, may permit migration of the shunt.[16] There is now an injector preloaded with the EX-PRESS™ shunt available to prevent this event. Regardless, using the correct needle size can minimize the likelihood of this complication

EROSION

When the EX-PRESS™ shunt is placed under a scleral flap, erosion is rare.[15] Erosions have been seen most frequently in patients with friable tissues, as is found in autoimmune diseases (such as rheumatoid arthritis and scleromalacia).[15] Another risk for erosion may be a keratoprosthesis. The EX-PRESS™ shunt is not contraindicated in patients who have had a penetrating keratoplasty. In fact, an EX-PRESS™ shunt may be preferable to a conventional tube shunt in these eyes because the EX-PRESS™ shunt has less than 2 mm of the tip in the anterior chamber and is rigid. Theoretically, if a patient with an EX-PRESS™ shunt rubs the eye, the tip is less likely to hit the corneal endothelium than with flexible silicone tubes. There is no data on endothelial cell counts after penetrating keratoplasty or Descemet stripping endothelial keratoplasty with EX-PRESS™ shunts.

REMOVING AN EX-PRESS™ SHUNT

Stein et al have reported a case series of exposure of the EX-PRESS™ shunt and described a technique for removal. In their case series, 8 eyes experienced exposure, with the average time to exposure of 8.5 months from the time of implantation. Conventional tube shunt surgery was performed concomitantly with removal of the EX-PRESS™ shunt. The device was removed by taking a sharp blade and making a stab incision against the shaft of the implant, which is necessary to remove the implant because of the spur (Figure 29.1). The implant was grasped with a forceps, pushed anteriorly to dislodge the spur, and then rotated and extracted.[11] The rotation allows for the spur to pass through the tract created by the blade.

Sometimes it is necessary to trephine the area around the sclerostomy to remove any fibrous tissue that may grow through the full-thickness scleral wound. After half-thickness trephining, underlying tissue can be removed with a Vannas scissor. A patch graft will be required to cover the hole. In most cases, trephination can be avoided by debridement of the surrounding tissue with absolute alcohol prior to explantation. After explantation, direct suture closure may be possible.

Typically, a patient with a failed EX-PRESS™ shunt will require another surgery to control IOP, and in most cases, the procedure would be a tube shunt to a reservoir. When combining the 2 surgeries (explantation with insertion of an anterior chamber tube shunt), a single oversized patch graft can be utilized to cover the tube and the site of the removed EX-PRESS™ shunt. However, if water-tight closure can be achieved by simple suture closure, then no tissue reinforcement graft is needed for the site of the explanted EX-PRESS™ shunt. It is important to remember that most cases of failed EX-PRESS™ shunts do not require removal.

CONCLUSION

The EX-PRESS™ Glaucoma Filtration Device directs aqueous from the anterior chamber to a space under a scleral flap and then to a filtering bleb, just as a trabeculectomy does. Any complication that can occur with a trabeculectomy can occur with an EX-PRESS™ shunt. Numerous procedure-specific devastating complications have been reported to occur if the EX-PRESS™ shunt is covered only by a conjunctival flap. Implantation under a scleral flap reduces the risk of most complications that are specific to the device/technique and is now considered the standard of care for EX-PRESS™ shunts. As with trabeculectomy, failure with the EX-PRESS™ shunt can occur. However, correct implantation of the EX-PRESS™ shunt using the current technique of implantation under a scleral flap is required to obtain potential benefits of the procedure.

Dr. Sarkisian is a consultant to Alcon, the manufacturer of the EX-PRESS™ Glaucoma Filtration Device. Dr. Sarkisian was supported by an Unrestricted Grant from Research to Prevent Blindness to the Dean McGee Eye Institute, University of Oklahoma College of Medicine.

COMMENTARY

NICHOLAS P. BELL

The EX-PRESS™ shunt procedure has become popular among glaucoma specialists and general ophthalmologists by modifying the trabeculectomy procedure with which we are all comfortable. It has simplified one of the more technically difficult steps of the trabeculectomy by eliminating the need to cut a block of scleral tissue with scissors or a punch. The EX-PRESS™ shunt can be easily inserted without employing the help of a surgical assistant to retract the scleral flap. A recent study by Good and Kahook has shown similar surgical success rates and bleb morphology as a trabeculectomy after more than 2 years average follow-up.[17] The EX-PRESS™ shunt has also been touted to decrease rates of postoperative hypotony due to flow limitation through the small caliber device. Hyphema and anterior chamber inflammation are less frequent because there is not a need to cut an iridectomy.

There are as many variations on the trabeculectomy procedure as there are glaucoma surgeons. What if your surgical technique does not commonly lead to hypotony? Through the use of careful intraoperative calibration of scleral flap suture tension and postoperative laser suture lysis or mechanical suture release, the surgeon modulates the flow of aqueous whether or not there is a metal stent connecting the anterior chamber and the sub-Tenon's space. In the traditional trabeculectomy, the relationship between the size of the sclerostomy and the size of the scleral flap (or rather the distance between the edges of them) can be used to titrate the "surgical dose" of the procedure, depending on how aggressively the surgeon wishes to lower the IOP.

Finally, in an era of skyrocketing national healthcare costs, is it fiscally responsible of us to increase the cost to society of a procedure that can achieve similar results whether or not an expensive device is added?

Dr. Bell was supported by a Challenge Grant from Research to Prevent Blindness to The University of Texas Medical School at Houston and the Hermann Eye Fund.

REFERENCES

1. Kaplan-Messas A, Traverso CE, Sellem E, Zagorsky ZF, Belkin M. The EX-PRESS™ miniature glaucoma implant in combined surgery with cataract extraction: Prospective Study [ARVO E-abstract 3348]. *Invest Ophthalmol Vis Sci.* 2002;43.

2. Gandolfi S, Traverso CF, Bron A, Sellem E, Kaplan-Messas A, Belkin M. Short-term results of a miniature draining implant for glaucoma in combined surgery with phacoemulsification. *Acta Ophthalmol Scand Suppl.* 2002;236:66.

3. Traverso CE, De Feo F, Messas-Kaplan A, et al. Long term effect on IOP of a stainless steel glaucoma drainage implant (EX-PRESS™) in combined surgery with phacoemulsification. *Br J Ophthalmol.* Apr 2005;89(4):425–429.

4. Wamsley S, Moster MR, Rai S, Alvim HS, Fontanarosa J. Results of the use of the EX-PRESS™ miniature glaucoma implant in technically challenging, advanced glaucoma cases: a clinical pilot study. *Am J Ophthalmol.* Dec 2004;138(6):1049–1051.

5. Wamsley S, Moster MR, Rai S, Alvim H, Fontanarosa J, Steinmann WC. Optonol EX-PRESS™ miniature tube shunt in advanced glaucoma [ARVO E-abstract 994]. *Invest Ophthalmol Vis Sci.* 2004;45.

6. Stewart RM, Diamond JG, Ashmore ED, Ayyala RS. Complications following EX-PRESS™ glaucoma shunt implantation. *Am J Ophthalmol.* Aug 2005;140(2):340–341.

7. Rivier D, Roy S, Mermoud A. EX-PRESS™ R-50 miniature glaucoma implant insertion under the conjunctiva combined with cataract extraction. *J Cataract Refract Surg.* Nov 2007;33(11):1946–1952.

8. Tavolato M, Babighian S, Galan A. Spontaneous extrusion of a stainless steel glaucoma drainage implant (EX-PRESS™). *Eur J Ophthalmol.* Sept-Oct 2006;16(5):753–755.

9. Garg SJ, Kanitkar K, Weichel E, Fischer D. Trauma-induced extrusion of an EX-PRESS™ glaucoma shunt presenting as an intraocular foreign body. *Arch Ophthalmol.* Sept 2005;123(9):1270–1272.

10. Filippopoulos T, Rhee DJ. Novel surgical procedures in glaucoma: advances in penetrating glaucoma surgery. *Curr Opin Ophthalmol.* Mar 2008;19(2):149–154.

11. Stein JD, Herndon LW, Brent Bond J, Challa P. Exposure of EX-PRESS™ miniature glaucoma devices: case series and technique for tube shunt removal. *J Glaucoma.* Dec 2007;16(8):704–706.

12. Dahan E, Carmichael TR. Implantation of a miniature glaucoma device under a scleral flap. *J Glaucoma.* Apr 2005;14(2):98–102.

13. de Jong LA. The EX-PRESS™ glaucoma shunt versus trabeculectomy in open-angle glaucoma: a prospective randomized study. *Adv Ther.* Mar 2009;26(3):336–345.

14. Maris PJ Jr., Ishida K, Netland PA. Comparison of trabeculectomy with EX-PRESS™ miniature glaucoma device implanted under scleral flap. *J Glaucoma.* Jan 2007;16(1):14–19.

15. Kanner EM, Netland PA, Sarkisian SR Jr., Du H. EX-PRESS™ miniature glaucoma device implanted under a scleral flap alone or combined with phacoemulsification cataract surgery. *J Glaucoma.* Aug 2009;18(6):488–491.

16. Teng CC, Radcliffe N, Huang JE, Farris E. EX-PRESS™ glaucoma shunt dislocation into the anterior chamber. *J Glaucoma.* Dec 2008;17(8):687–689.

17. Good TJ, Kahook MY. Assessment of bleb morphologic features and postoperative outcomes after EX-PRESS™ drainage device implantation versus trabeculectomy. *Am J Ophthalmol.* Mar 2011;151(3):507–513 e501.

PART FOUR

TUBE SHUNT COMPLICATIONS

A. INTRAOPERATIVE COMPLICATIONS

30

TUBE MISDIRECTION AND INADEQUATE TUBE LENGTH

OMAR PIOVANETTI

TUBE MISDIRECTION AND INADEQUATE TUBE LENGTH

Tube misdirection and inadequate tube length are 2 problems commonly seen by glaucoma surgeons. These complications can occur at the time of surgery or develop years later. Understanding the underlying causes for these problems and techniques to prevent and manage these issues is critical for successful outcomes.

TUBE MISDIRECTION

Anterior chamber tube placement

Tube placed too anteriorly. During anterior chamber tube shunt implantation, a 23-gauge needle is commonly used to make entry into the anterior chamber. The tube is then inserted through this track into the space between the corneal and iris planes. For most surgeons the anterior chamber depth has been altered prior to tube insertion from shallowing caused by loss of aqueous volume during creation of a paracentesis or deepening caused by filling the chamber with viscoelastic to create enough room for placement. As the intraocular pressure (IOP) becomes lower, the postoperative anterior chamber depth is not always equal to the preoperative depth. As a result, the iris may move slightly forward, or if the shunt is to be implanted in combination with lens extraction, the iris may move more posteriorly. The unpredictability of postoperative chamber depth prevents consistent intraoperative determination of the appropriate plane of entry. Minimizing steps that affect the anterior chamber depth prior to tube insertion may help avoid these issues.

However, despite limiting anterior chamber depth alterations, it is not uncommon for the tube to not end up in the desired anterior chamber plane. The correct plane is in front of the iris with just enough space to prevent iris contact. If the tube ends up too anteriorly, it may rub against the corneal endothelium[1] and result in endothelial cell loss with chronic corneal edema. Alternatively, if the tube is placed too posteriorly, it could rub against the iris and cause chronic low-grade inflammation, worsening glaucoma along with other iritis-related issues. In either case, a new track may be made to direct the tube into the anterior chamber.

Tube in iris stroma or in the posterior chamber. Occasionally the tube embeds in the iris stroma during its insertion.[2] Careful preoperative evaluation is important for prevention of this scenario. Gonioscopy may determine the anatomy of the anterior chamber angle and the presence of peripheral anterior synechiae (PAS) at the site of intended tube placement. PAS in the area where the tube enters the anterior chamber may make the appropriate placement of the tube difficult, and an alternative site may be indicated.

However, if the peripheral iris is captured by the needle tip during insertion of the tube into the anterior chamber, iridodialysis and/or hemorrhage may occur. Furthermore, the posterior point of the anteriorly beveled tube tip may become entrapped within the iris stroma and may result in tube occlusion. Either of these situations requires immediate tube repositioning. In a shallow chamber, balanced salt solution or viscoelastic inserted via a paracentesis or the scleral needle track can be useful to push the peripheral iris posteriorly and deepen the angle. When faced with high PAS, one pearl for facilitating tube insertion is to twist the tube so that the bevel faces posteriorly during placement. Once the tube is fully inside the anterior chamber, the bevel can be rotated back to its intended anteriorly facing orientation.

If the patient is phakic and the tube primarily enters the posterior chamber or becomes embedded in the iris stroma, a new, more anteriorly oriented track should be made to place the tube in the anterior chamber. Also, the tube may have impaled the crystalline lens, which may result in a cataract or an inflammatory response, both of which will possibly necessitate lens extraction.

If the eye is pseudophakic, the scleral tunnel can be revised to have its entry point behind the iris into the posterior chamber. The tube tip then must be recut to have a posteriorly oriented bevel to avoid occlusion by the iris pigment epithelium. Ideally the tip of the tube should be seen within the pupil. If the tube is too short to see within a normal pupil size, then an iridectomy can be created to visualize the end of the tube.

If any of these suggestions are unsuccessful, the original scleral tunnel can be abandoned altogether. Suture closure of the original needle track is usually not performed, as flow is generally not significant, and it may not be necessary, as it could serve as a temporary method of IOP lowering for a nonvalved tube. A new needle track may be created at a different clock hour where PAS are absent or less prominent. The new scleral tunnel can be made with an *ab interno* approach by inserting a 23-gauge needle through a paracentesis 180 degrees away from the intended entry site and making the track starting from inside the anterior chamber and coming out through the sclera. This track can be made with or without the help of an intraoperative gonioscopy lens for direct visualization. If necessary, the needle can be replaced by a rigid suture (e.g., 3–0 polypropylene) or a cannula, which can be used as a "guide wire" to facilitate tube placement. This technique is extremely useful when intentionally inserting the tube into the posterior chamber or if difficulty is encountered when inserting the tube of a valved device. When implanting a nonvalved tube shunt, a 3–0 polypropylene suture placed within the entire length of the tube eases insertion into the wound by acting as a stylet.

Preventing corneal damage from a migrating or eroding anterior tube. Over months or years tubes migrate anteriorly as the tube tends to straighten. This condition is more pronounced in children, as they have more malleable sclera,[3, 4] but occurs in adults, especially those with thin sclera (i.e., high myopes) or low sclera rigidity. The end result may be endothelial damage, or in extreme cases, the tube may fully erode through the cornea and become exposed.[5] Creating a new, more posteriorly oriented track should solve this problem. Unfortunately, corneal endothelial cells are extremely limited in their ability to replicate or regenerate (to the point where, clinically, endothelial cells can be considered nonreplicating). Instead, these cells enlarge and spread out to cover defects in response to focal damage.[6–10] If a tube is placed too anteriorly, over time it can act as a "sink" to which endothelial cells migrate to the entry site futilely trying to cover the area of cell loss. Corneal edema will persist after tube relocation if endothelial dysfunction continues.[11] If repositioning is necessary and the potential exists for future keratoplasty, it is prudent to move the tube to either the sulcus or pars plana to ease future corneal surgery.

Pars plana tube placement

When implanting a tube in the pars plana, the pass through the scleral wall should be angled radially and posteriorly toward the center of the posterior segment. The tip of the blade or needle used to make the pars plana entry must be observed through the pupil to ensure that the vitreous cavity has been entered. After the tube is inserted, visualization through the pupil will confirm localization and that there is no vitreous clogging the tube. As with tubes inserted into the posterior chamber, the bevel should be made posteriorly to prevent aspiration of ciliary processes or iris. If the eye has not already undergone adequate vitrectomy, this procedure should be planned with a vitreoretinal surgeon so that an adequate vitrectomy can performed, along with shaving of the vitreous base in the quadrant where the tube will be placed. For further discussion, see Chapter 46.

INADEQUATE TUBE LENGTH

Preventing inadequate tube length

Careful planning and a small repertoire of intraoperative techniques are crucial for preventing inadequate tube length. If not firmly secured to the sclera, the plate may move postoperatively, causing the tube to retract from the anterior chamber. A short tube cannot be untrimmed; it is better when cutting the tube to err on the side of leaving it too long and then trimming to a more appropriate length if necessary. One must make sure not to pull on the tube end, inadvertently stretching it while cutting, because when tension is released, the elastic properties of the tube may recoil so much that it may not be long enough to remain in the anterior chamber.

After intraocular insertion, the tube must be fastened to the sclera to prevent lateral or radial movement. Furthermore, when implanting a nonvalved device, extra care must be taken not to transect the tube if creating venting slits or when suturing the tube closed. Some surgeons prefer to suture the tube to the sclera in an S-fashion, or snake form, so there is extra slack in case additional length is needed postoperatively. If more length becomes necessary, a short or retracted tube can be easily revised by freeing it and repositioning it in a more radial orientation. Leaving extra length on the tube is especially important in pediatric cases, where growth of the globe and subsequent tube retraction is expected (see Chapter 48). However, it is important to avoid anterior-posterior and buckling forces on the tube, as they may predispose to tube extrusions.

Management of short tubes

The remainder of this chapter will present a variety of techniques for managing tubes that are too short. Replacement of the entire tube shunt at the time of implantation is rarely necessary. The following options are technically easy and generally cost-effective.

Resuturing the plate more anteriorly. In the case of cutting the tube too short intraoperatively, 1–2 mm of additional intraocular tube length can be achieved by resuturing the plate more anteriorly. However, it is advisable not to move the plate closer than 7 or 8 mm from the limbus, as the risk of conjunctival erosions will increase if the device is anterior enough that the upper eyelid rubs against it during blinking. If using a Baerveldt® Glaucoma Implant (Abbott Medical Optics, Inc., Santa Ana, California), the rectus muscles will limit anterior mobility (assuming the wings of the plate have been placed underneath the muscle bellies). If the tube retracts postoperatively, anterior repositioning of the plate is difficult

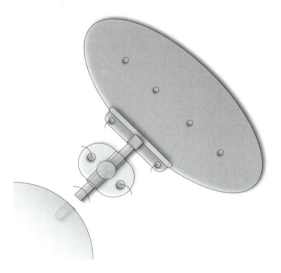

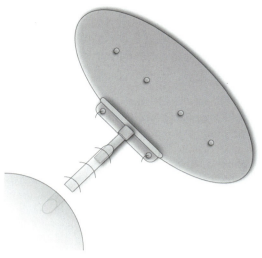

FIGURE 30.1 Tube Extender™ (New World Medical, Inc., Rancho Cucamonga, California)

FIGURE 30.2 Use of an angiocatheter to extend a short tube. The angiocatheter and its accompanying needle are inserted into the anterior chamber. The needle is then retracted, leaving the anterior end of the angiocatheter inside the anterior chamber. The posterior side of the catheter is then trimmed to the appropriate length, and the stump of the tube shunt is inserted onto the other end of the angiocatheter tube.

once the fibrous capsule develops around the plate.

Tube Extender™. The most popular technique for extending a tube, either during the initial tube shunt implantation or as a revision, is by using the commercially available Tube Extender™ (New World Medical, Inc., Rancho Cucamonga, California; Figure 30.1).[12, 13] This premade device is convenient because it comes long and can be trimmed to the desired length. It also has a plate with 2 loopholes for scleral fixation so the tube extender will not migrate. Making a bevel in the tip of the original tube's stump may be necessary to facilitate its insertion into the posterior end of the Tube Extender™. Additionally, with its large size and proximity to the limbus, the Tube Extender™ requires a patch graft cover to decrease the risk of conjunctival erosion and device extrusion.

Angiocatheters. A 22- or 23-gauge angiocatheter sleeve is a very economic alternative that can also be used as an extender.[14, 15] One way an angiocatheter can be used to extend a tube is in a procedure that mimics its use in phlebotomies. The angiocatheter and its accompanying needle are inserted into the anterior chamber. The needle is then retracted, leaving the anterior end of the angiocatheter inside the anterior chamber. The posterior side of the catheter is then trimmed

to the appropriate length, and the stump of the tube shunt is inserted (Figure 30.2). The catheter and tube must be tightly secured to the sclera[14, 15] to prevent migration into the anterior chamber[15] or into the vitreous in the case of an aphakic patient (Figure 30.3). Some

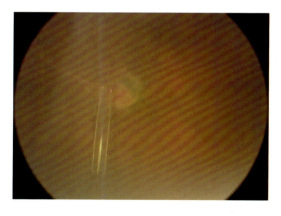

FIGURE 30.3 Unsecured tube migration into vitreous in an aphakic patient.

surgeons suture the 2 tubes together with a monofilament suture on a BV needle.[15]

To avoid slippage that occurs with the technique described above, a small segment of an angiocatheter can also be used as a sleeve extender to connect 2 pieces of tubing together (Figure 30.4).[14, 15] If the tube is transected inadvertently during surgery (most commonly as venting slits are being cut), this technique can be extremely useful. The short tube attached to the plate is cut in the middle of its length, and a segment of catheter is used as a bridge to connect the 2 halves of the original tube. The individual components must be tightly secured to the sclera to prevent migration.[15]

Canalicular repair tubes. If the free piece of tube cannot be salvaged, a Crawford tube can be inserted into the anterior chamber (Figure 30.5). Crawford tubes, silicone tubes used for canalicular and lacrimal drainage system surgery, have dimensions and properties similar to the tubes found on most common shunts. One individual Crawford tube can be used for a single patient, or one Crawford tube can be divided it into several pieces, packaged individually, sterilized, and then used for several patients.

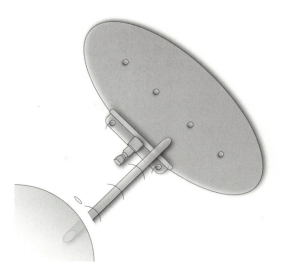

FIGURE 30.5   Use of a Crawford tube to extend a short tube. Only use a Crawford tube if there is a mature capsule over the plate of the tube shunt.

A Crawford tube can only be used for tube revisions once a mature capsule has formed around the plate, unless a technique is used for temporary occlusion, as is done routinely with nonvalved tube shunt devices (see Chapter 35). If used to revise a tube shunt that has a capsule present, the original tube should be cut close to the plate, and the capsule over the stump tied closed. Next, a small opening is made in the anterior aspect of the fibrous capsule over the plate, the new Crawford tube is inserted over the plate, and the capsule is tightly sutured closed around it. Alternatively, a 23-gauge needle can be used to enter the fibrous capsule with the tube and then inserted into the capsule in the same manner as it would be inserted into the anterior chamber. Either way, once the new tube is secured within the fibrous capsule, it is then inserted intraocularly and fastened to the sclera. Tightly securing the components to the sclera is extremely important to prevent migration, and the tube should not move or migrate as long as there is sufficient tension on these sutures. Finally, the anterior entry site should be covered with a patch graft, as is customarily done.

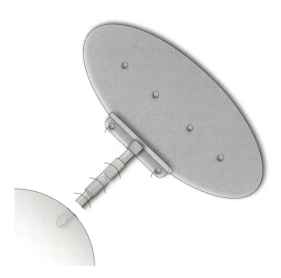

FIGURE 30.4   A second technique for using an angiocatheter to extend a short tube. The short tube attached to the plate is cut in the middle of its length, and a segment of catheter is used as a bridge to connect the 2 halves of the original tube.

Move to pars plana. Another approach to managing an intact but short tube is to move it to pars plana. See discussion above and Chapter 46 for further information.

CONCLUSION

Tube misdirection and inadequate tube length are likely to be encountered by every surgeon who implants enough tube shunts. The frequency of these problems can be lessened by routinely employing some of the surgical techniques recommended. Unfortunately, not every surgical complication can be avoided, so tube shunt surgeons should be familiar with techniques for managing tubes that do not remain in the intended location.

COMMENTARY

JEFFREY FREEDMAN

An alternative approach to dealing with tube misdirection and inadequate tube length

Prior to tube insertion, trim the tube to an appropriate length for the condition being treated; the usual length is 1–3 mm of tube in the anterior chamber. To prevent blockage of the tube in neovascular glaucoma, it should reach pupil margin. The tube should be cut while held over the cornea, not on the stretch, with bevel of tube opening up. A paracentesis is then made at the limbus with a microsharp blade, allowing for ability to maintain a consistent depth of the anterior chamber by balanced salt solution, or viscous gel, insertion prior to tube insertion. The paracentesis opening also allows for the insertion of an iris repositor, which can manipulate the tube during insertion, if the tip enters the iris. The 23- or 22-guage needle, used to enter the anterior chamber, is then inserted immediately behind the limbus. In the presence of peripheral anterior synechiae, the needle insertion should be moved forward to enter in front of the synechiae. The aim is to place the tube in mid-aqueous, midway between iris and cornea. The lip of the tunnel opening is grasped with a fine forceps, which opens the space and allows for easy insertion of the tube.

Management of inadequate tube length

An alternative approach to this problem is to use 2 tubes available from IOP, Inc. (Costa Mesa, California). The tubes are of 2 sizes. One is large and can fit snugly over the cut end of the silicone tube found in any of the glaucoma implants; the second smaller tube inserts snugly into the cut end of the larger tube. The tubes can be trimmed to the desired length, and after being connected to the shortened silicone tube, can be reinserted into the anterior chamber through the preexisting opening into the anterior chamber, if one exists, or by using a separate needle entry at the limbus.

COMMENTARY

RICHARD P. MILLS

I would like to provide a few additional tips to help achieve proper tube angulation in the anterior chamber. First, if using a nonvalved device, a temporary suture in the lumen stiffens the tube and produces a temporary moderate anterior angulation that will disappear when the suture is removed postoperatively. Second, if a first needle track has improper angulation, a second track can be placed just anterior or posterior to the original one, and the presence of the tube will close the unwanted track without a suture. Finally, if the anterior chamber shallows or there are peripheral anterior synechiae, a bimanual tube placement maneuver is very helpful. The anterior chamber at the point of tube entry is deepened with cohesive viscoelastic, and a cyclodialysis spatula through a paracentesis 90 degrees away is used to compress the iris root against the ciliary sulcus while the 23-gauge needle, and later the tube itself, passes easily through the obstruction without causing iridodialysis.

When the anterior chamber is absent peripherally, following multiple penetrating keratoplasty or trauma, tube placement in the posterior chamber is attractive. Often the anteriorly situated iris stands off the crystalline lens or pseudophakos, and this situation can be accentuated using focal introduction of viscoelastic during tube placement. I agree that leaving the tube long enough to visualize and cutting the bevel posteriorly to avoid iris incarceration are desirable maneuvers.

Prevention of short tube length is certainly preferable to dealing with it later, so it is better to err on the long side when placing one. Long tubes, even those near or even across the visual axis, seldom produce visual symptoms. One additional cause of short tube is intraoperative scleral collapse in a soft eye. The tube may seem to be long enough, but on reformation of the spherical globe shape, it may turn out to be too short. If it is necessary to lengthen a tube postoperatively, I have found that directly suturing the smaller tube ends to the overlapping splice with 10–0 nylon or polypropylene helps avoid disconnection. The tubes are slippery and can often slide under a suture, "anchoring" them to the sclera. Finally, I avoid the commercially available tube extender because it is rigid and bulky and tends to erode through even thick patch grafts with time.

REFERENCES

1. Tsai JC, Grajewski AL, Parrish RK 2nd. Surgical revision of glaucoma shunt implants. *Ophthalmic Surg Lasers.* Jan 1999;30(1):41–46.
2. Carrillo MM, Trope GE, Pavlin C, Buys YM. Use of ultrasound biomicroscopy to diagnose Ahmed™ valve obstruction by iris. *Can J Ophthalmol.* Aug 2005;40(4):499–501.
3. O'Malley Schotthoefer E, Yanovitch TL, Freedman SF. Aqueous drainage device surgery in refractory pediatric glaucomas: I. Long-term outcomes. *J AAPOS.* Feb 2008;12(1):33–39.
4. Ishida K, Mandal AK, Netland PA. Glaucoma drainage implants in pediatric patients. *Ophthalmol Clin North Am.* Sept 2005;18(3):431–442, vii.
5. Maki JL, Nesti HA, Shetty RK, Rhee DJ. Transcorneal tube extrusion in a child with a Baerveldt® glaucoma drainage device. *J AAPOS.* Aug 2007;11(4):395–397.
6. Hoppenreijs VP, Pels E, Vrensen GF, Treffers WF. Corneal endothelium and growth factors. *Surv Ophthalmol.* Sept-Oct 1996;41(2):155–164.
7. Doughman DJ, Van Horn D, Rodman WP, Byrnes P, Lindstrom RL. Human corneal endothelial layer repair during organ culture. *Arch Ophthalmol.* Oct 1976;94(10):1791–1796.
8. Van Horn DL, Hyndiuk RA. Endothelial wound repair in primate cornea. *Exp Eye Res.* Aug 1975;21(2):113–124.
9. Gipson IK, Joyce NC. Anatomy and cell biology of the cornea, superficial limbus, and conjunctiva. In: Albert DM, Jakobiec FA, eds. *Principles and Practice of Ophthalmology.* Vol 2: Conjunctiva, Cornea, and Sclera; Uveitis; Lens. Philadelphia: W.B. Saunders Company; 2000:612–629.
10. Waring GO 3rd, Bourne WM, Edelhauser HF, Kenyon KR. The corneal endothelium. Normal and pathologic structure and function. *Ophthalmology.* Jun 1982;89(6):531–590.
11. Dohlman CH, Klyce SD. Corneal edema. In: Albert DM, Jakobiec FA, eds. *Principles and Practice of Ophthalmology.* Vol 2: Conjunctiva, Cornea, and Sclera; Uveitis; Lens. Philadelphia: W.B. Saunders Company; 2000:646–657.
12. Merrill KD, Suhr AW, Lim MC. Long-term success in the correction of exposed glaucoma drainage tubes with a tube extender. *Am J Ophthalmol.* Jul 2007;144(1):136–137.
13. Sarkisian SR, Netland PA. Tube extender for revision of glaucoma drainage implants. *J Glaucoma.* Oct-Nov 2007;16(7):637–639.
14. Smith MF, Doyle JW. Results of another modality for extending glaucoma drainage tubes. *J Glaucoma.* Oct 1999;8(5):310–314.
15. Sheets CW, Ramjattan TK, Smith MF, Doyle JW. Migration of glaucoma drainage device extender into anterior chamber after trauma. *J Glaucoma.* Dec 2006;15(6):559–561.

31

SCLERAL PERFORATION

JORGE L. RIVERA-VELEZ

SCLERAL PERFORATION

Scleral perforation during tube shunt implantation is a rare complication.[1] In a recent publication of the Tube Versus Trabeculectomy Study, 3 out of 107 patients in the tube shunt group had scleral perforation during placement of a device.[2] Merino-de-Palacios et al reported scleral perforation during tube shunt surgery in 1 of 86 eyes.[3] The type of device used does not seem to be important in the incidence of scleral perforation. In the Tube Versus Trabeculectomy Study, Baerveldt® devices (Abbott Medical Optics, Inc., Santa Ana, California) were used exclusively, and Ahmed™ Glaucoma Valves (New World Medical, Inc., Rancho Cucamonga, California) and Molteno® implants (Molteno Ophthalmic, Ltd., Dunedin, New Zealand) were used in the study by Merino-de-Palacios et al. Serious sequelae, such as endophthalmitis or retinal detachment, have not been reported in recent literature following scleral perforation during tube shunt placement; nonetheless, this complication should be prevented and, if it does occur, managed promptly.

RISK FACTORS

Patients who are believed to have an increased risk for scleral perforation are myopic patients (>-6.00 D) and patients with previous extraocular muscle surgery.[4] Patients with previous scleral buckle surgery, autoimmune diseases, scleritis,[5] or any other conditions that cause or perpetuate thinning of the sclera potentially increase the risk. Patients with previous scleral buckling procedures who require tube shunt surgery will benefit from having the device anchored behind the buckle or directly over the buckle. No attempt should be made to dissect under the buckling device, as dissection may lead to the buckle anchoring sutures perforating the eye.[6]

PREVENTION

The most common site for tube shunt implantation is the superotemporal quadrant, between the superior and lateral rectus muscles. This location offers the benefit of having the implant hidden under the superior eyelid, no oblique muscles in the region, and better intraoperative exposure, allowing the surgeon to place the implant farther from the limbus. The plate of the implant is usually attached to the sclera approximately 8–10 mm posterior to the limbus. This is also the thinnest portion of the sclera. Exposure when implanting the tube shunt is probably the most important factor in avoiding scleral perforation. Good exposure means good visualization of the needle as it is passed. Although surgeons' choices of suture material may vary, most employ a spatulated needle. Care should be taken to ensure passage of the needle is through the superior third of the sclera because scleral thickness ranges from 0.3 mm at its thinnest point right behind the insertion of the rectus muscles to 0.4–0.5 mm at the equator.[7, 8] The needle must enter into the tissue flat and exit in the same way to prevent damage and tearing of the sclera. Direct visualization of the needle as it is passed through the sclera generally ensures proper depth placement of the suture to prevent perforation. Furthermore, if bluish choroid is visible through the sclera, this in an indication that the sclera is thin, and care should be taken to avoid perforation.

Recognizing when scleral perforation has occurred is essential to prevent further damage to the eye. Perforation of the sclera should be suspected if fluid, blood, vitreous, or pigment is seen oozing through the needle track. A soft globe during plate placement should also alert the surgeon that perforation might have occurred.

MANAGEMENT

The general consensus for treating scleral perforation during tube shunt implantation is application of cryotherapy.[2, 3] In this procedure, the probe is applied directly to the perforation site. Each application of cryotherapy is performed until a 1 mm ice crystal is created. If direct visualization through a dilated pupil is possible, then cryotherapy should be applied until blanching of the retina is seen. Transscleral diode laser might also be used to treat the perforation.

If perforation of the sclera has occurred, the patient should be informed, and symptoms related to a possible retinal detachment explained. Thorough examination of the affected area through a dilated pupil should be done during the postoperative period. If any signs of subretinal fluid or impending retinal detachment are detected, the patient should be referred to a vitreoretinal colleague for appropriate management. Although most surgeons would perform cryotherapy over the perforation site prophylactically, the literature contains no reports of retinal detachment related to scleral perforation with tube shunt procedures. There have, however, been reports of retinal detachment after perforation in strabismus surgery.[4, 9]

CONCLUSION

The tube shunt surgeon must have thorough understanding of the anatomy of the region where the shunt will be placed, understand who is at risk, and take care to recognize when scleral perforation has occurred. With careful surgical technique and awareness of the risk factors, this complication should continue to be exceedingly rare.

COMMENTARY

ROBERT J. NOECKER

Dr. Rivera's overview provides a very thorough description of a potentially serious complication of tube shunt placement. Perforation during plate fixation to the sclera can be vision threatening due to potential retinal detachment and/or endophthalmitis. Surgeons should ask themselves the following questions. First, does the risk of scleral perforation in at least some patients justify the benefit of plate fixation? Second, is plate fixation a necessary part of the procedure in order to achieve an effective, safe result?

For those patients who are at high risk, consideration needs to be given to using techniques that do not involve suturing the plate to the sclera posteriorly. Surgeons have already become comfortable with no longer placing sutures through all 4 holes of the Molteno® device, as was the norm with earlier implantations. It has become a generally accepted technique now to only suture the plate with the anterior 2 positioning holes—and indeed many new devices only have positioning holes on the anterior aspect of the plate. Fewer passes through the sclera in areas overlying the retina translates into less risk of perforation.

The next question is, does the plate need to be sutured at all? The plate is mobile in the first week or so after placement, but then fibrosis occurs through the positioning holes as well as any other holes in the body of the plate, such as those in the Baerveldt® implants. Once the plate is encapsulated around the perimeter and through the holes on the plate, the device is no longer mobile and indeed can be very difficult to remove once the fibrous bands have been established.

Some securing of the plate is necessary to prevent migration of the tube in the early post-operative period. This can often be accomplished by placing a suture over or through the tube and anchoring it to the underlying anterior sclera. This region is very safe for fixation given the thickness of the sclera and the absence of underlying retina 3 or 4 mm posterior to the limbus. The use of fixation sutures at the level of the tube is very effective in halting tube movement, and the plate also tends to remain in place in its position between the rectus muscles. New adhesives may also allow surgeons to avoid suture use around the plates of tube shunts and reduce the incidence of unnecessary complications associated with scleral perforation.

COMMENTARY

JEFFREY FREEDMAN

The author's description of this rare complication is very thorough. An additional helpful deterrent to this complication is the nature of the needle used for implant fixation. A needle with a severe curve allows the needle to exit the sclera very close to its insertion, which also decreases the subscleral passage of the needle, making it less likely to perforate the sclera. An 8–0 Ethilon suture TG175–8 spatula needle (Ethicon, Inc., Somerville, New Jersey) is an excellent needle for this purpose.

REFERENCES

1. Nguyen QH. Avoiding and managing complications of glaucoma drainage implants. *Curr Opin Ophthalmol.* Apr 2004;15(2):147–150.
2. Gedde SJ, Herndon LW, Brandt JD, Budenz DL, Feuer WJ, Schiffman JC. Surgical complications in the Tube Versus Trabeculectomy Study during the first year of follow-up. *Am J Ophthalmol.* Jan 2007;143(1):23–31.
3. Merino-de-Palacios C, Gutierrez-Diaz E, Chacon-Garces A, Montero-Rodriguez M, Mencia-Gutierrez E. [Intermediate-term outcome of glaucoma drainage devices]. *Arch Soc Esp Oftalmol.* Jan 2008;83(1):15–22.
4. Awad AH, Mullaney PB, Al-Hazmi A, et al. Recognized globe perforation during strabismus surgery: incidence, risk factors, and sequelae. *J AAPOS.* Jun 2000;4(3):150–153.
5. Okhravi N, Odufuwa B, McCluskey P, Lightman S. Scleritis. *Surv Ophthalmol.* Jul-Aug 2005;50(4):351–363.
6. Scott IU, Gedde SJ, Budenz DL, et al. Baerveldt® drainage implants in eyes with a preexisting scleral buckle. *Arch Ophthalmol.* Nov 2000;118(11):1509–1513.
7. Watson PG, Young RD. Scleral structure, organisation and disease. A review. *Exp Eye Res.* Mar 2004;78(3):609–623.
8. Norman RE, Flanagan JG, Rausch SM, et al. Dimensions of the human sclera: Thickness measurement and regional changes with axial length. *Exp Eye Res.* Feb 2010;90(2):277–284.
9. Wolf E, Wagner RS, Zarbin MA. Anterior segment ischemia and retinal detachment after vertical rectus muscle surgery. *Eur J Ophthalmol.* Jan-Mar 2000;10(1):82–87.

32

VITREOUS PROLAPSE

TONY REALINI AND ALBERT S. KHOURI

VITREOUS PROLAPSE

"I've never lost vitreous. However, I have found it on occasion."
—Robert D. Fechtner, MD

There are few absolutes in glaucoma surgery. Here is one: vitreous is bad. Anticipating and avoiding it are the best ways to avoid complications, but managing it is necessary when it rears its ugly head.

ANTICIPATE IT

There are several clinical settings in which vitreous anticipation is appropriate and expected. Recognizing these settings in advance will allow for a prepared surgical approach.

Aphakia

Aphakic eyes pose perhaps the highest risk of encountering vitreous during tube shunt placement. In an aphakic eye, the natural barrier holding the vitreous back—the lens and specifically its posterior capsule—is no longer present. These eyes typically have vitreous at or only just behind the pupil, bare millimeters from where the tip of the tube will rest. If vitreous is in the anterior chamber prior to surgery, judicious use of viscoelastics will typically keep the vitreous away from the tube; however, if the vitreous has breached the pupil, it would be wise to clean it up prior to tube insertion. (See below for surgical details.) With vitreous just peeking through the pupil, it might be tempting to try to slip the tube in quickly and get out without stirring things up, with possible success in the short term. Postoperatively, however, if the eye is cursed with a bout of hypotony or as vitreous syneresis progresses, vitreous will almost certainly find its way to the tube lumen, the operation will no longer be successful, and the vitreous will have to be dealt with anyway.

After complicated cataract surgery

Vitreous occasionally presents during cataract surgery, during which time a good clean-up yields a good visual outcome. An incomplete clean-up may also permit a good visual outcome, but leaves the equivalent of a landmine for the glaucoma surgeon who might follow in the cataract surgeon's wake. It behooves the glaucoma surgeon to review the operative reports for all pseudophakic eyes—particularly those with pseudoexfoliation that are prone to zonular dehiscence and subsequent vitreous laden complications during cataract surgery—so that any encounter with vitreous during tube shunt placement has been anticipated and planned for.

Traumatic eyes

The post-traumatic eye can offer a variety of unpleasant surprises for the unprepared surgeon. Subclinical disruption of the zonulo-capsular barrier can be difficult to appreciate on a routine examination, particularly in a phakic patient. The presence of phacodonesis is a good predictor of lack of zonulo-capsular integrity with unrecognized anteriorly prolapsed vitreous hidden behind the iris. A simple clinical test is to have the patient look quickly to the side and then straight ahead while observing in the slit lamp. Where there is a jiggly lens, there is often jiggly vitreous lurking about, waiting for an anterior decompression to leap forward into the void. A second test is to look for the same things while abruptly tapping the slit-lamp table. A careful inspection of the pupillary margin after dilation may also reveal peripheral vitreous. In these eyes, the surgeon might consider dilating the pupil (rather than constricting it) during surgery to provide better access to this vitreous for clean-up before tube insertion.

Eyes at risk for suprachoroidal hemorrhage

The worst of the worst case scenarios, an intra-operative expulsive suprachoroidal hemorrhage (SCH) will ruin everyone's day. SCH and vitreous prolapse share some of the same preoperative risk factors, such as aphakia/pseudophakia, traumatized eyes, vitrectomized eyes, and large eyes due to congenital glaucoma or pathological myopia. Systemic hypertension and bleeding disorders have also been associated with SCH, as well as rapid decompression from a highly elevated preoperative intraocular pressure (IOP). Vitreous can be propelled anteriorly by the sheer mass effect of the rapidly expanding choroid. This risk is higher with trabeculectomy than tube shunt surgery, but forward-moving vitreous can reach and occlude the tube tip in some cases. Should SCH occur during tube shunt surgery, the immediate goal is to tightly close the eye to raise the IOP, countering the rapid hemorrhage and prevent expulsion of intraocular contents. Vitreous clean-up and recovery of tube function should wait until the clot dissolves. Within 7–14 days drainage of the suprachoroidal space and any necessary vitrectomy to salvage tube function can usually safely be performed. The timing of this intervention can be guided by the appearance of yellow aqueous, which signifies clot dissolution. For more on suprachoroidal hemorrhage, see Chapter 6.

When planning pars plana tube placement

Pars plana insertion of the tube is occasionally preferred over anterior chamber placement, but is advised only if a prior (or concurrent) vitrectomy has been performed; otherwise the tube may become plugged by errant vitreous. So-called "limited" or "core" vitrectomies are often inadequate for this purpose, as they typically do not involve removal of the peripheral anterior vitreous near its base, where the tube will dwell. For more information, see Chapter 46.

When least expected

Unfortunately, it is not always possible to anticipate the appearance of vitreous. Like the tax man, it can appear anywhere, at any time, and no one is ever glad to see it.

AVOID IT

The single best way to avoid vitreous is to anticipate when it is most likely to appear, as just described, and (as with in-laws) take the appropriate steps to keep it far, far away. In some of the above cases, the prudent course is to plan removal of the potentially offending vitreous either in advance of your tube placement or immediately prior to tube insertion. In other cases, more conservative approaches may be warranted. For instance, if an eye is deemed at high risk for a suprachoroidal hemorrhage (Chapter 6), prophylactic sclerostomies may be advisable.[1]

An alternative approach is to consider the value of perioperative vitreous dehydration.[2] This state can be accomplished with external ocular compression devices, such as the Honan balloon (The Lebanon Corporation, Lebanon, Indiana), or with medications, such as mannitol. One consideration is that ocular compression will elevate IOP substantially in the perioperative period, which may be unacceptable in eyes with advanced glaucoma.

MAKE IT GO AWAY

If, despite anticipation and avoidance strategies, vitreous is still encountered during tube placement, surgical success depends largely on the thoroughness of clean-up. Here we share our approach to vitreous clean-up during tube surgery.

Operative considerations when vitreous is encountered

Once vitreous has gained access to the anterior chamber, the first priority is to prevent further vitreous prolapse by minimizing such factors as eyelid pressure and squeezing. It is important to ensure the patient's comfort with adequate anesthesia. Supplementing sub-Tenon's or peribulbar anesthesia may be necessary, keeping in mind that higher volumes of anesthetic will lead to a tighter orbit, potentially worsening vitreous prolapse.[3] Using the least required volume (we find 2–3 mL is usually sufficient) in combination with systemic sedation (midazolam or other agents) works well for most patients.

Once the patient is comfortable and everyone's pulses have returned to normal, the next priority is to prevent tube blockage with vitreous. Clean-up of the anterior chamber must be performed slowly, completely, and meticulously. The single port, coaxial anterior vitrectomy approach often further disrupts vitreous, inviting more of it to come forward. A 2-port anterior vitrectomy or anterior irrigation with single port pars plana vitrectomy is preferred as it separates irrigation from vitreous cutting, keeping the irrigating cannula in the anterior chamber while the cutter is more posterior. Maintaining anterior chamber depth with a low irrigation bottle height, using low vacuum, and high cut rates offer the best conditions to remove vitreous without excessive traction. For more information on tube shunts and vitreous complications, see Chapter 46.

Once clean-up appears complete, the anterior chamber should be diligently assessed for vitreous strands. The path of least resistance for outflow postoperatively is going to be through the tube. Even a few vitreous strands caught up in the tube are enough to obstruct flow and require another surgical intervention to reestablish tube function. Confirming that all vitreous is removed when viewing through the operating microscope's coaxial light can be challenging, as vitreous is generally clear in color and thus difficult to see within equally clear aqueous. It is helpful to observe for any iris movements while sweeping over the iris plane with a surgical spatula. Even the most subtle iris movement indicates residual vitreous. High-molecular-weight viscoelastics can be utilized to push the vitreous posteriorly behind the iris plane. Once all vitreous is removed, constricting the pupil with miotics may be useful to maintain additional separation from the posterior segment. Peaked or eccentric pupil constriction is another sign of persistent vitreous presence in the iris plane. Triamcinolone may be injected into the anterior chamber; the particulate matter will "stain" the vitreous strands, assisting visualization.

Tube placement

Consider tube placement carefully after an anterior vitrectomy. One encounter with vitreous may often lead to another. When trimming the tube prior to anterior chamber insertion, drape it over the cornea in order to visualize the length of the intraocular portion. The tube tip should be well into the anterior chamber, but not reaching over the pupil. Cut the tip bevel so it will face anteriorly rather than flat or posteriorly. Do not be overly cautious and trim the tube too short. Once intraoperative hypotony and postoperative inflammation resolve, the globe will assume its original configuration. A short tube may end up retracted into the scleral tunnel or iris root and need to be revised. When anticipating a posterior segment intervention for another retinal indication, or if operating in conjunction with a vitreoretinal surgeon who is performing a *complete* posterior vitrectomy, a pars plana tube may be inserted. This tube placement is preferred in eyes with shallow anterior chambers or compromised corneas.

POSTOPERATIVE CONSIDERATIONS

Alas, even after leaving the operating theater following a successful clean-up of vitreous, the evil humor may still have tricks up its sleeve. With attentive postoperative care, postoperative vitreous complications can be kept at bay. When using nonvalved devices, one should avoid early release of an occluding stent or suture, as outflow may pull vitreous strands anteriorly into the tube. Additionally, pharmacological miosis both shrinks the pupil and uses the iris as a shield between the posterior vitreous and the anterior tube tip. It is also wise to emphasize to patients the perils of eye rubbing, which may lead to forward expression of vitreous toward the tube tip during the early postoperative period.

Even after surviving the early postoperative period, the tube tip can become blocked at any time in the future.[4] Fibrin or blood clots are not uncommon in the early postoperative period. Sometimes vitreous strands are noted in the tube months to years after surgery. These late-appearing strands may lead to complete or partial obstruction, and by virtue of its miniscule internal diameter, even partial obstruction of the tube usually results in elevation of IOP, necessitating surgical clearance. For more information on obstruction, see Chapter 37.

The Nd:YAG laser can be used to lyse vitreous strands coming up through the tube. While it is attractive to attempt conservative measures before revisiting the operating theater, laser vitreolysis may result in an unsatisfying outcome. The vitreous is difficult to focus upon, and when hit with the Nd:YAG laser, tends to free up smaller parts that may then migrate even farther up the tube, blocking it more effectively and making later surgery more difficult. It is not imprudent to attempt this maneuver, but expectations for success should be low, and a reoperation should be anticipated.

CONCLUSIONS

In summary, vitreous prolapse during tube shunt surgery is a highly undesirable event. While it can often be anticipated, it can also appear seemingly at random. With appropriate attention to detail, a meticulous clean-up can provide a successful surgical outcome.

COMMENTARY

SHAN C. LIN

Drs. Realini and Khouri have written a very thorough and plainly spoken treatise on dealing with potential vitreous in the setting of tube surgery for glaucoma. As they point out, anyone who has significant experience with tube shunt surgery has likely had interaction with vitreous, sometimes in an unexpected fashion during or after the case. Suprachoroidal hemorrhage is one of the most feared complications, and this is addressed in detail by the authors.

Additional recommendations for eyes that have vitrectomy may include making the tube tip slightly longer in case there is tube retraction due to scleral collapse[5] and tying the tube tighter for nonvalved tubes to avoid hypotony.[5]

Dr. Lin was supported by an Unrestricted Grant from Research to Prevent Blindness to the University of California at San Francisco, National Eye Institute grant P30EY002162, and That Man May See, Inc.

COMMENTARY

PAUL A. SIDOTI AND MICHAEL R. BANITT

We agree that the best way to deal with vitreous is to anticipate and avoid it. When encountered, prolapsed vitreous is best visualized by injecting dilute unpreserved triamcinolone followed by a small volume of balanced salt solution. A pars plana vitrectomy is more efficient than an anterior vitrectomy in clearing vitreous that may cause or has caused tube occlusion. A 2-port approach can often be used, passing the vitreous cutter through a pars plana sclerotomy with infusion through a second pars plana sclerotomy or a corneal paracentesis track. More complete, posterior vitrectomy is sometimes advantageous in separating the posterior hyaloid and preventing future tube occlusion by prolapsed anterior vitreous.

When planning the entry site, the surgeon must anticipate the ultimate final placement of the tube's tip. In cases of aphakia or complicated cataract surgery where there could be vitreous ready to make friends with the tube, we typically try to avoid leaving the tip of the tube near a peripheral iridectomy. We also try to leave the tip of the tube more peripheral, which can be accomplished by cutting the tube shorter and/or inserting the tube at an oblique angle instead of radially.

Dr. Sidoti was supported by The David E. Marrus Glaucoma Research Fund. Dr. Banitt was supported by National Eye Institute grant P30EY014801, Department of Defense grant W81XWH-09–0675, and an Unrestricted Grant from Research to Prevent Blindness to the Bascom Palmer Eye Institute, Miller School of Medicine, University of Miami.

REFERENCES

1. Bellows AR, Chylack LT Jr., Epstein DL, Hutchinson BT. Choroidal effusion during glaucoma surgery in patients with prominent episcleral vessels. *Arch Ophthalmol.* Mar 1979;97(3):493–497.

2. Galin MA, Robbins R, Obstbaum S. Prevention of vitreous loss. *Br J Ophthalmol.* Aug 1971;55(8):533–537.

3. Sohn HJ, Moon HS, Nam DH, Paik HJ. Effect of volume used in sub-Tenon's anesthesia on efficacy and intraocular pressure in vitreoretinal surgery. *Ophthalmologica.* 2008;222(6):414–421.

4. Desatnik HR, Foster RE, Rockwood EJ, Baerveldt G, Meyers SM, Lewis H. Management of glaucoma implants occluded by vitreous incarceration. *J Glaucoma.* Aug 2000;9(4):311–316.

5. Van Aken E, Lemij H, Vander Haeghen Y, de Waard P. Baerveldt® glaucoma implants in the management of refractory glaucoma after vitreous surgery. *Acta Ophthalmol.* Feb 2010;88(1):75–79.

33

INADEQUATE CONJUNCTIVAL COVERAGE

SCOTT D. LAWRENCE AND PETER A. NETLAND

INADEQUATE CONJUNCTIVAL COVERAGE

Successful tube shunt surgery requires adequate coverage of the implant with conjunctiva. When a patient's conjunctiva is tight or scarred, preventing exposure of the large plate and tube becomes difficult. In these challenging cases, the glaucoma surgeon must modify the surgical approach and apply surgical techniques that may be more familiar to cornea and oculoplastic surgeons than glaucoma surgeons.

RISK FACTORS

Any patient who has undergone ocular surgery involving the conjunctiva (e.g., cataract extraction through a scleral tunnel, guarded filtration surgery, pars plana vitrectomy, penetrating keratoplasty, pterygium excision, strabismus surgery) is likely to have conjunctival scarring. Additionally, patients with a history of inflammation of the conjunctiva may have thin, friable tissue that is difficult to manipulate. Other conditions that may lead to inadequate conjunctiva for coverage are chronic conjunctivitis, chemical burns, ocular cicatricial pemphigoid, Stevens-Johnson syndrome, and rheumatoid arthritis.

SURGICAL INCISIONS AND DISSECTION

In cases with marginal conjunctiva, the required conjunctival incisions and dissection for implantation of the device are performed, followed by assessment of the amount and viability of tissue. Only when adequate tissue is found should the shunt be placed. If adequate tissue is not available, the procedure may be aborted for an alternate choice.

When a careful slit-lamp exam reveals conjunctival scarring to be localized, one may choose, preoperatively, to insert the tube shunt in an unaffected quadrant. However, in some instances, this approach is not possible due to diffuse scarring. Previous glaucoma surgery or posterior segment surgery (e.g., pars plana vitrectomy with silicone oil) may necessitate placement of the implant in a specific quadrant.

When scarring affects the limbus, it may be difficult to initiate dissection of a fornix-based conjunctival flap without creating conjunctival buttonholes. Alternatives include making a more posterior limbus-based conjunctival flap, creating a superficial partial-thickness scleral flap, or even removing the scarred conjunctiva/Tenon's layers and covering the defect with a conjunctival advancement flap. If upon examination the conjunctiva at the limbus cannot be easily mobilized with a sponge or blunt forceps, a limbus-based flap may be fashioned by making the initial incision 4–8 mm posterior to the limbus. The incision site should not be so far back as to overlay the intended site of reservoir placement.

If the scarring appears superficial, a #64 Beaver blade or sharp Wescott or Vannas scissors can be used to sharply dissect the affected conjunctiva and Tenon's capsule along a plane superficial to the sclera. If the conjunctiva is tightly adherent to the sclera, a thin lamellar scleral dissection is indicated. If the adhesion is limited to a few millimeters of the limbus, rather than dissecting the sclera other options include removing scarred conjunctiva using a combination of scraping, treatment with absolute alcohol and even light cautery. However, removal of conjunctiva should be minimized and avoided whenever possible, as the tissue may later be required for closure.

COVERAGE OF THE TUBE SHUNT

After placement of the tube shunt, the remaining conjunctiva should be assessed, and coverage of the shunt and the patch graft with tissue then planned. Small defects or tension on the wound may be treated with conjunctival relaxing incisions. Moderate-sized defects and areas with poor blood supply or inadequate subconjunctival tissue can be treated with conjunctival pedicle flaps.[1,2] Larger defects can be covered with autologous conjunctival patch grafts.[3–5]

Conjunctival advancement

As a result of tissue edema or the volume of the tube shunt plate, the conjunctiva may be too tight to achieve closure without compromising the integrity of the tissue. In such cases, fixation of the conjunctiva to the limbus can be particularly difficult, and conjunctival tears and buttonholes occur (see Chapter 4). Conjunctiva should cover the plate, tube, and patch graft, but areas of bare sclera away from the tube may be left exposed to heal primarily as long as the shunt is totally occluded. Small uncovered areas on the patch graft may eventually re-epithelialize but must be watched closely during the postoperative course in case additional revision becomes necessary. In some instances the patch may melt and lead to exposure of the tube. Alternatively, the patch graft may desiccate and cause enlargement of the defect with eventual exposure of the tube or plate.

Conjunctival advancement may be used to cover small conjunctival defects encountered during tube shunt surgery (Figure 33.1). If the coverage deficit is less than 2 or 3 mm, one can undermine the conjunctiva around the incisions and extend the incision toward an area with mobile conjunctiva. In some cases, these simple steps may allow advancement of conjunctiva towards the limbus. When more length is required, partial thickness relaxing incisions may be made in the direction of the fornix and can be accomplished using a blade or sharp scissors. It is important to remain in superficial conjunctiva without extending deeply into Tenon's capsule. Also, one should be careful to avoid incising extraocular muscle fibers. In most cases, 2–3 relaxing incisions can achieve the necessary additional tissue coverage.

Conjunctival pedicle flap

Vascularized conjunctival flaps are commonly utilized in eyelid reconstruction as well as in the treatment of severe corneal ulcers at risk for perforation.[2] The treatment objective in

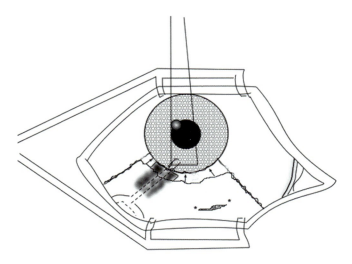

FIGURE 33.1 **Conjunctival advancement** The conjunctiva is advanced toward the limbus (arrows). A relaxing incision has been performed (asterisks).

these cases is to bring healthy, vascularized tissue into contact with ocular tissue that is deficient and devitalized. The flap, with its own blood supply, provides nutrients for tissue growth as well as scaffolding to aid in structural integrity of the tissue. Interpolated flaps incorporate nearby tissue that is not adjacent to the deficient area. The pedicle of the flap is rotated into position by passing above or below tissue that abuts the area of defect.[1]

This surgical method can be applied to exposed tube shunt plates or tubes and is particularly attractive in patients who have failed alternative therapies (Figure 33.2). Additionally, patients with recurrent tube erosions or localized disease of the conjunctiva may benefit from reestablishment of an adequate vascular network.

The pedicle flap is marked, and Wescott scissors are used to incise the conjunctiva and undermine Tenon's capsule. Prominent blood

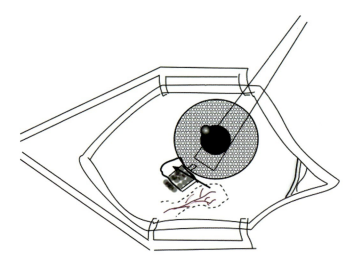

FIGURE 33.2 **Conjunctival pedicle flap** A conjunctival flap is prepared, then placed over the exposed area (arrow), connected to the original harvest site by a conjunctival pedicle.

vessels are identified, and the base of the flap is left attached to its original vascular supply. The pedicle is then rotated so that it covers the exposed area. The interpolated flap is then adjoined to neighboring conjunctiva using 9–0 polyglactin 910 (Vicryl™, Ethicon, Inc., Somerville, New Jersey) suture with a tapered needle. If the anterior edge of the flap reaches the limbus, this tissue can be sutured to the cornea using nylon sutures.[1]

Conjunctival patch graft

The use of autologous conjunctival patch grafts in bleb revision surgery is well described.[4] Autologous patch grafts may also be helpful in covering larger conjunctival defects encountered during tube shunt surgery (Figure 33.3). The size of the required conjunctival graft should be measured at the site of the tube shunt, and the graft oversized 1–2 mm. The globe is then rotated away from the site of the glaucoma drainage implant insertion—infero-medially if the implant is being placed in the traditional superotemporal location. In most cases a corneal traction suture is needed to achieve adequate exposure of the harvest site. The bulbar conjunctiva is then measured using calipers and marked with a surgical marking pen to outline the planned excision.

The harvested graft containing conjunctiva and Tenon's capsule is removed, leaving the episclera intact. Inclusion of Tenon's capsule adds tectonic support to the graft and reduces the risk of postoperative migration.[3] The epithelial surface should be kept upright and the limbal border noted so that the orientation can be maintained during the transplantation step. In most cases, large defects at the harvest site can be left uncovered.

After rotating the eye for optimal exposure during coverage of the tube shunt, the limbal border of the autograft is positioned at the limbus of the surgical site. The anterior corners of the graft are sutured to the peripheral cornea using 9–0 nylon or polyglactin 910 sutures on a tapered needle.[3] The graft is then joined to adjacent conjunctiva with a running or running mattress suture. A modification of this procedure involves posterior fixation of the autograft to forniceal conjunctiva with suturing in an anterior direction towards the limbus or scleral patch graft. In either case, the conjunctival graft will normally revascularize within 3–5 days, adhering to surrounding conjunctiva and sclera before removal of sutures, if nylon was used, in a few weeks.

CONCLUSION

While the surgeon performing tube shunt surgery may be surprised to find inadequate conjunctiva for coverage of the device, knowing how to anticipate and manage these complications is an important part of tube shunt surgery. Smaller defects may be covered by advancement of the adjacent conjunctiva, sometimes using relaxing incisions.

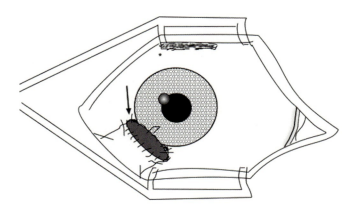

FIGURE 33.3 **Conjunctival patch graft** The autograft is harvested from a distant site (asterisk) and sutured into position over the patch graft (arrow).

Conjunctival pedicle flaps may be useful in some instances, for moderate-sized defects or for areas thought to have poor blood supply or inadequate subconjunctival tissue. Larger defects may be covered with autologous conjunctival patch grafts. Using these approaches, most conjunctival defects encountered during surgery can be adequately resolved.

COMMENTARY
ADAM C. REYNOLDS

Inadequate conjunctiva to cover classic tube shunt implants and the accompanying scleral reinforcement patch graft is a common problem confronting glaucoma surgeons. Even when there appears to be adequate mobile conjunctiva during preoperative assessment or in the early stages of the surgery itself, one can often be confronted unexpectedly with inadequate tissue for coverage usually from thinning, contraction, or scarring of conjunctiva from previous surgery in the area. There is always a need to be ready to employ the techniques so well delineated here by Drs. Lawrence and Netland. Whether during a full transfer autograft from the lower bulbar conjunctiva or a pedicle type transfer from adjacent areas, employing the patient's own tissue in these instances usually works very well. It should be noted that thus far no artificial tissue or other alternative, such as the various types of amniotic membrane tissue available for eye surgery, appears to work as well as using the patient's own conjunctiva in these instances.

Another alternative approach to dealing with this problem should be mentioned. Placement of classic tube shunts in the inferior nasal quadrant of the eye often avoids the potential problem of inadequate conjunctival tissue in the superior quadrants entirely. Anecdotal reports and a few abstracts on the subject[6] appear to show that placement of classic tube shunts in this fashion does not appear to decrease efficacy and, when compared to superior placement, also does not appear to increase the complications of corneal endothelial failure or strabismus . Some glaucoma surgeons actually prefer inferior nasal tube shunt placement, even in routine cases without superior conjunctival scarring that may indicate inadequate tissue for coverage or the need for some kind of tissue graft or transfer.

COMMENTARY
DETLEV SPIEGEL

As the authors stated above, most of these difficult cases of inadequate conjunctival coverage might be solved as described. However, a few of these cases still remain challenging in long-term follow-up, and alternative treatment might be required.

In my experience, patients with uveitic glaucoma seem to be predisposed to late tube exposure due to dissolving of the patch graft. I have observed 2 cases with dissolving patches over a period of 1–2 years. Before Baerveldt® tube shunt implantation in these patients, they underwent multiple filtering procedures and cyclophotocoagulations. In one of these 2 cases after the patch dissolved, the conjunctiva no longer covered the tube. An intervention of repatching with fascia lata and once again with pericardium with conjunctival covering was unsuccessful. A repeated patching and moving the tube, to a more posterior position just above the iris base, was undertaken. To support the healing process, the eye was constantly patched for 4 weeks postoperatively under the use of a 20 mm soft contact lens, which eventually led to wound closure.

If the tube were to become exposed again, I would recommend as a next step the use of an amniotic membrane procedure described by Ainsworth et al.[7] They report long-term success in similar cases using a double layer of amniotic membrane to cover the defect. In addition, the authors recommend using autologous serum to promote epithelial growth.

Late exposure of the tube might remain a challenging task, especially in cases with previous multiple scarring events or in patients with autoimmune diseases.

COMMENTARY
RICHARD K. PARRISH, II AND GABRIEL T. CHONG

Assessment of conjunctiva should take place prior to any tube shunt surgery. Inadequate closure can lead to complications such as endophthalmitis.[8] Prior to a primary tube shunt surgery, mobility of the conjunctiva can be assessed at the slit lamp using a moistened cotton tip applicator. All quadrants should be examined, because while tube shunts are generally placed superotemporally or inferonasally, the other 2 quadrants may offer fresh conjunctiva that can be utilized in a free conjunctival autograft or as a pedicle to be rotated into position elsewhere. During the actual procedure in the operating room, conjunctiva can be assessed again prior to the start of the case with a cotton tip or spear-shaped sponge. One technique that may free up more conjunctival "real estate" utilizes a superior corneal traction suture to rotate the eye upwards while simultaneously mobilizing superior conjunctiva downwards. This converging movement frees up additional conjunctiva for closure. The other previously stated techniques of conjunctival advancement through undermining techniques, conjunctival pedicle flaps, and conjunctival patch grafts are all useful techniques to ensure adequate closure during tube shunt surgery. It is important to note that attempting to close conjunctiva over the actual device is difficult due to a lack of underlying vascular support.[9] Such attempts will likely result in poor closure and wound dehiscence. A similar principle applies to attempts at closing tube exposure with a conjunctival autograft overlying a scleral or corneal patch graft.

The second area of conjunctiva assessment takes place during reoperations for an exposed tube shunt. Oftentimes, the exposed tube is epithelialized. This epithelium will need to be debrided to prevent complications. Once the epithelium has been removed, careful undermining of the surrounding conjunctiva to preserve remaining conjunctiva is essential to maximize the chances of an adequate closure at the end of the surgery. The exposed tube will need to be reinforced with a patch graft, which can be sclera, cornea, or pericardium. In cases of repeated exposure, it may be necessary to reroute the tube completely.[10] Once the new patch graft is in place, coverage with conjunctiva can be achieved with the previously stated techniques of conjunctival advancement and conjunctival pedicle flaps. It is important to note that a conjunctival autograft is less likely to survive when placed directly over the patch graft due to an inadequate vascular supply. This principle is similar to one found in full-thickness skin grafting techniques.[9]

Dr. Parrish was supported by National Eye Institute grant P30EY014801, Department of Defense grant W81XWH-09–0675, and an Unrestricted Grant from Research to Prevent Blindness to the Bascom Palmer Eye Institute, Miller School of Medicine, University of Miami.

REFERENCES

1. Godfrey DG, Merritt JH, Fellman RL, Starita RJ. Interpolated conjunctival pedicle flaps for the treatment of exposed glaucoma drainage devices. *Arch Ophthalmol.* Dec 2003;121(12):1772–1775.
2. Sandinha T, Zaher SS, Roberts F, Devlin HC, Dhillon B, Ramaesh K. Superior forniceal conjunctival advancement pedicles (SFCAP) in the management of acute and impending corneal perforations. *Eye.* Jan 2006;20(1):84–89.
3. Buxton JN, Lavery KT, Liebmann JM, Buxton DF, Ritch R. Reconstruction of filtering blebs with free conjunctival autografts. *Ophthalmology.* Apr 1994;101(4):635–639.
4. Harris LD, Yang G, Feldman RM, et al. Autologous conjunctival resurfacing of leaking filtering blebs. *Ophthalmology.* Sept 2000; 107(9):1675–1680.
5. Schnyder CC, Shaarawy T, Ravinet E, Achache F, Uffer S, Mermoud A. Free conjunctival autologous graft for bleb repair and bleb reduction after

trabeculectomy and nonpenetrating filtering surgery. *J Glaucoma.* Feb 2002;11(1):10–16.

6. Cortes, AD, WuDunn, D, Cantor, LB. Short term outcomes of interior versus superior placement of Baerveldt® tube shunts [ARVO e-abstract 3377]. *Invest Ophthalmol Vis Sci* 2002; 43: E-Abstract 3377.

7. Ainsworth G, Rotchford A, Dua HS, King AJ. A novel use of amniotic membrane in the management of tube exposure following glaucoma tube shunt surgery. *Br J Ophthalmol.* Apr 2006;90(4):417–419.

8. Gedde SJ, Scott IU, Tabandeh H, et al. Late endophthalmitis associated with glaucoma drainage implants. *Ophthalmology.* Jul 2001; 108(7):1323–1327.

9. Robson MC, Krizek TJ. Predicting skin graft survival. *J Trauma.* Mar 1973;13(3):213–217.

10. Heuer DK, Budenz D, Coleman A. Aqueous shunt tube erosion. *J Glaucoma.* Dec 2001;10(6):493–496.

B. POSTOPERATIVE COMPLICATIONS

34

EARLY HYPOTONY

PAUL A. SIDOTI AND MICHAEL R. BANITT

EARLY HYPOTONY

Ocular hypotony in the early postoperative period following tube shunt surgery is relatively common. The pressure level at which structural compromise of the eye and resultant secondary complications (e.g., shallow/flat anterior chamber, serous and/or hemorrhagic choroidal detachment, chorioretinal folds, corneal folds) occur varies considerably. Some patients may tolerate extremely low pressures well for extended periods of time. However, an increased amount of secondary complications is often seen with intraocular pressures (IOPs) below 6 mm Hg. For the purpose of the ensuing discussion, we will adopt a definition of hypotony based solely on this pressure criterion without regard to the clinical state of the eye. An understanding of the causes of hypotony is critical to its prevention as well as its treatment.

HOW HYPOTONY OCCURS

The etiologies of hypotony can be broken down into 2 broad categories: general (Table 34.1) and device-specific (Table 34.2). The device-specific causes can be further categorized into those that occur with valved devices and those that occur with non-valved devices.

Aqueous flow around the tube at the scleral insertion site may result in early postoperative hypotony regardless of the type of tube shunt used. A 23-gauge needle generally creates a tight track in an area of normal sclera with little potential for excess flow around the tube. Rarely, however, the scleral entry track can be significantly wider than the external diameter of the tube, resulting in peri-tube flow and a low IOP,[1] which are particularly likely to occur following excessive manipulation of the scleral opening as it is created or during tube insertion. The use of a 22-gauge or wider needle

Table 34.1. General Causes of Hypotony by Anatomic Site

CILIARY BODY

Aqueous hyposecretion secondary to ciliary body dysfunction

- Ciliary body detachment
- Intraocular inflammation (uveitis)
- Persistent effect from the use of an aqueous suppressant medication

RETINA

Retinal detachment

SCLERA

Leak around the tube at the scleral insertion site

- Abnormally thin sclera
- Excessive manipulation
- Intentional widening of a 23-gauge opening
- Use of a larger diameter needle to create the sclerostomy

Inadvertent opening of a scleral fistula from a prior surgery

Unused scleral entry

OTHER

Creation of a cyclodialysis cleft

Table 34.2. Device-specific Causes of Hypotony

NON-VALVED DEVICES

Incomplete ligation of the tube lumen

Early release of a tube ligature

- Spontaneously in children
- Intentionally via laser suture lysis or suture stent removal

Excessive outflow though a secondary "safety valve" used to control intraocular pressure while the tube is ligated

- Excessive flow through an "orphan" trabeculectomy
- Excessive flow through tube fenestrations
- Excessive flow through an oversized scleral fistula

VALVED DEVICES

Failure of the flow restricting mechanism to "close"

will increase the risk of peri-tube flow. Leak around the tube may also occur when a 23-gauge needle is used to create the fistula through an area of abnormally thin, ectatic sclera. Additionally, when 2 or more scleral openings are made in an effort to optimize tube placement, aqueous flow through an unused scleral entry site may result in overfiltration and early postoperative hypotony if the sclerostomy is not tightly closed.

Aqueous hyposecretion secondary to ciliary body dysfunction may also result in transient ocular hypotony in the early postoperative period. The causes of ciliary body shutdown are several. Excessive intraocular inflammation or ciliary body detachment secondary to supraciliary effusion may result in subnormal aqueous production.[2–6] Preexisting ciliary body

dysfunction secondary to chronic uveitis,[7,8] ocular ischemia,[3,9] or previous cycloablation with laser[10,11] or cryotherapy[12,13] may contribute in some patients. Persistent effects from the preoperative use of aqueous suppressant medications, particularly topical beta blockers, may also contribute to reduced aqueous production.[14–16] In some circumstances, a synergistic combination of these factors may act to produce profound and persistent hypotony. For example, marked, abrupt reduction of IOP following initiation of flow through a tube shunt may lead to supraciliary effusion and increased intraocular inflammation at a time when the effect of topical aqueous suppressant medication has not yet dissipated. In the setting of enhanced aqueous outflow through the newly functional shunt, these factors can lead to hypotony.

PREVENTION

Management of hypotony due to overfiltration through a scleral entry track is best directed at prevention. A 23-gauge needle should be used to create the scleral fistula, and areas of scleral thinning should be avoided. If the anteroposterior position of the initial opening is felt to be unacceptable, a new scleral entry site should be created just anterior or posterior to, but in the same meridian as, the initial track. Compression of the unused needle track caused by displacement of the walls of the adjacent scleral opening following insertion of the tube will facilitate closure and unwanted aqueous egress. Creation of a long intrascleral track with a 23-gauge needle, beginning 2–3 mm posterior to the limbus, also reduces the risk of both peri-tube leak and leak through an abandoned track.[17]

In the presence of multiple scleral openings, careful testing for unwanted aqueous drainage is critical. The use of fluorescein dye may be helpful in this regard. Closure of any leaking scleral fistulas with an absorbable suture can then be performed. An absorbable suture may be tied tightly, as any induced astigmatism will relax as the suture dissolves. Aqueous leak around a tube can be corrected by removal of the tube, closure of the original fistula, and creation of a new insertion site through an area of normal scleral integrity or using a larger gauge (smaller diameter) needle. Alternatively, the leaking fistula can be partially closed using an interrupted or mattress suture of 8–0 polyglactin 910 (Vicryl™, Ethicon, Inc., Somerville, New Jersey), tightening the scleral opening around the tube. Application of fibrin tissue adhesive around the tube at the scleral entry site may also be used to temporarily correct or prevent peri-tube leak.

Additionally, avoidance of inadvertent scleral perforation is critical. When very thin sclera with overlying immobile, scarred conjunctiva is identified preoperatively in the area of a prior trabeculectomy or full-thickness filtering procedure, it is sometimes best to direct the conjunctival opening around and posterior to the area of thin sclera or scarred conjunctiva. Prior to conjunctival closure at the conclusion of the case, the epithelial surface in the area of the preexisting filtering bleb or conjunctival scarring can be carefully denuded with a combination of light cautery and mechanical scraping. Posterior conjunctiva is then advanced to cover the site. Alternatively,

placement of the shunt in the inferonasal or inferotemporal quadrant should be considered when excessive scarring and scleral thinning from prior trabeculectomy are noted along the superior limbus (see Chapter 33).

Avoiding abrupt, profound reduction of IOP is generally beneficial in preventing the development of serous or hemorrhagic choroidal detachment, which can contribute to ciliary body shutdown and hypotony.[18] In patients at particular risk for hypotony, consideration should be given to prophylactic anterior chamber injection of viscoelastic or intravitreal injection of a long-acting gas at the time of surgery (for patients with valved tube shunts) or immediately following tube ligature release (for patients with nonvalved tube shunts). Two-stage insertion of non-valved tube shunts allows for the injection of fluid or viscoelastic at the time of second-stage tube insertion, thereby avoiding the abrupt, profound drop in pressure associated with ligature release after single-stage implantations.

A relatively small surface area tube shunt should be considered in patients with documented or suspected aqueous hyposecretion secondary to permanent ciliary body dysfunction, such as patients with chronic uveitis, chronic ocular ischemia, or previous ciliary body ablation.[19] Minimizing the capsular surface area available for aqueous outflow will help to limit the degree of IOP reduction in eyes with reduced aqueous production. Devices with flow-restricting mechanisms are not entirely protected from low IOP, as the "valves" in these devices tend to provide some resistance to aqueous flow but do not prevent IOP from dropping to very low levels.

MANAGEMENT

When hypotony does occur from peri-tube leak at the scleral entry site, it is best managed conservatively as the excessive aqueous flow will generally resolve within days to weeks due to fibrosis around the tube or at the site of a secondary scleral opening as part of the normal postoperative healing process. When secondary complications of hypotony (e.g., serous choroidal detachment, anterior chamber shallowing, maculopathy) necessitate intervention, treatment is best directed at temporizing measures to deepen the anterior chamber, internally tamponade the leak, and raise IOP. Anterior chamber injection of a viscoelastic agent for tubes positioned in the anterior segment or intravitreal injection of a long-acting gas for tubes placed through the pars plana in vitrectomized eyes are effective methods for stabilizing the globe. It is rarely necessary to intervene surgically during the postoperative period to close a leaking scleral entry site.

In patients who have undergone previous glaucoma filtering surgery, inadvertent opening of an old limbal fistula during dissection of the conjunctival/Tenon's capsular flap may result in a very low IOP in the early postoperative period. Unintended anterior scleral penetration is readily apparent and usually identified intraoperatively as fluid outflow with anterior chamber shallowing and softening of the globe (see Chapter 31). The defect may be difficult to close effectively, due to ectatic sclera, particularly in areas previously exposed to mitomycin-C. In-lay or superficial patching may facilitate watertight closure. Postoperatively, the source of the excessive fluid outflow may be identifiable as a localized bleb over the old filtering site, but more commonly, in the immediate postoperative period, diffusion of subconjunctival/sub-Tenon's fluid prevents precise localization of the site of aqueous outflow. Inadvertent scleral perforation sites will generally close with time due to scarring. Drainage of aqueous through the tube will ultimately shunt fluid away from the scleral opening and facilitate closure. Temporary stabilization of the eye in the setting of profoundly low IOP can be provided by an anterior chamber injection of a viscoelastic agent. Viscoelastic will both elevate the IOP and provide some internal tamponade of the scleral defect, reducing aqueous flow and facilitating healing.

Treatment of low pressure related to aqueous hyposecretion is directed at reversing the factors contributing to ciliary body shutdown. Aggressive treatment of intraocular inflammation with topical, systemic, intraocular, or periocular corticosteroids is essential. Additionally, aqueous suppressant medications should be discontinued. It is generally beneficial to stop some or all such medications several days or more prior to initiating flow through a tube shunt, as the IOP allows. Stopping topical beta-blockers in the other eye should be considered due to the potential for crossover effect[20–23] Furthermore, use of cycloplegic agents may be warranted to posteriorly rotate the ciliary body and the lens-iris diaphragm, thereby deepening the anterior chamber and reducing the risk of developing irido-corneal adhesions.[24]

Anterior chamber injection of a viscoelastic agent (for anterior segment tubes) or intravitreal injection of a long-acting gas (for pars plana tubes) should also be considered to treat early hypotony. These maneuvers will often provide transient elevation of IOP and allow for gradual reduction as the viscoelastic or gas dissipates over a period of days or weeks. In addition to replacing lost fluid volume in the eye, increased resistance to flow through the tube helps to maintain the IOP at a higher level. One or more injections may be required. The response to anterior chamber viscoelastic will vary depending on the particular patient and tube shunt as well as the postoperative interval and degree of fibrous encapsulation around the plate. It is generally best to start with a low viscosity agent and progress to higher viscosity agents depending on the magnitude and duration of IOP elevation achieved with the initial injection and the degree of instability of the eye.

The anterior chamber injection of viscoelastic fluids is rarely helpful for patients with tubes placed through the pars plana, due to the large volume of the vitreous cavity, the relatively poor accessibility of the proximal tube tip to substances injected in the anterior chamber, and the tendency of the vitrectomized eye to require higher volumes of fluid to restore structural integrity and elevate IOP. Intravitreal injection of a long-acting gas may help to reduce flow through the tube due to surface tension at the tube tip. A fluid-gas exchange may be necessary to allow for injection of an adequate amount of gas. An expansile concentration of C_3F_8 or SF_6 gas should be injected in sufficient quantity to completely surround the proximal tube tip. Intravitreal gas is not, however, uniformly successful in providing sustained elevation of IOP even when injected in sufficient quantity as there will be some egress of gas through the tube.

When additional surgical procedures, such as a pars plana vitrectomy or cataract extraction, are performed at the time of tube shunt surgery, aqueous leak from corneal or scleral incisions created as part of these procedures may result in early postoperative hypotony. The accidental creation of a cyclodialysis cleft, such as during the process of tube insertion (particularly posterior chamber) or following anterior chamber manipulations related to additional surgical procedures, can also lead to hypotony.[18,25–28] Rhegmatogenous retinal detachment is a potential complication of any intraocular surgical procedure and is commonly associated with a very low IOP.[3,18,29–31] Careful examination of the peripheral retina is warranted, particularly when there is no obvious cause for the hypotony.

DEVICE-SPECIFIC CAUSES OF HYPOTONY

The device-specific causes (Table 34.2) of hypotony can be further categorized into those that occur with valved devices and those that occur with non-valved devices.

Non-valved tube shunts

Tube shunts without a flow-restricting mechanism generally require some type of temporary occlusion of the tube lumen during the first 3–6 postoperative weeks while fibrous encapsulation of the drainage plate is taking place (see Chapter 35).[32] Incomplete ligation of the tube lumen or early, spontaneous release of a tube ligature can result in hypotony due to unimpeded flow of aqueous through the tube in the absence of a well-formed fibrous capsule. At the time of tube shunt placement, cannulation of the ligated tube with forceful injection of fluid is essential to confirm complete closure of the lumen. A 7-0 or 8-0 polyglactin 910 external ligature will generally release spontaneously 4–6 weeks postoperatively, although earlier release may occur in young children. A variety of methods to temporarily occlude the tube lumen (besides placement of a dissolvable external ligature) have been described. One technique involves placement of a 3-0 to 5-0 polypropylene or nylon suture (also known as a "ripcord") within the tube lumen or alongside the tube combined with a 7-0 or 8-0 polyglactin 910 or nylon external ligature. This method allow for opening the tube prior to spontaneous release of a dissolvable ligature without the need for laser lysis. When the fibrous capsule matures in 3–6 weeks, the ripcord suture can be removed in the office to establish flow.[33,34] The use of intravitreal gas for "pneumatic stenting" of pars plana tubes without an occlusive ligature[35] is unpredictable at best and may result in severe hypotony due to escape of gas through the unobstructed tube lumen.

A variety of methods may be employed to allow for some reduction in IOP and guard against massive postoperative pressure spikes during the period in which the tube is occluded. Excessive aqueous outflow via one of these "safety valves" may lead to early postoperative hypotony. An "orphan" trabeculectomy, tube fenestrations,[36,37] scleral fistulization with a 22-gauge needle, and incomplete ligation of the tube lumen[38] are some of the techniques used. Treatment directed at reducing aqueous flow through the overfiltering pathway may be difficult and require additional surgical intervention. Temporizing with anterior chamber injection of a viscoelastic agent or intravitreal injection of gas is a reasonable option to stabilize the eye while the normal healing process results in fibrosis at the filtering site, increased outflow resistance, and elevation of IOP.

Valved tube shunts

The "valve" mechanisms in several commercially available tube shunts act more as flow restrictors than true valves, providing some increased resistance to fluid flow without strict opening and closing pressures.[39,40] Early postoperative hypotony may result from overfiltration following uncomplicated insertion of a flow-restricted drainage device.[41–43] The secondary development of intraocular inflammation and serous choroidal detachment may lead to a component of ciliary body shutdown,[18] exacerbating the hypotony. Management is best directed at prevention. Prior to implantation, valved tube shunts should be "primed" to be certain that the valve is functional. Whereas this step is usually performed to *open* the valve, occasionally a defective valve is identified or excessively forceful priming may damage the valve and result in exuberant flow due to failure of the valve to close properly.[43] Additionally, particular care in grasping the device should be taken to avoid damage to the valve mechanism during implantation. Observation of the eye in the operating room after tube insertion should also be performed to assess flow, IOP, and anterior chamber stability as observation of these factors will sometimes permit the detection of overfiltration. Anterior chamber injection of a viscoelastic agent or intravitreal injection of a long-acting gas should be used to temporarily stabilize the eye in such situations. Partial or complete suture ligation of the tube may also be considered,[44] although there is some concern about the need to reprime the device following a period of complete interruption of flow through the system.[45]

Postoperative management of hypotony with valved tube shunts may initially involve observation. The IOP will gradually increase as the drainage plate becomes encapsulated. Should anterior chamber shallowing or choroidal effusions develop or progress, anterior chamber injection of a viscoelastic agent (for anterior or posterior chamber tubes) or intravitreal injection of a long-acting, expansile gas (for pars plana tubes) may be administered one or more times. The flow-restricting mechanism of the valve will often provide some resistance to outflow and tend to allow greater effect of intracameral agents relative to non-valved tube shunts. Complete obstruction of the flow-restricting mechanism in these devices may necessitate removal of retained viscoelastic or gas and repriming of the device by forceful injection of fluid.

In situations of extreme instability early in the postoperative course, particularly in patients at high risk for secondary complications of hypotony, suture ligation of the tube should be considered. Cannulation of the tube and repriming of the device may be necessary if flow does not spontaneously resume following release of the tube ligature.

CONCLUSION

Early, transient hypotony following aqueous shunt surgery is relatively common. The causes are varied and often multiple. Conservative management directed at stabilization of the eye to prevent or reverse secondary complications is generally preferred. IOP elevation occurs in most patients over a period of days to weeks as the plate of the tube shunt becomes encapsulated, aqueous production increases, and normal postoperative healing results in closure of leaky or inadvertent surgical wounds.

Dr. Sidoti was supported by The David E. Marrus Glaucoma Research Fund. Dr. Banitt was supported by National Eye Institute grant P30EY014801, Department of Defense grant W81XWH-09–0675, and an Unrestricted Grant from Research to Prevent Blindness to the Bascom Palmer Eye Institute, Miller School of Medicine, University of Miami.

COMMENTARY

RONALD L. GROSS

This chapter provides a superb, complete discussion of this topic. The most important idea is that as with all complications, it is better to anticipate, prevent, and avoid if possible. In the case of early hypotony after a tube shunt, it is generally preferable long-term to err on the side of elevated IOP rather than the side of hypotony. Adding medications and waiting a few weeks is more desirable than the potentially sight-threatening complications of hypotony. This is most commonly a consideration with the nonvalved implants where there may be a tendency to think that a small amount of flow is "just right" after occlusion. Unfortunately, sometimes that is not the case. A similar concern can also occur with valved devices where the "valve" does not perform as anticipated. This can be identified intraoperatively by no resistance to flow while priming the valve or by excessive fluid egress through the tube as evidenced by obvious flow over the plate after tube is inserted and a shallow or flat anterior chamber. Make sure an adequate IOP and chamber depth can be maintained at the end of the procedure.

In those cases where there is undue risk of elevated IOP over that time frame, the alternatives discussed include a trabeculectomy in a different quadrant at the same time as the first stage of tube shunt implantation or potentially a trabeculectomy alone. This is generally reserved for eyes with the most severe damage.

In eyes with severe glaucoma it may be difficult to determine if vision loss is due to hypotony, glaucoma progression, or postoperative structural change. To confirm hypotony is at least contributing, the presence of choroidal folds on fundus examination and/or optical coherence tomography (OCT) is invaluable. If present, although the hypotony may improve spontaneously, imaging facilitates better communication with and understanding by the patient so that all involved can have reasonable expectations going forward.

COMMENTARY

STEVEN R. SARKISIAN

In this excellent chapter on early hypotony in patients who have received tube shunts, I wholeheartedly agree that the key to addressing this problem is careful prevention. Despite the risk of hypotony caused by the use of a large needle (larger than 23-gauge), it seems to be a commonly performed technique due to the greater ease with which the tube can be inserted into the eye when using a 22-gauge or larger needle. With the use of the correct needle to make the wound for the tube, the need for intraoperative viscoelastics is usually eliminated.[46,47]

Typically, when faced with a patient with early hypotony, the first thing I do is to administer cycloplegics to deepen the chamber, thus preventing cornea-lenticular touch or tube-cornea touch. Early hypotony from overfiltration almost always resolves with cycloplegia alone, and the addition of viscoelastic is rarely needed but can be a useful tool to protect the corneal endothelium if necessary.

Finally, it seems clear from the Tube Versus Trabeculectomy data (TVT) that complications such as postoperative hypotony seem to be lower with tubes than with trabeculectomy. This should be considered when evaluating patients at particular risk.[48]

Dr. Sarkisian was supported by an Unrestricted Grant from Research to Prevent Blindness to the Dean McGee Eye Institute, University of Oklahoma College of Medicine.

REFERENCES

1. Garcia-Feijoo J, Cuina-Sardina R, Mendez-Fernandez C, Castillo-Gomez A, Garcia-Sanchez J. Peritubular filtration as cause of severe hypotony after Ahmed valve implantation for glaucoma. *Am J Ophthalmol.* Oct 2001;132(4):571–572.

2. Toris CB, Pederson JE. Aqueous humor dynamics in experimental iridocyclitis. *Invest Ophthalmol Vis Sci.* Mar 1987;28(3):477–481.

3. Liebmann JM, Sokol J, Ritch R. Management of chronic hypotony after glaucoma filtration surgery. *J Glaucoma.* Jun 1996;5(3):210–220.

4. Fine HF, Biscette O, Chang S, Schiff WM. Ocular hypotony: a review. *Compr Ophthalmol Update.* Jan-Feb 2007;8(1):29–37.

5. Dellaporta A, Obear MF. Hyposecretion hypotony: experimental hypotony through detachment of the uvea. *Am J Ophthalmol.* Nov 1964;58:785–789.

6. Chandler PA, Maumenee AE. A major cause of hypotony. *Am J Ophthalmol.* Nov 1961; 52:609–618.

7. Assaad MH, Baerveldt G, Rockwood EJ. Glaucoma drainage devices: pros and cons. *Curr Opin Ophthalmol.* Apr 1999;10(2):147–153.

8. Orengo-Nania S. Anterior and posterior chambers, iris and pupil, and lens. In: Gross RL, ed. *Clinical Glaucoma Management: Critical Signs in Diagnosis and Therapy*. Philadelphia: W.B. Saunders Company; 2001:347–363.

9. Hayreh SS, March W, Phelps CD. Ocular hypotony following retinal vein occlusion. *Arch Ophthalmol.* May 1978;96(5):827–833.

10. Devenyi RG, Trope GE, Hunter WS. Neodymium-YAG transscleral cyclocoagulation in rabbit eyes. *Br J Ophthalmol.* Jun 1987;71(6):441–444.

11. van der Zypen E, England C, Fankhauser F, Kwasniewska S. The effect of transscleral laser cyclophotocoagulation on rabbit ciliary body vascularization. *Graefes Arch Clin Exp Ophthalmol.* 1989;227(2):172–179.

12. Polack FM, De Roetth A Jr. Effect of freezing on the ciliary body (cyclocryotherapy). *Invest Ophthalmol.* Apr 1964;3:164–170.

13. Mastrobattista JM, Luntz M. Ciliary body ablation: where are we and how did we get here? *Surv Ophthalmol.* Nov-Dec 1996;41(3):193–213.

14. Spaeth GL. Indications for surgery. In: Spaeth GL, ed. *Ophthalmic Surgery: Principles and Practice.* 3rd ed. Philadelphia: Saunders; 2003:211–254.

15. Law SK. Procedural treatments: perioperative medication. In: Giaconi JA, Law SK, Caprioli J, eds. *Pearls of Glaucoma Management.* Heidelberg, Germany: Springer; 2010:279–284.

16. Motuz Leen M, Mills RP. Low postoperative intraocular pressure. In: Spaeth GL, ed. *Ophthalmic Surgery: Principles and Practice.* 3rd ed. Philadelphia: Saunders; 2003:379–387.

17. Ozdamar A, Aras C, Ustundag C, Tamcelik N, Ozkan S. Scleral tunnel for the implantation of glaucoma seton devices. *Ophthalmic Surg Lasers.* Sept-Oct 2001;32(5):432–435.

18. Pederson JE. Ocular hypotony. In: Ritch R, Shields MB, Krupin T, eds. *The Glaucomas.* Vol 1: Basic Sciences. 2nd ed. St. Louis: Mosby; 1996:385–395.

19. Wellemeyer ML, Price FW Jr. Molteno® implants in patients with previous cyclocryotherapy. *Ophthalmic Surg.* Jun 1993;24(6):395–398.

20. Dunham CN, Spaide RF, Dunham G. The contralateral reduction of intraocular pressure by timolol. *Br J Ophthalmol.* Jan 1994;78(1):38–40.

21. Zimmerman TJ, Kaufman HE. Timolol. A beta-adrenergic blocking agent for the treatment of glaucoma. *Arch Ophthalmol.* Apr 1977;95(4):601–604.

22. Zimmerman TJ, Kass MA, Yablonski ME, Becker B. Timolol maleate: efficacy and safety. *Arch Ophthalmol.* Apr 1979;97(4):656–658.

23. Radius RL, Diamond GR, Pollack IP, Langham ME. Timolol. A new drug for management of chronic simple glaucoma. *Arch Ophthalmol.* Jun 1978;96(6):1003–1008.

24. Wang T, Liu L, Li Z, Hu S, Yang W, Zhu X. Ultrasound biomicroscopic study on changes of ocular anterior segment structure after topical application of cycloplegia. *Chin Med J (Engl).* Mar 1999;112(3):217–220.

25. Maumenee AE, Stark WJ. Management of persistent hypotony after planned or inadvertent cyclodialysis. *Am J Ophthalmol.* Jan 1971;71(1 Pt 2):320–327.

26. Aminlari A, Callahan CE. Medical, laser, and surgical management of inadvertent cyclodialysis cleft with hypotony. *Arch Ophthalmol.* Mar 2004;122(3):399–404.

27. Meislik J, Herschler J. Hypotony due to inadvertent cyclodialysis after intraocular lens implantation. *Arch Ophthalmol.* Jul 1979;97(7):1297–1299.

28. Aminlari A. Inadvertent cyclodialysis cleft. *Ophthalmic Surg.* May 1993;24(5):331–335.

29. Schubert HD. Postsurgical hypotony: relationship to fistulization, inflammation, chorioretinal lesions, and the vitreous. *Surv Ophthalmol.* Sept-Oct 1996;41(2):97–125.

30. Jarrett WH 2nd. Rhematogenous retinal detachment complicated by severe intraocular inflammation, hypotony, and choroidal detachment. *Trans Am Ophthalmol Soc.* 1981;79:664–683.

31. Ringvold A. Evidence that hypotony in retinal detachment is due to subretinal juxtapapillary fluid drainage. *Acta Ophthalmol (Copenh).* Aug 1980;58(4):652–658.

32. Molteno AC, Polkinghorne PJ, Bowbyes JA. The Vicryl™ tie technique for inserting a draining implant in the treatment of secondary glaucoma. *Aust NZ J Ophthalmol.* Nov 1986;14(4):343–354.

33. Fechter HP, Lee PP, Walsh MM. Non-valved single-plate tube shunt procedures: Baerveldt and Molteno® implants. In: Chen TC, ed., *Surgical Techniques in Ophthalmology: Glaucoma Surgery.* Philadelphia, PA: Saunders; 2008:87–121.

34. Tanji TM, Heuer DK. Aqueous shunts. In: Spaeth GL, ed. *Ophthalmic Surgery: Principles and Practice.* 3rd ed. Philadelphia: Saunders; 2003:297–308.

35. Luttrull JK, Avery RL, Baerveldt G, Easley KA. Initial experience with pneumatically stented Baerveldt® implant modified for pars plana insertion for complicated glaucoma. *Ophthalmology.* Jan 2000;107(1):143–149; discussion 149–150.

36. Lim KS, Wells AP, Khaw PT. Needle perforations of Molteno® tubes. *J Glaucoma.* Oct 2002;11(5):434–438.

37. Trible JR, Brown DB. Occlusive ligature and standardized fenestration of a Baerveldt® tube with and without antimetabolites for

early postoperative intraocular pressure control. *Ophthalmology.* Dec 1998;105(12): 2243–2250.

38. Sherwood MB, Smith MF. Prevention of early hypotony associated with Molteno® implants by a new occluding stent technique. *Ophthalmology.* Jan 1993;100(1):85–90.

39. Eisenberg DL, Koo EY, Hafner G, Schuman JS. In vitro flow properties of glaucoma implant devices. *Ophthalmic Surg Lasers.* Sept-Oct 1999;30(8):662–667.

40. Prata JA Jr., Mermoud A, LaBree L, Minckler DS. In vitro and in vivo flow characteristics of glaucoma drainage implants. *Ophthalmology.* Jun 1995;102(6):894–904.

41. Coleman AL, Hill R, Wilson MR, et al. Initial clinical experience with the Ahmed™ Glaucoma Valve implant. *Am J Ophthalmol.* Jul 1995;120(1):23–31.

42. Fellenbaum PS, Almeida AR, Minckler DS, Sidoti PA, Baerveldt G, Heuer DK. Krupin disk implantation for complicated glaucomas. *Ophthalmology.* Jul 1994;101(7): 1178–1182.

43. Setabutr P, Bell NP, Feldman RM. Intraoperative management of nonfunctioning Ahmed™ glaucoma valve implant. *Ophthalmic Surg Lasers Imaging.* Jan-Feb 2006;37(1):62–64.

44. Kee C. Prevention of early postoperative hypotony by partial ligation of silicone tube in Ahmed™ glaucoma valve implantation. *J Glaucoma.* Dec 2001;10(6):466–469.

45. Feldman RM, el-Harazi SM, Villanueva G. Valve membrane adhesion as a cause of Ahmed glaucoma valve failure. *J Glaucoma.* Feb 1997;6(1):10–12.

46. Sarkisian SR Jr. Tube shunt complications and their prevention. *Curr Opin Ophthalmol.* Mar 2009;20(2):126–130.

47. Ishida K, Netland PA, Costa VP, Shiroma L, Khan B, Ahmed™, II. Comparison of polypropylene and silicone Ahmed Glaucoma Valves. *Ophthalmology.* Aug 2006;113(8):1320–1326.

48. Gedde SJ, Herndon LW, Brandt JD, Budenz DL, Feuer WJ, Schiffman JC. Surgical complications in the Tube Versus Trabeculectomy Study during the first year of follow-up. *Am J Ophthalmol.* Jan 2007;143(1):23–31.

35

ELEVATED IOP AND INTENTIONAL TUBE OCCLUSION

RONALD L. GROSS

ELEVATED IOP AND INTENTIONAL TUBE OCCLUSION

Intrinsic to glaucoma surgery using a tube shunt is the management of early postoperative hypotony.[1] This consideration is unavoidable in all cases when using a tube shunt without an intrinsic valve and must still be considered in tube shunts that contain a valve, as the valve may not function as anticipated.[2] Unfortunately, in the attempt to avoid hypotony and its associated complications, we are faced with elevated intraocular pressure (IOP) and its associated difficulties.[3] However, the attempt to control IOP is not the only consideration when anticipating intentional tube occlusion. Additional factors such as technical complexity of the procedure, predictability of IOP in the early postoperative period, potential to reverse occlusion either partially or completely, and the impact on the long-term function of the tube shunt must be considered.

HOW TO OCCLUDE A TUBE

The desired endpoint when occluding a tube intentionally is the complete prevention of flow to the tube shunt reservoir. The standard ways to occlude the tube are an external encircling ligature or an internal occluding suture, otherwise known as an "obturator" or a "ripcord,"[4] or some combination thereof. With the external suture technique, prior to placing the reservoir, a 7–0 or 8–0 polyglactin 910 (Vicryl™, Ethicon, Inc., Somerville, New Jersey) suture is tightly tied around the tube approximately 4–6 mm from the reservoir (Figure 35.1). It is anticipated that this suture will dissolve in about one month, opening the tube. However, the timing of opening may be highly variable between individuals, and that variability may be problematic. Alternatively, a 9–0 polypropylene suture can be placed around the tip of an anterior chamber tube with release performed by laser lysis.

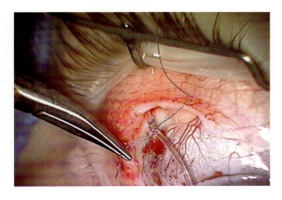

FIGURE 35.1 Encircling suture of 7–0 polyglactin 910 (Vicryl™, Ethicon, Inc., Somerville, New Jersey) completely closing off the tube lumen placed approximately midway between the reservoir and the limbal entry.

To prevent the polypropylene suture from floating freely in the anterior chamber after release, a pass should be made through the wall of the tube during placement.

Alternatively, with the "ripcord" technique, the end of a 3–0 polypropylene suture without the needle is threaded into the distal opening of the tube at the reservoir for a distance of 4–6 mm. A 7–0 or 8–0 polyglactin 910 or 9–0 or 8–0 nylon suture is then tied around the tube in where the 3–0 polypropylene obturator suture is in the lumen (Figure 35.2). The external suture is tied so as to prevent flow around the

obturator suture within the lumen. Just prior to conjunctival closure, the needle is passed subconjunctivally from the incision to a distal subconjunctival area about 120–180 degrees away and then externalized (Figure 35.3A). The suture should be cut flush with the conjunctiva, and its end should be placed no more than 5 mm posterior to the limbus (Figure 35.3B). Once the capsule around the reservoir has had ample time to mature, the 3–0 polypropylene suture can be removed at the slit lamp or in a minor procedure room. An advantage of this technique is that the polypropylene suture can be used as a stylet to ease tube entry into the anterior chamber. Following tube insertion and anchoring to the sclera, the suture can be easily retracted to its intended position.

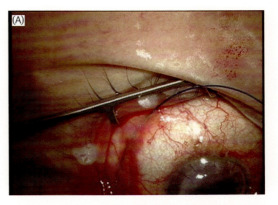

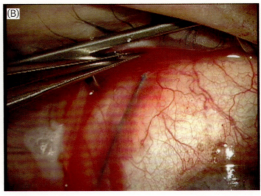

FIGURE 35.3 A. Externalization of the polypropylene suture in the inferior cul-de-sac, well away from the tube shunt reservoir. Some recommend externalizing this suture closer to the limbus to prevent loss of suture due to straightening from suture memory. B. The suture cut flush with the conjunctiva.

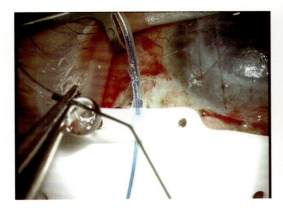

FIGURE 35.2 Placement of the 3–0 polypropylene suture within the distal tube and the encircling polyglactin 910 suture that is completely occluding the tube, preventing flow around the internal suture. Note the sausage crimping of the tube under the outer suture, a sign of good occlusion.

CONFIRMING TUBE OCCLUSION AND VENT INCISIONS

When using either technique, complete tube occlusion can be confirmed by cannulating the proximal end of the tube with a 30-gauge blunt cannula prior to tube insertion (Figure 35.4). The location of the tube occlusion in both techniques should allow adequate room between the entry site into the globe and the point of obstruction for vent incisions. These vents can be made by an incision through the wall of the tube with either a suture needle or a sharp knife[5,6] (Figure 35.5). In general, greater flow will occur during the early postoperative period with more needle holes, larger incisions (up to 1–2 mm), or by perforating both sides of the tube wall; however, the more aggressive the venting, the greater the risk of hypotony.[7–9]

Particularly when using a blade, care must be taken to prevent making an incision that is not parallel to the tube lumen. If an incision that is more perpendicular to the long axis of the lumen is made, excessive flow almost always occurs. If excessive flow is present, it is safest at this point to cut the tube to the reservoir side of the vent and use a tube extender to establish an intact lumen.[10] A more conservative vent incision is then possible. Alternatively, a nonabsorbable monofilament suture can be wrapped around the site of the vent in an attempt to decrease flow. Other techniques have been described, but appear to be less useful.[11] Under all circumstances, it is

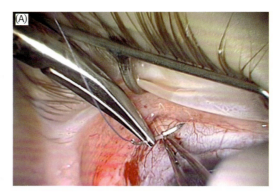

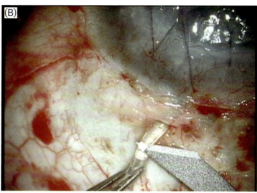

FIGURE 35.5 A. Needle vent incision being made. B. Slit knife vent incision being made.

advisable to fill the anterior chamber through the paracentesis site with balanced salt solution and test flow to assess the final level of IOP obtained (Figure 35.6). In general an IOP of 10–20 mm Hg is most desirable.

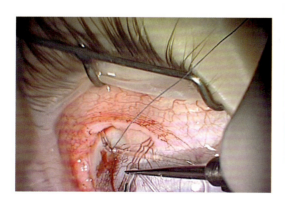

FIGURE 35.4 Tying off the tube.

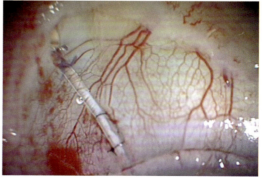

FIGURE 35.6 Testing flow after the vent incisions are made. Note the egress of fluid through the vent opening.

WHEN TO OPEN AN OCCLUDED TUBE

Realistically, most often the pressing decision is if or when to pull the ripcord or laser lyse the suture to open the tube.[4] A minimum period of 3–4 weeks (but in some cases up to 6 weeks) is required for formation of a mature enough capsule to provide adequate resistance to outflow of aqueous in the face of an open tube. Unfortunately, all too often the IOP is well above target in the early postoperative period, despite conservative measures. Most patients close to target IOP, or who are nearing the desired opening date, can tolerate some temporary elevation of IOP.

On the other hand, those eyes exceeding target by a wide margin very early in the postoperative period are more difficult. As a rule, the earlier the tube is opened, the greater the risk of hypotony. Hypotony is more likely in eyes that have undergone vitrectomy, are hyperopic, or have decreased aqueous production (as with uveitis). The immediate concern is serous or hemorrhagic choroidal detachments, flat anterior chamber, and subsequent sequelae.[3] (See Chapters 34 and 39 for more about hypotony with tube shunts.) Maintenance, increased frequency, or resumption of topical steroids may be required, as substantial inflammation may occur at the time of opening. This recurrent inflammation may be due to backflow of inflammatory debris within the encapsulated reservoir.

PREVENTING ELEVATED IOP WITH AN OCCLUDED TUBE

The presence of viscoelastic or hemorrhage can impede flow through the proximal tube and increase the risk of elevated IOP in the early postoperative period. Avoiding the use of viscoelastic agents, or thorough removal of them, can minimize this risk. The use of ranibizumab or bevacizumab preoperatively can aid regression of vessels in neovascular glaucoma[12,13] and minimize the risk of hemorrhage during surgery and postoperatively.[13,14]

To minimize the magnitude of IOP elevation postoperatively, institution of medical therapy immediately following surgery may be considered. In an appropriate patient, 500 mg of acetazolamide can be given intravenously or orally immediately following surgery and then again by mouth every 12 hours in the long-acting "sequel" form as needed. Topical drops to lower IOP can also be instituted once the patch can be removed, usually 4–6 hours after surgery. Prostaglandin analogs are usually avoided due to their delayed onset of action and the potential to increase intraocular inflammation.

In eyes with severe glaucoma damage where a substantial IOP rise could result in a catastrophic loss of vision, it is often desirable to check the IOP postoperatively on the day of surgery. Planning to perform these cases relatively early in the morning with an IOP check 3–6 hours later is a reasonable strategy to address this concern. If an elevated IOP is found, it can be treated in a timely fashion.

More commonly, an elevated IOP is found on the first postoperative day, and medical therapy is instituted. Patients should be made aware of this possibility prior to surgery as part of informed consent. It is easiest to reinstitute the topical glaucoma therapy that the patient was using preoperatively, as this therapy should be effective, safe, and well tolerated by the patient. Beta blockers, alpha agonists, and topical carbonic anhydrase inhibitors (CAIs) are the classes of medications used first, while prostaglandin analogs and oral CAIs are reserved for more severe cases. In general, treatment is indicated when the IOP is above the target IOP. The greater the IOP elevation and the more severe the glaucoma damage, the more aggressive the therapy indicated.

MANAGEMENT OF ELEVATED IOP WITH AN OCCLUDED TUBE

Unfortunately, all too often maximum tolerated medical therapy is inadequate preoperatively (thus the need for surgery) and when instituted for elevated IOP in the postoperative period, a similar result is possible with the IOP remaining above target. If the patient's previous medical regimen is inadequate, additional medical therapy may be considered.

The duration of therapy is not expected to be long, so considering additional medications is reasonable. Medications that have been suboptimally tolerated previously may be used. In general, safety concerns, particularly for beta-blockers, remain a contraindication. The use of oral CAIs may be considered for a few weeks in appropriate patients.

Additional interventions are also reasonable in the circumstance of marked elevation of IOP in the early postoperative period. The most common way to rapidly decrease the IOP is to perform an anterior chamber paracentesis. The use of an eyelid speculum, with topical anesthesia, and the instillation of povidine-iodine is appropriate. A 30-gauge sharp needle, either alone or attached to a syringe barrel without a plunger, can then be used to make a corneal paracentesis at the slit lamp or in a minor procedure area with an operating microscope. Begin just inside the limbus and travel parallel to the iris plane, tangential to the limbus for 1–2 mm within the corneal stroma until entering the anterior chamber. The needle should now be in an area of deep chamber away from other structures or vitreous. Using the 30-gauge needle that vents to the atmosphere equilibrates the IOP around 10 mm Hg due to resistance in the needle, minimizing the risk of profound hypotony. The needle should be removed slowly following the needle track to minimize leakage. Recently, the idea of using a needle to perform a trans-anterior chamber vent incision in the tube postoperatively has been proposed, although there is little data to allow evaluation of this alternative.[15] If a paracentesis was placed during surgery, this site can either be re-entered or "burped" at the slit lamp.

Paracentesis is not a long-term strategy to address elevated IOP; at most it may work for several hours. Therefore, paracentesis is generally viewed as a temporizing measure while instituting other interventions, including clearing the cornea in the presence of microcystic edema to allow visualization of the tube to make sure it is not occluded by iris, vitreous, or inflammatory debris. Alternatively, when reintroducing medical therapy, topical medications will diffuse more readily into the eye without a marked IOP elevation.

In cases where an elevation of IOP even for a few weeks is likely to be catastrophic, a valved tube shunt may be more appropriate, even though there may be some less desirable long-term implications (i.e., IOP control, hypertensive phase). Alternatively, a 2-staged insertion of the tube whereby the reservoir is placed initially and then, at a second procedure at least 3–4 weeks later, the tube is inserted after the encapsulation of the reservoir provides adequate resistance so that no tube occlusion is required. It is possible to combine this technique with a trabeculectomy, if technically possible, in another quadrant to control IOP until the tube is inserted. The trabeculectomy can also be performed in a typical one-stage tube shunt insertion to immediately control IOP, but in this circumstance, if the filter works long-term, no opening of the tube is necessary. And permanent encircling sutures or an internal obturator (ripcord) suture may be used and remain in place indefinitely.

CONCLUSION

Elevated IOP in the first month following implantation of a intentionally occluded non-valved tube shunt is expected. Both the surgeon and the patient should be aware of the possibility and of what may be necessary to control IOP during this period. Generally, the patient can tolerate slightly elevated IOP for the few weeks until the capsule surrounding the reservoir matures, and tube occlusion is relieved. Balancing the risk of progressive damage from elevated IOP against the potential sequelae of ocular hypotony can be one of the most difficult dilemmas facing the glaucoma surgeon.

COMMENTARY
ROBERT M. FELDMAN

Dr. Gross presents an excellent summary of elevated IOP occurring in the first few weeks after tube shunt surgery. It is important to emphasize that although the reservoir capsule may, in most cases, be mature enough at 3 or 4 weeks postoperatively, there are cases where persistent hypotony can still occur upon release. Of more than 1500 shunts, I have personally not seen a suprachoroidal hemorrhage in a case in which I left the ripcord in for at least 6 weeks. Sometimes the suture may not ever need to be removed, as there may be adequate flow with natural loosening of the suture surrounding the tube.

More typically, upon removing a ripcord there is a temporary hypotony that may last from one to 3 days. This may be followed by a high-pressure phase, as is commonly seen in valved shunts. I theorize that this is due to compression of collagen that mechanically occurs upon bleb expansion. The hypertensive phase typically lasts just a few weeks and is best treated by observation if possible. If intervention is needed aqueous suppression seems most efficacious, according to my personal observation, although on occasion combination drug therapy may be required. Over time these hypertensive phases will generally resolve without further surgical intervention, but patience is important and removal medications may not be possible for 6–12 months.

Dr. Feldman was supported by a Challenge Grant from Research to Prevent Blindness to The University of Texas Medical School at Houston and the Hermann Eye Fund.

COMMENTARY
STEVEN J. GEDDE

All modern tube shunts (a.k.a. aqueous shunts, glaucoma drainage implants, and setons) consist of a silicone tube that shunts aqueous to an endplate located in the equatorial region of the globe. Fibrous encapsulation of the endplate produces a reservoir into which aqueous pools. The major resistance to aqueous flow through tube shunts occurs across the fibrous capsule around the plate.[16] Commercially available shunts are either nonvalved or valved, depending on whether a valve mechanism that limits aqueous flow if the IOP becomes too low is incorporated into their design. Nonvalved shunts require a temporary restriction of flow by tube ligation or occlusion at the time of surgical implantation, or alternatively the device may be implanted in two stages. These maneuvers allow a capsule to develop around the endplate before the tube shunt is functional, thereby providing resistance to aqueous outflow and minimizing the risk of hypotony. Valved shunts do not require temporary flow restriction and offer the advantage over nonvalved shunts of providing immediate IOP reduction postoperatively.

Dr. Gross offers an excellent review of techniques for temporary flow restriction and methods to provide early IOP reduction when using nonvalved shunts. I generally prefer to ligate the tube with a 7–0 polyglactin 910 suture near the tube-plate junction to achieve a watertight closure. This suture will reliably lyse approximately 4–6 weeks after surgery. I will frequently open a tube after adequate time has elapsed to allow encapsulation of the plate (a minimum of 4 weeks) with multiple argon laser applications to the polyglactin 910 suture using a Hoskins lens. (I use the same laser settings as with laser suture lysis after trabeculectomy.) Tube fenestration is an effective way of providing IOP lowering in the early postoperative period.[17] Tube fenestration is generally performed intraoperatively, but the procedure may also be done postoperatively applying a similar technique as is used with bleb needling (i.e., passing a needle subconjunctivally, then through the tube at a location posterior to the patch graft and anterior to the polyglactin 910 ligature). Unfortunately, fenestrations frequently begin failing after a couple of weeks— (usually before the tube has opened), —and medical therapy is reinstituted in response to the upward drift in IOP. An orphan trabeculectomy at the time of tube shunt placement is a more reliable means of providing early IOP reduction and offers the surgeon the ability to titrate down the IOP with sequential laser suture lysis (which may be especially desirable in patients with markedly elevated IOP at the time of surgery to minimize the risk of a suprachoroidal hemorrhage).

Dr. Gedde was supported by National Eye Institute grant P30EY014957, Department of Defense grant W81XWH-09-1-0675, and an Unrestricted Grant from Research to Prevent Blindness to the Bascom Palmer Eye Institute, Miller School of Medicine, University of Miami.

REFERENCES

1. Minckler DS, Francis BA, Hodapp EA, et al. Aqueous shunts in glaucoma: a report by the American Academy of Ophthalmology. *Ophthalmology.* Jun 2008;115(6):1089–1098.

2. Setabutr P, Bell NP, Feldman RM. Intraoperative management of nonfunctioning Ahmed™ glaucoma valve implant. *Ophthalmic Surg Lasers Imaging.* Jan-Feb 2006;37(1):62–64.

3. Valimaki J, Tuulonen A, Airaksinen PJ. Outcome of Molteno® implantation surgery in refractory glaucoma and the effect of total and partial tube ligation on the success rate. *Acta Ophthalmol Scand.* Apr 1998;76(2):213–219.

4. Sherwood MB, Smith MF. Prevention of early hypotony associated with Molteno® implants by a new occluding stent technique. *Ophthalmology.* Jan 1993;100(1):85–90.

5. Breckenridge RR, Bartholomew LR, Crosson CE, Kent AR. Outflow resistance of the Baerveldt® glaucoma drainage implant and modifications for early postoperative intraocular pressure control. *J Glaucoma.* Oct 2004;13(5):396–399.

6. Gilbert DD, Bond B. Intraluminal pressure response in Baerveldt® tube shunts: a comparison of modification techniques. *J Glaucoma.* Jan 2007;16(1):62–67.

7. Brooks SE, Dacey MP, Lee MB, Baerveldt G. Modification of the glaucoma drainage implant to prevent early postoperative hypertension and hypotony: a laboratory study. *Ophthalmic Surg.* May 1994;25(5):311–316.

8. Kansal S, Moster MR, Kim D, Schmidt CM Jr., Wilson RP, Katz LJ. Effectiveness of nonocclusive ligature and fenestration used in Baerveldt® aqueous shunts for early postoperative intraocular pressure control. *J Glaucoma.* Feb 2002;11(1):65–70.

9. Lim KS, Wells AP, Khaw PT. Needle perforations of Molteno® tubes. *J Glaucoma.* Oct 2002; 11(5):434–438.

10. Sarkisian SR, Netland PA. Tube extender for revision of glaucoma drainage implants. *J Glaucoma.* Oct-Nov 2007;16(7):637–639.

11. Stewart W, Feldman RM, Gross RL. Collagen plug occlusion of Molteno® tube shunts. *Ophthalmic Surg.* Jan 1993;24(1):47–48.

12. Horsley MB, Kahook MY. Anti-VEGF therapy for glaucoma. *Curr Opin Ophthalmol.* Mar 2010;21(2):112–117.

13. Takihara Y, Inatani M, Kawaji T, et al. Combined intravitreal bevacizumab and trabeculectomy with mitomycin C versus trabeculectomy with mitomycin C alone for neovascular glaucoma. *J Glaucoma.* Mar 2011;20(3):196–201.

14. Saito Y, Higashide T, Takeda H, Ohkubo S, Sugiyama K. Beneficial effects of preoperative intravitreal bevacizumab on trabeculectomy outcomes in neovascular glaucoma. *Acta Ophthalmol.* Feb 2010;88(1):96–102.

15. Campbell RJ, Buys YM, McIlraith IP, Trope GE. Internal glaucoma drainage device tube fenestration for uncontrolled postoperative intraocular pressure. *J Glaucoma.* Sept 2008;17(6):494–496.

16. Minckler DS, Shammas A, Wilcox M, Ogden TE. Experimental studies of aqueous filtration using the Molteno® implant. *Trans Am Ophthalmol Society.* 1987;85:368–392.

17. Emerick GT, Gedde SJ, Budenz DL. Tube fenestrations in Baerveldt® Glaucoma Implant surgery: 1-year results compared with standard implant surgery. *J Glaucoma.* Aug 2002; 11(4):340–346.

36

ENCYSTED BLEB

JEFFREY FREEDMAN

ENCYSTED BLEB

The formation of a true *pathologic encysted bleb* is characterized by intraocular pressure (IOP) elevation that generally starts around 6 weeks postoperatively. An encysted bleb has lost the ability to adequately reduce IOP in the presence of a patent tube, implying that aqueous permeability of the bleb wall has decreased (Figure 36.1). *Physiologic encapsulation* around the tube shunt plate differs from that of the pathologic encysted bleb. The normal postoperative encapsulation develops through several steps. Initially, edema and inflammation occur around the shunt's plate during the first 7 days postoperatively. Next the edema subsides, and the bleb begins to become defined by a fibrous wall. The connective tissue forming this wall thickens over the next 3 weeks.[1] During wall thickening the IOP may rise for about 4–6 weeks. This expected physiologic change is sometimes referred to as the hypertensive phase; however, not all patients will have elevated IOP. After 6 weeks the bleb typically becomes pale, thinner, and less congested, while the IOP stabilizes at a lower level over the next 6 months. Understanding why *pathologic encysted blebs* develop and how they are identified is important in prevention of their occurrence and in management once they do occur.

ETIOLOGY

Prostaglandin E_2 (PGE_2) and transforming growth factor-beta (TGF-β) have been shown to be present in glaucomatous aqueous. These proinflammatory substances stimulate a tissue reaction culminating in the production of excessive amounts of collagen and other contractile proteins. Excessive collagen and proteins may result in a thick and relatively impermeable bleb wall.[2]

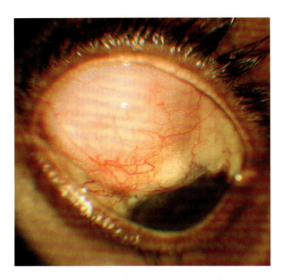

FIGURE 36.1   A thick and vascularized encysted bleb.

This hypertensive phase usually resolves in 6–8 weeks, and any persistence of high IOP after this time is suggestive of an encysted bleb. Encysted blebs may also occur after a period of good IOP control and may be either vascular or avascular in appearance.

To evaluate whether a bleb is encysted, a 30-gauge needle attached to a 3-mL syringe can be inserted into the bleb. Aspiration of aqueous, with a drop in IOP, will confirm unobstructed flow from the anterior chamber to the bleb. On the contrary, the more bulky tube shunts may have an elevation over the plate, suggestive of a bleb, with an elevated IOP. This elevation may just be fibrous tissue and the plate, which can be mistaken for an encysted bleb. Tapping the bleb with a fine needle and syringe will reveal the absence of aqueous, confirming tube obstruction.

PREVENTION

Encysted blebs may be prevented by adopting a program aimed primarily at modifying an expected tissue reaction. The choice of surgery and postoperative care will depend on an assessment of the patient and the nature of the glaucoma being managed. Important patient parameters include ethnicity, age, history of previous eye surgery, and use of ocular medications. Tube shunt procedures in eyes with previous filtration failure are also more likely to exhibit a stronger postoperative wound-healing response, which may lead to the development of a cystic bleb. Additionally, uveitic and neovascular glaucoma are the most likely types of glaucoma to develop encysted blebs. These risk factors require modification of the surgical approach and postoperative care.

Tube shunts without valves require occlusion of the tube for the first 3–6 postoperative weeks to prevent hypotony until the capsule matures around the plate of the tube shunt. Different techniques for tube occlusion are available (see Chapter 35), but they all have in common that the proinflammatory aqueous does not reach the plate surface, potentially reducing the likelihood of an aggressive tissue reaction, a thick bleb wall, and an encysted bleb. Keeping the IOP under control from the time of surgery until the time of tube opening

Various predisposing factors are suspected to potentially enhance this excessive fibrotic tissue reaction. Black patients have been identified as having a more rigorous tissue reaction to glaucoma surgical procedures[3, 4] and are therefore at a higher risk of developing encysted blebs. A history of keloid formation may indicate a greater tendency for a bleb to encyst due to an overly aggressive healing process.[3] Pediatric patients are likely to have a stronger tissue response to surgery than older patients, most likely due to a stronger wound healing response. Additionally, prior surgical procedures with conjunctival scarring in the region of the implant may predispose the patient to a more rapid and exuberant postoperative wound healing response.[3,5] Eyes with higher preoperative IOP may also have a greater intraocular concentration of the proinflammatory substances TGF-β and PGE$_2$.[2] Prior use of steroids and long-term treatment with IOP-lowering medications, in particular sympathomimetics, may predispose to encysted blebs.[6, 7] Finally, blebs can encyst without obvious predisposition, probably as a result of individual tissue reaction.

IDENTIFICATION

Tube shunts may exhibit enlarged blebs with elevated IOP 4–6 weeks postoperatively.

is important and can be accomplished with slits or vent holes in the tubing anterior to the point of occlusion (see Chapter 35). My preferred technique is to create 1–2 slits of approximately 2 mm in length with a 15 degree blade to allow the passage of aqueous to assist in normalizing IOP until the occluding stent is removed 3–6 weeks postoperatively.[8]

The use of a valved implant does allow aqueous to reach the plate surface, and it has been reported that the hypertensive phase in valved implants is more aggressive and results in a thicker bleb capsule than in non-valved implants, often requiring the use of IOP-lowering medications to assist in pressure control.[9] A recent report describes the use of intraoperative mitomycin-C (MMC), 0.5 mg/mL, given over the plate beneath the Tenon's-conjunctival flap for an average time of 8 minutes, followed by postoperative use of 5 weekly doses of subconjunctival 5-fluorouracil (5-FU). This regimen resulted in a marked decrease in the hypertensive phase seen in these patients, with long-term thinner capsules and better IOP control.[10] However, prior studies had shown that using only MMC intraoperatively, for a shorter duration, did not improve the pressure lowering effect of glaucoma implants.[11,12]

The hypertensive phase may still occur in some eyes and needs to be treated aggressively to prevent the possible development of a future encysted bleb. Persistent high pressure in a bleb will stimulate further production of additional proinflammatory substances, resulting in more inflammation and a thicker bleb capsule.[2] Traditionally, the hypertensive phase has been treated with glaucoma medications. This method is usually sufficient in controlling the IOP. The elevated IOP may persist despite medicinal therapy and can be managed either by the use of a regimen of topical and systemic antiinflammatory medications, as described by Molteno,[13] by the removal of aqueous from the bleb, or by a combination of both regimens. Aqueous may be removed from the bleb cavity by using a 30-gauge needle and syringe in a procedure that can easily be performed in the office using topical anesthesia. Aqueous removal can be repeated at weekly intervals if necessary until the pressure is normalized. By normalizing the intrableb tension the production of proinflammatory substances by the bleb wall is decreased, preventing the development of a thick capsule and ultimately lessening the probability of the bleb becoming encysted. The use of at least 6 weeks of systemic antiinflammatory medications during the early development of the encysted bleb has been recommended as well by Molteno,[13] but complications have led to this recommendation not becoming widely followed.[14,15]

MANAGEMENT

After the hypertensive phase has passed, the management of encysted blebs may be medical or surgical. Nonsurgical management, which may be tried when the IOP rises in the presence of a previously well-functioning bleb, includes the use of antiinflammatory medications, pressure-lowering medications, and digital massage. Both steroidal and nonsteroidal medications can be administered topically, systemically, or as a combination of both.

Sometimes, surgical intervention will be required. The easiest surgical procedure is transconjunctival needling of the bleb, which can be done at the slit lamp in a fashion similar to a post-trabeculectomy filtering bleb. (See Chapter 28.) Subconjunctival injection of 5-FU adjacent to the bleb after successful needling has been reported in blebs resulting from both trabeculectomy and tube shunt implantation[16,17]; MMC has been used as a subconjunctival injection prior to successful bleb needling in trabeculectomy blebs.[16] The successful use of bevacizumab (Avastin®, Genentech, Inc., South San Francisco, California), given as a subconjunctival injection in association with bleb needling, has also been reported following needle revision of encysted trabeculectomy filtering blebs, but not after tube shunts.[18] An intravitreal injection of bevacizumab at the time of opening the occluding stent of the implant tube, resulting in a decrease of the hypertensive phase as well as thinner blebs, has also been anecdotally reported. Needling may need to be repeated before adequate IOP is obtained in some cases.[16, 19]

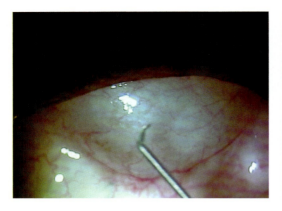

FIGURE 36.2 Needle with bent tip used to tear inner bleb lining in encysted bleb.

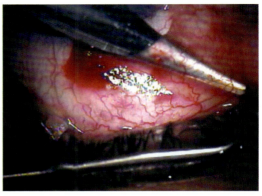

FIGURE 36.3 Separation of conjunctiva from underlying Tenon's capsule.

Another method of needling the bleb consists of entering the bleb with a 27-gauge needle in which the tip has been bent to form a small hook. After entering the bleb cavity, the needle is rotated so that the point of the needle is now facing the bleb wall. The needle can now be used to tear gaps in the thick bleb wall inner lining, allowing aqueous to escape into the conjunctival covering of the bleb (Figure 36.2). This maneuver can be repeated at different sites in the bleb wall, allowing multiple new sites to be opened for aqueous to reach the subconjunctival space. This needling procedure can also be accompanied by injection of 5-FU or MMC. For more information on bleb needling, please see Chapter 28.

Failure of these needling procedures may then require the insertion of a second implant in a different quadrant of the eye. Should the encysted bleb be large and uncomfortable, the bleb may be aspirated and the tube tied off, or the implant may be removed. The site of removal should not be reused to insert another implant, as the tissue will almost certainly form another encysted bleb. The second implant can be placed in a supra-Tenon's pocket, as has been described[20] (Figures 36.3, 36.4, and 36.5). The elimination of Tenon's from participating in the bleb formation may result in a thinner bleb, which is less likely to encyst (Figure 36.6).

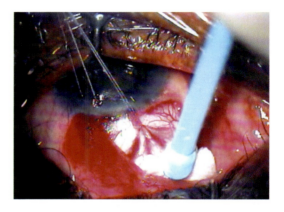

FIGURE 36.4 Cellular sponge used to form pocket above Tenon's capsule (pulled forward with suture) for placement of implant.

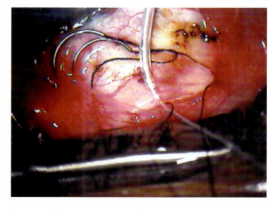

Figure 36.5 Implant in position above Tenon's capsule. Tenon's capsule has been removed anterior to the implant to facilitate attachment of the implant to the sclera.

CONCLUSION

Bleb fibrosis remains a significant problem associated with tube shunts. With recognition of the probability of bleb fibrosis occurring, adoption of preventive measures, and subsequent treatment, the success of tube shunt surgery can be markedly improved.

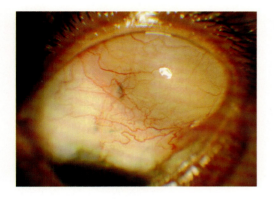

FIGURE 36.6 Thin-walled bleb over supra-Tenon's implant.

COMMENTARY
STEVEN T. SIMMONS

Encysted filtering blebs following tube shunt surgery frustrate all glaucoma surgeons. In high-risk patients the "Molteno cocktail" and antimetabolites can be helpful but are not always tolerated and may increase early postoperative complications. In high-risk patients using either a large single plate or a double plate, increasing the filtration surface area is probably the most effective way to control the IOP postoperatively. Postoperative massage is very valuable following "valved" tube shunts. It is usually initiated 2–3 weeks postoperatively when the IOP reaches between 15 and 20 mm Hg. Massage with nonvalved tube shunts has little or no value. In aphakic and pseudophakic patients with an uncontrolled ocular hypertensive phase on maximum tolerated medical therapy, a limited cycloablative procedure can work extremely well.

COMMENTARY
PHILIP P. CHEN

This chapter summarizes well the findings and associations of encysted blebs and the hypertensive phase after glaucoma drainage implant surgery. A few points to add:

1. The hypertensive phase occurs 4–6 weeks after the tube is open. For an Ahmed™ implant (New World Medical, Inc., Rancho Cucamonga, California), this is 4–6 weeks immediately postoperative. For a nonvalved device such as a Molteno® (Molteno Ophthalmic Ltd., Dunedin, New Zealand) or Baerveldt® implant (Abbott Medical Optics, Santa Ana, California), the hypertensive phase occurs 4–6 weeks after the ligature suture dissolves, is lysed via green laser application, or the "ripcord" is pulled, allowing aqueous flow into the implant capsule.
2. Patients who undergo a hypertensive phase may have an IOP as high as or higher than preoperatively, much to the chagrin of the patient and surgeon. Medications even beyond those needed preoperatively may be necessary to control IOP during this phase. Nouri-Mahdavi and Caprioli found that eyes with Ahmed™ implants that had a hypertensive phase ultimately did worse (had higher long-term mean IOP, needed more medications for long-term IOP control) than eyes that did not have a hypertensive phase.[9]

3. In my experience with Baerveldt® implants, I have found that striving to keep IOP low (low teens or lower) after the tube is open by using medications, including oral acetazolamide, as necessary seems to help prevent the hypertensive phase from developing at all.

Dr. Chen was supported by an Unrestricted Grant from Research to Prevent Blindness to the University of Washington and the University of Washington Glaucoma Research Fund.

REFERENCES

1. Lloyd MA, Baerveldt G, Nguyen QH, Minckler DS. Long-term histologic studies of the Baerveldt® implant in a rabbit model. *J Glaucoma.* Oct 1996;5(5):334–339.

2. Freedman J, Goddard D. Elevated levels of transforming growth factor beta and prostaglandin E$_2$ in aqueous humor from patients undergoing filtration surgery for glaucoma. *Can J Ophthalmol.* Jun 2008; 43(3):370.

3. Broadway DC, Chang LP. Trabeculectomy, risk factors for failure and the preoperative state of the conjunctiva. *J Glaucoma.* Jun 2001;10(3): 237–249.

4. Broadway D, Grierson I, Hitchings R. Racial differences in the results of glaucoma filtration surgery: are racial differences in the conjunctival cell profile important? *Br J Ophthalmol.* Jun 1994;78(6):466–475.

5. Broadway DC, Grierson I, Hitchings RA. Local effects of previous conjunctival incisional surgery and the subsequent outcome of filtration surgery. *Am J Ophthalmol.* Jun 1998; 125(6):805–818.

6. Broadway D, Grierson I, Hitchings R. Adverse effects of topical antiglaucomatous medications on the conjunctiva. *Br J Ophthalmol.* Sept 1993; 77(9):590–596.

7. Loftfield K, Ball SF. Filtering bleb encapsulation increased by steroid injection. *Ophthalmic Surg.* Apr 1990;21(4):282–287.

8. Sherwood MB, Smith MF. Prevention of early hypotony associated with Molteno® implants by a new occluding stent technique. *Ophthalmology.* Jan 1993;100(1):85–90.

9. Nouri-Mahdavi K, Caprioli J. Evaluation of the hypertensive phase after insertion of the Ahmed™ Glaucoma Valve. *Am J Ophthalmol.* Dec 2003;136(6):1001–1008.

10. Alvarado JA, Hollander DA, Juster RP, Lee LC. Ahmed™ valve implantation with adjunctive mitomycin C and 5-fluorouracil: long-term outcomes. *Am J Ophthalmol.* Aug 2008;146(2): 276–284.

11. Cantor L, Burgoyne J, Sanders S, Bhavnani V, Hoop J, Brizendine E. The effect of mitomycin C on Molteno® implant surgery: a 1-year randomized, masked, prospective study. *J Glaucoma.* Aug 1998;7(4):240–246.

12. Trible JR, Brown DB. Occlusive ligature and standardized fenestration of a Baerveldt® tube with and without antimetabolites for early postoperative intraocular pressure control. *Ophthalmology.* Dec 1998;105(12):2243–2250.

13. Molteno ACB, Dempster AG. Methods of controlling bleb fibrosis around draining implants. In: Mills KB, ed. *Glaucoma: Proceedings of the Fourth International Symposium of the Northern Eye Institute Manchester, UK, 14–16 July 1988.* Oxford, UK: Pergamon Press; 1989:192–211.

14. Huang WH, Hsu CW, Yu CC. Colchicine overdose-induced acute renal failure and electrolyte imbalance. *Ren Fail.* 2007;29(3):367–370.

15. Abdel-Tawab M, Zettl H, Schubert-Zsilavecz M. Nonsteroidal anti-inflammatory drugs: a critical review on current concepts applied to reduce gastrointestinal toxicity. *Curr Med Chem.* 2009;16(16):2042–2063.

16. Feldman RM, Tabet RR. Needle revision of filtering blebs. *J Glaucoma.* Oct-Nov 2008;17(7): 594–600.

17. Chen PP, Palmberg PF. Needling revision of glaucoma drainage device filtering blebs. *Ophthalmology.* Jun 1997;104(6):1004–1010.

18. Kahook MY, Schuman JS, Noecker RJ. Needle bleb revision of encapsulated filtering bleb with bevacizumab. *Ophthalmic Surg Lasers Imaging.* Mar-Apr 2006;37(2):148–150.

19. Solish AM, Solish SP. Treatment of leaking filtration blebs using mitomycin-C. *J Glaucoma.* Feb 1999;8(1):S20.

20. Freedman J, Chamnongvongse P. Supra-Tenon's capsule placement of a single-plate Molteno® implant. *Br J Ophthalmol.* May 2008;92(5): 669–672.

37

OBSTRUCTION OF THE TUBE/VALVE

PHILIP P. CHEN

OBSTRUCTION OF THE TUBE/VALVE

Tube shunt obstruction is a relatively common complication, with reported rates up to 15%.[1,2] Tube obstructions can be divided into 2 basic types: 1) distal tube obstruction in the anterior chamber, ciliary sulcus, or pars plana; and 2) proximal tube obstruction at the tube-plate junction. Occasionally tube obstruction may lead the surgeon and patient to believe that the tube shunt was never successful at controlling intraocular pressure (IOP) postoperatively.[3] This complication generally has a high impact on the patient's postoperative course. Preoperative planning and careful surgical technique can avoid many cases of obstruction.

DISTAL TUBE OBSTRUCTION

Anterior chamber and sulcus tube shunts

Distal tube obstruction is typically a serious postoperative complication, with a sudden elevation in IOP resulting in pain, inflammation, and worsened vision. The distal end of the tube may be obstructed by blood, fibrin, iris, vitreous, lens material, silicone oil, and/or viscoelastic.[3-12] Treatment is tailored to the immediate cause. No matter what the cause of obstruction, if tube repositioning becomes necessary, the use of tube extenders, available either commercially[13] or created with readily available 22-gauge angiocatheter sleeves and silicone tubing (used for nasolacrimal duct intubation),[13] facilitate this procedure if the tube is too short to reposition (see Chapter 30).

If a blood clot or fibrin is present, observation with use of ocular hypotensive agents and frequent (every 1–2 hours) application of topical prednisolone acetate, 1% may be sufficient. Tissue plasminogen activator (tPA) also may be injected into the anterior chamber to rapidly resolve the clot.[14] The usual dose of tPA is 12.5 μg in 0.1 cc (0.1 mL) and is readily available from most hospital pharmacies. Multiple injections may be required,[15] but concerns about cost have lessened with the advent of a recombinant form of tPA.[16] In one series of 36 patients treated with tPA after tube shunt surgery, severe hyphema, flat anterior chamber, and profound hypotony were seen after 11% (6 of 55) tPA injections.[15] Blood in the tube may be flushed out with balanced saline solution, using a 27-gauge cannula inserted into the eye through a paracentesis wound.[4]

If the tube is buried in the iris, pilocarpine may pull the iris out of the tube.[12] If not, laser iridoplasty and/or iridotomy techniques are usually helpful in relieving the obstruction, using either a green wavelength laser (argon or diode) to perform iridoplasty and/or Nd:YAG lasers to perform iridotomy.[8] In some cases these procedures will be unsuccessful or the condition may recur and repositioning the tube or incisional iridectomy may be required. This complication can generally be prevented by ensuring placement of the tube away from the iris.

Lens material has also been reported to obstruct tube shunts.[8,10] The Nd:YAG laser may be used to remove the obstructing tissue, although incisional revision using an automated vitrector may be necessary. Theoretically, intraocular lens (IOL) haptics or optics could also obstruct the tube. The tube should be situated to avoid anterior chamber IOL haptics and optics when possible. If an IOL shifts position and blocks the tube, a 30-gauge needle or cannula at the slit lamp could be used to lift the tube out of the position that results in blockage. If sulcus placement of the tube is performed and the IOL-capsular bag complex obstructs the tube tip, surgical repositioning of the tube or revision of the tube length or tip configuration may be necessary.

Tube obstruction by viscoelastic can occur intraoperatively during subsequent ocular surgery. Irrigation of the viscoelastic out of the eye and tube was curative in one report.[9] Whenever high-molecular-weight viscoelastic is injected in the anterior chamber in the setting of prior placement of a tube shunt, it may be prudent to irrigate the tube via its distal (intracameral) end at the end of the procedure, even if the tube shunt is already functioning.

Vitreous may also obstruct tubes placed in the anterior chamber in aphakic eyes or in pseudophakic eyes in which an open posterior capsule[17] and/or a surgical iridectomy from a previous trabeculectomy allow vitreous to come forward into the anterior chamber. The Nd:YAG laser may be used to lyse such anterior strands, using a high power lens, such as an Abraham iridotomy lens (Ocular Instruments, Redmond, Washington) and low power settings (< 1.0 mJ) with anterior offset. In some cases vitreous will return to obstruct the tube again, and a return to the operating room to perform an automated anterior vitrectomy may be necessary.

Pars plana tube shunts

Tube obstruction with vitreous may occur when the distal tube is placed in the pars plana, despite previous or concurrent pars plana vitrectomy. If the tube tip can be visualized, a Nd:YAG laser may be used to lyse the vitreous obstruction, but often vitreolysis is only a temporary solution. Usually this situation requires further pars plana vitrectomy to completely remove all vitreous from the posterior segment, with special attention to the vitreous skirt at the pars plana. Tubes placed in the pars plana may become kinked at the junction of the extraocular and intraocular portions of the tube, where the tube makes a sharp turn from the scleral surface into the pars plana.[18] Surgical repositioning is necessary to correct the kinking.

Ultrasound biomicroscopy

Tube shunt tubes in the anterior chamber may become obstructed in eyes without a clear cornea. Similarly, tubes placed in the pars plana may also be obstructed by kinking of the tube as it enters the pars plana from the scleral surface and are also difficult to visualize directly. In these cases, use of ultrasound biomicroscopy (UBM)[19] may be helpful in determining the presence and nature of the tube obstruction.

PROXIMAL TUBE OBSTRUCTION

Proximal tube obstruction due to fibrosis of the tube opening at the tube shunt plate might be considered to be a relatively unrecognized cause of late failure of the device. One postoperative complication seen specifically with the Ahmed™ (New World Medical, Inc., Rancho Cucamonga, California) tube shunt is obstruction of the silicone valve complex that restricts aqueous outflow.[20] This complication occurred in 4% of 160 eyes (6 eyes) and was felt to be due to inadvertent intraoperative disruption of the plastic valve cover from the valve body junction (caused by handling the implant with forceps along the center line, which allowed fibrovascular ingrowth into the resulting gap). Of the 6 cases identified, 2 were initially amenable to transcameral tube irrigation, but ultimately 5 required exchange of the drainage implant.[20]

However, Trigler et al disputed mishandling of the valve as a cause of failure in a series of Ahmed™ shunts in a pediatric population.[21] They found that fibrovascular ingrowth into the valve complex caused failure in 6% of Model S2 implants (4 of 63) and 14% of Model S3 implants (1 of 7). The authors did not consider intraoperative disruption of the valve cover to be likely, as the implants were not handled along the midline. Failure instead was attributed to the enhanced healing reaction seen in children.[21] It is also possible that these shunts were faulty because silicone sheets that make up the valve mechanism might not reopen once closed.

Proximal tube obstruction is perhaps most common with the use of an anterior chamber tube shunt to a preexisting episcleral encircling band (also known as ACTSEB,[22–24] or Schocket procedure). One report noted this complication, which the authors termed distal obstruction of the tube, in 31% of patients (4 of 13) who underwent the procedure, which is one reason this procedure is not frequently performed.[10] Perkins et al reported a similar condition in Baerveldt® implant (Abbott Medical Optics, Inc., Santa Ana, CA) surgery and found irrigation of the tube successfully reestablished flow.[23]

PREVENTION OF TUBE OBSTRUCTION

Careful intraoperative tube placement may play a role in preventing obstruction. Prior to tube shunt surgery, the surgeon should carefully examine the eye with consideration given to the site of tube placement. Gonioscopy should be used to assess the depth of the angle and the anterior chamber and to determine the location of peripheral anterior synechiae, peripheral iridectomies (and possible vitreous prolapse through them), previous trabeculectomy sites that might be best avoided, and IOL haptics, if present in the anterior chamber.

During surgery, the placement of the tube should be considered among the most critical steps of the procedure, requiring high magnification and an unobstructed view of the placement site and anterior chamber whenever possible. When a 23- or 25-gauge needle is used to create the track for the tube to enter the eye, simply bending the needle at the hub, bevel up, and mounting the needle on a syringe allows for greater ease of handling when penetrating the sclera with the needle. When placing the tube in the anterior chamber, I measure 1.5–2.0 mm posterior to the conjunctival insertion to ensure a tube track that is not situated too anteriorly but that will also avoid inadvertent placement in or behind the iris. Unfortunately, gauging depth of the anterior chamber through the operating microscope is more difficult than at the slit lamp, especially if peripheral anterior synechiae are present. Also, since a preplaced paracentesis is generally used and aqueous may escape the paracentesis during construction, the anterior chamber depth might be altered from its native state. Additionally, I avoid use of viscoelastic in the anterior chamber prior to tube placement, since it may distort the anterior chamber depth and lead to poor tube positioning.

When trimming the tube to an appropriate length for intraocular placement, consideration should be given to the narrowness of the angle, anterior chamber depth, and presence of possible obstructions, such as iris, vitreous, or lens material. The tube should be trimmed to create a bevel at the tip at least 1 mm long, which presents a greater surface area for aqueous passage than perpendicular truncation and thereby lessens the risk of postoperative tube obstruction. Additionally, the bevel also facilitates passage of the tube into the eye through the needle track. The bevel should be oriented so that the most likely surface (usually the iris) to obstruct the tube is opposite the bevel. Therefore, tubes in the anterior chamber should have anteriorly created bevels, and tubes placed through the ciliary sulcus (and pars plana in aphakic patients) should have posterior bevels.

If the tube appears excessively long after intraocular placement, it should be removed and retrimmed to an appropriate length. Notably, for tubes placed in the pars plana without using an implant or tube clip designed specifically for pars plana implantation or for those placed in the ciliary sulcus, the tube should be left sufficiently long to allow for direct visualization of the tube at the slit lamp, using a gonioprism or a Goldmann 3-mirror lens if necessary. This longer tube will allow easier identification of tube obstruction and allow for surgical planning, should it occur.

CONCLUSION

Tube obstruction can result in failure of tube shunt surgery. When this complication is recognized, a previously nonfunctional device can be resuscitated and IOP control can be regained. Careful intraoperative surgical technique is vital to preventing potential tube occlusion, both distally and proximally. Astute diagnosis of postoperative tube obstruction with subsequent medical and/or laser interventions or manipulation of the tube at the slit lamp or in the operating room can result in positive outcomes.

Dr. Chen was supported by an Unrestricted Grant from Research to Prevent Blindness to the University of Washington and the University of Washington Glaucoma Research Fund.

COMMENTARY

SILVIA D. ORENGO-NANIA

Obstruction of the tube can be easily and conservatively treated in some cases and in others may require a return to the operating room. The treatment plan is primarily determined once the distinction is made regarding the etiology and location of the obstruction. It is important to make the distinction between failure of the surgery with too much scarring at the plate versus obstruction of the distal or proximal end of the tube. This distinction can be easily made if one observes blood, inflammation, vitreous, haptic, IOL, or debris at the tip of the tube positioned in the anterior chamber. It becomes much more difficult if the tube is positioned in the posterior chamber or vitreous cavity where direct visualization of the distal end of the tube is difficult. In these cases UBM or anterior segment imaging techniques can be used to help make the diagnosis.

This chapter nicely describes various techniques to eliminate the obstruction depending on the cause. With blood, inflammation, or debris, conservative treatments such as time, steroids, or blood clot dissolvers may easily solve the problem. With haptic, IOL, or vitreous obstruction, more aggressive means are necessary, which includes laser treatment or a trip back to the operation room to reposition the tube or eliminate the obstruction. Meticulous surgical technique, especially with attention to tube placement, can prevent most problems. To prevent vitreous obstruction into the tube placed in the vitreous cavity, a vitrectomy performed by a skilled surgeon is necessary to remove all the vitreous, including the vitreous base, and the tube should be longer to avoid any residual vitreous not removed from the vitreous base.

Distal tube obstruction or valve obstruction is the most difficult diagnosis to make as a reason for tube shunt failure. If one visualizes that the tube is open, then one must assume that the obstruction is at the proximal end of the tube. If it is due to excessive scarring, time may lead to thinning of the scar tissue and better pressure control. In most cases medical treatment will be necessary, and if this does not achieve the desired goal, surgical revision is necessary.

COMMENTARY

STEVEN D. VOLD

Meticulous surgical technique optimizes the chance of surgical success in complex glaucoma patients undergoing tube shunt surgery. In my clinical experience, distal tube obstruction is largely preventable with proper tube placement and clearance of potentially tube-occluding material such as vitreous, silicone oil, iris, and lens material from the area of tube placement. Surgeons must be aware that any material near the distal end of the tube may be drawn into the tube due to the osmotic forces present within the eye.

Vitreous is notorious for finding its way into tubes even when present in only small amounts. Utilizing a pars plana vitrectomy approach may be especially helpful in keeping vitreous out of the anterior chamber. With pars plana tube placement, careful removal of posterior vitreous and the vitreous skirt by a skilled vitreoretinal surgeon is commonly recommended. When removing vitreous from the tube, spatulas or cannulas may be helpful for pulling vitreous out of the tube. Amputating a vitreous strand without removing the retained vitreous within the tube must be avoided. In eyes with blood or fibrin clots occluding the tube, the value of tPA cannot be underestimated. The utilization of topical difluprednate (Durezol, Alcon Laboratories, Fort Worth, Texas) may also be beneficial in rapidly dissolving fibrin clots in this setting.[25] Distal tube retraction from the eye can be avoided with proper implant and tube placement. In children, tube migration may understandably be more common due to eye enlargement over time and less scleral rigidity.

Proximal tube or valve obstructions also can be problematic. In these cases, placement of a second tube shunt in a different quadrant rather than revising the entire tube shunt procedure may potentially offer better surgical outcomes.[26] However, in some cases, revising the shunt procedure by removing the valve may offer benefit. When a valve appears to be malfunctioning, surgeons frequently remove the valve by exposing and then excising the valve over the tube shunt plate. Cannulation of the tube with the stylet of a 25- or 27-gauge spinal needle and punching out the valve from an *ab interno* approach potentially may offer another effective surgical alternative in this situation. In cases where sutures have been placed around or within the tube, their removal may provide for excellent surgical outcomes when removed at the proper time.

Dr. Vold is a consultant to Alcon.

REFERENCES

1. Gedde SJ, Herndon LW, Brandt JD, Budenz DL, Feuer WJ, Schiffman JC. Surgical complications in the Tube Versus Trabeculectomy Study during the first year of follow-up. *Am J Ophthalmol.* Jan 2007;143(1):23–31.

2. Heuer DK, Lloyd MA, Abrams DA, et al. Which is better? One or two? A randomized clinical trial of single-plate versus double-plate Molteno® implantation for glaucomas in aphakia and pseudophakia. *Ophthalmology.* Oct 1992; 99(10):1512–1519.

3. Melamed S, Cahane M, Gutman I, Blumenthal M. Postoperative complications after Molteno® implant surgery. *Am J Ophthalmol.* Mar 15 1991;111(3):319–322.

4. Coleman AL, Hill R, Wilson MR, et al. Initial clinical experience with the Ahmed™ Glaucoma Valve implant. *Am J Ophthalmol.* Jul 1995;120(1):23–31.

5. Friberg TR, Fanous MM. Migration of intravitreal silicone oil through a Baerveldt®

tube into the subconjunctival space. *Semin Ophthalmol.* Sept-Dec 2004;19(3–4):107–108.

6. Hodkin MJ, Goldblatt WS, Burgoyne CF, Ball SF, Insler MS. Early clinical experience with the Baerveldt® implant in complicated glaucomas. *Am J Ophthalmol.* Jul 1995;120(1):32–40.

7. Krishna R, Godfrey DG, Budenz DL, et al. Intermediate-term outcomes of 350-mm(2) Baerveldt® glaucoma implants. *Ophthalmology.* Mar 2001;108(3):621–626.

8. Molteno AC. The use of draining implants in resistant cases of glaucoma. Late results of 110 operations. *Trans Ophthalmol Soc NZ.* 1983; 35:94–97.

9. Ressiniotis T, Dowd T. Molteno tube obstruction due to viscoelastic after penetrating keratoplasty. *Eye.* Dec 2005;19(12):1342–1343.

10. Sidoti PA, Minckler DS, Baerveldt G, Lee PP, Heuer DK. Aqueous tube shunt to a preexisting episcleral encircling element in the treatment of complicated glaucomas. *Ophthalmology.* Jun 1994;101(6):1036–1043.

11. Siegner SW, Netland PA, Urban RC Jr., et al. Clinical experience with the Baerveldt® glaucoma drainage implant. *Ophthalmology.* Sept 1995;102(9):1298–1307.

12. Valimaki J, Tuulonen A, Airaksinen PJ. Outcome of Molteno® implantation surgery in refractory glaucoma and the effect of total and partial tube ligation on the success rate. *Acta Ophthalmol Scand.* Apr 1998;76(2):213–219.

13. Smith MF, Doyle JW. Results of another modality for extending glaucoma drainage tubes. *J Glaucoma.* Oct 1999;8(5):310–314.

14. Lundy DC, Sidoti P, Winarko T, Minckler D, Heuer DK. Intracameral tissue plasminogen activator after glaucoma surgery. Indications, effectiveness, and complications. *Ophthalmology.* Feb 1996;103(2):274–282.

15. Zalta AH, Sweeney CP, Zalta AK, Kaufman AH. Intracameral tissue plasminogen activator use in a large series of eyes with valved glaucoma drainage implants. *Arch Ophthalmol.* Nov 2002; 120(11):1487–1493.

16. Activase® [package insert]. South San Francisco, CA: Genetech, Inc.2005.

17. Gomez Ledesma I, Gutierrez Diaz E, Montero Rodriguez M, Mencia Gutierrez E, Redondo Marcos I. [Glaucoma drainage device obstruction]. *Arch Soc Esp Oftalmol.* Jul 2004; 79(7):341–346.

18. Rothman RF, Sidoti PA, Gentile RC, et al. Glaucoma drainage tube kink after pars plana insertion. *Am J Ophthalmol.* Sept 2001; 132(3):413–414.

19. Carrillo MM, Trope GE, Pavlin C, Buys YM. Use of ultrasound biomicroscopy to diagnose Ahmed™ valve obstruction by iris. *Can J Ophthalmol.* Aug 2005;40(4):499–501.

20. Hill RA, Pirouzian A, Liaw L. Pathophysiology of and prophylaxis against late Ahmed™ glaucoma valve occlusion. *Am J Ophthalmol.* May 2000;129(5):608–612.

21. Trigler L, Proia AD, Freedman SF. Fibrovascular ingrowth as a cause of Ahmed™ glaucoma valve failure in children. *Am J Ophthalmol.* Feb 2006; 141(2):388–389.

22. Schocket SS, Lakhanpal V, Richards RD. Anterior chamber tube shunt to an encircling band in the treatment of neovascular glaucoma. *Ophthalmology.* Oct 1982;89(10):1188–1194.

23. Schocket SS, Nirankari VS, Lakhanpal V, Richards RD, Lerner BC. Anterior chamber tube shunt to an encircling band in the treatment of neovascular glaucoma and other refractory glaucomas. A long-term study. *Ophthalmology.* Apr 1985;92(4):553–562.

24. Schocket SS. Investigations of the reasons for success and failure in the anterior shunt-to-the-encircling-band procedure in the treatment of refractory glaucoma. *Trans Am Ophthalmol Soc.* 1986;84:743–798.

25. Foster CS, Davanzo R, Flynn TE, McLeod K, Vogel R, Crockett RS. Durezol (Difluprednate Ophthalmic Emulsion 0.05%) compared with Pred Forte 1% ophthalmic suspension in the treatment of endogenous anterior uveitis. *J Ocul Pharmacol Ther* Oct 2010;26(5):475–483.

26. Shah AA, WuDunn D, Cantor LB. Shunt revision versus additional tube shunt implantation after failed tube shunt surgery in refractory glaucoma. *Am J Ophthalmol.* Apr 2000;129(4):455–460.

38

LATE EXTRUDING SHUNTS AND CONJUNCTIVAL EROSIONS

STEVEN D. VOLD

LATE EXTRUDING SHUNTS AND CONJUNCTIVAL EROSIONS

A serious complication associated with tube shunt surgery is conjunctival erosion and late extrusion of the implant. This postoperative complication has been estimated to occur in 2%–7% of eyes following tube shunt surgery.[1–8] In these eyes, the risk of subsequent intraocular infection is significantly increased.[9–11] With increasing tube shunt utilization, understanding etiologies, prevention, diagnosis, and management of this complication become essential.

POTENTIAL ETIOLOGIES AND RISK FACTORS

Although our understanding of this problem is limited, a number of key factors are believed to play important roles in the development of late tube shunt extrusion and conjunctival erosion. Possible etiologies include both patient- and surgeon-dependent factors. Conjunctival health and viability should be carefully assessed preoperatively in eyes requiring tube shunt surgery. Eyes that have undergone previous conjunctival surgery, such as trabeculectomy (especially when performed with antifibrotic agents), other incisional glaucoma surgeries, large incision cataract surgery, scleral buckling, and penetrating keratoplasty, may potentially be at increased risk for developing this complication.[12–14] Conjunctival limbal stem cell loss resulting from chronic topical glaucoma medication use, keratoconjunctivitis sicca, chemical burns, pterygia, trauma, and systemic inflammatory conditions may also serve as predisposing factors.[15] Pediatric patients also appear predisposed to tube migration (see Chapter 48) and tube shunt complications.[9,16–19]

Surgical technique is also assumed to play a significant role in the development of this complication. Proper positioning of the tube shunt, adequate tissue reinforcement over the tube, and meticulous conjunctival closure may impact long-term surgical outcomes.

PREVENTION

Maximizing conjunctival health prior to tube shunt surgery is often encouraged, but not always possible. For patients with significant ocular surface disease, anti inflammatory medications and lubricants may assist in improving the health of corneal and conjunctival limbal stem cells and epithelium preoperatively. Proper management of systemic diseases such as rheumatoid arthritis and diabetes mellitus might also favorably impact long-term surgical outcomes. Unfortunately, prospective studies validating the assumption that a healthy conjunctiva prevents tube shunt extrusion and conjunctival erosion are currently lacking. Furthermore, no evidence-based perioperative or long-term medical regimen can be recommended at this time.

Surgical technique is also widely believed to impact the incidence of late tube shunt extrusion and conjunctival erosion. In my opinion, 3 key elements of surgical technique should be kept in mind when performing tube shunt surgery: proper tube shunt placement, tissue reinforcement over the tube, and meticulous conjunctival closure (Table 38.1).

Proper tube shunt placement

Placement of the implant at least 8–10 mm behind the limbus is generally recommended. With a more anterior tube shunt placement, the anterior edge of the implant plate and tube may place more pressure on the overlying patch graft material and conjunctiva.

Table 38.1. Keys to Successful Tube Shunt Outcomes

KEYS TO SUCCESSFUL TUBE SHUNT OUTCOMES
• Proper implant and tube positioning
• Tissue reinforcement over the tube
• Meticulous conjunctival closure

Good upper and lower eyelid coverage of the tube and plate has been recommended as well. Securing both the implant plate and tube to the underlying sclera helps prevent migration of the tube shunt and minimizes tissue tension on superficial tissue over time. Nylon, polyglactin 910 (Vicryl™, Ethicon, Inc., Somerville, New Jersey), and polyethylene terephthalate (MERSILENE™, Ethicon, Inc.) sutures have all been successfully utilized to secure tube shunts and tubes to underlying sclera. However, recent data from Huddleston and coauthors has shown that polyethylene terephthalate may lead to an overly large number of erosions, potentially due to either the large size of the knot (resulting in an inability of the knot to rotate into the anchoring hole of the plate, leaving it in contact with the soft tissue) or an inherent physical property of the material.[20] Although controversial, surgeon selection of specific tube shunts has yet to be clearly identified as a contributing factor to the development of late tube shunt extrusion and conjunctival erosion.[21,22]

Careful tube placement can reduce torque and stress on the overlying patch graft and conjunctival tissues. In eyes with previous encircling bands used in retinal detachment repair, surgeons may consider removing part of the scleral buckle or performing a modified Schocket procedure[23] in order to avoid highly elevated implants. Pars plana tube placement or utilization of scleral tube tracks longer than 3 mm before entering the anterior chamber have been suggested to reduce the incidence of late shunt extrusion and conjunctival erosion.[24]

Tissue reinforcement over the tube

Tissue reinforcement over the tube can be performed successfully with a variety of tissues. Autologous or donor sclera, donor glycerin-preserved cornea, and donor pericardium are the most commonly used sources of tissue for patch grafts over the tube.[25,26] Autologous tensor fascia lata,[27,28] dermis,[29] dura mater,[30] tarsal plate, Tenon's layer, and bioengineered porcine lamellar patch graft (keraSys™, IOP, Inc., Costa Mesa, California) have been used successfully as well; however, dura mater is no longer available due to infectious prion concerns.[31,32]

Placement of tissue reinforcement over the length of the tube has been demonstrated to dramatically reduce the risk of late tube shunt exposure.[3] Although compelling clinical data is lacking, my clinical impression is that cornea and sclera provide better long-term tube coverage than pericardium.[33–35] Using a double-layered pericardial patch graft may reduce the advantages of corneal or scleral patch grafts.[36] Again, no long-term studies are currently available to either validate or disprove these hypotheses.

Conjunctival closure

Quality conjunctival closure is the third important element of surgical technique to help avoid late extrusion and conjunctival erosion (Table 38.2). In patients with extensive conjunctival scarring, achieving good conjunctival closure may be challenging. Fornix-based conjunctival incisions are preferred to minimize any loss of tissue needed for conjunctival closure, especially in eyes that have extensive conjunctival scarring. Conjunctival stretching with bandage forceps can be a very effective means of reducing conjunctival tissue tension

Table 38.2. Surgical Pearls for Obtaining Quality Conjunctival Closure

SURGICAL PEARLS FOR OBTAINING QUALITY CONJUNCTIVAL CLOSURE

- Fornix-based conjunctival incisions minimize tissue loss.
- Conjunctival stretching with bandage forceps helps maximize conjunctival coverage.
- Relaxing incisions in conjunctiva and Tenon's layer reduce conjunctival tissue tension.
- Suture fixation of Tenon's layer to host sclera anterior to globe equator facilitates anterior conjunctival closure.
- Rotational conjunctival flaps and autologous conjunctival grafts may be necessary in eyes with severe conjunctival scarring.
- Amniotic membrane and tube extenders may have roles in eyes with severe conjunctival tissue loss.

and providing adequate conjunctival coverage over tube shunts. Posterior or peripheral relaxing incisions in the conjunctiva and/or Tenon's layer may be necessary to achieve good conjunctival coverage of tube shunts and their patch grafts in some cases. Securing deep Tenon's layer to the host sclera with 2 polyglactin 910 mattress sutures, one on each side of the tube just anterior to the equator, can also relieve conjunctival tension and facilitate closure anteriorly. Conjunctiva and Tenon's layer are typically secured at the limbus with polyglactin 910 or nylon sutures. When adequate conjunctiva is simply unavailable, rotational conjunctival flaps or autologous conjunctival grafts from either the ipsilateral or contralateral eye may be considered. Amniotic membrane may serve a role in managing these types of cases, especially when limbal stem cells are present.[37,38] Surgeons should not underestimate the importance of a meticulous conjunctival closure in tube shunt surgery. For further information, please see Chapter 33.

DIAGNOSIS

As one might expect, early detection of any complication is advantageous in maintaining good tube shunt surgical outcomes. Surgeons want to intervene prior to the development of significant shunt extrusion, conjunctival erosion, and endophthalmitis. When following post-tube shunt patients, physicians should closely monitor tube and implant position, bleb configuration, and health of both conjunctiva and patch graft material. Slow migration of the tube shunt over months to years may predispose eyes to conjunctival erosion or an extruded shunt. Bleb configuration may provide clues to tube shunt function and potential points of focal contact. Thinning of the patch graft material commonly occurs prior to true conjunctival erosion. These clues may assist surgeons in intervening before sight-threatening complications occur.

Patients with tube shunt extrusion and conjunctival erosion commonly present with foreign body sensation, ocular redness, irritation, and potentially with decreased vision. (Figures 38.1 and 38.2) Once extrusion or conjunctival erosion has occurred,

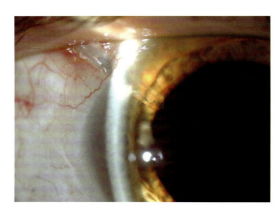

FIGURE 38.1 Limbal conjunctival erosion with exposure of tube at lid margin.

clinical diagnosis is rather straightforward. Fluorescein dye can be used to confirm conjunctival erosion over the tube shunt. Once the diagnosis has been made, prompt intervention is indicated.

MANAGEMENT

The management of this challenging complication is generally surgical, but not always straightforward. A thorough and thoughtful assessment of the clinical situation is required to achieve good patient outcomes. Factors such as the type and severity of glaucoma, intraocular pressure (IOP) control, presence of infection, extent of tube shunt extrusion and

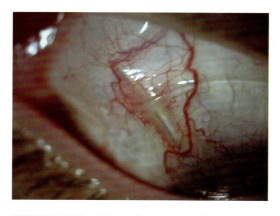

FIGURE 38.2 Thinned patch graft with tube exposure in eye with keratoprosthesis. Contact lens wear utilized for patient comfort prior to tube shunt revision surgery.

conjunctival erosion, and scarring all must be considered in developing a management strategy. Furthermore, if surface epithelium grows along the conjunctival wound and onto the scleral surface of the globe, thorough removal of this epithelium is essential to surgical success. Although a variety of medical and surgical techniques have been attempted with some success, each complication must be handled on an individual basis.

In the setting of infection, aggressive topical antibiotic therapy may be warranted. If endophthalmitis is present, vitreous surgery with intravitreal antibiotics may be indicated (see Chapter 42). When tube shunt extrusion and conjunctival erosion are present without infection, topical antibiotic is also recommended, followed by prompt surgical intervention. No data is currently available regarding the preferred timing of surgery.[9–11]

Removal of the extruded tube shunt and placement of a second tube shunt in another quadrant is an effective way to fix this problem.[39] Most initial tube shunts are placed in the superotemporal quadrant. Second tube shunt placement is usually performed in the inferonasal, inferotemporal, or superonasal quadrants. Larger tube shunts are probably best suited in one of the inferior quadrants in order to avoid the superior oblique muscle.[40]

If a tube shunt is functioning well, surgeons may be reluctant to remove the tube shunt and may prefer to place reinforcing tissue over the tube and repair the conjunctival wound. In this kind of repair, several critical surgical steps must be followed. First, complete removal of conjunctival epithelium along the surface of the globe is needed for surgical success; this goal can be achieved with careful dissection and cautery of the scleral surface. Localized and precise administration of absolute alcohol may be beneficial in achieving complete epithelial removal along the scleral surface. Removal of additional conjunctiva, fibrotic tissue, and Tenon's layer are often required as well.

Second, additional reinforcement over the tube is indicated. Although donor scleral or glycerin-preserved corneal grafts remain my most common selections, a variety of other tissues have been used with some success (as detailed above). Graft tissue should be trimmed and placed in such a manner that the tube does not place significant tension on the graft. Furthermore, low-lying patch grafts well covered by the eyelids are preferred to avoid pressure points and the development of corneal dellen. Repositioning of the tube utilizing at least a 3 mm scleral tunnel may assist in this endeavor.[24] Some surgeons have successfully performed partial thickness scleral dissections to provide reinforcement over tube shunt tubes.[25]

Third, as described before, meticulous conjunctival closure is vital to preventing further recurring episodes of tube shunt extrusion and conjunctival erosion. Maintaining healthy conjunctiva is likely also important in preventing conjunctival erosion recurrence. In the setting of significant ocular surface disease, long-term vigorous lubrication may be indicated.

Tube extenders and lateral tarsorrhaphy may also have a role in treatment of certain challenging cases with exposure problems.[41] Lastly, surgeons must not overlook systemic management of underlying systemic immunologic or collagen vascular disorders.

CONCLUSION

Late tube shunt extrusion and conjunctival erosion are serious complications associated with tube shunt surgery. Good surgical and perioperative medical management go a long way in preventing these complications. However, if faced with this challenging complication, early diagnosis, determination of etiology, and assessment of glaucoma status can provide guidance on how to best manage the problem. With prompt and meticulous intervention, patient outcomes can be favorable.

COMMENTARY

DONALD L. BUDENZ

Extrusion of tube shunt tubes and plates is a rare complication that should be addressed to avoid endophthalmitis. Very little is known about the risk factors for extrusion, probably because it is a rare complication and may be multifactorial. There are many theories regarding the predisposing factors for erosion (besides the obvious surgical causes).

To prevent tube erosion, I like to place the limbal entry into the anterior chamber as far posteriorly as possible. Tubes placed through the sulcus or pars plana may have the lowest risk of exposure. To prevent plate erosion, in addition to the techniques already mentioned in this chapter, ensuring that none of the conjunctival incisions are placed in the vicinity of the plate is important. Burying the sutures used to fix the implant to the globe can prevent holes and erosion later and is an important surgical step.

While some have proposed observation of exposed tubes unless there is a Seidel positive leak,[42] I prefer to fix the exposure (although this does not need to be done urgently). I always combine recovering the tube (using a different patch graft material than used initially) with removing the tube from the anterior chamber and placing it farther posteriorly in the anterior chamber, sulcus, or pars plana. In my experience, recovering the tube alone often only solves the problem temporarily.

In my experience, exposed plates are not worth attempting to repair because repeat exposure almost always occurs, and removal with placement of another implant in a different quadrant is a definitive approach. There are some patients who have poor tissue turgor and the second plate erodes as well, in which case I remove the second tube and use alternate therapies to control IOP (such as cyclophotocoagulation).

COMMENTARY

MICHAEL R. BANITT AND PAUL A. SIDOTI

With regard to tube exposure, our general philosophy is to attempt a repair once in the same quadrant by utilizing a wide limbal peritomy with extensive undermining of the surrounding tissue. If re-exposure occurs, we typically remove the tube and re-exposure; culture the sclera surface to exclude atypical, slow-growing infections as a cause of re-exposure, and either implant a new tube in another quadrant or consider a cyclodestructive procedure.

Repairing exposures can be challenging. The difficulty comes in freeing enough conjunctiva to achieve a conjunctival closure that is not on tension at the end of the case. We agree that the epithelial edges of the defect, as well as the sclera surface, should be debrided to reduce the potential for epithelial ingrowth. This may, however, reduce the amount of conjunctiva available. A natural tendency is to use a large patch graft since the first one eroded. However, this may make the conjunctival closure more difficult. A wider limbal peritomy and blunt dissection freeing up a large area will aid in wound closure.

Also important is an evaluation of the tube's entry site. If very anterior, we consider suturing closed or filling the original entry site with patch graft and moving the tube more posteriorly within the anterior chamber, sulcus, or pars plana.

When a plate becomes exposed, we generally remove the entire implant and either place a new device in another quadrant or consider a cyclodestructive procedure.

Dr. Banitt was supported by National Eye Institute grant P30EY014801, Department of Defense grant W81XWH-09–0675, and an Unrestricted Grant from Research to Prevent Blindness to the Bascom Palmer Eye Institute, Miller School of Medicine, University of Miami. Dr. Sidoti was supported by The David E. Marrus Glaucoma Research Fund.

REFERENCES

1. Ayyala RS, Zurakowski D, Smith JA, et al. A clinical study of the Ahmed™ glaucoma valve implant in advanced glaucoma. *Ophthalmology*. Oct 1998;105(10):1968–1976.

2. Coleman AL, Mondino BJ, Wilson MR, Casey R. Clinical experience with the Ahmed™ Glaucoma Valve implant in eyes with prior or concurrent penetrating keratoplasties. *Am J Ophthalmol*. Jan 1997;123(1):54–61.

3. Heuer DK, Budenz D, Coleman A. Aqueous shunt tube erosion. *J Glaucoma*. Dec 2001;10(6):493–496.

4. Heuer DK, Lloyd MA, Abrams DA, et al. Which is better? One or two? A randomized clinical trial of single-plate versus double-plate Molteno® implantation for glaucomas in aphakia and pseudophakia. *Ophthalmology*. Oct 1992; 99(10):1512–1519.

5. Huang MC, Netland PA, Coleman AL, Siegner SW, Moster MR, Hill RA. Intermediate-term clinical experience with the Ahmed™ Glaucoma Valve implant. *Am J Ophthalmol*. Jan 1999;127(1):27–33.

6. Lim KS, Allan BD, Lloyd AW, Muir A, Khaw PT. Glaucoma drainage devices; past, present, and future. *Br J Ophthalmol*. Sept 1998;82(9): 1083–1089.

7. Palmer DJ, Klein CS, Edward DP. Scleral patch graft calcification and erosion following Molteno® implant surgery. *Ophthalmic Surg Lasers Imaging*. May-Jun 2008;39(3):230–231.

8. Siegner SW, Netland PA, Urban RC Jr., et al. Clinical experience with the Baerveldt® glaucoma drainage implant. *Ophthalmology*. Sept 1995; 102(9):1298–1307.

9. Al-Torbak AA, Al-Shahwan S, Al-Jadaan I, Al-Hommadi A, Edward DP. Endophthalmitis associated with the Ahmed™ glaucoma valve implant. *Br J Ophthalmol*. Apr 2005;89(4): 454–458.

10. Gedde SJ, Scott IU, Tabandeh H, et al. Late endophthalmitis associated with glaucoma drainage implants. *Ophthalmology*. Jul 2001;108(7):1323–1327.

11. Krebs DB, Liebmann JM, Ritch R, Speaker M. Late infectious endophthalmitis from exposed glaucoma setons. *Arch Ophthalmol*. Feb 1992; 110(2):174–175.

12. Alvarado JA, Hollander DA, Juster RP, Lee LC. Ahmed™ valve implantation with adjunctive mitomycin C and 5-fluorouracil: long-term outcomes. *Am J Ophthalmol*. Aug 2008;146(2):276–284.

13. Azuara-Blanco A, Moster MR, Wilson RP, Schmidt CM. Simultaneous use of mitomycin-C with Baerveldt® implantation. *Ophthalmic Surg Lasers*. Dec 1997;28(12):992–997.

14. Broadway DC, Iester M, Schulzer M, Douglas GR. Survival analysis for success of Molteno® tube implants. *Br J Ophthalmol*. Jun 2001; 85(6):689–695.

15. Merino-de-Palacios C, Gutierrez-Diaz E, Chacon-Garces A, Montero-Rodriguez M, Mencia-Gutierrez E. [Intermediate-term outcome of glaucoma drainage devices]. *Arch Soc Esp Oftalmol*. Jan 2008; 83(1):15–22.

16. Al-Torbak A, Edward DP. Transcorneal tube erosion of an Ahmed™ valve implant in a child. *Arch Ophthalmol*. Oct 2001;119(10):1558–1559.

17. Beck AD, Freedman S, Kammer J, Jin J. Aqueous shunt devices compared with trabeculectomy with Mitomycin-C for children in the first two years of life. *Am J Ophthalmol*. Dec 2003; 136(6):994–1000.

18. Maki JL, Nesti HA, Shetty RK, Rhee DJ. Transcorneal tube extrusion in a child with a Baerveldt® glaucoma drainage device. *J AAPOS*. Aug 2007;11(4):395–397.

19. Rolim de Moura C, Fraser-Bell S, Stout A, Labree L, Nilfors M, Varma R. Experience with the Baerveldt® glaucoma implant in the management of pediatric glaucoma. *Am J Ophthalmol*. May 2005;139(5):847–854.

20. Huddleston SM, Feldman RM, Budenz DL, et al. Aqueous shunt exposure: a retrospective review of repair outcome. *J Glaucoma*. Jun 13 2011, *forthcoming*.

21. Ayyala RS, Harman LE, Michelini-Norris B, et al. Comparison of different biomaterials for glaucoma drainage devices. *Arch Ophthalmol*. Feb 1999;117(2):233–236.

22. Ayyala RS, Michelini-Norris B, Flores A, Haller E, Margo CE. Comparison of different biomaterials for glaucoma drainage devices: part 2. *Arch Ophthalmol*. Aug 2000;118(8):1081–1084.

23. Sherwood MB, Joseph NH, Hitchings RA. Surgery for refractory glaucoma. Results and complications with a modified Schocket technique. *Arch Ophthalmol*. Apr 1987;105(4): 562–569.

24. Ollila M, Falck A, Airaksinen PJ. Placing the Molteno® implant in a long scleral tunnel to prevent postoperative tube exposure. *Acta Ophthalmol Scand*. Jun 2005;83(3):302–305.

25. Aslanides IM, Spaeth GL, Schmidt CM, Lanzl IM, Gandham SB. Autologous patch graft in tube shunt surgery. *J Glaucoma*. Oct 1999; 8(5):306–309.

26. Raviv T, Greenfield DS, Liebmann JM, Sidoti PA, Ishikawa H, Ritch R. Pericardial patch grafts in glaucoma implant surgery. *J Glaucoma*. Feb 1998;7(1):27–32.

27. Tanji TM, Lundy DC, Minckler DS, Heuer DK, Varma R. Fascia lata patch graft in glaucoma tube surgery. *Ophthalmology*. Aug 1996;103(8): 1309–1312.

28. Gutierrez-Diaz E, Montero-Rodriguez M, Mencia-Gutierrez E, Cabello A, Monescillo J. Long-term persistence of fascia lata patch graft in glaucoma drainage device surgery. *Eur J Ophthalmol*. May-Jun 2005;15(3):412–414.

29. Kalenak JW. Revision for exposed anterior segment tubes. *J Glaucoma*. Jan 2010;19(1): 5–10.

30. Brandt JD. Patch grafts of dehydrated cadaveric dura mater for tube-shunt glaucoma surgery. *Arch Ophthalmol*. Oct 1993;111(10): 1436–1439.

31. Hamaguchi T, Noguchi-Shinohara M, Nozaki I, et al. Medical procedures and risk for sporadic Creutzfeldt-Jakob disease, Japan, 1999–2008. *Emerg Infect Dis*. Feb 2009;15(2):265–271.

32. Noguchi-Shinohara M, Hamaguchi T, Kitamoto T, et al. Clinical features and diagnosis of dura mater graft associated Creutzfeldt Jakob disease. *Neurology*. Jul 24 2007;69(4):360–367.

33. King AJ, Azuara-Blanco A. Pericardial patch melting following glaucoma implant insertion. *Eye*. Apr 2001;15(Pt 2):236–237.

34. Lama PJ, Fechtner RD. Tube erosion following insertion of a glaucoma drainage device with a pericardial patch graft. *Arch Ophthalmol*. Sept 1999;117(9):1243–1244.

35. Smith MF, Doyle JW, Ticrney JW Jr. A comparison of glaucoma drainage implant tube coverage. *J Glaucoma*. Apr 2002;11(2):143–147.

36. Lankaranian D, Reis R, Henderer JD, Choe S, Moster MR. Comparison of single thickness and double thickness processed pericardium patch graft in glaucoma drainage device surgery: a single surgeon comparison of outcome. *J Glaucoma*. Jan-Feb 2008;17(1):48–51.

37. Ainsworth G, Rotchford A, Dua HS, King AJ. A novel use of amniotic membrane in the management of tube exposure following glaucoma tube shunt surgery. *Br J Ophthalmol*. Apr 2006;90(4):417–419.

38. Rai P, Lauande-Pimentel R, Barton K. Amniotic membrane as an adjunct to donor sclera in the repair of exposed glaucoma drainage devices. *Am J Ophthalmol*. Dec 2005;140(6):1148–1152.

39. Ayyala RS, Zurakowski D, Monshizadeh R, et al. Comparison of double-plate Molteno® and

Ahmed™ glaucoma valve in patients with advanced uncontrolled glaucoma. *Ophthalmic Surg Lasers*. Mar-Apr 2002;33(2):94–101.

40. Puustjarvi T, Ronkko S, Terasvirta M. A novel oculoplastic surgery for exposed glaucoma drainage shunt by using autologous graft. *Graefes Arch Clin Exp Ophthalmol*. Jun 2007;245(6):907–909.

41. Merrill KD, Suhr AW, Lim MC. Long-term success in the correction of exposed glaucoma drainage tubes with a tube extender. *Am J Ophthalmol*. Jul 2007;144(1):136–137.

42. Rosenberg LF, Krupin T. Implants in glaucoma surgery. In: Ritch R, Shields MB, Krupin T, eds. *The Glaucomas*. Vol 3: Glaucoma Therapy. St. Louis: Mosby; 1996:1783–1807.

39

LATE HYPOTONY

MATTHEW G. MCMENEMY

LATE HYPOTONY

As with all surgeries, numerous complications can occur with tube shunts; one particular complication is hypotony. Early hypotony is defined as intraocular pressure (IOP) of less than 6 mm Hg and occurs before maturation of the fibrotic capsule around the tube shunt plate. The physiologic development of the capsule typically occurs during the first postoperative 4–6 weeks after implantation. Late hypotony can be defined as IOP of less than 6 mm Hg that occurs after the plate is encysted. Hypotony in and of itself may not require treatment unless secondary complications develop (see Chapter 10 and 34). Untreated, hypotony can result in shallowing or flattening of the anterior chamber, corneal decompensation (see Chapter 40), peripheral anterior synechiae, cataract, maculopathy (see Chapter 22), optic nerve edema, choroidal effusion or hemorrhage (see Chapter 6), and even endophthalmitis (see Chapter 42). Although hypotony is common in the early postoperative period, it is less common as a late complication.[1] Knowing how to prevent and manage late hypotony is essential for long-lasting surgical success.

INCIDENCE

Persistent hypotony is less common with tube shunts than with trabeculectomy.[2] In the Tube Versus Trabeculectomy Study, of the 107 eyes in the tube group, none had persistent hypotony, whereas of the 105 eyes in the trabeculectomy group, 3 developed persistent hypotony.[2] A pediatric population study comparing trabeculectomy with mitomycin-C (24 eyes) with Ahmed™ (New World Medical, Inc., Rancho Cucamonga, California) or Baerveldt® (Abbott Medical Optics, Inc., Santa Ana, California) shunts (46 shunts total) had one eye in the trabeculectomy group with late hypotony, while no eyes in shunt group developed persistent hypotony.[3] WuDunn et al implanted 250 mm[2] Baerveldt® devices in 108 patients, with 5 failing due to persistent hypotony.[4] In all likelihood, late hypotony in the WuDunn et al study was due to either progression of underlying disease resulting in less aqueous production or secondary to another complication of shunt surgery.

However, across the different types of shunts, the incidences of early and late hypotony are not significantly different. Hong et al, in a literature review of multiple tube shunt studies, compared various implants, including the Molteno® (Molteno Ophthalmic Ltd., Dunedin, New Zealand) with or without surgical modification to restrict outflow, Baerveldt®, Ahmed™, and Krupin (Eagle Vision, Inc., Memphis, Tennessee) implants. Hong et al found that there were no statistically significant differences in the overall incidence of transient hypotony in the immediate postoperative period or in the incidence of chronic hypotony among the different types of tube shunts.[1]

Unlike shunt type, plate design, to an extent, does appear to affect the incidence of hypotony. With respect to the Molteno® plate, the incidence of chronic hypotony was 5 out of 234 patients using a single plate without modification, 5 out of 571 patients using a single plate with modification, and 5 out of 165 patients using a double plate with modification. A higher incidence of hypotony was seen with double plates. It is important to realize that this was not a randomized trial and that selection bias of which eyes received which shunts may play a large role.[1] Heuer et al, comparing single to double plate Molteno® implants, found that double plate implants resulted in significantly lower IOPs in both the early and late postoperative periods.[5] However, Lloyd et al found no difference in IOP control between 350 mm[2] and 500 mm[2] Baerveldt® implants.[6]

ETIOLOGY AND MANAGEMENT

A systematic approach should be undertaken to ascertain the etiology of the hypotony.

Understanding that hypotony may result from hyposecretion, overfiltration, or most commonly a combination of each is essential in management. Hypotony may be due to egress of fluid from an eye that is inadequately restricted, as in cases of wound leakage or overfiltration. Hyposecretion of aqueous may result from progression of underlying diseases, such ocular ischemia in diabetics with neovascular glaucoma or ciliary shutdown with exacerbation of uveitis[7,8] (see Chapter 34 for more information about hyposecretion). These underlying diseases are also often the initial cause of the glaucoma that necessitated shunt implantation in the first place. Additionally, intercurrent causes of hypotony may include new vascular events,[9] retinal detachments,[10-12] and endophthalmitis. Care must be taken in interpreting the literature on shunt comparisons as most is retrospective, and many surgeons have their own preferences for various types of glaucoma.

Leakage

Leakage is the most common cause of late hypotony and generally occurs years after implantation. It should be the first item on the differential diagnosis of late hypotony after a tube shunt. Generally, by the time hypotony is detected, a hole will be seen in the conjunctiva overlying the plate. Extrusion of the tube itself rather than the plate generally does not result in hypotony. In cases where no hole is easily seen, leakage may be detected by painting the tube and plate areas with a fluorescein strip followed by inspection using the Cobalt blue light at the slit lamp, in the same way that filtering bleb leaks are detected.

If a leak is discovered, it should be repaired. A small pinhole in the overlying conjunctiva may be closed with direct suturing of the defect. Due to the location of the plate posteriorly, care must be taken not to confuse the orifices of the lacrimal gland laterally, near the conjunctival fornix.

Overfiltration

Overfiltration may result from large surface area shunts combined with too thin a capsule or abnormally low aqueous production. In their 4-year study of Ahmed™ and Baerveldt® implants, Tsai et al concluded that the IOP reductions were similar, but there was a greater risk of hypotony with the Baerveldt® implant, likely owing to its large plate size.[13] When chronic hypotony results from too large of an implant, the plate can be surgically modified (wing removal) to allow a smaller surface area of filtration and result in a higher, more stable intraocular pressure.[14]

Inflammation and ciliary body hyposecretion

Hypotony may also result from reduced aqueous production. The low aqueous output may be secondary to iridocyclitis with consequent reduction of aqueous production by the ciliary body,[15] an inflammatory cyclitic membrane, or the effect from hypotensive therapy in the fellow eye, particularly reported with beta blockers.[16,17] Hyposecretion can also occur when the ciliary body is damaged by prior cyclodestruction[18–20] or chemicals, including toxic medications, most commonly mitomycin-C administered during previous glaucoma surgery[21] (see Chapter 34 for more information). History of several prior retinal surgeries may also be an indicator of low aqueous production. Chronic traction on the anterior vitreous base, as may occur in cases of proliferative vitreoretinopathy, may also result in hyposecretion from an annular choroidal detachment.[22]

If the glaucoma surgeon suspects that the eye is at risk for low aqueous production, implantation of a smaller device should be considered. For example, a 350 mm^2 Baerveldt® implant might be too large in a uveitic eye; a 250 mm^2 implant might be more appropriate. As for management, removal of oral or topical aqueous suppressant medications (including oral beta blockers), even from the nonhypotonous eye, should be an initial consideration. Untreated inflammation can result in phthisis bulbi. Thus, inflammation should be treated early and aggressively. Surgical removal of epiciliary membranes, if possible, may be indicated if complications of hypotony develop.

Tube and plate exposure

Wound dehiscence or conjunctival erosion may result in tube or implant exposure in the late postoperative period. Timely closure of the wound or defect is important to minimize the risk of hypotony and endophthalmitis. Treatment of tube or plate exposure involves covering the defect with a patch graft and conjunctiva. Chapter 38 discusses the management of such conjunctival erosions in more detail. Quadrant placement has been suggested as a risk factor for tube extrusion, but in a study of superior versus inferior tube implantation, Pakravan et al found no cases of hypotony at one month or later in 106 study eyes undergoing either superior or inferior Ahmed™ tube insertion.[23] However, the average follow-up period of approximately one year in this study may not be long enough to detect late extrusions, as these may occur multiple years later.

The tissues over the tube and plate are more likely to become thin and melt when implantation is combined with antifibrotic administration.[24] The thinning may ultimately be followed by erosion of the tube or plate through the conjunctiva. Loss of conjunctival capillaries over the tube, typically within 3 mm from the corneo-scleral junction, is an indication of impending erosion through the conjunctiva and should prompt close observation. Several studies have demonstrated an increased incidence of hypotony, flat chamber, and choroidal effusion when mitomycin-C is used during tube shunt implantation.[25–27] Currently, there is no strong evidence to support the use of antifibrotic agents as adjuncts to tube shunts,[28,29] and their use should be avoided to prevent these late complications.

Implant removal

Severe hypotony may require removal of the implant. Papadaki et al removed 4 of 60 Ahmed™ implants due to severe hypotony. In their study, severe hypotony and associated conditions including hypotony maculopathy, flat anterior chamber, and choroidal effusion, had an incidence of 1.2%/person-years.[30] Souza et al explanted one of 64 Ahmed™ valves due to chronic hypotony.[31] Spiegel et al explanted 3 of 42 Schocket implants (tube from anterior chamber to an encircling band) because of long-term hypotony.[32] Explantation may consist of removal and truncation of the tube or complete removal of the implant. When hypotony is due to an extrusion or hyposecretion, if the plate is well covered there is no reason to remove it. More simply remove the tube itself from its insertion site and amputate it.

CONCLUSION

Late hypotony is an uncommon occurrence following tube shunt surgery and in many cases can be prevented by proper preoperative planning, choosing the correct location away from previous mitomycin-C administration or dense conjunctival scarring, and selecting the appropriate-sized implant for the underlying condition. Unfortunately, late hypotony can occur despite the best planning, surgical technique, and postoperative management. Fortunately, complications of late hypotony can generally be successfully managed when not associated with permanent ciliary shutdown.

COMMENTARY

JAMES C. TSAI

Although late hypotony is an uncommon common complication of glaucoma tube shunt implants, it should be recognized and treated appropriately when it occurs. In my clinical experience, the occurrence is more commonly observed in the setting of 1) acute exacerbation of uveitis in an eye with a nonvalved implant and 2) implantation of a larger size shunt in an eye with prior cyclodestruction (i.e., aqueous hyposecretion). Other likely etiologies include undiagnosed retinal detachment, annular choroidal detachment and/or ciliary body detachment secondary to proliferative vitreoretinopathy, recalcitrant iridocyclitis with or without inflammatory cyclitic membrane, or pharmacologic aqueous suppression.

Depending on the exact cause of the late hypotony, judicious surgical revision should be pursued. Late-onset conjunctival holes may prove difficult to close surgically, especially if surface epithelium has grown in through the wound and around the implant. In an eye with a larger than desired plate size, surgical modification (with wing removal) may prove successful. To avoid this situation, a smaller size implant (e.g., 250 mm² Baerveldt® implant) should be strongly considered in eyes with a history of cyclodestruction procedures. Finally, I agree with the author that there is currently no strong evidence to support the use of antifibrotic agents as adjuncts to tube shunt procedures, though there is ongoing research on devices that allow for sustained release of these agents.

Dr. Tsai was supported by a Departmental Challenge Grant from Research to Prevent Blindness, Inc.

COMMENTARY

PAUL J. HARASYMOWYCZ

Hypotony after tube shunt implantation may been seen in up to 12% of cases in uveitic patients, depending on the type of implant used.[33] Preoperative or postoperative assessment with UBM may be useful to document the status of the ciliary body and help with management of hypotony. Atrophy of ciliary processes may indicate hyposecretion of aqueous, and cyclitic membranes may sometimes be seen causing tractional ciliary body detachment. Before implant revision is planned, a trial of steroid drops or subconjunctival injection may help in increasing IOP. Similarly a trial of viscoelastic injection into the anterior chamber may be attempted and may sometimes result in a prolonged rise in IOP. Finally, autologous subconjunctival blood injections may also be tried when hyposecretion is suspected.

Dr. Harasymowycz was supported by the Quebec Glaucoma Foundation.

REFERENCES

1. Hong CH, Arosemena A, Zurakowski D, Ayyala RS. Glaucoma drainage devices: a systematic literature review and current controversies. *Surv Ophthalmol.* Jan-Feb 2005;50(1):48–60.

2. Gedde SJ, Schiffman JC, Feuer WJ, Herndon LW, Brandt JD, Budenz DL. Treatment outcomes in the Tube Versus Trabeculectomy Study after one year of follow-up. *Am J Ophthalmol.* Jan 2007;143(1):9–22.

3. Beck AD, Freedman S, Kammer J, Jin J. Aqueous shunt devices compared with trabeculectomy with mitomycin-C for children in the first two years of life. *Am J Ophthalmol.* Dec 2003;136(6):994–1000.

4. WuDunn D, Phan AD, Cantor LB, Lind JT, Cortes A, Wu B. Clinical experience with the Baerveldt® 250-mm2 Glaucoma Implant. *Ophthalmology.* May 2006;113(5):766–772.

5. Heuer DK, Lloyd MA, Abrams DA, et al. Which is better? One or two? A randomized clinical trial of single-plate versus double-plate Molteno® implantation for glaucomas in aphakia and pseudophakia. *Ophthalmology.* Oct 1992;99(10):1512–1519.

6. Lloyd MA, Baerveldt G, Fellenbaum PS, et al. Intermediate-term results of a randomized clinical trial of the 350- versus the 500-mm2 Baerveldt® implant. *Ophthalmology.* Aug 1994;101(8):1456–1463; discussion 1463–1454.

7. Assaad MH, Baerveldt G, Rockwood EJ. Glaucoma drainage devices: pros and cons. *Curr Opin Ophthalmol.* Apr 1999;10(2):147–153.

8. Orengo-Nania S. Anterior and posterior chambers, iris and pupil, and lens. In: Gross RL, ed. *Clinical Glaucoma Management: Critical Signs in Diagnosis and Therapy.* Philadelphia: W.B. Saunders Company; 2001:347–363.

9. Hayreh SS, March W, Phelps CD. Ocular hypotony following retinal vein occlusion. *Arch Ophthalmol.* May 1978;96(5):827–833.

10. Jarrett WH 2nd. Rhematogenous retinal detachment complicated by severe intraocular inflammation, hypotony, and choroidal detachment. *Trans Am Ophthalmol Soc.* 1981;79:664–683.

11. Pederson JE. Ocular hypotony. In: Ritch R, Shields MB, Krupin T, eds. *The Glaucomas.* Vol 1: Basic Sciences. 2nd ed. St. Louis: Mosby; 1996:385–395.

12. Ringvold A. Evidence that hypotony in retinal detachment is due to subretinal juxtapapillary fluid drainage. *Acta Ophthalmol (Copenh).* Aug 1980;58(4):652–658.

13. Tsai JC, Johnson CC, Kammer JA, Dietrich MS. The Ahmed™ shunt versus the Baerveldt® shunt for refractory glaucoma II: longer-term outcomes from a single surgeon. *Ophthalmology.* Jun 2006;113(6):913–917.

14. Minckler DS, Francis BA, Hodapp EA, et al. Aqueous shunts in glaucoma: a report by the American Academy of Ophthalmology. *Ophthalmology.* Jun 2008;115(6):1089–1098.

15. Toris CB, Pederson JE. Aqueous humor dynamics in experimental iridocyclitis. *Invest Ophthalmol Vis Sci.* Mar 1987;28(3):477–481.

16. Dunham CN, Spaide RF, Dunham G. The contralateral reduction of intraocular pressure by timolol. *Br J Ophthalmol.* Jan 1994;78(1):38–40.

17. Radius RL, Diamond GR, Pollack IP, Langham ME. Timolol. A new drug for management of chronic simple glaucoma. *Arch Ophthalmol.* Jun 1978;96(6):1003–1008.

18. Devenyi RG, Trope GE, Hunter WS. Neodymium-YAG transscleral cyclocoagulation in rabbit eyes. *Br J Ophthalmol.* Jun 1987;71(6):441–444.

19. van der Zypen E, England C, Fankhauser F, Kwasniewska S. The effect of transscleral laser cyclophotocoagulation on rabbit ciliary body vascularization. *Graefes Arch Clin Exp Ophthalmol.* 1989;227(2):172–179.

20. Wellemeyer ML, Price FW Jr. Molteno® implants in patients with previous cyclocryotherapy. *Ophthalmic Surg.* Jun 1993;24(6):395–398.

21. Mietz H. The toxicology of mitomycin C on the ciliary body. *Curr Opin Ophthalmol.* Apr 1996;7(2):72–79.

22. Arevalo JF, Garcia RA, Fernandez CF. Anterior segment inflammation and hypotony after posterior segment surgery. *Ophthalmol Clin North Am.* Dec 2004;17(4):527–537, vi.

23. Pakravan M, Yazdani S, Shahabi C, Yaseri M. Superior versus inferior Ahmed™ glaucoma valve implantation. *Ophthalmology.* Feb 2009;116(2):208–213.

24. Ayyala RS, Zurakowski D, Smith JA, et al. A clinical study of the Ahmed™ glaucoma valve implant in advanced glaucoma. *Ophthalmology.* Oct 1998;105(10):1968–1976.

25. Perkins TW, Cardakli UF, Eisele JR, Kaufman PL, Heatley GA. Adjunctive mitomycin C in Molteno® implant surgery. *Ophthalmology.* Jan 1995;102(1):91–97.

26. Perkins TW, Gangnon R, Ladd W, Kaufman PL, Libby CM. Molteno® implant with mitomycin C: intermediate-term results. *J Glaucoma.* Apr 1998;7(2):86–92.

27. Susanna R Jr., Nicolela MT, Takahashi WY. Mitomycin C as adjunctive therapy with glaucoma implant surgery. *Ophthalmic Surg.* Jul 1994;25(7):458–462.

28. Cantor L, Burgoyne J, Sanders S, Bhavnani V, Hoop J, Brizendine E. The effect of mitomycin C on Molteno® implant surgery: a 1-year randomized, masked, prospective study. *J Glaucoma.* Aug 1998;7(4):240–246.

29. Costa VP, Azuara-Blanco A, Netland PA, Lesk MR, Arcieri ES. Efficacy and safety of adjunctive mitomycin C during Ahmed™ Glaucoma Valve implantation: a prospective randomized clinical trial. *Ophthalmology.* Jun 2004;111(6):1071–1076.

30. Papadaki TG, Zacharopoulos IP, Pasquale LR, Christen WB, Netland PA, Foster CS. Long-term results of Ahmed™ glaucoma valve implantation for uveitic glaucoma. *Am J Ophthalmol.* Jul 2007;144(1):62–69.

31. Souza C, Tran DH, Loman J, Law SK, Coleman AL, Caprioli J. Long-term outcomes of Ahmed™ glaucoma valve implantation in refractory glaucomas. *Am J Ophthalmol.* Dec 2007; 144(6):893–900.

32. Spiegel D, Shrader RR, Wilson RP. Anterior chamber tube shunt to an encircling band (Schocket procedure) in the treatment of refractory glaucoma. *Ophthalmic Surg.* Dec 1992;23(12):804–807.

33. Ceballos EM, Parrish RK 2nd, Schiffman JC. Outcome of Baerveldt® glaucoma drainage implants for the treatment of uveitic glaucoma. *Ophthalmology.* Dec 2002;109(12):2256–2260.

40

VISUAL LOSS

JESS T. WHITSON

VISUAL LOSS

Tube shunt surgery use has increased significantly in recent years.[1,2] Once reserved as a treatment option for more refractory types of disease, such as uveitic[3] or neovascular glaucoma,[4] or for eyes that had failed one or more trabeculectomies,[5] tube shunts are now being used by some surgeons in place of trabeculectomy as a first-line surgical alternative in eyes with other less aggressive or less difficult to control forms of glaucoma.[6–9] Visual loss can occur following tube shunt implantation as a result of complications during the postoperative period or from the progression of underlying disease (see Table 40.1). Although tube shunt implantation is associated with similar postoperative complications as trabeculectomy surgery, such as hypotony, hemorrhage, and failure to control IOP, there are several unique complications that may develop with the use of tube shunts, many of which may result in vision loss.

INCIDENCE OF VISUAL LOSS FOLLOWING TUBE SHUNT SURGERY

Visual loss following tube shunt surgery is not uncommon. A large, systematic literature review of tube shunts by Hong and coworkers[10] reported rates of vision loss following tube shunt surgery (defined as loss of 2 or more lines of visual acuity at last follow-up) ranging from (mean [SD]) 24 (7)% with the Ahmed™ Glaucoma Valve (New World Medical, Inc., Rancho Cucamonga, California) to 33 (18)% with the Molteno® implant (Molteno Ophthalmic Ltd., Dunedin, New Zealand). In the Tube Versus Trabeculectomy (TVT) Study, an ongoing, prospective, randomized clinical trial that is comparing the Baerveldt® 350 mm² tube shunt (Abbott Medical Optics, Inc., Santa Ana, California) to trabeculectomy with mitomycin-C (MMC) in eyes with previous trabeculectomy and/or cataract

Table 40.1. Common Causes of Visual Loss Following Tube Shunt Surgery

COMMON CAUSES OF VISUAL LOSS FOLLOWING TUBE SHUNT SURGERY

Anterior Segment Complications

- Corneal decompensation[10,12,14,15]
- Corneal graft failure[16–21]
- Cataract[11,23]

Hypotony and Posterior Segment Disorders

- Choroidal effusion[28,29]
- Suprachoroidal hemorrhage[29–31]
- Vitreous hemorrhage[25]
- Retinal detachment[25,32]
- Chorioretinal folds[33]

Endophthalmitis (Chapter 43)

surgery,[7] vision loss (defined as loss of 2 or more lines of Snellen visual acuity) occurred in 31 of the 107 patients (29%) in the tube shunt group. The occurrence of any postoperative complication significantly increased the risk of vision loss (p < 0.001), and this risk correlated to the number of complications.[11]

ANTERIOR SEGMENT COMPLICATIONS ASSOCIATED WITH VISUAL LOSS

Corneal decompensation has been reported to occur in up to 30% of patients during long-term follow-up after tube shunt surgery.[12] This complication is especially serious in patients who have undergone penetrating keratoplasty (PKP), with reported rates of graft failure ranging from 10% to 51%.[10] The mechanism of corneal decompensation following tube shunt surgery is not clear. Tube-cornea touch can lead to localized loss of endothelial cells.[13] Progressive endothelial cell loss can also result from repeated, intermittent tube-cornea touch, as occurs with blinking or inadvertent eye rubbing.[14] Immunologic factors and breakdown of the blood-aqueous barrier may play a role as well.[15]

The optimal sequence and time for PKP and tube shunt surgery is controversial. Studies by

Beebe et al[16] and Rapuano et al[17] showed higher rates of graft failure when the tube shunt was placed after the PKP. Conversely, Kwon and colleagues[18] reported the lowest rates of graft survival in patients who underwent tube shunt surgery prior to PKP. Some authors have recommended vitrectomy and placement of the tube shunt in the pars plana as a way to improve long-term graft survival.[19,20] Sidoti et al,[21] however, found comparable rates of graft survival and higher rates of posterior segment complications, such as retinal detachment (6%; 2 of 34 patients), epiretinal membrane formation (9%; 3 of 34 patients), and cystoid macular edema (3%; 1 of 34 patients), with the pars plana approach. Insertion of the tube through the pars plana is probably best suited for patients who are undergoing simultaneous vitrectomy for associated retinal pathology, such as neovascular glaucoma with vitreous hemorrhage, or for those with significant posterior synechiae and very shallow anterior chambers.[22]

In addition to corneal complications, tube-lens touch may lead to the development of a focal cataract[23] or even possibly hasten the onset of age-related cataractous changes. In the TVT Study, cataract progression was reported as the cause of decreased vision in 8 out of 24 (33%) phakic patients who underwent tube shunt surgery.[11] However, research has shown that cataract surgery can be performed safely and without loss of intraocular pressure (IOP) control in patients with a functioning tube shunt.[24] For more information, see Chapters 44 and 45.

HYPOTONY AND POSTERIOR SEGMENT DISORDERS

Hypotony may result in a flat or shallow anterior chamber leading to corneal decompensation or cataract formation (see above) and is also associated with an increased risk of choroidal effusion, suprachoroidal hemorrhage, and other retinal complications. Early reports placed the incidence of early postoperative hypotony and flat anterior chambers following tube shunt surgery at over 40%.[4] Since the advent of valved devices and techniques to limit early aqueous flow, this incidence has dropped significantly, ranging from 3.5% to 27% for both valved and nonvalved devices.[25] Various methods to prevent hypotony with nonvalved tube shunts in the early postoperative period have been described, including tube ligature[26] and internal tube occlusion.[27] Early IOP elevation in these eyes can be temporized by placing fenestrations in the tube at the time of surgery and with the use of IOP-lowering medications postoperatively. After 4–6 weeks, fibrous encapsulation of the plate occurs, allowing for more controlled egress of aqueous humor. Absorbable stitches will typically dissolve by 6 weeks postoperatively; if not, argon laser suture lysis of the tube ligature can be performed. For more information on hypotony with tube shunts, see Chapters 34 and 39.

Choroidal effusion is associated with hypotony and occurs in up to 37% of eyes following tube shunt surgery[28] with an average reported incidence of 18.6%[29] (see Figure 40.1). Most choroidal effusions are small, localized, and not visually significant; these types of effusions will typically resolve spontaneously as IOP returns to normal. Should an extensive choroidal effusion block the visual axis or cause apposition of retinal tissue, surgical drainage may be necessary (see Chapter 6). Hypotony maculopathy occurs in 1.3% of eyes following tube shunt surgery and can lead to persistent decreased

vision postoperatively.[14] Should this condition develop, measures to elevate IOP, including temporary ligature of the tube, should be instituted (see Chapter 22).

Suprachoroidal hemorrhage is potentially more serious and vision-threatening than choroidal effusion and occurs with an average incidence of 4.2% after tube shunt surgery.[29] In a large review of 422 tube shunt surgeries, Tuli and colleagues[30] reported an incidence of suprachoroidal hemorrhage in 2.8% of valved tube shunts (2 of 72 implantations) and in 7.1% of nonvalved tube shunts (25 of 350 implantations). Visual outcomes in these eyes were poor, decreasing from logMAR visual acuity of 0.72 (20/105) preoperatively to 1.36 (20/460) at last follow-up ($P < 0.0001$).[30] Risk factors for suprachoroidal hemorrhage include aphakia/anterior chamber intraocular lens, intraoperative vitrectomy, elevated preoperative IOP, atherosclerosis, and prolonged hypotony.[30,31] Suprachoroidal hemorrhage occurs in a bimodal fashion: immediately postoperatively, especially with valved devices, and then 4–6 weeks later in nonvalved implants when the tube is no longer occluded. A 23-gauge needle should be used during surgery to create a water-tight seal for tube insertion, thus helping prevent early overfiltration and hypotony. Moreover, opening of the tube ligature in a nonvalved tube shunt early in the postoperative period before

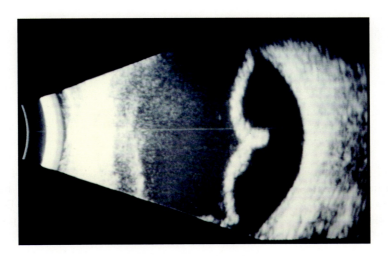

FIGURE 40.1   B-scan ultrasound showing a serous choroidal effusion from hypotony following tube shunt implantation surgery.

encapsulation of the plate has occurred should be avoided (see Chapter 35).

Reported rates of vitreous hemorrhage following tube shunt surgery range from 1.3% to 7%.[25] Sources of blood include retinal tears, breakthrough bleeding from suprachoroidal hemorrhage, and scleral perforation while suturing the plate to the globe. Management includes observation and excluding associated retinal pathology. Extensive or persistent vitreous hemorrhage may require surgical removal to restore vision. Retinal detachment occurs in 3.5%–5% of eyes undergoing tube shunt implantation,[25] typically within a few months after surgery.[32] Risk factors include peripheral retinal pathology, trauma, uveitis, scleral perforation, and retinal dialysis after pars plana tube insertion.[32] Additionally, chorioretinal folds, corresponding to the size and location of the episcleral plate, have been reported as a potential cause of decreased visual acuity after tube shunt surgery.[33]

Postoperative hemorrhagic complications, such as hyphema, intraretinal hemorrhage, and suprachoroidal hemorrhage, are more common in patients who are on oral anticoagulation (ACT) or antiplatelet (APT) therapy. Law and coworkers[34] reported that 347 patients who were on ACT or APT prior to glaucoma surgery had a higher rate of hemorrhagic complications than age-matched controls (10.1% [35 of 347 patients] vs. 3.7% [13 of 347 patients], respectively, $P = 0.002$). Vision loss (defined as a decrease of 2 or more lines of Snellen visual acuity) occurred in 29.2% of eyes (10 patients) with hemorrhagic complications. Severe vision loss (defined as a decrease of 4 or more lines of Snellen visual acuity or final visual acuity of 20/200 or less) occurred in 17.1% of patients with hemorrhagic complications (6 patients), compared to 5.9% of patients without hemorrhagic complications (19 patients; $P = 0.018$).[34] Since discontinuation of ACT or APT therapy may predispose patients to a transient, but dangerous, hypercoagulable state,[35] the decision to reduce or stop anticoagulants or antiplatelet medication prior to surgery should be made only after consultation with the patient's internist or medical subspecialist. For more information on hyphemas, see Chapters 5 and 23.

OTHER COMPLICATIONS

Many other complications that may result in vision loss (e.g., endophthalmitis, Chapter 42) are discussed elsewhere in this book. Please see Part Four, Tube Shunt Complications.

CONCLUSION

Tube shunt surgery is a valuable and effective treatment option for patients with refractory glaucoma. Despite recent advances in implant design and surgical technique, visual loss remains an important potential complication of tube shunt surgery. Prompt recognition and appropriate management of factors that can lead to visual loss following tube shunt surgery will help improve final outcomes for these patients.

Dr. Whitson was supported by an Unrestricted Grant from Research to Prevent Blindness to The University of Texas Southwestern Medical School.

COMMENTARY
JONATHAN S. MYERS

Vision loss may follow tube shunt surgery, or other glaucoma surgery, as the result of inadequate control of IOP. Postoperative loss of fixation, so-called "snuff," is a rare but devastating complication of glaucoma surgery that may be seen in very advanced disease, such as split fixation. Tube shunt surgery sometimes presents the special challenge of elevated IOP in the first 2 months after surgery. In nonvalved shunts, the pressure may be high for up to 6 weeks while awaiting dissolution of the ligature suture, even if venting slits were made in the tube, as these slits often close by 3 weeks. Additionally, in rare cases, the sudden release of this suture may lead to hypotony with subsequent suprachoroidal hemorrhage. The elevated IOP or the hypotony and suprachoroidal hemorrhage may lead to vision loss, especially in eyes with far advanced damage.

Some surgeons will use valved tubes to allow for better control of IOP in the first 6 weeks. This approach is often effective, but valved tubes are more likely to be associated with a hypertensive phase, requiring medications and possibly leading to higher than tolerated IOP. Although this resolves with time in most cases, there is the potential for additional glaucomatous progression. It has been suggested that valved shunts do not achieve quite as low IOPs as nonvalved shunts.[36]

A concurrent trabeculectomy has been used to help manage early IOP control with nonvalved shunts in select patients. This is more labor intensive and may not be possible in some scarred eyes. It can be effective in controlling eye pressure before the ligature suture dissolves. Some surgeons will use nondissolving ligatures coupled with ripcord sutures to allow planned opening of the tube only if the trabeculectomy fails. An additional concern is the exposure of the patient to the potential complications of a trabeculectomy in addition to those of the tube shunt.

REFERENCES

1. Joshi AB, Parrish RK, 2nd, Feuer WF. 2002 survey of the American Glaucoma Society: practice preferences for glaucoma surgery and antifibrotic use. *J Glaucoma*. Apr 2005;14(2):172–174.

2. Ramulu PY, Corcoran KJ, Corcoran SL, Robin AL. Utilization of various glaucoma surgeries and procedures in Medicare beneficiaries from 1995 to 2004. *Ophthalmology*. Dec 2007; 114(12):2265–2270.

3. Molteno AC, Bevin TH, Herbison P, Houliston MJ. Otago glaucoma surgery outcome study: long-term follow-up of cases of primary glaucoma with additional risk factors drained by Molteno® implants. *Ophthalmology*. Dec 2001;108(12):2193–2200.

4. Molteno AC, Van Rooyen MM, Bartholomew RS. Implants for draining neovascular glaucoma. *Br J Ophthalmol*. Feb 1977;61(2):120–125.

5. Mills RP, Reynolds A, Emond MJ, Barlow WE, Leen MM. Long-term survival of Molteno® glaucoma drainage devices. *Ophthalmology*. Feb 1996;103(2):299–305.

6. Gedde SJ, Schiffman JC, Feuer WJ, Herndon LW, Brandt JD, Budenz DL. Treatment outcomes in the Tube Versus Trabeculectomy Study after one year of follow-up. *Am J Ophthalmol*. Jan 2007; 143(1):9–22.

7. Gedde SJ, Schiffman JC, Feuer WJ, Parrish RK 2nd, Heuer DK, Brandt JD. The Tube Versus Trabeculectomy Study: design and baseline characteristics of study patients. *Am J Ophthalmol*. Aug 2005;140(2):275–287.

8. Wilson MR, Mendis U, Paliwal A, Haynatzka V. Long-term follow-up of primary glaucoma surgery with Ahmed™ glaucoma valve implant versus trabeculectomy. *Am J Ophthalmol*. Sept 2003;136(3):464–470.

9. Wilson MR, Mendis U, Smith SD, Paliwal A. Ahmed™ glaucoma valve implant vs trabeculectomy in the surgical treatment of glaucoma: a randomized clinical trial. *Am J Ophthalmol*. Sept 2000;130(3):267–273.

10. Hong CH, Arosemena A, Zurakowski D, Ayyala RS. Glaucoma drainage devices: a systematic literature review and current controversies. *Surv Ophthalmol*. Jan-Feb 2005; 50(1):48–60.

11. Gedde SJ, Herndon LW, Brandt JD, Budenz DL, Feuer WJ, Schiffman JC. Surgical complications in the Tube Versus Trabeculectomy Study during the first year of follow-up. *Am J Ophthalmol*. Jan 2007;143(1):23–31.

12. Topouzis F, Coleman AL, Choplin N, et al. Follow-up of the original cohort with the Ahmed™ glaucoma valve implant. *Am J Ophthalmol*. Aug 1999;128(2):198–204.

13. McDermott ML, Swendris RP, Shin DH, Juzych MS, Cowden JW. Corneal endothelial cell counts after Molteno® implantation. *Am J Ophthalmol*. Jan 1993;115(1):93–96.

14. Guerrero AH, Latina MA. Complications of glaucoma drainage implant surgery. *Int Ophthalmol Clin*. Winter 2000;40(1):149–163.

15. Classen L, Kivela T, Tarkkanen A. Histopathologic and immunohistochemical analysis of the filtration bleb after unsuccessful glaucoma seton implantation. *Am J Ophthalmol*. Aug 1996;122(2):205–212.

16. Beebe WE, Starita RJ, Fellman RL, Lynn JR, Gelender H. The use of Molteno® implant and anterior chamber tube shunt to encircling band for the treatment of glaucoma in

keratoplasty patients. *Ophthalmology.* Nov 1990;97(11):1414–1422.

17. Rapuano CJ, Schmidt CM, Cohen EJ, et al. Results of alloplastic tube shunt procedures before, during, or after penetrating keratoplasty. *Cornea.* Jan 1995;14(1):26–32.

18. Kwon YH, Taylor JM, Hong S, et al. Long-term results of eyes with penetrating keratoplasty and glaucoma drainage tube implant. *Ophthalmology.* Feb 2001;108(2):272–278.

19. Arroyave CP, Scott IU, Fantes FE, Feuer WJ, Murray TG. Corneal graft survival and intraocular pressure control after penetrating keratoplasty and glaucoma drainage device implantation. *Ophthalmology.* Nov 2001; 108(11):1978–1985.

20. Ritterband DC, Shapiro D, Trubnik V, et al. Penetrating keratoplasty with pars plana glaucoma drainage devices. *Cornea.* Oct 2007; 26(9):1060–1066.

21. Sidoti PA, Mosny AY, Ritterband DC, Seedor JA. Pars plana tube insertion of glaucoma drainage implants and penetrating keratoplasty in patients with coexisting glaucoma and corneal disease. *Ophthalmology.* Jun 2001; 108(6): 1050–1058.

22. Hodkin MJ, Goldblatt WS, Burgoyne CF, Ball SF, Insler MS. Early clinical experience with the Baerveldt® implant in complicated glaucomas. *Am J Ophthalmol.* Jul 1995;120(1):32–40.

23. Rosenberg LF, Krupin T. Implants in glaucoma surgery. In: Ritch R, Shields MB, Krupin T, eds. *The Glaucomas.* Vol 3: Glaucoma Therapy. 2nd ed. St. Louis: Mosby; 1996:1783–1807.

24. Bhattacharyya CA, WuDunn D, Lakhani V, Hoop J, Cantor LB. Cataract surgery after tube shunts. *J Glaucoma.* Dec 2000;9(6):453–457.

25. Lim KS, Allan BD, Lloyd AW, Muir A, Khaw PT. Glaucoma drainage devices; past, present, and future. *Br J Ophthalmol.* Sept 1998;82(9):1083–1089.

26. Trible JR, Brown DB. Occlusive ligature and standardized fenestration of a Baerveldt® tube with and without antimetabolites for early postoperative intraocular pressure control. *Ophthalmology.* Dec 1998;105(12):2243–2250.

27. Latina MA. Single stage Molteno® implant with combination internal occlusion and external ligature. *Ophthalmic Surg.* Jun 1990; 21(6):444–446.

28. Wirostko WJ, Mieler WF, Levin DS, et al. Hypotony and retinal complications after aqueous humor shunt implantation: the 1999 Dohlman Lecture. *Int Ophthalmol Clin.* Winter 2000;40(1):1–12.

29. Law SK, Kalenak JW, Connor TB, Jr., Pulido JS, Han DP, Mieler WF. Retinal complications after aqueous shunt surgical procedures for glaucoma. *Arch Ophthalmol.* Dec 1996;114(12):1473–1480.

30. Tuli SS, WuDunn D, Ciulla TA, Cantor LB. Delayed suprachoroidal hemorrhage after glaucoma filtration procedures. *Ophthalmology.* Oct 2001;108(10):1808–1811.

31. Nguyen QH, Budenz DL, Parrish RK 2nd. Complications of Baerveldt® glaucoma drainage implants. *Arch Ophthalmol.* May 1998; 116(5):571–575.

32. Waterhouse WJ, Lloyd MA, Dugel PU, et al. Rhegmatogenous retinal detachment after Molteno® glaucoma implant surgery. *Ophthalmology.* Apr 1994;101(4):665–671.

33. Sibayan SA, Latina MA. Chorioretinal folds following glaucoma valve implantation. *Ophthalmic Surg Lasers.* Mar 1998;29(3):242–243.

34. Law SK, Song BJ, Yu F, Kurbanyan K, Yang TA, Caprioli J. Hemorrhagic complications from glaucoma surgery in patients on anticoagulation therapy or antiplatelet therapy. *Am J Ophthalmol.* Apr 2008;145(4):736–746.

35. Konstantatos A. Anticoagulation and cataract surgery: a review of the current literature. *Anaesth Intensive Care.* Feb 2001;29(1):11–18.

36. Budenz DL, Barton K, Feuer WJ, et al. Treatment outcomes in the Ahmed™ Baerveldt® Comparison Study after 1 year of follow-up. *Ophthalmology.* Mar 2011;118(3):443–452.

41

AXIAL LENGTH CHANGES

OSMAN ORAM

AXIAL LENGTH CHANGES

The biometric changes of the human eye with lowered intraocular pressure (IOP), like those observed after glaucoma surgery, have been investigated by *in vivo* studies.[1,2] Leydolt et al demonstrated IOP-dependent axial eye length changes in human eyes. An axial eye length decrease of 2 µm/mm Hg with short-term reduction of IOP was observed. They suggested that this concomitant shortening of axial length and IOP reduction could be a result of a decrease in scleral length owing to the reduced IOP or an increase in choroidal blood flow compensating the reduced ocular fundus pulsations during the increased IOP phase.[1] In another *in vivo* study, Read et al showed that axial length underwent significant variation over a 24-hour period in normal human eyes, and a significant association existed between the change in axial length and the change in IOP, as measured by dynamic contour tonometry. The association observed between IOP

and axial length was found to be consistent with the hypothesis of passive expansion and contraction of the globe in response to IOP.[2]

Studies on trabeculectomy patients, performed with or without cataract extraction, have shown a significant decrease of axial length after surgery, correlated with IOP reduction.[3–7] Similarly, IOP lowering after tube shunt surgery may produce a decrease in axial length that is dependent on the amount of IOP lowering.[4] Understanding how axial length changes impact clinical decisions, such as lens power choice for cataract surgery, is important for treating patients after glaucoma surgery or patients who have had previous glaucoma surgery.

AXIAL LENGTH CHANGES AFTER GLAUCOMA FILTERING SURGERY

Table 41.1 summarizes reported axial length changes following different types of trabeculectomy procedures. Nemeth and Horoczi

Table 41.1. Reported Axial Length Changes after Trabeculectomy and Tube Shunt Implantation

AXIAL LENGTH CHANGES AFTER SURGERY

AUTHORS	PROCEDURE	MEAN INTERVAL AFTER SURGERY	MEAN CHANGE IN AXIAL LENGTH (MM)
Cashwell and Martin[3]	Trabeculectomy with or without 5-Fu or MMC	Various	−0.423
Kook et al[5]	Trabeculectomy with MMC	1 wk	−0.54
		1 mo	−1.15
		3 mo	−0.83
		6 mo	−0.80
		12 mo	−0.91
Law et al[6]	Combined cataract surgery and trabeculectomy with MMC	7.3 mo	−0.12
Francis et al[4]	Trabeculectomy with 5-Fu or MMC	1 wk	−0.15
		1 mo	−0.17
		> 3 mo	−0.05
	Baerveldt® Glaucoma Implant (Abbot Medical Optics, Santa Ana, California)	1 wk	−0.15
		1 mo	−0.30
		> 3 mo	−0.13

5-Fu: 5-Fluorouracil; MMC: Mitomycin-C

noted decreased axial length and increased thickness and volume of the ocular wall 4 days after trabeculectomy.[7] In a retrospective study, Cashwell and Martin found a significant decrease in axial length (mean: 0.423 mm, range: 2.8 to +0.5 mm) after successful initial trabeculectomy in 62 patients using ultrasound biometry. Preoperative factors found to be associated with a greater decrease in axial length were young age, myopia, exposure to an antimetabolite, and a post-trabeculectomy IOP drop greater than 30 mmHg.[3] Kook et al prospectively evaluated the short-term effect of trabeculectomy with adjunctive mitomycin-C (MMC) on axial length in 18 eyes using ultrasound biometry. The mean change in axial length was -1.15 mm at 1 month, -0.80 mm at 6 months, and -0.91mm at 12 months. In this study, the mean axial length at each follow-up was significantly shorter than preoperatively. Axial length continued to change over 6 months and did not fully recover even at 12 months. There was a positive correlation between postoperative axial length and IOP. Eyes with higher preoperative IOP had a greater decrease in axial length after trabeculectomy.[5]

Law et al evaluated the effect of combined cataract surgery and trabeculectomy with MMC on axial length using noncontact optical coherence biometry. The study demonstrated a significant reduction in the axial length after a combined operation, and the magnitude of axial length reduction correlated significantly with the postoperative IOP. However, the mean change in axial length (-0.12 mm) was lower than the previous studies, which may be explained by use of a noncontact measurement technique.[6] Francis et al measured axial length changes following trabeculectomy with 5-fluorouracil or MMC using noncontact optical biometry and found a mean decrease of -0.15 mm at 1 week, -0.17 mm at 1 month, and -0.05 mm at ≥3 months. Axial length decrease was statistically significant again at all time points.[4] Together, these studies show that axial length consistently decreases after glaucoma filtering surgery, although the magnitude of change may be related to the device used to acquire the measurement.

AXIAL LENGTH CHANGES AFTER TUBE SHUNT SURGERY

Francis et al[4] also examined axial length changes after tube shunt implantation. The mean postoperative change in axial length was -0.15 mm at 1 week, -0.30 mm at 1 month, and -0.13 mm at ≥3 months (Table 41.1). To my knowledge, this report is the only published study about axial length changes after tube shunt implantation, and it demonstrated a small but statistically significant decrease in axial length postoperatively at all time points. This reduction was related to postoperative IOP and the amount of IOP reduction, but not to age, race, sex, type of surgery (trabeculectomy or tube shunt surgery), preoperative axial length, or lens status.[4]

IMPACT OF AXIAL LENGTH CHANGES

The importance of a decrease in the axial length after tube shunt surgery or trabeculectomy is in its impact on the patient's future vision. Because axial length is a primary determinant of intraocular lens (IOL) implant power, patients who undergo cataract extraction before, combined with, or following tube shunt implantation or trabeculectomy can undergo clinically significant changes in their refractive error. In fact, a variance of just

1 mm in the axial length can affect the IOL power calculation and postoperative refraction by 2.5–3 diopters.[8]

Several situations exist in which clinical decision making may be impacted by the axial length changes after surgery. The most important scenario is a combined cataract extraction and tube shunt surgery/trabeculectomy, where the axial length decrease can result in a significant postoperative hyperopic error. Combined cataract and tube shunt implantation is now performed more frequently, and the results are more comparable to those of combined phacotrabeculectomy.[9,10] The axial length change would be especially important in complicated or refractory glaucoma patients with cataract in whom large alteration in IOP is observed postoperatively. The surgeon should anticipate a change in the axial length, and IOL calculations should be performed accounting for this combined surgery or performed after the IOP is stable, in cases where cataract surgery follows implant surgery. Additionally, Francis et al suggested that axial length reduction after tube shunt implantation could be predicted after 3 months by the formula: Axial length reduction (mm) = −1.99 + (0.006 x IOP reduction) + (0.008 x final IOP).[4] A postoperative change in spectacle correction may become necessary to refine visual acuity.

CONCLUSION

In summary, although IOP lowering surgery may successfully control the progression of glaucoma, it may surgically alter axial length and affect future intraocular surgery and postoperative central vision. To achieve the best refractive outcome, cataract extraction and IOL implantation should be delayed, when possible, until axial length measurements are stable, which should occur when the IOP is stable. Patients should be warned of these changes before having IOP lowering surgery, as many will have persistent refractive changes.

COMMENTARY
ANGELO P. TANNA

Axial lengths do often decrease after trabeculectomy, resulting in a change in refraction. Every patient who undergoes trabeculectomy or tube shunt surgery should undergo refraction once IOP is stable. The most common scenario in which axial length reduction comes into play is when cataract surgery is planned, either in conjunction with or after incisional glaucoma surgery. Reasonable goals to aim for in these cases include 1) avoiding clinically significant anisometropia, unless monovision is the goal or fellow eye cataract surgery is anticipated in the not too distant future and 2) avoiding hyperopia, unless this is in conflict with the aim of avoiding anisometropia.

Technicians should be told to, where possible, avoid ultrasonic biometry with immersion in eyes that have had incisional glaucoma surgery. The use of biometry with optical coherence tomography is preferred to ultrasonic axial length determinations in eyes that have had glaucoma surgery. If axial length discrepancy between the 2 eyes is detected with optical biometry, confirmatory ultrasonic biometry may show an even lower axial length in eyes that have functioning trabeculectomies. In such cases, the noncontact techniques are usually more accurate.

IOL selection in an eye with previous glaucoma surgery or in an eye about to undergo combined glaucoma and cataract surgery are situations where the surgeon should prepare the patient for all possible outcomes. It is the surgeon's responsibility to gather information regarding the patient's preferences regarding the refractive outcome and to fully inform him/her of the possibility of a refractive surprise and ways in which that may be handled. Always set appropriate and realistic expectations. The usual considerations in planning the target refraction, including the refraction and lens status of the fellow eye, ocular dominance, and the possible goal of monovision, should be taken into account.

For eyes about to undergo combined glaucoma and cataract surgery, I anticipate a 0.3 mm reduction in axial length for each of the following factors: 1) age < 50 years; 2) axial length > 24 mm; and 3) > 15 mm Hg difference between the baseline and target IOP. For example, in a 45-year-old patient with axial myopia and an axial length 24.5 mm, with a baseline IOP of 35 mm Hg and target IOP of 17 mm Hg, I anticipate an axial length reduction of 0.9 mm and select the IOL power accordingly. If none of these factors is present, I still typically aim for a target refraction of − 0.5 to -1.0 D unless this carries an unacceptable risk of anisometropia when the fellow eye is either already pseudophakic or not likely to undergo cataract surgery in the near future. This is based purely on clinical experience but has worked well for my patients.

Dr. Tanna was supported by an Unrestricted Grant from Research to Prevent Blindness to Northwestern University.

REFERENCES

1. Leydolt C, Findl O, Drexler W. Effects of change in intraocular pressure on axial eye length and lens position. *Eye*. May 2008;22(5):657–661.
2. Read SA, Collins MJ, Iskander DR. Diurnal variation of axial length, intraocular pressure, and anterior eye biometrics. *Invest Ophthalmol Vis Sci*. Jul 2008;49(7):2911–2918.
3. Cashwell LF, Martin CA. Axial length decrease accompanying successful glaucoma filtration surgery. *Ophthalmology*. Dec 1999; 106(12):2307–2311.
4. Francis BA, Wang M, Lei H, et al. Changes in axial length following trabeculectomy and glaucoma drainage device surgery. *Br J Ophthalmol*. Jan 2005;89(1):17–20.
5. Kook MS, Kim HB, Lee SU. Short-term effect of mitomycin-C augmented trabeculectomy on axial length and corneal astigmatism. *J Cataract Refract Surg*. Apr 2001;27(4):518–523.
6. Law SK, Mansury AM, Vasudev D, Caprioli J. Effects of combined cataract surgery and trabeculectomy with mitomycin C on ocular dimensions. *Br J Ophthalmol*. Aug 2005; 89(8):1021–1025.

7. Nemeth J, Horoczi Z. Changes in the ocular dimensions after trabeculectomy. *Int Ophthalmol*. Sept 1992;16(4–5):355–357.

8. Shammas HJ. *Intraocular Lens Power Calculation: Avoiding the Errors*. Glendale, CA: The News Circle Publishing House; 1996.

9. Hoffman KB, Feldman RM, Budenz DL, Gedde SJ, Chacra GA, Schiffman JC. Combined cataract extraction and Baerveldt® glaucoma drainage implant: indications and outcomes. *Ophthalmology*. Oct 2002;109(10):1916–1920.

10. Minckler DS, Francis BA, Hodapp EA, et al. Aqueous shunts in glaucoma: a report by the American Academy of Ophthalmology. *Ophthalmology*. Jun 2008;115(6):1089–1098.

42

ENDOPHTHALMITIS

WON I. KIM AND DONALD L. BUDENZ

ENDOPHTHALMITIS

Tube shunts have become an important part of the surgical armamentarium for controlling intraocular pressure (IOP). Once reserved for use only in refractory cases, they are rapidly gaining popularity as an effective alternative to trabeculectomy and cyclodestruction for lowering IOP in patients who are not satisfactorily controlled on medications.

Although trabeculectomy remains the most commonly performed glaucoma surgery, tube shunts offer some significant advantages. One of these advantages is a theoretically reduced risk of one of the most feared complications of any penetrating ocular surgery—endophthalmitis. The incidence of late-onset infections such as blebitis and endophthalmitis after trabeculectomy with antifibrotic agents is alarmingly high compared to other penetrating intraocular surgeries, perhaps as

high as 5% over 3–5 years.[1] Trabeculectomies produce a perilimbal bleb that may be made thinner and more ischemic by the concomitant use of antifibrotics such as 5-fluorouracil and mitomycin-C (MMC). These anteriorly placed blebs are more exposed, more fragile, and more prone to become infected than the robust, thicker, and more posteriorly located blebs overlying a tube shunt plate. Gedde and associates reported a 1% (1 of 107 eyes) incidence of endophthalmitis after Baerveldt® Glaucoma Implant (BGI) placement compared to a 5% (5 out of 105 eyes) incidence after trabeculectomy with MMC after 5 years of follow-up.[2] However, despite this potential advantage, endophthalmitis still does occur in association with shunts, and it is essential to understand the risk factors for its occurrence and the proper steps to take to prevent, recognize, and treat this potentially devastating complication.

INFECTIOUS VS. NONINFECTIOUS ENDOPHTHALMITIS

Distinguishing sterile from infectious endophthalmitis can be difficult. Signs suggestive of an *infectious* endophthalmitis include marked inflammation, hypopyon, fibrinoid anterior chamber reaction, corneal edema, marked conjunctival congestion, eyelid edema, vitritis, and retinal periphlebitis. Signs suggestive of a *noninfectious* etiology are a gradual onset of symptoms, such as pain, redness, and inflammation, in the absence of tube or plate erosion.[3,4] Sterile endophthalmitis one month after discontinuation of corticosteroid therapy postoperatively has been reported.[5] Possible causes for noninfectious (sterile) endophthalmitis include exacerbated preexisting uveitis, iris trauma, and toxicity from foreign substances introduced during surgery.[3,6] These scenarios must also be differentiated from rebound inflammation after discontinuation of topical corticosteroids.

Causative organisms for infectious endophthalmitis associated with tube shunts are similar to those causing endophthalmitis after other forms of penetrating ocular surgery.[3] *Staphylococcus* species both coagulase-positive and coagulase-negative (commonly *Staphylococcus aureus*),[7] *Streptococcus* species (commonly *Streptococcus pneumoniae*),[7,8] *Propionibacterium acnes*,[9] *Pseudomonas aeruginosa*,[7] and *Mycobacterium chelonae*[7] have all been reported as pathogens in adults.[3,10,11] The microorganisms reported for endophthalmitis in children include *Propionibacterium acnes*,[12] *Haemophilus influenzae*,[7,10,13,14] and *S pneumoniae*.[3,10] Gedde and colleagues suggested from their series of 4 patients that the organisms that cause late-onset endophthalmitis associated with tube exposure are similar to those that cause late bleb-associated endophthalmitis after filtering surgery, such as gram-negative organisms and *S pneumoniae*, although definitive conclusions are hard to draw from such small numbers.[7]

OCCURRENCE

The incidence of endophthalmitis in association with tube shunts has been reported to be 0.8%–6.3%.[3] Topouzis and colleagues reported that 1.73% (27 of 1563) of Medicare patients who received tube shunts in 1994 were also treated for endophthalmitis.[15] Unfortunately, the authors did not have access to information on laterality in the Medicare database and identified laterality as a potential source of error in some cases where the shunt may have followed successful treatment of an infected bleb. Al-Torbak and associates reported a 1.7% (9 eyes) incidence of endophthalmitis in a large series of 542 eyes implanted with the Ahmed™ Glaucoma Valve (AGV™) followed over a 9-year period.[10] The Krupin Eye Valve Filtering Surgery Study Group reported a 2% incidence of endophthalmitis (1 out of 50 eyes) over 16–36 months of follow-up.[16] Nguyen and colleagues reported a 1% rate of endophthalmitis (1 out of 107 eyes) over 4 years after BGI implantation.[17] Price and Wellemeyer reported a 1.4% incidence of endophthalmitis after Molteno® implantation (1 of 72 eyes) over 18 months of follow-up.[18] The reported rates of endophthalmitis among the various implants are similar, and at this time there is no evidence to suggest that one type of implant is more predisposed to infection than another.[3]

Endophthalmitis associated with tube shunt surgery can occur at any time in the postoperative course.[3] Isolated cases of endophthalmitis occurring in the early postoperative course, within the first few weeks of surgery (ranging from 2 to 30 days), have been reported.[11,17,19-24] Such early-onset endophthalmitis may occur without any obvious risk factors (such as tube exposure), as reported by Nguyen and associates,[17] and is probably related to direct contamination at the time of surgery or via access through the conjunctival wound before it is healed. Additionally, tube shunt associated endophthalmitis can occur months to years after surgery. Gedde and colleagues reported 4 cases of late endophthalmitis after BGI surgery,[7] and Krebs and associates reported 2 cases of late-onset endophthalmitis occurring after Krupin implantation.[25] Endophthalmitis has been reported to occur as far out as 4 years after BGI implantation[8] and as late as 6 years after Krupin valve surgery.[25] (Figure 42.1)

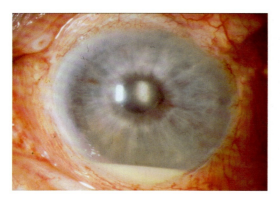

FIGURE 42.1 Hypopyon from tube shunt related endophthalmitis, courtesy Steven J. Gedde, MD.

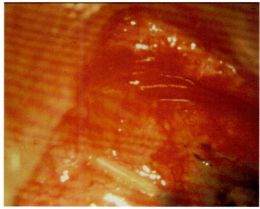

FIGURE 42.2 Erosion of conjunctiva over a tube that places a patient at high risk for infection, courtesy Steven J. Gedde, MD.

RISK FACTORS

Several factors have been identified as increasing the risk of endophthalmitis after tube shunt surgery. Exposure of the tube or plate with erosion of the overlying conjunctiva is a major risk factor for postoperative endophthalmitis[3] (Chapter 38). Multiple regression analysis in Al-Torbak and associates' study of 542 eyes implanted with AGV™ found that conjunctival erosion over the tube was significantly associated with the development of endophthalmitis ($P < 0.01$).[10] Additionally, all 4 of the patients Gedde and colleagues reported to have developed endophthalmitis after BGI surgery had exposed tubes.[7] The reports of late endophthalmitis by Krebs and associates[25] and Francis and associates[8] also were all associated with conjunctival erosion over an implant (Figure 42.2).

Al-Torbak and colleagues also found by regression analysis that an age of less than 18 years was significantly associated with endophthalmitis after AGV™ implantation. They reported a 5-fold higher rate of endophthalmitis in pediatric patients compared with adults (4.4% versus 0.9%).[10] Similar rates of endophthalmitis in children following AGV™ implantation have been reported, ranging from 2.9% to 5.0%.[3,26,27] These higher rates of endophthalmitis may be related to the higher rates of tube exposure in children. Morad and associates reported an astonishing 13% rate of tube exposure (8 of 60 eyes) in

children implanted with tube shunts.[26] Chen and associates reported a 5.8% rate of tube exposure (3 eyes) in 52 pediatric eyes.[28] Rates of tube exposure in adults are thought to be lower, with one study reporting a 2.4% rate (1 of 41 eyes) after Molteno® implantation[29] and another reporting a 2.7% rate (2 of 73 eyes) of plate exposure, with one eye developing endophthalmitis (1.4%), after BGI implantation.[23] Also it is possible that violation of the orbital septum during surgery in young children may predispose to preseptal infections entering the orbit and the eye via the shunt. Such infections often begin in the sinuses. Frequent examination of the tubes for anterior migration and extrusion/exposure is critical in the long-term care of children with shunts.

Manipulating an implanted tube shunt can also lead to endophthalmitis. Needling revision to improve functioning of the bleb overlying a BGI,[30] surgical tube repositioning of a Molteno®,[31] and capsulectomy to improve functioning of an AGV™[27] have all been reported to have resulted in endophthalmitis. Endophthalmitis due to these procedures probably occurs due to intraoperative seeding of the implant from the conjunctiva.

PREVENTION

Preventing tube exposure is a major priority in the intraoperative and postoperative management of tube shunts. Standard surgical technique includes shielding the overlying conjunctiva from direct contact with the tube of the implant, especially anteriorly near the limbus. Most commonly, patch grafts are used to cover the tube with materials such as glycerin-preserved cornea,[3,7] donor human sclera,[3,7] processed pericardium,[32] dura mater,[33] and fascia lata.[34] Placing the tube under a partial thickness scleral flap or under a long scleral tunnel are alternative options if patching materials are unavailable.[35] Additional measures that can be applied to prevent tube exposure in appropriate cases include routing the tube to enter the anterior chamber at the 12-o'clock position, which may help by permanently leaving the affected area covered by the upper eyelid and preventing the repetitive mechanical trauma of the eyelid margin moving over conjunctiva and the underlying tube.[36] Also, when appropriate, a pars plana insertion can be considered, placing the tube farther posterior and away from exposure and mechanical trauma. However, it is important to note that pars plana tubes can also become exposed.

Postoperatively, it is important at each follow-up visit to carefully inspect for evidence of tube exposure and conjunctival erosion. When such a defect is found, prompt surgical repair is recommended to prevent infection. Some authors have suggested that in the absence of symptoms or when there is no concomitant aqueous leakage, exposed tubes may be observed.[37] However, given the high association with endophthalmitis and the potentially devastating consequences of this complication, surgical repair of all exposed tubes is strongly recommended.[7] Repair of exposed tubes should involve placement of a patch graft using one of the aforementioned materials. Consideration can also be given to rerouting the tube to the 12-o'clock position or a pars plana insertion, when possible, to place the tube in a more protected environment. It is important that the tube be well-anchored so that there is no movement. Surrounding healthy conjunctiva should then be mobilized and used to cover the tube and graft.[3,7] If the surrounding conjunctiva is inadequate, amniotic membrane sewn over the patch graft to encourage epithelialization can be considered.[9] However, inadequate conjunctival coverage of an implant can result in recurrent erosions and thus lead to the recurrent risk for endophthalmitis.[7] If satisfactory closure is not possible, one can consider removing the entire glaucoma implant and placing a new one in an alternative quadrant.[3] For more information on inadequate conjunctival closure, see Chapter 33.

MANAGEMENT

The treatment of tube shunt associated endophthalmitis is generally the same as for any other form of postoperative endophthalmitis. The treatment of most cases will start with a 0.2 mL pars plana vitreous aspirate and anterior chamber paracentesis for cultures and smears. Immediate pars plana vitrectomy is recommended for cases with light perception vision or worse, extrapolating from the Endophthalmitis Vitrectomy Study.[38] Pars plana vitrectomy may also be beneficial in select cases of tube shunt associated endophthalmitis to reduce bacterial load and provide material for culture. Intravitreal antibiotics that can be used include vancomycin (1 mg/0.1 mL) for gram positive coverage and ceftazidime (2.25 mg/0.1 mL) for gram negative coverage injected through the pars plana.[5] Other treatments that can be considered are systemic antibiotics, topical fortified antibiotics, intense topical corticosteroids, and cycloplegia for comfort.[39]

As expected, treatment for sterile endophthalmitis differs from infectious etiologies. Corticosteroid therapy alone should be successful in most cases of sterile endophthalmitis and have a better prognosis for visual recovery. When the diagnosis is in question, such as in eyes with mild to moderate inflammation without hypopyon, intense topical corticosteroids can be tried initially with very close follow-up. Rapidly worsening clinical signs would indicate infectious endophthalmitis, and the patient should then be treated accordingly. However, infection caused by less virulent organisms, such as coagulase-negative staphylococci, may have less exuberant inflammation that can make distinguishing between infectious and noninfectious etiologies difficult.[6] When an infectious process cannot be ruled out, vitreous tap for culture and intravitreal antibiotic injection to cover for the possibility of infection may be necessary.[3]

Visual prognosis after successful treatment is strongly associated with the type of infecting organism, with results being significantly poorer for infection with species other than gram-positive coagulase-negative species.[7,40] Outcomes with *Pseudomonas aeuruginosa* infections may be particularly poor with 64% of cases resulting in evisceration or enucleation at one institution despite prompt treatment with antibiotics to which the organisms were sensitive.[41] For severe uncontrollable infections resulting in blind painful eyes, enucleation or evisceration may be necessary.

TO REMOVE OR NOT TO REMOVE THE IMPLANT?

The main topic of controversy in the management of endophthalmitis associated with tube shunt surgery is whether or not it is necessary to remove the implant itself as an adjunct to antibiotic therapy. There have been reports of successful treatment with retention of the device.[17,25,42] Al-Torbaq and associates also reported successful resolution of endophthalmitis with retention of an AGV™ in a 6-year-old child but later had to remove the implant due to anterior migration.[13]

Even so, there is evidence that glaucoma implants can sequester microorganisms and prevent resolution of infection. Hollander and colleagues[43] reported a case of *P acnes* endophthalmitis after cataract surgery in a 7-year-old girl with a preexisting Molteno® implant that required explantation of the implant to achieve resolution. Fanous and Cohn reported a case of *P acnes* endophthalmitis that occurred after tube repositioning for corneal touch in a Molteno® implant. Tube removal and intracameral vancomycin resolved the inflammation, and the eye remained quiet over 3 months. However, endophthalmitis recurred when the tube was reinserted for elevated IOP, and explantation of the device was necessary to obtain complete resolution of the infection.[9] *P acnes* endophthalmitis

in association with tube shunts appears to behave similarly to *P acnes* endophthalmitis after cataract extraction and intraocular lens implantation, which often requires capsulectomy and lens removal to completely eradicate the infection.[44]

Park and Rabowsky reported a case of endophthalmitis that occurred 4 days after an AGV™ placement that had initial improvement with intravitreal and intravenous antibiotics but developed new purulent discharge draining through the peritomy 10 days after the initial diagnosis. The AGV™ was removed with resolution of all signs of infection.[45] Gedde and associates, in their series of 4 cases of late-onset endophthalmitis after BGI, removed the implant at the time of vitrectomy in 3 of the patients because of concerns that the implant was seeded by the infectious organism. In all cases where the implants were removed, cultures of the implants grew organisms very commonly associated with postoperative endophthalmitis that also matched the cultured organisms from intraocular aspirates in 2 of 3 cases.[7] Perkins suggested that explantation may be beneficial not only for the purpose of removing a foreign body that could be contaminated but also as a means of extending the retention of intravitreal antibiotics inside the eye.[19] (Figure 42.3)

An additional consideration is the possibility of an intraocular infection spreading into the orbital compartment or vice versa with the tube acting as the conduit. Although there

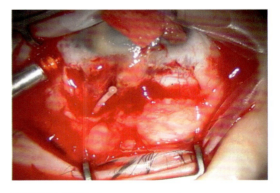

FIGURE 42.3 Endophthalmitis with purulent material draining from tube, courtesy Mark Werner, MD.

are no reported cases of endophthalmitis and orbital cellulitis occurring simultaneously in conjunction with a tube shunt, there are several case reports of orbital cellulitis, some in conjunction with an exposed tube.[46–49] In Chaudry and colleagues' report of 2 cases, one patient was diagnosed early and was successfully treated with systemic antibiotics alone without the need for implant removal whereas the second patient had a delayed presentation and required explantation of the implant for complete resolution of the infection.[46]

There is currently no consensus on whether or not to remove an implant in the setting of an infection, and clinical judgment will have to be exercised with each individual case. One can take into consideration the severity of the infection, evidence of localized inflammation or purulence of the tissues surrounding the implant, and type of infectious organism (such as *P acnes* or *P aeruginosa*) as guidelines in the decision on whether or not to remove an implant during an episode of endophthalmitis. It may be prudent, however, to maintain a very low threshold for removing glaucoma implants in cases of endophthalmitis to ensure resolution and minimize recurrences and additional morbidity.[43] Because of the rarity of this complication and the relatively low

volume of this type of surgery, generating a prospective randomized trial to provide guidance on this matter is difficult, and none have been conducted to date.

CONCLUSIONS

Endophthalmitis after implantation of a tube shunt is an uncommon but serious complication that can occur at any point in the postoperative course. The major risk factor associated with endophthalmitis is tube or plate exposure by erosion of the overlying conjunctiva. Therefore, the clinician should always check for such erosions and promptly repair them when found. Younger patients (under 18 years old) may be at increased risk for developing implant exposure and appear to have higher rates of endophthalmitis. Any surgical intervention to improve the functioning of an implant should be done with the awareness that endophthalmitis can occur as a result. Endophthalmitis following tube shunt surgery is treated as any other case of postoperative endophthalmitis. Although there is no definitive study defining the need for explanting a tube shunt as an adjunct to antibiotic therapy, a low threshold for tube removal is justified.

COMMENTARY
LEONARD K. SEIBOLD AND MALIK Y. KAHOOK

This detailed review by Dr. Budenz clearly outlines several key points regarding endophthalmitis after tube shunt surgery. Although the reported incidence of this complication is low, the severe consequences can have a profound impact on patients. In the adult population, tube exposure is clearly a key risk factor for infection. Therefore, it is crucial to routinely examine these patients for evidence of compromised conjunctiva at every visit. Any evidence of exposure should be promptly addressed.

As the authors mention, a key debate surrounding this topic involves the need for surgical management of the infection. In principle, most physicians would agree that an infection in the presence of a surgical implant likely involves colonization of the hardware. Thus, the implant should be removed to fully eradicate bacteria from the tissue. However, given the scarcity of cases, there is no strong clinical evidence available to prove this. Anecdotal reports such as those from Fanous and Cohn and from Hollander and colleagues are the most meaningful data we have to support this concept of microorganism sequestration in devices.[31,43] Therefore, we strongly recommend removal of any tube shunts in the setting of endophthalmitis. This may prove troublesome in the setting of eyes with more than one device and in advanced disease where IOP control will be difficult without the tube shunt. In addition, the removal of a tube shunt that has been in place for an extended period of time can lead to significant local tissue disruption and even injury to adjacent muscles due to the encapsulation of tissue surrounding the plate.

Perhaps useful to this discussion is a debate involving a similar clinical scenario of endophthalmitis in the setting of an intraocular lens (IOL) implant. Most glaucoma surgeons would likely have a low threshold for removing a tube shunt in the setting of endophthalmitis, as it is easily identifiable as a potential focus for sequestration of bacteria. However, an IOL can easily be overlooked as another potentially contaminated foreign body within the eye. A review of postoperative *P acnes* endophthalmitis after cataract surgery by Aldave et al found that none (0/13) of the patients undergoing IOL removal or exchange required retreatment. This is in stark contrast to the 10 out of 21 (48%) patients initially treated by other means (intraocular antibiotics, pars plana vitrectomy, partial capsulectomy) who required retreatment.[44] Although these cases of infection occurred in a different postoperative setting and with a specific type of bacteria, we feel these findings can be translated to any ocular infection in the setting of implanted hardware that contacts intraocular fluid. Therefore, in the setting of endophthalmitis we would recommend removal of tube shunts with strong consideration of an IOL removal as well, if present.

COMMENTARY
RONALD L. FELLMAN

The disadvantage of any procedure that diverts aqueous externally is the long-term risk of infection. Late endophthalmitis after filtration surgery is a well-known and well-understood event. A pale, thin, leaking bleb is a set up for blebitis, a well-appreciated scenario. But what are the causes of long-term infection following drainage implant surgery? As tube shunt implantation has become a common procedure, eye care professionals need to focus on the predisposing factors for infection in this hardware group just as they learned to for patients with blebs.

As the authors note, it is incumbent on the physician to recognize who is at highest risk for late-onset endophthalmitis, a lifetime task. Patients who appear to be at high risk should always be warned of this event and be prescribed an appropriate antibiotic to have at home for emergencies. They should be instructed to call promptly and be evaluated in a timely fashion.

Since exposure of the tube appears to be the most common culprit causing long-term infection, consideration should be given to what is the best tissue to cover the tube in order to prevent long-term erosion. Patch melt over the tube is serious business. The recent introduction of split thickness glycerin preserved corneal tissue appears to be an advantage; however, long-term data is lacking. One helpful intraoperative trick regarding any type of patch that appears thin is to double it over the tube, creating 2 layers.[50] This decreases the likelihood of long-term erosion. In addition, keeping the patch flush with the cornea at the limbus will reduce the chance of a dellen and other types of irritation at the limbus that degrade the anatomy at this juncture.

The increased risk of infection in children with tubes is especially worrisome. This should prompt the surgeon to exercise special precautions in the operating room along with a lifetime of vigilance concerning perilimbal tube coverage.

One ever-present dilemma is what to do about patch tissue that slowly thins over the tube, a long-term risk for infection. If the conjunctiva directly over the tube appears vascularized, it is probably less likely to erode than pale avascular conjunctiva. Surgeons should be aggressive in children with replacing patch grafts that appear to thin over the tube.

The authors' information and knowledge regarding removal of infected plates is cogent advice and should be followed closely.

In addition, consider interpolated conjunctival pedicle flaps to cover tubes, especially when there is a shortage of tissue. This usually requires the teamwork of the oculoplastic and glaucoma services.[51]

REFERENCES

1. Nguyen QH. Avoiding and managing complications of glaucoma drainage implants. *Curr Opin Ophthalmol.* Apr 2004;15(2): 147–150.
2. Gedde SJ, Schiffman JC, Feuer WJ, Herndon LW, Brandt JD, Budenz DL, and the Tube Versus Trabeculectomy Study Group. Postoperative Complications in the Tube Versus Trabeculectomy (TVT) Study During Five Years of Follow-up. *Am J Ophthalmol.* May 2012;153(5):804–814.
3. Wentzloff JN, Grosskreutz CL, Pasquale LR, Walton DS, Chen TC. Endophthalmitis after glaucoma drainage implant surgery. *Int Ophthalmol Clin.* Spring 2007;47(2):109–115.
4. Recchia FM, Busbee BG, Pearlman RB, Carvalho-Recchia CA, Ho AC. Changing trends in the microbiologic aspects of postcataract endophthalmitis. *Arch Ophthalmol.* Mar 2005;123(3):341–346.
5. Heher KL, Lim JI, Haller JA, Jampel HD. Late-onset sterile endophthalmitis after Molteno® tube implantation. *Am J Ophthalmol.* Dec 15 1992;114(6):771–772.
6. Flynn HW, Jr., Scott IU, Brod RD, Han DP. Current management of endophthalmitis. *Int Ophthalmol Clin.* Fall 2004;44(4):115–137.
7. Gedde SJ, Scott IU, Tabandeh H, et al. Late endophthalmitis associated with glaucoma drainage implants. *Ophthalmology.* Jul 2001;108(7):1323–1327.
8. Francis BA, DiLoreto DA Jr., Chong LP, Rao N. Late-onset bacteria endophthalmitis following glaucoma drainage implantation. *Ophthalmic Surg Lasers Imaging.* Mar-Apr 2003;34(2):128–130.
9. Fechter HP, Parrish RK 2nd. Preventing and treating complications of Baerveldt® Glaucoma Drainage Device surgery. *Int Ophthalmol Clin.* Spring 2004;44(2):107–136.
10. Al-Torbak AA, Al-Shahwan S, Al-Jadaan I, Al-Hommadi A, Edward DP. Endophthalmitis associated with the Ahmed™ glaucoma valve implant. *Br J Ophthalmol.* Apr 2005;89(4):454–458.
11. Law SK, Kalenak JW, Connor TB Jr., Pulido JS, Han DP, Mieler WF. Retinal complications after aqueous shunt surgical procedures for glaucoma. *Arch Ophthalmol.* Dec 1996;114(12):1473–1480.
12. Gutierrez-Diaz E, Montero-Rodriguez M, Mencia-Gutierrez E, Fernandez-Gonzalez MC, Perez-Blazquez E. Propionibacterium acnes endophthalmitis in Ahmed™ glaucoma valve. *Eur J Ophthalmol.* Oct-Dec 2001;11(4):383–385.
13. Al-Torbaq AA, Edward DP. Delayed endophthalmitis in a child following an Ahmed™ glaucoma valve implant. *J AAPOS.* Apr 2002;6(2): 123–125.
14. Trzcinka A, Soans FP, Archer SM, Moroi SE. Late-onset Haemophilus Influenzae endophthalmitis in an immunized child after Baerveldt® implant. *J AAPOS.* Aug 2008;12(4):412–414.
15. Topouzis F, Yu F, Coleman AL. Factors associated with elevated rates of adverse outcomes after cyclodestructive procedures versus drainage device procedures. *Ophthalmology.* Dec 1998;105(12):2276–2281.
16. Krupin eye valve with disk for filtration surgery. The Krupin Eye Valve Filtering Surgery Study Group. *Ophthalmology.* Apr 1994;101(4): 651–658.
17. Nguyen QH, Budenz DL, Parrish RK 2nd. Complications of Baerveldt® glaucoma drainage implants. *Arch Ophthalmol.* May 1998;116(5): 571–575.
18. Price FW Jr., Wellemeyer M. Long-term results of Molteno® implants. *Ophthalmic Surg.* Mar-Apr 1995;26(2):130–135.
19. Perkins TW. Endophthalmitis after placement of a Molteno® implant. *Ophthalmic Surg.* Oct 1990;21(10): 733–734.
20. Munoz M, Tomey KF, Traverso C, Day SH, Senft SH. Clinical experience with the Molteno® implant in advanced infantile glaucoma. *J Pediatr Ophthalmol Strabismus.* Mar-Apr 1991;28(2):68–72.
21. Smith MF, Doyle JW, Sherwood MB. Comparison of the Baerveldt® glaucoma implant with the double-plate Molteno® drainage implant. *Arch Ophthalmol.* Apr 1995;113(4):444–447.
22. Chihara E, Kubota H, Takanashi T, Nao-i N. Outcome of White pump shunt surgery for neovascular glaucoma in Asians. *Ophthalmic Surg.* Oct 1992;23(10):666–671.
23. Lloyd MA, Baerveldt G, Fellenbaum PS, et al. Intermediate-term results of a randomized clinical trial of the 350- versus the 500-mm2 Baerveldt® implant. *Ophthalmology.* Aug 1994;101(8):1456–1463; discussion 1463–1454.
24. Molteno AC. The use of draining implants in resistant cases of glaucoma. Late results of 110 operations. *Trans Ophthalmol Soc N Z.* 1983;35:94–97.
25. Krebs DB, Liebmann JM, Ritch R, Speaker M. Late infectious endophthalmitis from exposed glaucoma setons. *Arch Ophthalmol.* Feb 1992;110(2):174–175.
26. Morad Y, Donaldson CE, Kim YM, Abdolell M, Levin AV. The Ahmed™ drainage implant in

the treatment of pediatric glaucoma. *Am J Ophthalmol.* Jun 2003;135(6):821–829.

27. Djodeyre MR, Peralta Calvo J, Abelairas Gomez J. Clinical evaluation and risk factors of time to failure of Ahmed™ Glaucoma Valve implant in pediatric patients. *Ophthalmology.* Mar 2001;108(3):614–620.

28. Chen TC, Bhatia LS, Walton DS. Ahmed™ valve surgery for refractory pediatric glaucoma: a report of 52 eyes. *J Pediatr Ophthalmol Strabismus.* Sept-Oct 2005;42(5):274–283; quiz 304–275.

29. Melamed S, Cahane M, Gutman I, Blumenthal M. Postoperative complications after Molteno® implant surgery. *Am J Ophthalmol.* Mar 15 1991;111(3):319–322.

30. Chen PP, Palmberg PF. Needling revision of glaucoma drainage device filtering blebs. *Ophthalmology.* Jun 1997;104(6):1004–1010.

31. Fanous MM, Cohn RA. Propionibacterium endophthalmitis following Molteno® tube repositioning. *J Glaucoma.* Aug 1997;6(4): 201–202.

32. Raviv T, Greenfield DS, Liebmann JM, Sidoti PA, Ishikawa H, Ritch R. Pericardial patch grafts in glaucoma implant surgery. *J Glaucoma.* Feb 1998;7(1):27–32.

33. Brandt JD. Patch grafts of dehydrated cadaveric dura mater for tube-shunt glaucoma surgery. *Arch Ophthalmol.* Oct 1993;111(10): 1436–1439.

34. Dresner SC, Boyer DS, Feinfield RE. Autogenous fascial grafts for exposed retinal buckles. *Arch Ophthalmol.* Feb 1991;109(2):288–289.

35. Ozdamar A, Aras C, Ustundag C, Tamcelik N, Ozkan S. Scleral tunnel for the implantation of glaucoma seton devices. *Ophthalmic Surg Lasers.* Sept-Oct 2001;32(5):432–435.

36. Heuer DK, Budenz D, Coleman A. Aqueous shunt tube erosion. *J Glaucoma.* Dec 2001;10(6): 493–496.

37. Rosenberg LF, Krupin T. Implants in glaucoma surgery. In: Ritch R, Shields MB, Krupin T, eds. *The Glaucomas.* Vol 3. 2nd ed. St. Louis: Mosby; 1996:1783–1807.

38. Doft BH, Barza M. Optimal management of postoperative endophthalmitis and results of the Endophthalmitis Vitrectomy Study. *Curr Opin Ophthalmol.* Jun 1996;7(3):84–94.

39. Ehlers JP, Shah CP, Fenton GL, Hoskins EN, Shelsta HN. Postoperative endophthalmitis. *The Wills Eye Manual: Office and Emergency Room Diagnosis and Treatment of Eye Diseases.* 5th ed. Baltimore: Lippincott Williams & Wilkins; 2008:358–359.

40. Microbiologic factors and visual outcome in the endophthalmitis vitrectomy study. *Am J Ophthalmol.* Dec 1996;122(6):830–846.

41. Eifrig CW, Scott IU, Flynn HW Jr., Miller D. Endophthalmitis caused by Pseudomonas aeruginosa. *Ophthalmology.* Sept 2003;110(9): 1714–1717.

42. Ellis BD, Varley GA, Kalenak JW, Meisler DM, Huang SS. Bacterial endophthalmitis following cataract surgery in an eye with a preexisting Molteno® implant. *Ophthalmic Surg.* Feb 1993;24(2):117–118.

43. Hollander DA, Dodds EM, Rossetti SB, Wood IS, Alvarado JA. Propionibacterium acnes endophthalmitis with bacterial sequestration in a Molteno®'s implant after cataract extraction. *Am J Ophthalmol.* Nov 2004;138(5):878–879.

44. Aldave AJ, Stein JD, Deramo VA, Shah GK, Fischer DH, Maguire JI. Treatment strategies for postoperative Propionibacterium acnes endophthalmitis. *Ophthalmology.* Dec 1999; 106(12):2395–2401.

45. Park SS, Rabowsky J. Early postoperative endophthalmitis after pars plana Ahmed™ valve placement with persistent extraocular infection. *Ophthalmic Surg Lasers Imaging.* Sept–Oct 2007;38(5):404–405.

46. Chaudry IA, Shamsi FA, Morales J. Orbital cellulitis following implantation of aqueous drainage devices. *Eur J Ophthalmol.* Jan-Feb 2007;17(1):136–140.

47. Marcet MM, Woog JJ, Bellows AR, Mandeville JT, Maltzman JS, Khan J. Orbital complications after aqueous drainage device procedures. *Ophthal Plast Reconstr Surg.* Jan 2005; 21(1):67–69.

48. Lavina AM, Creasy JL, Tsai JC. Orbital cellulitis as a late complication of glaucoma shunt implantation. *Arch Ophthalmol.* Jun 2002; 120(6):849–851.

49. Karr DJ, Weinberger E, Mills RP. An unusual case of cellulitis associated with a Molteno® implant in a 1-year-old child. *J Pediatr Ophthalmol Strabismus.* Mar-Apr 1990;27(2):107–110.

50. Godfrey DG, Merritt JH, Fellman RL, Starita RJ. Interpolated conjunctival pedicle flaps for the treatment of exposed glaucoma drainage devices. *Arch Ophthalmol.* Dec 2003;121(12): 1772–1775.

51. Lankaranian D, Reis R, Henderer JD, Choe S, Moster MR. Comparison of single thickness and double thickness processed pericardium patch graft in glaucoma drainage device surgery: a single surgeon comparison of outcome. *J Glaucoma.* Jan-Feb 2008;17(1):48–51.

43

DIPLOPIA AND OCULAR MOTILITY DISTURBANCES

AMIR A. PIROUZIAN

DIPLOPIA AND OCULAR MOTILITY DISTURBANCES

Strabismus and diplopia have been reported with tube shunt implants in glaucoma surgery in several case series. Overall, the reports of strabismus (vertical and horizontal) as a potentially disabling surgical complication widely range from 5% to 100% depending on the type of tube shunt used.[1-12] The challenge in determining the exact incidence of strabismus after tube shunt implantation arises from a lack of accurate preoperative strabismus evaluation and documentation in the published studies, as well as a higher incidence of reduced peripheral fusion and visual acuity in these selected groups of patients.

The mechanism of postoperative strabismus is likely due to one of the following: 1) the size and the height of the device inserted and the resulting mass effect (bleb size); 2) the technique of surgical placement; 3) postoperative surgical adhesion, scar formation, and restriction; 4) probable muscle ischemia in conjunction with antifibrotic agents; 5) fat adherence syndrome; and 6) muscle-tendon stretching. Understanding the mechanism of strabismus is important for prevention and treatment of this condition.

PATHOPHYSIOLOGY FOR MOTILITY DISORDER DEVELOPMENT

Mass effect

The mass effect following tube shunt implantation has been noted in multiple studies[2,4,5,7,11,12]; however, the true pathophysiology remains unclear. A proposed mechanism of postoperative ocular dysmotility suggests a direct mass effect on the extraocular muscles (EOM) from the implant or the encapsulated cystic bleb surrounding the device.[3,13] Use of a large device or creation of a highly elevated bleb may shift an EOM pulley from its original anatomical pathway, thus creating a heterotopic pulley phenomenon. Therefore extreme caution and thorough preoperative counseling should be exercised in those patients with an already restricted peripheral sensory fusion because even a minor shift in extraocular muscle alignment may compromise the patient's ability to maintain fusion and trigger the development of a secondary strabismus. Selection of the smallest device for an appropriate reduction of intraocular pressure (IOP) is also strongly advised in such patients. The newer generation of Baerveldt® implants with fenestrated plates (Abbot Medical Optics, Inc., Santa Ana, California) and flexible plate Ahmed™ valves (New World Medical, Inc., Rancho Cucamonga, California) may result in a lower bleb height, which will decrease the compressive effect on an individual EOM and its pulley system. Unfortunately, no prospective comparative trial has been published to support a reduction in postoperative strabismus.

Scar tissue, fibrosis, and adhesions

A significant number of glaucoma patients have had numerous previous filtering and/or shunt procedures, which have resulted in conjunctival, Tenon's layer, and scleral scarring.[2,7] Additionally, fat adherence syndrome has been reported as an etiology of progressive ocular dysmotility following Molteno® (Molteno Ophthalmic, Ltd., Dunedin, New Zealand) device implantation.[7] Postoperative inflammation in cases of multiple prior procedures leads to a higher incidence of tissue adhesions to the muscles, which leads to a restrictive postoperative phenomenon (i.e., EOM pulley hindrance).[2,7] Formation of posterior fixation (i.e., Faden effect) has been described.[2] In my experience, in this select group of patients who have already undergone one surgical site procedure, thorough removal of previously formed scar tissues, as well as an injection of long acting steroids, likely results in resolution of the adhesions and diplopia. This treatment must be balanced against the possibility of a steroid-induced rise in IOP.

Leash effect

The postoperative leash effect has been proposed as another etiology of ocular dysmotility.[14–17]

With this mechanism, the device leads to the limitation of passive duction movement in the field where it is located. However, studies have not conclusively determined whether strabismus is linked to the quadrant where the device is implanted.[14,16,17]

Muscle etiology

Direct trauma, muscle ischemia (from high dose antimetabolite application), or muscle stretching as a result of positioning of a shunt device under the muscle belly may lead to strabismus.[9] Caution should be the rule when considering the use of antifibrotic agents with tube shunts. Given that there is little evidence of improved outcomes when antifibrotic agents are administered,[18] their use should be limited.

Although all of the above factors are possible etiologies of ocular dysmotility following tube shunt surgery, no single etiology has been proven to be the definitive cause of ocular motility, which makes the management of these problems difficult.

ANTICIPATION AND DIAGNOSIS

While accurately predicting which patients will experience strabismus following tube shunt implantation is challenging, a preoperative strabismus evaluation may assist in determining a surgical plan. The preoperative considerations potentially associated with induced strabismus following tube shunt implantation are listed in Table 43.1.

Anticipating strabismus prior to tube shunt implantation may be difficult, but making a postoperative strabismus diagnosis is simple. There is typically a relatively short period of time to the onset of strabismus following a glaucoma operation. Generally the patient will report diplopia (if asked) in at least one field of gaze. Restriction in the field of action is frequently observed in passive duction testing; however, a forced duction test may not be positive. Saccadic velocity as well as forced generation should also be evaluated and documented. Additionally, clinical evaluation of bleb height and ultrasonography should be done to assess the posterior extension of the

Table 43.1. Factors Potentially Associated With Postoperative Strabismus Following Tube Shunt Implantation

FACTOR	MECHANISM/PATHOPHYSIOLOGY
Previous ocular surgery with conjunctival incisions, particularly in the same quadrant	Scar tissue and fibrosis
Use of double-plated implants	Mass effect Muscle-tendon stretching
Significant restriction of peripheral visual field with resultant reduced preoperative peripheral sensory fusion	Mass effect (can disturb the already compromised ability of the patient to maintain motor fusion)
Direct violation of an extraocular muscle-pulley system	Mass effect Leash effect
History of previous preoperative strabismus	Scar tissue and fibrosis
Application of a high dose/long duration antimetabolite intraoperatively (e.g., mitomycin-C > 2 min in close proximity to an extraocular muscle)	Muscle ischemia

bleb and location of the plate and its wings, depending on implant type, to ensure the plate has not migrated. It may be helpful in surgical repair planning to obtain high resolution orbital magnetic resonance imaging (MRI) with gadolinium contrast to determine precisely the anatomical location of the implant, bleb size, and the EOM pulley system, as well as the relative position of the implant and the bleb to an EOM (Figure 43.1).[25]

Ocular dysmotility in pediatric glaucoma tube shunt surgeries

The rate of postoperative strabismus following pediatric glaucoma tube shunt implantation has been reported to be up to 15%,[19-22] with one study reporting a rate as high as 57%.[23] Glaucoma surgeons are advised to avoid placement of primary tube shunts in the inferior quadrants and consider superotemporal placement of a shunt rather than superonasal placement.[23-25] Additionally, if ocular dysmotility is noted, attention should be directed to the bleb size and the exact location of the implant through orbital MRI or possibly ultrasound assessment during an examination under anesthesia for consideration of the optimal surgical approach for correction of strabismus.[25]

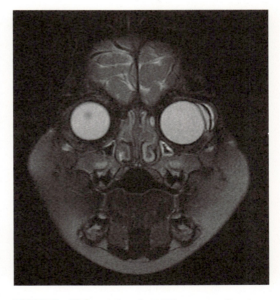

FIGURE 43.1 Orbital MRI, coronal view: Glaucoma tube shunt in superotemporal quadrant of the left eye with impingement on the lateral rectus muscle.

PREVENTION

In order to reduce the risk of postoperative ocular dysmotility, several factors should be entertained. First, a smaller shunt size with a decreased plate surface area should be considered. Creation of minimal bleb height should also be taken into account. Proper placement of the shunt device between the EOM and shunning away from the EOM-pulley pathway are additional key factors. Placement of the shunt in the superotemporal quadrant is preferable over the superonasal quadrant due to large anatomical space in the superotemporal quadrant and avoidance of the superior oblique muscle.[8] Some surgeons avoid inferior placement if possible, but recent reports have shown diplopia unusual after Baerveldt® shunt implantation in the inferonasal quadrant.[26,27]

Modification of how the rectus muscles are handled intraoperatively may decrease the risk of strabismus. Schmidt et al proposed placement of a polyglactin 910 net (Vicryl™, Ethicon, Inc., Somerville, New Jersey) between Tenon's capsule and the muscle or between the muscle and sclera.[28] Consideration of a nylon (Supramid®, S. Jackson, Inc., Alexandria, Virginia) sleeve around the muscle at the time of Molteno® implantation has also been proposed.[28]

In cases with an already compromised binocular fusion and a higher likelihood of postoperative diplopia, other surgical techniques should be considered.

TREATMENT

Nonsurgical management

Conservative, nonsurgical management of strabismus following glaucoma shunt procedures consists of observation and prism. However, prism use is often not adequate due to the incomitant nature of the strabismus. Prisms may reduce or collapse diplopia in central primary gaze; however peripheral diplopia and reading or driving diplopia typically persist and are often debilitating. Botulinum toxin may also improve alignment but has not been rigorously clinically tested.[29]

Surgical management

Surgical management of strabismus would ideally not jeopardize the shunt site, as there would be risk of loss of IOP control with further loss of vision and/or peripheral visual fields. Ipsilateral recession or resection of an EOM away from the quadrant of the shunt site or surgery on the contralateral yoke EOM should be contemplated as the primary surgical approach for the collapse of the greater part of diplopia, though some patients will continue to have diplopia in the specific field where the shunt is implanted. In persistent strabismus conditions, direct EOM exploration should be considered with surgical debulking of the primary shunt site for both the bleb revision and for removal of adhesions and fibrotic capsules once a proper preoperative high resolution orbital MRI and assessment are performed.[23,25] In strabismus cases where the direct bulk of an implant impinges on a rectus muscle evidenced either by direct visualization or on the MRI, replacement or modification of the tube shunt by size reduction should be performed.[23,25,30]

CONCLUSION

Due to a potential risk of developing strabismus following glaucoma tube shunts, the following final recommendations are made: 1) selection of smallest plate for an appropriate IOP reduction; 2) proper anatomical placement and minimal intraoperative tissue manipulation; and 3) judicious application of adequate antiinflammatories. Although most tube shunt procedures are not complicated by postoperative strabismus, incorporation of these premises into routine cases may potentially prevent diplopia following the implantation of glaucoma drainage devices.

COMMENTARY

CHARLOTTE AKOR

Patients who undergo tube shunt placement have to be counseled about the potential of diplopia. Incomitant strabismus is the most difficult type of strabismus to treat because single binocular vision is often obtained in a few head positions and fields of gaze. The patient must be counseled that they may have to move their eyes and/or head to obtain single binocular vision in primary or reading position even after strabismus surgery.

The surgical plan to correct strabismus in patients with tube shunts is difficult because many patients have asymmetric vision and refuse to have surgery on their better seeing eye or have the device removed. Moreover, strabismus in these patients can be horizontal and vertical. Muscle transposition procedures can be performed to avoid the area of the bleb and limit surgery to a single eye; however this technique again limits the relief of diplopia in a few fields of gaze.[31] Additionally, limiting strabismus surgery to one eye can lead to more complication of strabismus surgery. A muscle that the strabismus surgeon normally recesses would have to resected, which could lead to abnormalities in lid position and cause lid retraction.

Nonsurgical methods of diplopia treatment also have limited success because the strabismus caused by tube shunts is incomitant and multiplanar. Prism glasses can treat diplopia in certain primary gaze and reading position, but the amount of deviation must be the same in these fields of gaze. Spectacles have been used to blur vision in amblyopia therapy and may be useful in glaucoma patients with poor vision before complete occlusion with a patch has to be used to blur the second image. Strabismus from tube shunts may sometimes be amenable to bleb shrinkage procedures or to plate trimming if a large plate device has been implanted and negate the need for traditional muscle surgery.

There is not a single plan that can be applied to treat patients with diplopia from tube shunt surgery. Nevertheless, with individualized surgical and nonsurgical planning, the condition can be improved.

COMMENTARY

MALCOLM L. MAZOW

The development of strabismus following tube shunt for glaucoma is covered very well in this chapter, including the various mechanisms for this complication. Diplopia as a result of incomitant strabismus is definitely a problem that should be avoided.

Mass effect from the shunt has become less, as the sizes of mechanical shunts have been made smaller. Adherence syndrome with scarring still remains a major cause of restrictive strabismus from any orbital ocular surgery. Careful dissection and discretionary placement of the implant, as the authors suggest, may help avoid the development of strabismus.

The author has done an admirable job of covering diplopia as a complication. Emphasis on pre-existing strabismus should not be underplayed, and the author has expressed the ideal way of measuring for such a problem before embarking on a tube shunt.

Complete orthoptic strabismus evaluation is not practical, but basic measurements should be attempted. In those patients with significant visual field loss, deviations may occur even with excellent surgical techniques.

By reminding the glaucoma surgeon of diplopia as a postoperative complication, adjustment of surgical techniques to avoid this difficult problem is the main take-home point made in this chapter.

REFERENCES

1. Krupin eye valve with disk for filtration surgery. The Krupin Eye Valve Filtering Surgery Study Group. *Ophthalmology.* Apr 1994;101(4):651–658.
2. Christmann LM, Wilson ME. Motility disturbances after Molteno® implants. *J Pediatr Ophthalmol Strabismus.* Jan-Feb 1992;29(1): 44–48.
3. Coleman AL, Hill R, Wilson MR, et al. Initial clinical experience with the Ahmed™ Glaucoma Valve implant. *Am J Ophthalmol.* Jul 1995;120(1):23–31.
4. Dobler-Dixon AA, Cantor LB, Sondhi N, Ku WS, Hoop J. Prospective evaluation of extraocular motility following double-plate Molteno® implantation. *Arch Ophthalmol.* Sept 1999;117(9):1155–1160.
5. Heuer DK, Lloyd MA, Abrams DA, et al. Which is better? One or two? A randomized clinical trial of single-plate versus double-plate Molteno® implantation for glaucomas in aphakia and pseudophakia. *Ophthalmology.* Oct 1992;99(10):1512–1519.
6. Lloyd MA, Baerveldt G, Fellenbaum PS, et al. Intermediate-term results of a randomized clinical trial of the 350- versus the 500-mm2 Baerveldt® implant. *Ophthalmology.* Aug 1994;101(8):1456–1463; discussion 1463–1454.
7. Munoz M, Parrish R. Hypertropia after implantation of a Molteno® drainage device. *Am J Ophthalmol.* Jan 15 1992;113(1):98–100.
8. Munoz M, Parrish RK 2nd. Strabismus following implantation of Baerveldt® drainage devices. *Arch Ophthalmol.* Aug 1993;111(8):1096–1099.
9. Sidoti PA, Baerveldt G. Glaucoma drainage implants. *Curr Opin Ophthalmol.* Apr 1994; 5(2):85–98.
10. Smith SL, Starita RJ, Fellman RL, Lynn JR. Early clinical experience with the Baerveldt® 350-mm2 glaucoma implant and associated extraocular muscle imbalance. *Ophthalmology.* Jun 1993;100(6):914–918.
11. Wilson-Holt N, Franks W, Nourredin B, Hitchings R. Hypertropia following insertion of inferiorly sited double-plate Molteno® tubes. *Eye.* 1992;6 (Pt 5):515–520.
12. Astle WF, Lin DT, Douglas GR. Bilateral penetrating keratoplasty and placement of a Molteno® implant in a newborn with Peters' anomaly. *Can J Ophthalmol.* Oct 1993;28(6): 276–282.
13. Rhee DJ, Casuso LA, Rosa RH Jr., Budenz DL. Motility disturbance due to true Tenon cyst in a child with a Baerveldt® glaucoma drainage implant. *Arch Ophthalmol.* Mar 2001;119(3):440–442.
14. Ball SF, Ellis GS, Jr., Herrington RG, Liang K. Brown's superior oblique tendon syndrome after Baerveldt® glaucoma implant. *Arch Ophthalmol.* Oct 1992;110(10):1368.
15. Coats DK, Paysse EA, Orenga-Nania S. Acquired Pseudo-Brown's syndrome immediately following Ahmed™ valve glaucoma implant. *Ophthalmic Surg Lasers.* May 1999;30(5): 396–397.
16. Dobler AA, Sondhi N, Cantor LB, Ku S. Acquired Brown's syndrome after a double-plate Molteno® implant. *Am J Ophthalmol.* Nov 15 1993;116(5):641–642.
17. Prata JA Jr., Minckler DS, Green RL. Pseudo-Brown's syndrome as a complication of glaucoma drainage implant surgery. *Ophthalmic Surg.* Sept 1993;24(9):608–611.
18. Minckler DS, Francis BA, Hodapp EA, et al. Aqueous shunts in glaucoma: a report by the American Academy of Ophthalmology. *Ophthalmology.* Jun 2008;115(6):1089–1098.
19. Fellenbaum PS, Sidoti PA, Heuer DK, Minckler DS, Baerveldt G, Lee PP. Experience with the Baerveldt® implant in young patients with complicated glaucomas. *J Glaucoma.* Apr 1995; 4(2):91–97.
20. Englert JA, Freedman SF, Cox TA. The Ahmed™ valve in refractory pediatric glaucoma. *Am J Ophthalmol.* Jan 1999;127(1):34–42.
21. Morad Y, Donaldson CE, Kim YM, Abdolell M, Levin AV. The Ahmed™ drainage implant in the treatment of pediatric glaucoma. *Am J Ophthalmol.* Jun 2003;135(6):821–829.
22. Beck AD, Freedman S, Kammer J, Jin J. Aqueous shunt devices compared with trabeculectomy with Mitomycin-C for children in the first two years of life. *Am J Ophthalmol.* Dec 2003; 136(6):994–1000.
23. O'Malley Schotthoefer E, Yanovitch TL, Freedman SF. Aqueous drainage device surgery in refractory pediatric glaucoma: II. Ocular motility consequences. *J AAPOS.* Feb 2008; 12(1):40–45.
24. Hiles DA, Watson BA. Complications of implant surgery in children. *J Am Intraocul Implant Soc.* Jan 1979;5(1):24–32.
25. Pirouzian A, Scher C, O'Halloran H, Jockin Y. Ahmed™ glaucoma valve implants in the pediatric population: the use of magnetic resonance imaging findings for surgical approach to reoperation. *J AAPOS.* Aug 2006;10(4): 340–344.
26. Harbick KH, Sidoti PA, Budenz DL, et al. Outcomes of inferonasal Baerveldt® glaucoma

drainage implant surgery. *J Glaucoma.* Feb 2006; 15(1):7–12.

27. Rachmiel R, Trope GE, Buys YM, Flanagan JG, Chipman ML. Intermediate-term outcome and success of superior versus inferior Ahmed™ Glaucoma Valve implantation. *J Glaucoma.* Oct-Nov 2008;17(7):584–590.

28. Schmidt T, Hofmann H, Spiessl S. [Polyglactin 910 implants in muscle revision surgery for the reconstruction of physiologic limits in Tenon's capsule]. *Klin Monatsbl Augenheilkd.* Sept 1988;193(3):271–274.

29. Dawson EL, Sainani A, Lee JP. Does botulinum toxin have a role in the treatment of secondary strabismus?*. *Strabismus.* Jun 2005;13(2):71–73.

30. Roizen A, Ela-Dalman N, Velez FG, Coleman AL, Rosenbaum AL. Surgical treatment of strabismus secondary to glaucoma drainage device. *Arch Ophthalmol.* Apr 2008;126(4):480–486.

31. Coats DK, Olitsky SE. Unexpected and atypical anatomy. *Strabismus Surgery and Its Complications.* Berlin, Germany: Springer; 2007:267–284.

44

TUBE SHUNT RELATED COMPLICATIONS OF THE CORNEA

NAN WANG

TUBE SHUNT RELATED COMPLICATIONS OF THE CORNEA

Tube shunts can be placed in the anterior chamber, the ciliary sulcus, or the pars plana. However, if the eye is phakic, the choice is limited to the anterior chamber; ciliary sulcus placement is likely to result in cataract formation, and pars plana placement will likely complicate removal of the cataract that will likely develop.

Most corneal complications of tube shunt surgery result from tubes that are too anterior. Loss of vision may result due to these complications. If the tube is inadvertently inserted too close to the cornea, a loss of endothelial cells will result in edema and require transplantation to restore vision.

FREQUENCY OF CORNEAL COMPLICATIONS DUE TO TUBE SHUNT IMPLANTATION

Reported rates of corneal complications range from 2% to 33% and consist mostly of corneal edema/decompensation and corneal graft failure.[1–9] In a cohort of patients implanted with the Ahmed™ Glaucoma Valve (New World Medical, Inc., Rancho Cucamonga, California), postoperative corneal abrasions occurred in 5 of 60 (8%) eyes.[2] Another study reported the rate of corneal drying/dellen later in the postoperative course (8 of 59 eyes; 13.6%).[10] Contact between the tube and the cornea has been noted at a rate of up to 5%.[1,3,4,11] As the rate of tube shunt implantation has increased,[12] the incidence of corneal edema in patients with tube shunts has also increased.[13] Some of these cases develop corneal opacification with decreased vision and may require corneal transplantation to clear the visual axis. One large study of patients with Ahmed tube shunts (159 eyes total) reported corneal graft failure resulting in repeat penetrating keratoplasty (PKP) in 11 of 31 (35%) eyes with corneal grafts.[1]

INTRAOPERATIVE CORNEA COMPLICATIONS

Improper anterior chamber tube entry may damage the cornea. If the entry angle is not parallel to the iris and aims anteriorly, the needle used to create the tunnel may tear or detach Descemet's membrane. Entry through the cornea (rather than the sclera) may also predispose to epithelial downgrowth[14] or tube extrusion.[15] To avoid such a complication, full-thickness entry into the anterior chamber should be as far posterior as possible.

POSTOPERATIVE CORNEA COMPLICATIONS

As the eye heals postoperatively, scarring may result in tube retraction or even a change in the tube's directional angle in both the anterior-posterior direction and laterally. To prevent problems related to tube misdirection, at least 2 millimeters of tube length should be placed in the anterior chamber (see Chapter 30). Other directional changes can be avoided by direct radial entry of the tube with proper plate positioning so that the tube to the entry site is straight without bend. If a bend is required, multiple nonabsorbable sutures should be used to secure the tube tightly to the sclera. However, memory in the tube will still lend toward straightening over time (see Chapter 48).

On the other hand, a long tube may be predisposed to touch the cornea with blinking or eye rubbing. An anterior chamber tube pivots around its entry site, as there is no internal fixation of the tube and little rigidity of the tube. Any rubbing against the globe may result in an unpredictably wide range of movements, including corneal touch with resulting loss of corneal endothelial cells. Consequently, repeated episodes may lead to corneal edema and decompensation, rupture of Descemet's membrane by the tip of the tube, or even erosion of the tube through the corneal stroma to the point of extrusion.[15]

When localized cornea edema develops around the tube entry site (Figure 44.1), surgical revision is required to prevent the entire cornea from decompensating (Figure 44.2). Endothelial cells may migrate towards the entry site to try to fill in the defect in the endothelium, eventually resulting in insufficient cell density to keep the cornea from swelling (see Chapter 30 for more information). Tear or detachment of Descemet's membrane can also occur in these settings but is more likely with a flattening of the anterior chamber. We have seen patients who have rubbed their eyes after tube shunt implantation, to the point of causing exposure of the plate (see Chapter 38 for information about repair) with aqueous leakage and flattening of the anterior chamber. This may result in localized Descemet's membrane detachment (Figure 44.3; see also Chapter 8). Management of this complication requires tube removal, an alternate method of IOP control, and Descemet stripping automated endothelial keratoplasty (DSAEK) to rehabilitate the eye.

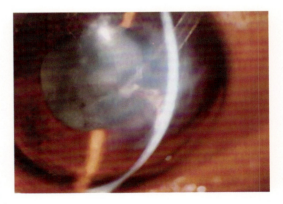

FIGURE 44.1 Localized cornea edema near the tip of the anterior chamber tube shunt.

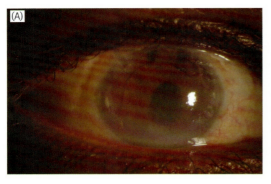

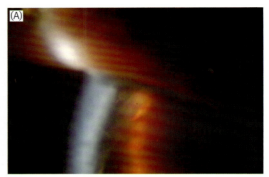

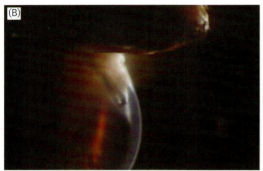

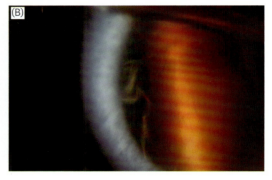

FIGURE 44.2 A) Diffuse cornea edema after anterior chamber tube shunt implantation in a patient with an anterior chamber intraocular lens. B) Notice that the tip of the tube is in contact with the cornea.

FIGURE 44.3 An 80-year-old female with tube shunt plate exposure resulting in hypotony with recent anterior chamber flattening and localized Descemet's membrane detachment due to contact of the tube with the cornea (courtesy of Robert Feldman, MD). A) End of tube shunt and Descemet's membrane detachment. B) Full extent of Descemet's membrane detachment

SPECIAL CONSIDERATIONS WITH ANTERIOR CHAMBER TUBE SHUNTS AND CORNEAL TRANSPLANT

Patients in need of both a tube shunt for control of glaucoma and a corneal transplant are at risk for developing complications associated with the combination of these 2 procedures. Reports in the literature indicate that presence of a tube shunt is a risk factor for corneal graft failure after PKP.[16,17]

Most cases of PKP after tube shunts are caused by a loss of corneal endothelial cells, possibly related to the tube rather than underlying disease. These cases are generally amenable to DSAEK, and this procedure has replaced a large number of PKP procedures for the treatment of endothelial disease. Eyes that have undergone DSAEK present special challenges for placement of tube shunts, and tube shunts may also make subsequent DSAEK more difficult. DSAEK requires an air bubble to hold the graft in place for the first hours after transplantation, and the preexisting tube may allow egress of the air bubble too quickly; also the size of the graft may need to be reduced to prevent touching the tube. A large graft may actually occlude the shunt or result in graft dehiscence (Figure 44.4). To prevent this, tube repositioning (Figure 44.5) or shortening may be required either prior to or during DSAEK.[18] New research in Descemet's membrane endothelial keratoplasty (DMEK) will possibly resolve some of these problems in the near future.[19]

To prevent similar problems with preexisting corneal grafts, differing approaches to tube shunts need to be applied in grafted eyes.

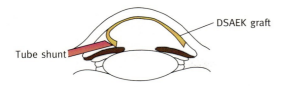

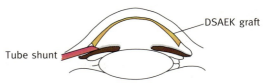

FIGURE 44.4 Schematic diagram showing impaired unfolding of the DSAEK graft as well as tube shunt occlusion.

FIGURE 44.5 Schematic diagram showing contact between the DSAEK graft and tube shunt with possible occlusion of tube by the DSAEK graft.

The key concept is to stay as far away from the cornea as possible. In pseudophakic eyes this may mean ciliary sulcus placement[20] or combined pars plana vitrectomy and pars plana tube placement. However, it is possible that corneal failure is not only due to mechanical properties but also decreased nutrition of the cornea. If this is the case, redirecting aqueous more posteriorly towards a sulcus or pars plana tube may limit the amount of fresh new aqueous that can nourish the corneal endothelium. To the best of our knowledge, no studies have been reported comparing corneal effects of pars plana or ciliary sulcus placement of shunts to anterior placement with regard to corneal endothelium.

Combined surgery with lens extraction and posterior tube placement may also be indicated in phakic patients. Alternatives include lens extraction alone or combined with cyclophotocoagulation (CPC) by either the endoscopic or transscleral approaches. Data available regarding the effects of CPC on corneal endothelium in the grafted eye are conflicting,[21-24] but CPC also may alter the nutritional status of the cornea by decreasing aqueous production, potentially contributing to graft failure.

CONCLUSION

In summary, endothelial loss and edema remain the most common corneal complications of tube shunt surgery. Despite employment of intraoperative methods aimed at protecting the cornea, decompensation is sometimes unavoidable. Current corneal transplantation techniques allow effective management of this problem.

Dr. Wang was supported by a Challenge Grant from Research to Prevent Blindness to The University of Texas Medical School at Houston and the Hermann Eye Fund.

COMMENTARY

MICHAEL R. BANITT AND FRANCISCO E. FANTES†

In our experience, corneal complications after tube shunts typically involve damage to the endothelium. Surface disease in the form of dellen may also occur. A result of local dehydration, dellen are initially treated with preservative-free artificial tears and ointments. Dellen unresponsive to these measures may resolve with patching or placement of a bandage contact lens (see Chapter 19 for more information on dellen). Large diameter lenses (16 mm or larger) are used so that the lens sits well over the patch graft.

It is exceedingly uncommon for a tube to cause corneal perforation. However, we have successfully treated this by performing a pars plana vitrectomy through a temporary keratoprosthesis followed by penetrating keratoplasty and tube repositioning to the pars plana.

Anterior chamber tubes can lead to corneal decompensation, particularly when placed anterior to the trabecular meshwork. Peripheral contact between the endothelial cells and the tube can be exacerbated by blinking and eye rubbing. Correcting the position of the tube is the best surgical option for these patients. Descemet's stripping endothelial keratoplasty (DSEK) is indicated in eyes where the cornea has failed and can successfully be performed in eyes after penetrating glaucoma surgery.[25-28] DSEK surgeons need to carefully plan for surgery in these patients and note the position of the tube(s), proximity of the tube(s) to the cornea, and the length of the tube(s) in the eye. Tubes that are too long should be shortened prior to insertion of the DSEK lenticule. Anteriorly placed tubes should be repositioned within the anterior chamber or to the sulcus or pars plana.

Dr. Banitt was supported by National Eye Institute grant P30EY014801, Department of Defense grant W81XWH-09–0675, and an Unrestricted Grant from Research to Prevent Blindness to the Bascom Palmer Eye Institute, Miller School of Medicine, University of Miami.

REFERENCES

1. Huang MC, Netland PA, Coleman AL, Siegner SW, Moster MR, Hill RA. Intermediate-term clinical experience with the Ahmed™ Glaucoma Valve implant. *Am J Ophthalmol.* Jan 1999;127(1):27–33.

2. Topouzis F, Coleman AL, Choplin N, et al. Follow-up of the original cohort with the Ahmed™ glaucoma valve implant. *Am J Ophthalmol.* Aug 1999;128(2):198–204.

3. Irak I, Moster MR, Fontanarosa J. Intermediate-term results of Baerveldt® tube shunt surgery with mitomycin C use. *Ophthalmic Surg Lasers Imaging.* May-Jun 2004;35(3):189–196.

4. Britt MT, LaBree LD, Lloyd MA, et al. Randomized clinical trial of the 350-mm2 versus the 500-mm2 Baerveldt® implant: longer term results: is bigger better? *Ophthalmology.* Dec 1999;106(12):2312–2318.

5. Gedde SJ, Schiffman JC, Feuer WJ, Herndon LW, Brandt JD, Budenz DL. Three-year follow-up of the Tube Versus Trabeculectomy Study. *Am J Ophthalmol.* Nov 2009;148(5):670–684.

6. Broadway DC, Iester M, Schulzer M, Douglas GR. Survival analysis for success of Molteno® tube implants. *Br J Ophthalmol.* Jun 2001;85(6): 689–695.

7. WuDunn D, Phan AD, Cantor LB, Lind JT, Cortes A, Wu B. Clinical experience with the Baerveldt® 250-mm2 Glaucoma Implant. *Ophthalmology.* May 2006;113(5):766–772.

8. Nguyen QH, Budenz DL, Parrish RK 2nd. Complications of Baerveldt® glaucoma drainage implants. *Arch Ophthalmol.* May 1998;116(5): 571–575.

9. Hau S, Barton K. Corneal complications of glaucoma surgery. *Curr Opin Ophthalmol.* Mar 2009;20(2):131–136.

10. Wilson MR, Mendis U, Paliwal A, Haynatzka V. Long-term follow-up of primary glaucoma surgery with Ahmed™ glaucoma valve implant versus trabeculectomy. *Am J Ophthalmol.* Sept 2003;136(3):464–470.

11. Krishna R, Godfrey DG, Budenz DL, et al. Intermediate-term outcomes of 350-mm(2) Baerveldt® glaucoma implants. *Ophthalmology.* Mar 2001;108(3):621–626.

12. Ramulu PY, Corcoran KJ, Corcoran SL, Robin AL. Utilization of various glaucoma surgeries and procedures in Medicare beneficiaries from 1995 to 2004. *Ophthalmology.* Dec 2007; 114(12):2265–2270.

13. Stein JD, Ruiz D Jr., Belsky D, Lee PP, Sloan FA. Longitudinal rates of postoperative adverse outcomes after glaucoma surgery among medicare beneficiaries 1994 to 2005. *Ophthalmology.* Jul 2008;115(7):1109–1116 e1107.

14. Rosenberg LF, Krupin T. Implants in glaucoma surgery. In: Ritch R, Shields MB, Krupin T, eds. *The Glaucomas.* Vol 3: Glaucoma Therapy. St. Louis: Mosby; 1996:1535–1548.

15. Maki JL, Nesti HA, Shetty RK, Rhee DJ. Transcorneal tube extrusion in a child with a Baerveldt® glaucoma drainage device. *J AAPOS.* Aug 2007;11(4):395–397.

16. Alvarenga LS, Mannis MJ, Brandt JD, Lee WB, Schwab IR, Lim MC. The long-term results of keratoplasty in eyes with a glaucoma drainage device. *Am J Ophthalmol.* Aug 2004; 138(2):200–205.

17. Kwon YH, Taylor JM, Hong S, et al. Long-term results of eyes with penetrating keratoplasty and glaucoma drainage tube implant. *Ophthalmology.* Feb 2001;108(2):272–278.

18. Banitt MR, Chopra V. Descemet's stripping with automated endothelial keratoplasty and glaucoma. *Curr Opin Ophthalmol.* Mar 2010; 21(2):144–149.

19. Bersudsky V, Trevino A, Rumelt S. Management of endothelial decompensation because of glaucoma shunt tube touch by Descemet membrane endothelial keratoplasty and tube revision. *Cornea.* Jun 2011;30(6):709–711.

20. Weiner A, Cohn AD, Balasubramaniam M, Weiner AJ. Glaucoma tube shunt implantation through the ciliary sulcus in pseudophakic

eyes with high risk of corneal decompensation. *J Glaucoma.* Aug 2010;19(6):405–411.

21. Beiran I, Rootman DS, Trope GE, Buys YM. Long-term results of transscleral Nd:YAG cyclophotocoagulation for refractory glaucoma postpenetrating keratoplasty. *J Glaucoma.* Jun 2000;9(3):268–272.

22. Threlkeld AB, Shields MB. Noncontact transscleral Nd:YAG cyclophotocoagulation for glaucoma after penetrating keratoplasty. *Am J Ophthalmol.* Nov 1995;120(5):569–576.

23. Ocakoglu O, Arslan OS, Kayiran A. Diode laser transscleral cyclophotocoagulation for the treatment of refractory glaucoma after penetrating keratoplasty. *Curr Eye Res.* Jul 2005;30(7):569–574.

24. Sood S, Beck AD. Cyclophotocoagulation versus sequential tube shunt as a secondary intervention following primary tube shunt failure in pediatric glaucoma. *J AAPOS.* Aug 2009;13(4):379–383.

25. Banitt M, Arrieta-Quintero E, Parel JM, Fantes F. Technique for air bubble management during endothelial keratoplasty in eyes after penetrating glaucoma surgery. *Cornea.* Feb 2011;30(2):184–188.

26. Duarte MC, Herndon LW, Gupta PK, Afshari NA. DSEK in eyes with double glaucoma tubes. *Ophthalmology.* Aug 2008;115(8):1435, 1435 e1431.

27. Esquenazi S, Rand W. Safety of DSAEK in patients with previous glaucoma filtering surgery. *J Glaucoma.* Apr 2009;94(4):558–559.

28. Vajaranant TS, Price MO, Price FW, Gao W, Wilensky JT, Edward DP. Visual acuity and intraocular pressure after Descemet's stripping endothelial keratoplasty in eyes with and without preexisting glaucoma. *Ophthalmology.* Sep 2009;116(9):1644–1650.

45

TUBE SHUNT RELATED COMPLICATIONS OF THE ANTERIOR CHAMBER

PARAG A. GOKHALE

TUBE SHUNT RELATED COMPLICATIONS OF THE ANTERIOR CHAMBER

Postoperative complications in the anterior chamber can affect both glaucoma progression and vision. Preoperative considerations and surgical technique are important to reduce and prevent these complications.[1]

FLAT ANTERIOR CHAMBER DUE TO HYPOTONY

A flat anterior chamber is one of the most common complications following tube shunt surgery, occurring at a rate of 3.5%–27%.[2–4] Although often associated with hypotony and choroidal effusions and usually due to increased outflow after surgery, it may also be related to decreased aqueous production, especially in eyes with previous ciliary body ablation.[5,6] Increased outflow could result from leakage around the tube or overfiltration either before fibrous capsule formation over the plate or through tube fenestrations.[7]

Diagnosis

Diagnosis of the cause of hypotony can be made with a careful slit-lamp examination. Leakage around the tube can be viewed internally by gonioscopy, though a flat or shallow anterior chamber can make seeing potential leakage difficult. The location of overfiltration can be determined by looking at areas of conjunctival elevation. Conjunctival bleb formation at the limbus could help identify leakage around the tube at its scleral tunnel insertion. Early elevation of a bleb over the reservoir of a tube shunt is also seen with incomplete occlusion in the nonvalved (or sometimes valved) tube. Elevation near the tube-plate junction could also indicate overflow at a fenestration but is unusual. Intracameral irrigation of fluorescein can help identify the source of leakage.[8]

Management

A flat anterior chamber associated with hypotony can have serious sequelae, including corneal edema, cataract, and failure of the procedure. Medical treatment to deepen the anterior chamber with cycloplegics and reduction of wound healing inhibitors should be tried first but is often insufficient, as this treatment will not quickly eliminate the source of leakage. More aggressive intervention will be needed if there is central flattening (Grade 2 or 3 flat chamber).

Identifying the source of leakage is important in determining management. If there is leakage at the site of the tube's entry into the sclera, viscoelastic may be needed to fill the anterior chamber. Air injection is an alternative that allows for continued visualization of the leak if desired.

Although time may be an adequate solution, a chamber flat enough to require intervention due to leakage around the tube may be simply repaired. A small conjunctival peritomy should be made at the limbus over the tube insertion site. Sutures of 10–0 nylon should be placed on either side of the tube. The conjunctiva should be closed with a water-tight closure.

If hypotony is due to overfiltration (due to inadequate occlusion or improper functioning of the valve), then the tube should be occluded. Viscoelastic can be injected into the anterior chamber to impede flow through the tube and raise the intraocular pressure (IOP).[1] Some glaucoma specialists inject a viscoelastic to reform the anterior chamber and occlude the tube without other intervention.[9] Most would proceed further to occlude the tube, either internally or externally. To place an external ligature, a conjunctival incision should be made posterior to the patch graft, and the tube should be mobilized enough to pass a 7–0 polyglactin 910 (Vicryl™, Ethicon, Inc., Somerville, New Jersey) suture around the tube. The suture is then tied tightly around the tube to occlude it, and the conjunctival incision is closed. If the tube can be easily seen, as with a corneal patch graft, it may be externally ligated without conjunctival incision. For more information on intentional tube occlusion, see Chapter 35. For more information on hypotony after tube shunt implantation, see Chapters 34 and 39.

FLAT ANTERIOR CHAMBER DUE TO PUPILLARY BLOCK

Diagnosis

This complication would be recognized as a flat or shallow anterior chamber with elevated IOP and iris bombé in the absence of a patent peripheral iridotomy. This scenario is unusual because often a tube shunt is performed after a failed trabeculectomy, which typically has an iridectomy already present. However, with the increasing numbers of primary tube shunts, it may become more common. Pupillary block may also result if a seemingly patent iridectomy is blocked by an inflammatory membrane in uveitic glaucoma or silicone oil after retinal detachment repair.

Management

In the situation where an inflammatory membrane is occluding both the pupil and the previous iridotomy, a new laser iridotomy or surgical iridectomy should be made in a location less likely to become blocked (e.g., inferiorly in silicone oil related glaucoma). When a fibrinous uveitic membrane is occluding the existing iridectomy, laser or incisional techniques can be employed to reestablish patency,

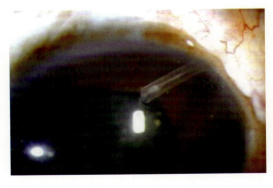

FIGURE 45.1 Obstruction of an anterior chamber tube by a strand of fibrin.

or a new hole can be created. Aggressive postoperative steroid dosing should be utilized by topical, periocular, oral, and/or intraocular routes to prevent development of a new inflammatory membrane.

FLAT ANTERIOR CHAMBER SECONDARY TO MALIGNANT GLAUCOMA

Malignant glaucoma (also known as aqueous misdirection syndrome) is more commonly seen after trabeculectomy but occurs after tube shunts in 0.5%–2.7% of cases,[10] depending on the type of implant. It can occur days to months after surgery but seems to be related to an initial leak with overfiltration and shallowing of the anterior chamber, leading to a rotation of the lens-iris diaphragm and posterior diversion of aqueous.[11]

Diagnosis

Diagnosis is made by the presence of the flat anterior chamber and patent iridotomy. The intraocular pressure (IOP) can be high, but it may start out normal or even low, so it may be difficult to distinguish this complication from hypotony secondary to overfiltration. However, in malignant glaucoma, there will be no elevation of conjunctiva over the shunt plate. If ultrasound biomicroscopy (UBM) is available, it will show anterior rotation of the ciliary body with ciliary block at the peripheral lens.[11]

Management

Treatment of malignant glaucoma is discussed in detail in Chapter 11, but in short, medical treatment includes cycloplegia, aqueous suppression, and topical steroids. An Nd:YAG hyaloidotomy may be successful, though vitrectomy and lens extraction may be necessary.

FLAT ANTERIOR CHAMBER SECONDARY TO SUPRACHOROIDAL HEMORRHAGE

Suprachoroidal hemorrhage occurs in 0.5%–4.2% of tube shunts.[7,8] Risk factors include older age, prolonged hypotony, choroidal effusions,

hypertension, and atherosclerosis.[12,13] If the IOP is lower than the perfusion pressure of the choroidal vasculature, rupture of choroidal vessels may also result in suprachoroidal hemorrhage.

Diagnosis

A suprachoroidal hemorrhage is recognized as a sudden, painful shallowing of the anterior chamber and may also be associated with Valsalva exertion. The IOP is elevated, and the red reflex may be lost. B-scan ultrasonography is also helpful in diagnosis. Postoperative suprachoroidal hemorrhage can be seen at the time of the spontaneous release of the ligating suture[1] or following planned removal of an obturator suture.

Management

Treatment will be determined based on the visual potential of the eye, the IOP, and the level of pain. Medical pressure control and observation is an option, but careful surgical drainage of the hemorrhage may be needed. For more information about choroidal hemorrhages and treatment, see Chapter 6.

TUBE OCCLUSION

Tube occlusion, which occurs about 6%–11% of the time,[8] can be due to iris, blood, fibrin, posterior capsule, or vitreous obstructing the tube. Tube occlusion by the iris can occur if the tube is misdirected toward the iris or in the presence of peripheral anterior synechiae (PAS) enveloping a short tube. Anterior chamber shallowing (as discussed above) can also lead to iris occlusion.

Diagnosis

Tube occlusion usually can be recognized by slit-lamp examination. In situations where the tube cannot be visualized (e.g., corneal edema or scarring), the occlusion sometimes can be identified by UBM.[14]

Management

A first attempt at dislodging an occlusion can be done by pumping pressure over the plate.[1]

If the occlusion can be visualized, it can be treated by stretching the iris out of the tube using the argon laser or cutting the iris with the Nd:YAG laser.[8] If these procedures are unsuccessful, it may be necessary to reposition the tube, either within the anterior chamber or into the ciliary sulcus. If the occlusion is also related to anterior chamber shallowing or PAS, it may be beneficial to place the tube into a vitrectomized posterior segment.[4] Diagnosis and management of occlusion by specific substances are discussed below. For further information on tube occlusion, also see Chapter 37.

TUBE OCCLUSION BY BLOOD OR FIBRIN

Tube occlusion by blood or fibrin occurs most commonly in neovascular or inflammatory glaucoma.[15]

Diagnosis

Tube occlusion by blood or fibrin can be recognized by elevated IOP and direct slit-lamp visualization of the occluding material. Figure 45.1 shows obstruction of an anterior chamber tube by a strand of fibrin. As mentioned above, if the cornea is edematous and/or opacified and the tube is not easily seen, UBM can assist in diagnosing tube occlusion.

Management

If the occlusion is by fibrin, aggressive treatment with corticosteroids in combination with aqueous suppressants for elevated IOP may be sufficient for resolution. In cases where the IOP cannot be controlled or the occlusion is not clearing, the tube can be flushed with balanced salt solution on a 27-gauge needle or a 30-gauge cannula via a corneal paracentesis wound made 6 clock hours away from the tube. Injection of intracameral tissue plasminogen activator (tPA) has been shown to be successful with one or more injections.[15] Surgery ultimately may be required to clear the blood and fibrin and perhaps reposition the tube.

TUBE OCCLUSION BY VITREOUS

Diagnosis

Tube occlusion by vitreous can be recognized by slit-lamp visualization. Care should be taken to identify the path of the vitreous, the presence of vitreous traction, and the status of the posterior capsule. Thorough dilated fundus examination should also be performed to evaluate for retinal breaks or detachment.

Management

Nd:YAG vitreolysis can be attempted but is largely unsuccessful. Vitrectomy, preferably via the pars plana, is usually required.[1]

TUBE MIGRATION

Tubes can migrate farther into the anterior chamber or out of the anterior chamber altogether. Migration can occur with growth of the eye in pediatric glaucoma or from eye rubbing, scleral thinning, PAS formation, or wound dehiscence. Additionally, the whole implant can migrate with subsequent tube extrusion.[4]

Management

If the tube migrates forward and the plate is encapsulated, or the tube moves back but not out, no intervention may be required. If the tube moves into the visual axis, is related to wound dehiscence, involves movement of the plate away from the sclera, or results in tube/plate extrusion, surgical revision will be necessary. Trimming of the tube may be sufficient if the tube is in the visual axis, but usually the plate will need to be reattached to the sclera, perhaps at a different location. If the tube moves out of the chamber (i.e., becomes too "short"), then the tube might need to be extended after refastening the plate. A tube extender can be used or a "connector" can be fashioned with an angiocatheter.[7] See Chapters 30 and 48 for more information about tube migration and extending a tube.

CHRONIC IRITIS OR UVEITIS

Chronic postoperative iritis or uveitis occurs at a rate of 0.5%–9.3%, depending on the type of shunt,[10] and is often related to chronic preoperative iritis. However, a tube that chronically touches the iris can cause this complication as well. [8]

Management

If the inflammation worsens or does not resolve with aggressive perioperative and postoperative antiinflammatory treatment, the tube may need to be trimmed or repositioned. Tube revision may be handled with the argon or Nd:YAG laser in a manner similar to how they can be used to manage occlusion, though laser treatment applied to the iris could risk a flare of the uveitis. See Chapters 13 and 20 for more information about iritis and uveitis.

OTHER ANTERIOR SEGMENT COMPLICATIONS

Dyscoria secondary to a tuft of peripheral iris stuck to the tube entry site has been recognized most commonly in pediatric patients.[16] Close observation is adequate, as no additional long-term sequelae occur. Migration of a polypropylene obturator stent into the anterior chamber may require premature removal of the suture with subsequent risk of hypotony.[16] Later shallowing of the anterior chamber could be due to progressive cataract and may require cataract removal and/or repositioning of the tube in the anterior chamber, ciliary sulcus, or posterior segment.[17]

PREVENTING TUBE SHUNT COMPLICATIONS IN THE ANTERIOR CHAMBER

Preoperative evaluation

Preoperative evaluation and appropriate surgical technique are helpful in reducing anterior chamber complications. Uveitis should be treated as aggressively as possible before, during, and after surgical intervention to reduce tube occlusion. Neovascularization should be pretreated with panretinal photocoagulation and/or vascular endothelial growth factor (VEGF) inhibitors to reduce the risk of bleeding and failure of the procedure. Anterior chamber depth, PAS, and lens status may influence a decision to primarily position the tube into the ciliary sulcus or posterior segment. The status of the posterior capsule and presence of vitreous in the anterior chamber will determine the need for vitrectomy at the time of tube insertion. Controlling hypertension and reducing anticoagulation can decrease the risk of bleeding. Evaluating the visual potential of the eye can help determine the initial procedure as well as how to deal with complications.

Surgical technique

A 23-gauge needle should be used to create the scleral tunnel so that the tube fit is tight.[7] Leakage around the tube should be recognized and repaired intraoperatively. The tube should be positioned level and anterior to the iris, and the bevel of the tube should be away from the iris (forward if in the anterior chamber, backward if in the sulcus or the vitreous).[1] Additionally, contact between the tube and the iris, cornea, or lens should be avoided.

When possible the tube should be placed into the anterior chamber at a clock hour that is free of PAS.[1] Injection of an air bubble, balanced salt solution, or viscoelastic may facilitate positioning the tube in the anterior chamber[7] but may also lead to a false sense of the depth where the tube is located in the anterior chamber. Artificial deepening of the anterior chamber may result in iris-tube touch, even though the tube appeared in good position at the end of surgery. Similarly a shallow chamber may result in too anterior of tube placement. When implanting tube shunts in pediatric patients, the tube should be left long to allow for growth of the eye.[7] Snaking of the tube to the entry site may assist in later extension in these cases (see Chapter 30 and 48). Also, initial patency of the tube or valve must be confirmed. Completely occlude nonvalved tubes and attempt to confirm some resistance to flow in valved tubes (after the valve is "primed"). Tube fenestrations may be necessary for early control of IOP in nonvalved tubes.[18] (See Chapter 35 for intentional tube occlusion.) Lastly, patients must be sternly warned to avoid heavy lifting, bending, and straining to prevent suprachoroidal hemorrhage.

CONCLUSION

Anterior segment complications can be reduced by careful preoperative assessment and surgical technique. Many anterior chamber complications can be recognized by slit-lamp examination and relationship to IOP. However, complications of the anterior segment can have serious consequences for vision and the treatment of glaucoma. Management of these complications can sometimes be performed at the slit lamp, but will often need additional surgical intervention.

COMMENTARY

STEVEN T. SIMMONS

A little prevention is worth a lot of cure. Location of the tube shunt is critical in many of these cases and should be determined preoperatively after thorough slit-lamp examination and gonioscopy. It is important to avoid areas of PAS, neovascularization, and previous scleral incisions. Tube shunts placed through previous scleral incisions or in areas of previous filtration surgery always tend to leak in the early postoperative period. Also, in patients with relatively thin sclera, extended "tunneling" the 23-gauge needle paracentesis may reduce or prevent leakage around the tube entry site.

To avoid migration of the plate, it is helpful to place one of the 8–0 nylon sutures through the edge of the superior rectus muscle tendon. This allows for a "deep" scleral placement of the suture, usually approximately 8 mm off the limbus, ideal for either the superior temporal or nasal quadrant placement. Placing a 4–0 silk suture under the superior rectus muscle helps identify this landmark and facilitates the suture placement. I secure the tube shunt to the sclera with a 10–0 polypropylene suture. Late migration may occur when nylon sutures lose their tensile strength. Slow migration may occur even after encapsulation.

Vitreous will always find the tube shunt if given the opportunity. In all aphakic patients and patients with anterior chamber lenses or known zonular dehiscence, a complete pars plana vitrectomy is required prior to or in association with the placement of a tube shunt. If the vitrectomy is done the same day, it is vital to check the sclerostomies closely to make sure there is no leak that can result in early hypotony.

Lastly, if using a valved tube shunt, surgeons should check the valve function with balanced salt solution and a 30-gauge cannula as there have been intermittent quality issues with some devices. If little or no resistance exists, then the surgeon should use another tube shunt. Having done this for many years, it is extremely helpful to avoid "surprise" overfiltration. The use of a viscoelastic at the time of surgery with these valved procedures is also helpful to minimize hypotony.

COMMENTARY

CYNTHIA MATTOX

Anterior-chamber-related complications from tube shunt implantation can be divided into those that can be observed and those that need early and urgent intervention, utilizing the techniques outlined in this chapter (Table 45.1).

Table 45.1   Complications Requiring Observation or Urgent Intervention

COMPLICATIONS REQUIRING OBSERVATION OR URGENT INTERVENTION

Urgent

- Flat Anterior chamber with corneal touch centrally by lens, intraocular lens, tube, or vitreous needs urgent intervention to correct the underlying mechanism and reform the anterior chamber.
- Cornea-tube touch needs urgent correction to prevent eventual corneal decompensation that will inevitably occur if left untreated. Early intervention may save the patient from additional future surgery of endothelial or penetrating keratoplasty.
- Total iris-tube obstruction will need urgent treatment because the IOP will be extremely high.
- Fibrin formation in the anterior chamber following tube shunt implantation should be vigorously and promptly treated whether or not it is causing tube obstruction. Subconjunctival or systemic corticosteroids are mandatory, as even frequent topical steroids are usually not sufficient.
- Complete tube occlusion by vitreous will need urgent surgical intervention, preferably by performing a complete pars plana vitrectomy.

Observation

- Shallow anterior chamber from choroidal effusions/aqueous shutdown can be observed if mild or may require anterior chamber reformation, possibly repeated, with viscoelastic as a temporizing measure until the intraocular pressure rises to reverse or stabilize the effusions.
- Iris-tube touch, even with small amounts of iris incarceration, can be observed, assuming the lumen is mostly unobstructed and nothing indicates there will be rapid worsening of the tube touch.
- Milder anterior chamber inflammation should be treated aggressively with topical medications in the early to midterm postoperative periods, or if it develops late postoperatively, patients often do well with low-dose topical steroid if low-grade iritis persists.
- Small strands of vitreous may not completely occlude the tube and could be watched or treated with vitreolysis, but the eye should be watched closely for more movement of the vitreous into the tube that completely obstructs it.

REFERENCES

1. Fechter HP, Parrish RK 2nd. Preventing and treating complications of Baerveldt® Glaucoma Drainage Device surgery. *Int Ophthalmol Clin.* Spring 2004;44(2):107–136.

2. Gedde SJ, Herndon LW, Brandt JD, Budenz DL, Feuer WJ, Schiffman JC. Surgical complications in the Tube Versus Trabeculectomy Study during the first year of follow-up. *Am J Ophthalmol.* Jan 2007;143(1):23–31.

3. Gedde SJ, Schiffman JC, Feuer WJ, Herndon LW, Brandt JD, Budenz DL. Treatment outcomes in the Tube Versus Trabeculectomy Study after one year of follow-up. *Am J Ophthalmol.* Jan 2007;143(1):9–22.

4. Lai JS, Poon AS, Chua JK, Tham CC, Leung AT, Lam DS. Efficacy and safety of the Ahmed™ glaucoma valve implant in Chinese eyes with complicated glaucoma. *Br J Ophthalmol.* Jul 2000;84(7):718–721.

5. Devenyi RG, Trope GE, Hunter WS. Neodymium-YAG transscleral cyclocoagulation in rabbit eyes. *Br J Ophthalmol.* Jun 1987;71(6):441–444.

6. van der Zypen E, England C, Fankhauser F, Kwasniewska S. The effect of transscleral laser cyclophotocoagulation on rabbit ciliary body vascularization. *Graefes Arch Clin Exp Ophthalmol.* 1989;227(2):172–179.

7. Nguyen QH. Avoiding and managing complications of glaucoma drainage implants. *Curr Opin Ophthalmol.* Apr 2004;15(2):147–150.

8. Guerrero AH, Latina MA. Complications of glaucoma drainage implant surgery. *Int Ophthalmol Clin.* Winter 2000;40(1):149–163.

9. Noecker R, Kahook M. Glaucoma drainage devices. *Techniques in Ophthalmology.* Jun 2006;4(2):69–73.

10. Lim KS, Allan BD, Lloyd AW, Muir A, Khaw PT. Glaucoma drainage devices; past, present, and future. *Br J Ophthalmol.* Sept 1998;82(9): 1083–1089.

11. Greenfield DS, Tello C, Budenz DL, Liebmann JM, Ritch R. Aqueous misdirection after glaucoma drainage device implantation. *Ophthalmology.* May 1999;106(5):1035–1040.

12. Law SK, Kalenak JW, Connor TB, Jr., Pulido JS, Han DP, Mieler WF. Retinal complications after aqueous shunt surgical procedures for glaucoma. *Arch Ophthalmol.* Dec 1996;114(12):1473–1480.

13. Nguyen QH, Budenz DL, Parrish RK 2nd. Complications of Baerveldt® glaucoma drainage implants. *Arch Ophthalmol.* May 1998;116(5): 571–575.

14. Carrillo MM, Trope GE, Pavlin C, Buys YM. Use of ultrasound biomicroscopy to diagnose Ahmed™ valve obstruction by iris. *Can J Ophthalmol.* Aug 2005;40(4):499–501.

15. Zalta AH, Sweeney CP, Zalta AK, Kaufman AH. Intracameral tissue plasminogen activator use in a large series of eyes with valved glaucoma drainage implants. *Arch Ophthalmol.* Nov 2002;120(11):1487–1493.

16. van Overdam KA, de Faber JT, Lemij HG, de Waard PW. Baerveldt® glaucoma implant in paediatric patients. *Br J Ophthalmol.* Mar 2006;90(3):328–332.

17. Joos KM, Lavina AM, Tawansy KA, Agarwal A. Posterior repositioning of glaucoma implants for anterior segment complications. *Ophthalmology.* Feb 2001;108(2):279–284.

18. Trible JR, Brown DB. Occlusive ligature and standardized fenestration of a Baerveldt® tube with and without antimetabolites for early postoperative intraocular pressure control. *Ophthalmology.* Dec 1998;105(12):2243–2250.

46

TUBE SHUNT RELATED COMPLICATIONS OF THE RETINA AND VITREOUS

JUDIANNE KELLAWAY AND GARVIN H. DAVIS

TUBE SHUNT RELATED COMPLICATIONS OF THE RETINA AND VITREOUS

Tube shunt complications of the retina and vitreous can threaten vision. It is important to understand how to recognize, prevent, and manage these complications.

INCIDENCE OF RETINAL COMPLICATIONS WITH TUBE SHUNTS

While many retrospective studies regarding retinal complications of tube shunts are in the literature, there are now 2 major prospective studies that can be looked to for the incidence of retinal complications. In the Tube Versus Trabeculectomy (TVT) Study, at 3 years of follow-up, 4 eyes out of 107 total eyes (4%) with tube shunts had required pars plana

vitrectomies due to a retinal complication (e.g., vitreous occlusion of the tube, retinal detachment, choroidal detachment). Drainage of a choroidal effusion was performed in 2 patients. Early postoperative retinal complications (onset at 1 month or less after tube shunt implantation) included choroidal effusion (15 eyes; 14%), suprachoroidal hemorrhage (2 eyes; 2%), and vitreous hemorrhage (1 eye; 1%). Late postoperative retinal complications (onset more than 1 month after tube shunt implantation) included choroidal effusion (2 eyes; 2%) and retinal detachment (1 eye; 1%).[1]

In the Ahmed Baerveldt Comparison (ABC) Study, at one year of follow-up, one eye of 276 total eyes (0.4%) required a pars plana vitrectomy to clear a postoperative hemorrhage and one eye (0.4%) required reoperation for drainage of a suprachoroidal hemorrhage. Early postoperative retinal complications (3 months of less after implantation of the tube shunt) reported included choroidal effusion (34 eyes; 12%), suprachoroidal hemorrhage (2 eyes; 1%), endophthalmitis (1 eye; 0.4%), and vitreous hemorrhage (5 eyes; 2%). Late retinal postoperative complications (more than 3 months after tube shunt implantation) included choroidal effusion (3 eyes; 1%), endophthalmitis (2 eyes; 1%), vitreous hemorrhage (3 eyes; 1%), and retinal detachment (2 eyes; 1%).[2] Both of these studies indicate a similar incidence of retinal complications after tube shunt implantation.

INDICATIONS FOR PARS PLANA TUBE SHUNT

Tube shunt surgery is performed in cases of uncontrolled glaucoma where medications are inadequate. A pars plana tube is most often indicated for anatomic reasons, such as a small eye, or an eye that already has coexisting corneal disease. Eyes with Fuchs' dystrophy, low endothelial cell count, posterior dystrophy of the cornea, a previous penetrating keratoplasty, or an anterior chamber intraocular lens (IOL) are examples of eyes that may benefit from a pars plana tube shunt over an anterior chamber tube shunt to protect the already diseased cornea. Additionally, a tube may already be in the anterior chamber but may be moved to the pars plana due to occlusion by fibrin or the iris, inflammatory processes such as uveitis, or because the tube itself is causing corneal problems. If the anterior tube shunt is in contact with the corneal endothelium, this may lead to edema, opacification, and even corneal decompensation. Contraindications to pars plana tube shunt (PPTS) surgery include an opaque cornea (because poor visualization will preclude safe vitrectomy) and retinal detachment that is not simultaneously repairable. Potentially, in the case of a retinal detachment, the tube shunt may need to be staged in order to manage the retinal detachment first.

SURGICAL GOALS

Several surgical goals should be kept in mind when a vitrectomy is required. The most important goal of a vitrectomy is to provide an adequate area free of vitreous so the PPTS can function efficiently. Any vitreous that might get into the tube should be cleared; for example, any strands of vitreous that can move in proximity to the tube should be removed. Not all of the anterior-to-posterior fibers have to be removed, just those in the anterior half of the globe. Unless careful and complete removal is performed, care should be taken to avoid creating a posterior vitreous detachment or peeling of the internal limiting membrane, which could create free vitreous with the potential for moving into the tube. Additionally, scleral depression should be used to clear as much of the vitreous base as possible. We usually remove vitreous base approximately 180 degrees within the proximity of the location of the tube. Finally, any other elements in the vitreous that may occlude the tube should be cleared. This would include vitreous hemorrhage, clots, and membranes left after cataract extraction.

Providing a guide to performing a vitrectomy is beyond the scope of this chapter, but there are several key principles to remember when performing a vitrectomy for PPTS placement. There are 3 general phases to inserting a PPTS: 1) placement of the tube shunt plate by the glaucoma surgeon; 2) preparation of the vitreous space for the tube shunt and addressing any other concomitant posterior segment disease by the retina surgeon; and 3) completion of the tube shunt procedure by the glaucoma surgeon. A few guidelines are presented here to assist in this procedure.

1. We strongly suggest using the binocular indirect ophthalmo microscope (BIOM; Oculus, Wetzlar, Germany) or similar noncontact visualization system for vitrectomy. It makes complete removal of the anterior vitreous easier, and the scleral indentation can more easily visualized. Contact lens type systems can be more difficult to use to get an adequate view of the anterior vitreous and vitreous base anatomy.

2. Make sure the pupil is widely dilated. This will allow direct visualization of the internal sclerostomy with scleral indentation.

If necessary, iris hooks or other pupil dilating device should be used to maximize visualization.

3. During the core vitrectomy the posterior hyaloid face does not usually need to be elevated and removed, unless there is concurrent macular pathology that needs to be addressed.

4. Commonly there is retinal disease also present, which needs to be treated at the time of the PPTS procedure. Vitreous hemorrhage, retinal neovascularization, proliferative diabetic retinopathy, and central and branch retinal vein occlusion can all be managed easily during PPTS implantationwith the customary vitrectomy procedures.

5. After the posterior vitrectomy and posterior problems are attended to, the next procedure is an anterior vitrectomy with scleral indentation. Under ideal conditions, it is relatively straightforward to perform a vitreous base dissection. In addition, capsular opacities may also be removed during the vitrectomy.

6. Careful inspection should be performed to identify any vitreous strands that may still remain.

7. *Testing the proposed site for tube placement.* When the preceding steps have been accomplished, and it is time to place the tube in the pars plana, a test of the proposed site can be performed. Prepare a DORC brush (Dutch Ophthalmic Research Center [D.O.R.C.] BV, Zuidland, The Netherlands) by making a 5 mm mark from the end of the instrument. This will approximate the length of the PPTS, and its position in the vitreous. The mark can be made with a surgical marking pen or by etching a line on the instrument at the 5 mm distance. Next, insert the instrument to this 5 mm point, and watch for flow out of the tube. If fluid is flowing freely through the DORC brush, you can be more certain that the site has been adequately prepared for the PPTS. Also, the fluid dynamics should be changed to simulate more natural conditions (i.e. lower the infusion pressure). If fluid is not flowing freely, then vitreous strands may still be present, obstructing the flow through the DORC brush, which may predict limited flow after placement of the tube.

SURGICAL TECHNIQUES FOR SPECIAL PROBLEMS

Cornea

An opaque cornea is a relative contraindication for performing a PPTS, although in extreme circumstances we have attempted to perform the procedure with limited visualization when no other alternative is available, with some success. When corneal opacities are present, the retinal surgeon needs to decide if a PPTS implantation can be performed safely. The decision should take into account the level of difficulty for both the retina surgeon performing the vitrectomy and, to a lesser degree, the glaucoma surgeon placing the shunt. If corneal edema is present, a hypertonic ophthalmic solution may help in the preoperative and postoperative setting.

Pupil

If the pupil is small, it can be usually dilated several ways. Button hooks can be used to gently dilate the opening. We prefer prolene iris hooks to enlarge the pupil. These can be revised with the plate during surgery. Beware especially of neovascularization of the iris and membranes. Caution must be used when manipulating the iris, as hemorrhage can occur in the setting of neovascularization of the iris.

Lens

If the patient is phakic, caution must be used during the vitrectomy to prevent touching or traumatizing the lens. In pseudophakic patients, we usually use an anterior chamber maintainer. An IOL can move in this setting, so be cautious during the dissection to avoid collapsing the anterior chamber. Hinged IOLs are especially mobile when performing a vitrectomy using an anterior chamber maintainer or larger gauge infusion ports, and removal should be considered. Capsular opacifications can be addressed with a blade or with the vitrector.

Neovascular disease

When neovascularization is present, this procedure can be particularly challenging. The risk of hyphema is quite high with the presence of active vessels (Chapters 5 and 23) and can make visualization difficult. A high viscosity viscoelastic can be used to temporize this problem and improve visualization.

OTHER COMPLICATIONS

Retinal complications with tube shunts can occur with either a PPTS or an anterior chamber tube shunt. Some retinal complications that occur with tube shunt surgery have been discussed elsewhere in this book but are repeated here for emphasis.

Hypotony

Hypotony is a potentially serious complication. The intraocular pressure must be elevated immediately to prevent more serious sequelae. For more information on how to handle this complication, see Chapters 34 and 39.

Choroidal effusion and choroidal hemorrhage

These complications can lead to secondary hypotony, secondary retinal detachment, or fibrosis. Drainage may be required to resolve the effusion or hemorrhage. For more information, see Chapter 6.

Scleritis

In the setting of inflammatory diseases, the integrity of the patch graft may be compromised; a replacement patch or suture may be necessary.

Endophthalmitis

See Chapter 42.

Occlusion of the tube

If possible, the tube should be examined to determine the cause of the occlusion. Inflammatory membranes, fibrin, vitreous, and inflammatory debris can cause occlusions. This will sometimes require return to the operating suite to try to cannulate and irrigate the tube with balanced salt solution. For more information on this complication, see Chapter 37.

Retinal detachment or tear

Macular and retinal detachments should be repaired within a reasonable time period. Recent macular detachments should be repaired as soon as possible and typically within 72 hours. If the macula is already detached, retinal detachment should be repaired within one week.

Cause One of the common causes of retinal tears/detachments is incomplete vitrectomy. The vitreous can occlude the tube, and traction from peripheral vitreous to peripheral retina can create a tear, which can then lead to a detachment

Prevention As previously stated, a careful vitrectomy with depression 360 degrees and removal of the vitreous base should be done to prevent this complication. We prefer to also place a soft tip needle through the wound that will house the tube and provide active suction, looking carefully for any vitreous that may become entrapped in the soft tip during the aspiration.

In the case of a PPTS, the retinal periphery should be carefully examined 360 degrees prior to placing the tube and any retinal tears addressed during surgery. With an anterior tube shunt, movement of the vitreous and collapse of the vitreous can lead to retinal breaks but is less likely if the patient has had a posterior vitreous detachment. Examining the vitreous prior to any type of tube surgery, particularly looking for evidence of a posterior vitreous detachment, is an important preoperative step.

Management In the presence of an inferior detachment, the preferred management is a scleral buckle and vitrectomy, although the placement of an encircling band is challenging in the presence of the PPTS plate. With a superior detachment, either a scleral buckle and a vitrectomy or a primary vitrectomy, is usually used to manage the detachment.

Vitreous Hemorrhage

This is managed by repeat vitrectomy. In the setting of neovascular disease, recurrent vitreous hemorrhage can be a challenge.

Causes Neovascularization can lead to vitreous hemorrhage (e.g., diabetes, radiation, central retinal vein occlusion). Trauma to ciliary body or iris during placement of tube can also lead to hemorrhage. Patients should have an ultrasound in the setting of vitreous hemorrhage to identify or rule out retinal tear.

Prevention Careful attention to hemostasis during the procedure can minimize this complication. Preoperative bevacizumab may be useful.

Management We usually prefer observation in the setting of vitreous hemorrhage. After vitrectomy, a vitreous hemorrhage should resolve more quickly. If patient has neovascular glaucoma, removing the vitreous may decrease the vascular endothelial growth factor (VEGF) load,[3,4] with the blood more likely to clear. Small hemorrhages from a hyphema or iris damage are often self-limited. Observation of a postoperative vitreous hemorrhage for 1–2 months is generally recommended, as long as there are not any problems with IOP and if blood has not occluded the tube. A repeat vitrectomy would then be indicated.

CONCLUSION

Pars plana tube shunts can provide a successful solution to severe and complicated glaucoma disease when the glaucoma and retinal specialists plan together. The procedure is relatively straightforward, and management of complications is within the realm of conscientious surgeons in these specialties.

Dr. Kellaway and Dr. Davis were supported by a Challenge Grant from Research to Prevent Blindness to The University of Texas Medical School at Houston and the Hermann Eye Fund.

REFERENCES

1. Gedde SJ, Schiffman JC, Feuer WJ, et al. Three-year follow-up of the Tube Versus Trabeculectomy Study. *Am J Ophthalmol.* Nov 2009;148(5):670–684.
2. Budenz DL, Barton K, Feuer WJ, et al. Treatment outcomes in the Ahmed Baerveldt Comparison Study after 1 year of follow-up. *Ophthalmology.* Mar 2011;118(3):443–452.
3. Citirik M, Kabatas EU, Batman C, Akin KO, Kabatas N. Vitreous vascular endothelial growth factor concentrations in proliferative diabetic retinopathy versus proliferative vitreoretinopathy. *Ophthalmic Research.* 2012; 47(1):7–12.
4. Shirasawa M, Arimura N, Otsuka H, Sonoda S, Hashiguchi T, Sakamoto T. Intravitreous VEGF-A in eyes with massive vitreous hemorrhage. *Graefes Arch Clin Exp Ophthalmol.* Dec 2011;249(12):1805–1810.

47

TUBE SHUNT RELATED COMPLICATIONS OF THE ORBIT

MARC R. CRIDEN

TUBE SHUNT RELATED COMPLICATIONS OF THE ORBIT

Orbital complications during or after glaucoma filtering or tube shunt surgery are relatively rare but may pose a significant treatment challenge or threat to vision. The incidence of complications is highly variable,[1] and transient events may not be reported as frequently as those that persist.

A variety of orbital complications occur following glaucoma surgery. Complications may be categorized as mechanical, infectious, neurogenic, or myogenic. However, each complication may be multimodal and fall into more than one category.

MECHANICAL

Mechanical complications are the most frequent type of orbit complication related to glaucoma surgery and more specifically to tube shunt implantation. Mechanical complications include ptosis,[2] lid retraction,[3] strabismus,[4] and proptosis.[5]

Ptosis

Several theories address why ptosis may occur after ocular surgery and why it may be either transient or permanent. The levator muscle may be damaged or dehisced by an eyelid speculum, leading to a lid droop.[6,7] Bridle sutures, which are often used during glaucoma surgery, have also been implicated as they apply counter traction against the superior rectus muscle.[8] Prolonged eyelid edema and local anesthesia have each been more strongly associated with postoperative ptosis.[7,9] For more information on ptosis, see Chapter 25.

Strabismus

Strabismus after tube shunt implantation is most commonly related to either the device itself or to scarring and fibrosis that develop postoperatively.[4] Transient strabismus may be related to swelling or edema of local tissues and may also follow retrobulbar injection.[9,10] The strabismus is usually incomitant and does not present with a characteristic pattern of deviation; thus, prisms and other nonsurgical treatments are seldom adequate.[11] Although strabismus following tube shunt surgery is usually transient, persistent diplopia may occur.[1,4]

The type of implant, size, location, and material each play a role. Implants with larger surface areas have a higher incidence of motility disturbance due to mass effect.[12] Tube shunt plates that require placement below the rectus muscles risk direct muscle injury or adhesion scarring to the implant.[4,11] In addition, a pseudo-Brown's syndrome may be created by a superonasal implant due to interference with the superior oblique muscle function.[13, 14]

The bleb that develops around the tube shunt reservoir can also act as a mass. A large encapsulation resulting from aqueous expansion of the capsule may displace the globe or the rectus muscles, with resultant proptosis with or without an ocular motility disturbance.[5]

Considerations for treating strabismus complications related to the implant should include revising the implant to a smaller size by cutting off a wing of the plate, moving the implant to a different quadrant, or revising its positioning within its original location. Roizen et al suggested that the Ahmed™ (New World Medical, Inc., Racho Cucamonga, California) valve may have a lower incidence of strabismus due to its smaller size (184 mm) compared to the Baerveldt® (350mm; Abbott Medical Optics, Santa, Ana, California) or double-plate Molteno® valve (270 mm; Molteno Ophthalmic, Ltd., Dunedin, New Zealand).[11] However, there is little comparative data. Strabismus surgery on the contralateral eye may be appropriate if the deviation is small and comitant. Additionally, contralateral surgery may be technically less challenging and provide a more predictable outcome with less risk of disturbing the tube shunt. For more on strabismus and tube shunts, see Chapter 43.

Scarring and fibrosis

Scarring and fibrosis are the primary causes of strabismus related to tube shunts, and it

is imperative to verify etiology with forced duction testing. Capsular fibrosis between the implant and rectus muscles may be quite extensive and involve more than one muscle.[4,11] The large extent of these adhesions poses several challenges for the strabismus surgeon. When attempting surgical lysis of adhesions, both the tube shunt and the rectus muscles should be directly visualized. After scarring is released, forced duction testing should be performed to demonstrate treatment of the restrictive strabismus. It should be noted that it is often not possible to completely excise the scar tissue. In this event, dissection should be continued until forced ductions return to normal or until the limit of safe dissection has been reached. Scarring is also the presumed mechanism behind the pseudo-Brown's syndrome seen with a superonasal tube shunt.[13] Adhesions between the rectus muscle and sclera on the posterior aspect of the implant mimic posterior fixation and limit the mechanical advantage of the muscle.

During repair, caution should be undertaken to avoid entering the fibrous capsule surrounding the shunt reservoir because aqueous will be released and hypotony may ensue. In addition, extensive scar dissection or conjunctival excision may not only cause problems during closure but may adversely affect the long-term function of the tube shunt. Thus, the availability of a glaucoma specialist during these procedures is advised. As with any strabismus procedure, there is a risk of further scarring, endophthalmitis, pain, and the need for revision. Intraoperative steroid injections into the scarred area may limit the degree of recurrence of these complications but should be used with care. Adjustable suture techniques for strabismus surgery are often advantageous in these cases as well. For more information, see Chapter 43.

Proptosis

Proptosis is a very uncommon consequence of glaucoma surgery. It may be due to large encapsulation or a pseudocyst that forms posteriorly off the main loculation. Large encapsulations, especially with Ahmed™ implants, generally become smaller over time, and the proptosis resolves.[1, 5]

As with any ophthalmic surgical procedure where a retrobulbar or peribulbar anesthetic block is administered, orbital hemorrhage may occur.[10] If recognized prior to starting the scheduled surgery, the surgeon should strongly consider aborting the glaucoma surgery and treating any resultant elevated intraocular pressure (IOP) by performing a lateral canthotomy. Although the patient is likely using maximum tolerated medical therapy already, canthotomy would relieve the external pressures exerted on the globe by the orbital congestion.

Delayed retrobulbar hematoma has been reported to occur as late as one week after blepharoplasty,[15] and it could likewise occur following implantation of a tube shunt. When the quadrant where the tube is to be placed is dissected open, the surgeon must be careful to cauterize any ruptured blood vessels. However, increased intravascular pressure (as can be created by the Valsalva maneuver) or diminished platelet and clotting factor function may cause the vessel to reopen a few days after surgery. Conservative measures are typically appropriate in managing this unusual postoperative complication.

INFECTIOUS

Orbital cellulitis

Orbital cellulitis is a rare complication of tube shunt surgery and may be primary or secondary. Only a few cases are reported in the literature,[1,12,16,17] but early diagnosis and aggressive treatment are critical to prevent further complications. The presentation is similar to other types of orbital cellulitis with pain, tenderness, injection, proptosis, dysmotility, and periorbital edema. The implant may be an identifiable primary nidus for the infection, or the infection may begin elsewhere and extend to the implant (e.g., secondary to sinus disease or following trauma). Evaluation should include emergent CT imaging and blood work. Intravenous and possibly periocular and/or topical antibiotics should be initiated promptly to prevent further progression. Because the tube establishes a direct communication between the intraocular and extraocular spaces, close attention should also be paid to the presence of endophthalmitis and functioning of the tube shunt and IOP. Early cases may respond well to antibiotic therapy; however, more advanced cases or those recalcitrant to therapy may require implant removal or drainage of any orbital abscesses. An inherent increase in infection risk exists with any implant device or foreign body. In the presence of these, even early cases of preseptal cellulitis should be observed closely and managed aggressively to prevent progression. An implant should only be replaced after the infection has cleared completely to prevent further seeding of the infection into otherwise undisturbed areas of the orbit. However, bacteria may move in a retrograde fashion from the orbit into the eye via the tube itself, turning orbital cellulitis into endophthalmitis. In this situation, prompt removal of at least the intraocular portion of the tube shunt is necessary. After the device is removed, elevated IOP should be managed in the usual fashion with any appropriate intervention. Just as orbital cellulitis may secondarily cause endophthalmitis, a primary intraocular infection may theoretically spread through the tube into the orbit.

MYOGENIC AND NEUROGENIC

Myogenic complications of glaucoma surgery include direct muscle or nerve damage, pressure necrosis, or ischemia. These conditions are often transient,[18] and conservative management is most appropriate. Surgical manipulation of extraocular muscles may lead to damage or dysfunction.[2,6] Inadvertent transection, partial or complete, of the muscle should be identified and repaired immediately.

Local injection of anesthetic is also likely to cause muscle injury and occurs with direct muscle infiltration.[1,9,10] The ensuing paresis may or may not recover. This complication is seen with both retrobulbar and frontal blocks.[19] Transient muscle paresis following retrobulbar injection is not unusual. The lateral rectus muscle is most commonly affected, but any muscle or combination of muscles may become paretic after retrobulbar anesthesia.

Pressure necrosis or muscle ischemia may result from a malpositioned or migrated tube shunt.[11] If suspected, early revision of the implant along with release of adhesions should be pursued. At least 3 months should elapse to allow for recovery, and the deviation should be stable prior to any strabismus surgery.

CONCLUSION

It is fortunate that orbital complications following tube shunt implantation are rare, considering the frequency and variety of glaucoma surgery. Many of these complications may be managed conservatively and often resolve over time. When they do not, significant disability or morbidity may occur, and deterioration may progress rapidly. Once a complication has been identified, the patient should be carefully counseled and followed closely. A balance must be established between further intervention and management of the glaucoma.

REFERENCES

1. Sarkisian SR Jr. Tube shunt complications and their prevention. *Curr Opin Ophthalmol.* Mar 2009;20(2):126–130.
2. Alpar J. Acquired ptosis following cataract and glaucoma surgery. *Glaucoma.* 1982;4:66–68.
3. Awwad ST, Ma'luf RN, Noureddin B. Upper eyelid retraction after glaucoma filtering surgery and topical application of mitomycin C. *Ophthal Plast Reconstr Surg.* Mar 2004;20(2):144–149.
4. Rauscher FM, Gedde SJ, Schiffman JC, Feuer WJ, Barton K, Lee RK. Motility disturbances in the tube versus trabeculectomy study during the first year of follow-up. *Am J Ophthalmol.* Mar 2009;147(3):458–466.
5. Danesh-Meyer HV, Spaeth GL, Maus M. Cosmetically significant proptosis following a tube shunt procedure. *Arch Ophthalmol.* Jun 2002;120(6):846–847.
6. Paris G, Quickert M. Disinsertion of the levator aponeurosis superioris muscle after cataract surgery. *Am J Ophthalmol.* 1976;81:337.
7. Deady J, Price N, Sutton G. Ptosis following cataract and trabeculectomy surgery. *Br J Ophthalmol.* 1989;73:283–285.
8. Kaplan LJ, Jaffe NS, Clayman HM. Ptosis and cataract surgery. A multivariant computer analysis of a prospective study. *Ophthalmology.* Feb 1985;92(2):237–242.
9. Ropo A, Ruusuvaara P, Nikki P. Ptosis following periocular or general anaesthesia in cataract surgery. *Acta Ophthalmol (Copenh).* Apr 1992;70(2):262–265.
10. Ropo A, Ruusuvaara P, Paloheimo M, Maunuksela EL, Nikki P. Periocular anaesthesia: technique, effectiveness and complications with special reference to postoperative ptosis. *Acta Ophthalmol (Copenh).* Dec 1990;68(6):728–732.
11. Roizen A, Ela-Dalman N, Velez FG, Coleman AL, Rosenbaum AL. Surgical treatment of strabismus secondary to glaucoma drainage device. *Arch Ophthalmol.* Apr 2008;126(4):480–486.
12. Marcet MM, Woog JJ, Bellows AR, Mandeville JT, Maltzman JS, Khan J. Orbital complications after aqueous drainage device procedures. *Ophthal Plast Reconstr Surg.* Jan 2005;21(1): 67–69.
13. Ball SF, Ellis GS Jr., Herrington RG, Liang K. Brown's superior oblique tendon syndrome after Baerveldt® glaucoma implant. *Arch Ophthalmol.* Oct 1992;110(10):1368.
14. Ventura MP, Vianna RN, Souza Filho JP, Solari HP, Curi RL. Acquired Brown's syndrome secondary to Ahmed™ valve implant for neovascular glaucoma. *Eye (Lond).* Feb 2005;19(2):230–232.
15. Cruz AA, Ando A, Monteiro CA, Elias J Jr. Delayed retrobulbar hematoma after blepharoplasty. *Ophthal Plast Reconstr Surg.* Mar 2001;17(2):126–130.
16. Chaudhry IA, Shamsi FA, Morales J. Orbital cellulitis following implantation of aqueous drainage devices. *Eur J Ophthalmol.* Jan-Feb 2007;17(1):136–140.
17. Lavina AM, Creasy JL, Tsai JC. Orbital cellulitis as a late complication of glaucoma shunt implantation. *Arch Ophthalmol.* Jun 2002; 120(6): 849–851.
18. Wolfort FG, Poblete JV. Ptosis after blepharoplasty. *Ann Plast Surg.* Mar 1995; 34(3):264–266; discussion 266–267.
19. Rainin EA, Carlson BM. Postoperative diplopia and ptosis. A clinical hypothesis based on the myotoxicity of local anesthetics. *Arch Ophthalmol.* Sept 1985;103(9):1337–1339.

48

TUBE SHUNT RELATED COMPLICATIONS IN PEDIATRICS

MEGAN M. GELONECK, ROBERT M. FELDMAN AND NICHOLAS P. BELL

TUBE SHUNT RELATED COMPLICATIONS IN PEDIATRICS

Although medical therapy is usually an excellent therapeutic option in the adult population, in children it is often ineffective or associated with an undesirable risk:benefit ratio. Therefore, surgical intervention is frequently required for adequate control of glaucoma in young patients.[1-3] The initial surgical approach for management of glaucoma in children includes goniotomy and trabeculotomy, each with a high success rate.[4,5] When these interventions fail or have a high likelihood of failure (i.e., in patients with Sturge-Weber syndrome, aniridia, anterior chamber dysgenesis, or congenital glaucoma), tube shunt procedures are often required. Tube shunts were first used in the pediatric population by Molteno and colleagues in 1973[6] and have since grown in popularity and secured

an integral role in the treatment of refractory glaucoma in infants and children. Possible complications and causes for failure of tube shunt devices in children are very similar to those in adults; however, issues such as tube migration and retraction must be anticipated in the child's growing eye.

INCIDENCE

One of the most frustrating, and unfortunately the most common, complications is tube malposition. While tube malposition is not entirely specific to the pediatric population, it occurs far more frequently in children than in adults.[7-13] (See Chapter 30 for information about tube malposition in adults.) Incidence of tube malposition in pediatric patients ranges from 3% to 35%.[7-12,14,15] In infants and young children, the tube tends to retract from the eye and/or migrate towards the cornea in the anterior chamber. The initial presentation of tube migration is often tube-cornea touch at the proximal end of the tube near the insertion site.[13] In severe cases, tube migration can lead to transcorneal extrusion of the tube. Secondary complications, including corneal decompensation, cataract, iris abnormalities, and endophthalmitis, can result from these initial insults if tube malposition is not identified early and appropriately addressed.[7,13,16]

ETIOLOGY

The cause of tube migration and retraction is likely multifactorial, but there are 2 basic mechanisms thought to be at fault: 1) somatic growth causing concomitant tube migration and 2) elasticity of the buphthalmic eye, allowing shrinkage as intraocular pressure (IOP) decreases and tube straightening due to "memory." The somatic growth of the infant eye is an expected mechanism of tube migration, which must be anticipated and accounted for by the surgeon when inserting the tube to try to prevent potential tube retraction and migration. During the first 2 years of life, the eye enlarges from 66% of the diameter of an adult eye to near full adult size.[2] Specifically, growth in the axial length causes complications with tube malposition. As the eye enlarges axially, the tube retracts posteriorly with the expanding sclera. As the tube is pulled toward the angle, the distal end of the tube subsequently pushes forward in the anterior chamber towards the corneal endothelium.[13] Several studies have discussed the possibility of somatic growth of the eye contributing to tube malposition in young children.[13,16]

However, growth alone is unlikely to account for most cases of tube malposition as the buphthalmic eye grows at a variable rate compared to normal. At birth, the infant sclera is half the thickness of that of an adult.[2] The thin sclera confers significant elasticity to the sclera not found in an adult eye. The relative elastic recoil pulls inwards on the stretched sclera and globe, causing shrinkage. As the eye shrinks, the anterior chamber shallows,

thereby shortening the distance between the tube and corneal endothelium. If the eye shrinks in such a way to change the angle at which the drainage tube penetrates the globe or if the tube was initially inserted at an angle other than parallel to the iris, it may then come in contact with the iris or cornea.[8,10,13]

We agree with Ishida and colleagues that the reduced rigidity of the infant eye may enable the bent silicone tubing to return to its straight "memory."[13] At the time of surgery, a bend is introduced into the tubing where it enters the globe. However, as the tube tries to return to its initial straightened state, it may push forward in the anterior chamber, thereby coming in contact with the cornea.[13] It is more likely that the tissue surrounding the tube entry turns over faster in children and would decrease thickness in an area of pressure, filling in behind the tube and forcing it forward over time with tissue regeneration.

There are a couple of other factors thought to be responsible for some cases of tube migration in children. One, as described by O'Malley Schotthoefer and colleagues, is the tendency of children to rub their eyes. The rubbing of the eye may cause the tube to push forward into the cornea and backwards into the iris and lens, causing transient tube malposition. This mechanism was suggested after examining children with peaked pupils and focal cataracts in which the tube was well-positioned at the time of exam.[16] This proposed contributing factor seems likely, and repeated episodes of eye rubbing may actually cause small tears and erosions around the insertion site of the tube, thereby enabling the tube to move more easily against an immature sclera.

MANAGEMENT

Early identification of tube retraction and anterior migration is essential to prevent secondary complications, such as corneal decompensation from prolonged tube-cornea touch.[17,18] Therefore, proper postoperative management of the pediatric patient begins with close monitoring. Children, especially infants and the very young, should be monitored very attentively for several years for any signs of tube migration or retraction. While the majority of cases of tube migration occur within the first few years after surgery, we have seen tube malposition occur in children 10 years after implantation. There is no restriction as to when tube migration may occur, so it is important to evaluate the position of the tube at every examination. Furthermore, patients must also be monitored closely during the first few years after any tube repositioning or other revision performed for tube malposition.[17]

Surgical revision is necessary when the tube changes position, extends farther into the anterior chamber, or retracts from the anterior chamber. Often, the first sign of tube migration is tube-cornea touch at the most proximal end, near the insertion site.[13] When these signs of tube migration are present, the tube must be repositioned in the operating room and trimmed appropriately. It is crucial to reposition the tube as close to the iris as possible and at an appropriate angle. The tube should then be trimmed to an appropriate length, generally 2–3 mm beyond the limbus, with the bevel facing the cornea. Tube repositioning and trimming are usually all that are required for successful revision, with maintenance of good IOP thereafter.[7,13] (For more information on surgical techniques for repositioning tubes, see Chapter 30.) If transcorneal extrusion or exposure of the implanted device is present, the overlying patch graft must be revised as well. In severe cases of implant exposure in which a simple graft revision is futile, the tube shunt should be extracted as quickly as possible to prevent secondary endophthalmitis. In these rare, but severe cases, a different surgical avenue or perhaps a different quadrant placement of the tube shunt should then be pursued.

PREVENTION

It is very difficult, if not impossible, to prevent tube migration and retraction. However, there are several measures that can be taken at the time of surgery to reduce the risk for this frustrating complication. The initial positioning of the tube is crucial. It is important to position the tube as close to the iris as possible.[7,8,13] Equally important as posterior positioning is the angle of insertion of the tube into the anterior chamber.[13] The tube should be inserted as parallel to the iris as possible to further increase the distance between tip of the tube and corneal endothelium. As previously mentioned, this angle will also help to reduce the likelihood of tube-cornea touch in buphthalmic eyes likely to shrink with postoperative normalization of IOP.

In anticipation of tube retraction, as is most common in infants and very young patients, some slack or an "S" shaped pathway used before entering the chamber should be left in the tubing. Leaving this extra tubing at the time of surgery makes dealing with later retraction easier. This extra segment of tube must be well secured to prevent spontaneous straightening and subsequent further advancement into the anterior chamber. If the growth of the eye causes the tube to pull out of the anterior chamber, surgical revision to remove the "S" curve can be performed. The tube and reservoir plate should also be properly secured in place to reduce any potential movement of the shunt contributing to tube migration and retraction.[8] It has also been suggested that the surgeon should avoid placement of the tube near any areas of Haab's striae, which are often found in patients with congenital glaucoma. In a case study of the rare, but dreaded complication of transcorneal extrusion, Maki and colleagues observed the tube extrude through an area of Haab's striae. They hypothesized that this area of weakness in the cornea combined with the potential for formation of peripheral anterior synechiae around the striae may predispose to transcorneal extrusion of the tube.[17] We have seen this complication without Haab's striae.

CONCLUSION

Although there may be many advances yet to come in the management of pediatric glaucoma, tube shunt devices are currently a very important tool. As with any surgical intervention, risks and complications may arise.

Management of children with glaucoma can be especially frustrating since they have a higher incidence of complications, with tube migration and retraction being the most common. However, with full understanding of the complications, we can orchestrate a proper surgical approach and postoperative plan to help reduce the incidence of tube malposition and lessen the burden of secondary complications on our youngest patients.

Dr. Geloneck, Dr. Feldman, and Dr. Bell were supported by a Challenge Grant from Research to Prevent Blindness to The University of Texas Medical School and the Hermann Eye Fund.

COMMENTARY

SHARON F. FREEDMAN

This chapter details the common problem of tube malposition following glaucoma drainage device (tube shunt) implantation in children with glaucoma. The authors discuss the complications of tube malposition including tube elongation, shortening, and transcorneal erosion, providing suggested mechanisms as well as modifications of surgical technique intended to decrease their incidence, as well as to resolve these tube-related problems once they present.

The authors do not address the myriad other problems that can and unfortunately do occur in eyes of children after glaucoma drainage device surgery. Most of these complications are not unique to the pediatric population and are discussed elsewhere in this book; however, some occur with increased frequency in children, so I will briefly outline them below. Tube-related problems have been pretty well covered, except to note that the tube may rarely become blocked by iris, residual cortex, or vitreous (if placed pars plana without complete vitrectomy; also see Chapter 37). Reservoir-related problems may include encapsulation of the reservoir with elevation of intraocular pressure, blockage of the valve chamber (specific to devices such as the Ahmed™ Glaucoma Valve [New World Medical, Inc., Rancho Cucamonga, California] and requiring their replacement), erosion of the plate (Chapter 38), or eye movement limitation (Chapter 43). Needling or bleb revision rarely provides long-term resolution for encapsulated blebs, and a second drainage device or limited cycloablation may be helpful. The presence of a fluid-filled bleb overlying a fairly large drainage device plate can cause eye movement limitations and sometimes even severe misalignment of the eye(s). Although young children usually do not complain of diplopia, very extreme limitation of movement usually requires surgical intervention, with bleb revision in cases of an overly large bleb, and sometimes with plate removal and additional extraocular muscle surgery. The later should usually be undertaken by the strabismus surgeon in conjunction with the glaucoma surgeon, unless he/she is very familiar with the placement of these devices in children (Chapter 43).

As mentioned in this chapter, infection in the setting of glaucoma drainage device surgery is happily quite rare, and often relates to exposure of the drainage device tube or plate. Aggressive intervention is needed to save the vision and the eye (including vitreoretinal intervention with intravitreal antibiotics and sometimes vitrectomy), often requiring removal of the drainage device to prevent an intraocular infection from becoming a life-threatening orbital cellulitis (Chapter 47). Additional severe complications including retinal detachment and/or phthisis may occur early or late after glaucoma drainage device surgery, usually in aphakic eyes, which may have preexisting peripheral retinal pathology. Prompt intervention by an experienced vitreoretinal surgeon may rescue the eye and sometimes the vision, but is complex, often requiring silicone oil and scleral buckle placement.

Glaucoma drainage device implantation remains a reasonable option for management of pediatric glaucoma refractory to medication and other surgical interventions but must be considered in light of the many complications that may present.[16,19,20]

REFERENCES

1. deLuise VP, Anderson DR. Primary infantile glaucoma (congenital glaucoma). *Surv Ophthalmol.* Jul-Aug 1983;28(1):1–19.

2. Friedman NJ, Kaiser PK, Trattler WB. Pediatrics/Strabismus. *Review of Ophthalmology.* Philadelphia: Elsevier Saunders; 2005:89–158.

3. Maris PJ Jr., Mandal AK, Netland PA. Medical therapy of pediatric glaucoma and glaucoma in pregnancy. *Ophthalmol Clin North Am.* Sept 2005;18(3):461–468, vii.

4. Anderson DR. Trabeculotomy compared to goniotomy for glaucoma in children. *Ophthalmology.* Jul 1983;90(7):805–806.

5. Shaffer RN. Prognosis of goniotomy in primary infantile glaucoma (trabeculodysgenesis). *Trans Am Ophthalmol Soc.* 1982;80:321–325.

6. Molteno ACB, Ancer E, Biljon GV. Children with advanced glaucoma treated by draining implants. *S Afr J Ophthalmol.* 1973;1:55–61.

7. Beck AD, Freedman S, Kammer J, Jin J. Aqueous shunt devices compared with trabeculectomy with mitomycin-C for children in the first two years of life. *Am J Ophthalmol.* Dec 2003;136(6):994–1000.

8. Djodeyre MR, Peralta Calvo J, Abelairas Gomez J. Clinical evaluation and risk factors of time to failure of Ahmed™ Glaucoma Valve implant in pediatric patients. *Ophthalmology.* Mar 2001;108(3):614–620.

9. Eid TE, Katz LJ, Spaeth GL, Augsburger JJ. Long-term effects of tube-shunt procedures on management of refractory childhood glaucoma. *Ophthalmology.* Jun 1997;104(6):1011–1016.

10. Englert JA, Freedman SF, Cox TA. The Ahmed™ valve in refractory pediatric glaucoma. *Am J Ophthalmol.* Jan 1999;127(1):34–42.

11. Fellenbaum PS, Sidoti PA, Heuer DK, Minckler DS, Baerveldt G, Lee PP. Experience with the Baerveldt® implant in young patients with complicated glaucomas. *J Glaucoma.* Apr 1995;4(2):91–97.

12. Hill RA, Heuer DK, Baerveldt G, Minckler DS, Martone JF. Molteno® implantation for glaucoma in young patients. *Ophthalmology.* Jul 1991;98(7):1042–1046.

13. Ishida K, Mandal AK, Netland PA. Glaucoma drainage implants in pediatric patients. *Ophthalmol Clin North Am.* Sept 2005;18(3):431–442, vii.

14. Morad Y, Donaldson CE, Kim YM, Abdolell M, Levin AV. The Ahmed™ drainage implant in the treatment of pediatric glaucoma. *Am J Ophthalmol.* Jun 2003;135(6):821–829.

15. Netland PA, Walton DS. Glaucoma drainage implants in pediatric patients. *Ophthalmic Surg.* Nov 1993;24(11):723–729.

16. O'Malley Schotthoefer E, Yanovitch TL, Freedman SF. Aqueous drainage device surgery in refractory pediatric glaucomas: I. Long-term outcomes. *J AAPOS.* Feb 2008;12(1):33–39.

17. Maki JL, Nesti HA, Shetty RK, Rhee DJ. Transcorneal tube extrusion in a child with a Baerveldt® glaucoma drainage device. *J AAPOS.* Aug 2007;11(4):395–397.

18. Topouzis F, Coleman AL, Choplin N, et al. Follow-up of the original cohort with the Ahmed™ glaucoma valve implant. *Am J Ophthalmol.* Aug 1999;128(2):198–204.

19. Freedman SF, Johnston S. Glaucoma in infancy and early childhood. In: Wilson EM, Saunders W, Rupal T, eds. *Pediatric Ophthalmology: Current Thought and a Practical Guide.* Heidelberg, Germany: Springer Press; 2009:345–374.

20. O'Malley Schotthoefer E, Yanovitch TL, Freedman SF. Aqueous drainage device surgery in refractory pediatric glaucoma: II. Ocular motility consequences. *J AAPOS.* Feb 2008;12(1):40–45.

PART FIVE

ANGLE SURGERY COMPLICATIONS

A. COMPLICATIONS SPECIFICALLY RELATED TO TRABECULOTOMY IN ADULTS

49

COMPLICATIONS SPECIFICALLY RELATED TO TRABECULOTOMY IN ADULTS

ADAM C. REYNOLDS AND RONALD L. FELLMAN

COMPLICATIONS SPECIFICALLY RELATED TO TRABECULOTOMY IN ADULTS

Disruptive or ablative surgeries involving the trabecular meshwork and Schlemm's canal, which have traditionally been applied to the developmental and congenital glaucomas, are currently receiving renewed interest in adult open-angle glaucoma because of the development of new technologies. The Trabectome® (NeoMedix Corporation, Tustin, California) procedure,[1] canaloplasty with or without stent,[1] direct trabecular bypass,[2] excimer laser trabeculotomy (ELT),[3, 4] and other techniques in development are all based in their surgical approaches on classic trabeculotomy. Some of the proposed mechanisms of action, as well as the potential complications that occur in classic angle surgeries, are also likely quite similar.

It is prudent to note that in some specific limited populations, adult trabeculotomy *ab externo* has long been employed. For example, in Japan trabeculotomy has been used in adult open-angle glaucoma,[5–9] and even in North America there have been studies of trabeculotomy combined with cataract surgery.[10, 11] It is well accepted that any and all of the complications related to these procedures in congenital glaucoma can occur when applied to the adult eye, and mitigation and avoidance of them are likely very similar. Some specific complications may be more likely in adult eyes.

HYPHEMA

By far the most common complication related to trabeculotomy, whether in adults or children, is hyphema. In fact it is expected, and some bleeding should be considered a sign that the procedure was done correctly rather than a complication. However, in several large clinical series from Japan, rates of clinically significant postoperative hyphema in adult trabeculotomy often approach 20%.[5–8, 12] It is thought that hyphema occurs due to disruption of the trabecular meshwork, as a barrier between retrograde flow of blood from the collector channel system into the anterior chamber is removed at least temporarily. Once the trabecular meshwork is disrupted, if the intraocular pressure (IOP) is lower than the episcleral venous pressure (EVP), retrograde flow of blood into the anterior chamber may result. One commonly employed technique to avoid significant hyphema in trabeculotomy is to temporarily "tamponade" the anterior chamber with viscoelastic. Leaving viscoelastic in the anterior chamber at the end of the case to prevent hyphema must be balanced with the substantial risk for a significant postoperative IOP spike from residual viscoelastic. However, an IOP spike is not as likely as in an eye with a normal trabecular meshwork because there is less obstruction to outflow. On the other hand, raising IOP to physiologic levels once the entry sites are closed usually will stop bleeding. However, if viscoelastic is left at the end of the case, use of topical and systemic temporizing IOP-lowering measures in the immediate postoperative period would be prudent to prevent a significant, immediate IOP elevation. If significant hyphema occurs during surgery but is cleared with tamponade and irrigation, it is likely to recur in the immediate postoperative period.

Most hyphemas in adult trabeculotomy are self-limited and resolve spontaneously with conservative treatment, such as topical steroids and cycloplegia. However, rarely they can be severe, recurrent, and require surgical removal similar to a traumatic hyphema.[13] (Figure 49.1) See Chapters 5 and 23 for more information about hyphema.

DESCEMET'S MEMBRANE DETACHMENT AND IRIDODIALYSIS

Accidental iridodialysis or Descemet's membrane detachment (Figure 49.2) are common risks of trabeculotomy *ab externo*. The key to preventing these common and potentially troublesome complications is correct surgical technique. When using the classic Harms trabeculotomes, it is critical that the

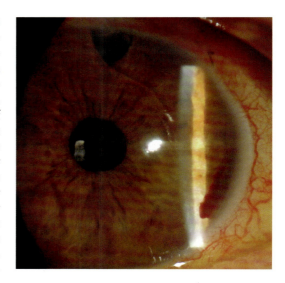

FIGURE 49.1   Blood clot in the anterior chamber after trabeculotomy.

posterior probe is correctly inserted into Schlemm's canal and rotated into the anterior chamber, tearing through the trabecular meshwork. During the breakage into the anterior chamber, the trabeculotome should be parallel to the iris plane in the midchamber. Deepening the anterior chamber with viscoelastic can widen the angle, making more room and a more forgiving space. Other techniques to prevent these problems should include

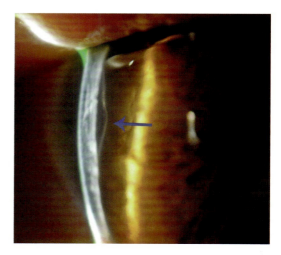

FIGURE 49.2   Descemet's detachment (arrow) after trabeculotomy.

slow rotation and visualization of the probe as it pulls through the trabecular meshwork. Undue traction and movement of the iris root or the start of a Descemet's membrane detachment can usually be avoided by early identification and repositioning of the probe in a more correct position. However, these complications are more likely with a more hyperopic and/or shallow anterior chamber. Small Descemet's membrane detachments in the periphery, which occur in up to 15%[8, 12] of clinical series, do not usually require treatment and resolve spontaneously. However, if a Descemet's membrane detachment impinges upon the visual axis or is large (more than 4–5 clock hours), it needs to be managed by repositioning and partial air tamponade in the anterior chamber with correct head positioning for 24–48 hours to maximize the likelihood for reattachment. Viscoelastic must be evacuated from between Descemet's membrane and the underlying corneal stroma for reattachment to quickly occur. (See Chapter 8 for more information on Descemet's membrane detachment.) A small iridodialysis can also be managed with observation only, but if it is large or visually significant, it may need surgical repair.

Suture- or catheter-guided trabeculotomy techniques probably greatly decrease the likelihood of either of these complications, as a flexible suture or catheter being pulled centrally through the trabecular meshwork likely seeks a path of least resistance through the meshwork from Schlemm's canal in a "self-guiding" fashion. Although these techniques are being currently explored in developmental glaucomas,[14, 15] they could easily be adapted to adult trabeculotomy techniques.

SHALLOW ANTERIOR CHAMBER, TRANSIENT HYPOTONY, PERIPHERAL ANTERIOR SYNECHIAE, BLEB FORMATION

Careful surgical technique and watertight closures in trabeculotomy should be used to prevent subsequent hypotony and flat or shallow anterior chambers. However, hypotonic and shallowing are potential complications, even without unexpected aqueous egress. In published series, rates of these problems are much lower than associated with trabeculectomy, but still occur at 2%–5%.[5–8, 16]

In the early postoperative period following trabeculotomy, reforming the anterior chamber with viscoelastic through a paracentesis is likely to be effective. In trabeculectomy, such maneuvers used in isolation without correcting the underlying overfiltration of aqueous may actually increase the risk of serious complications, such as choroidal effusions and hemorrhage. With trabeculotomy, however, hypotony often is truly transient, as aqueous outflow likely decreases with fibrin formation and tissue proliferation at the level of the collector channels and Schlemm's canal within a few days after surgery. Use of cycloplegics during this period without other contraindications, such as increased likelihood of optic edge capture in combined cases, is indicated. If hypotony extends beyond 2 weeks without an aqueous leak or a bleb formation, a cyclodialysis cleft should be suspected, and careful exploration for one should be done with appropriate treatment. Inadvertent bleb formation, although not the goal of trabeculotomy, can be managed conservatively as long as hypotony and shallowing do not occur. For low IOP, a compression contact lens, compression sutures, or other bleb reduction techniques could be employed, as well as surgical closure. (See Chapter 10 for more information on treating early hypotony.)

Peripheral anterior synechiae (PAS) formation post-trabeculotomy is unusual but does occur in up to 5% of cases[6,8,16]. Shallowing of the anterior chamber postoperatively and significant hyphema are both risk factors. Appropriate cycloplegia postoperatively is preventative, and goniosynechiolysis for significant PAS could be employed once IOP is stabilized, with potential improvement of the ultimate IOP outcomes.[17]

EARLY PERFORATION INTO THE ANTERIOR CHAMBER

Techniques that allow identification and exposure of Schlemm's canal using an external approach are helpful in facilitating adult trabeculotomy and other canal-related techniques. Whether using a one or 2 scleral flap technique, it is important to make the plane of dissection deep enough to see through the sclera to the choroid without unroofing the choroid.

Once Schlemm's canal is unroofed and the trabeculotomes are passed, care must be taken to prevent premature penetration into the anterior chamber. In adults the sclera, the scleral spur, and the trabecular meshwork itself are much less flexible and elastic than in the newborn eye. Whereas Schlemm's canal can be accessed with the trabeculotome via a simple cut down through the sclera without much difficulty in pediatric cases, this type of approach is often very difficult to achieve in the adult eye. Any posterior angulation of the probes in the canal can easily result in premature perforation.

The Japanese literature describes formation of a large (4–5 mm across) and deep (4/5 scleral thickness) flap.[6,8,9,18] At least 3 mm of the canal can then be unroofed, facilitating insertion of the probes. Other techniques, when used alone or in combination, that can decrease the risk of early perforation include the following: 1) using viscoelastic to dilate the canal; 2) dilating the canal with a 5–0 or 6–0 suture; 3) lowering the IOP to minimize compression of the canal; and 4) initiating probe insertion along the posterior, rather than anterior, edge of the canal. If early perforation occurs, it does not necessarily mean that access with the trabeculotome is impossible. In particular, if the lateral edge of the perforation through the meshwork can be identified, further lateral deroofing of the canal can be achieved, and the surgery can proceed as planned. Also if access from one side of the canal cannot be accomplished, access to the other side should proceed. One of the advantages of suture- or catheter-guided access to the canal is that often a large portion of the canal can be accessed while having good anatomical identification of the canal from only one side.

CYCLODIALYSIS, CHOROIDAL HEMORRHAGE AND DETACHMENT, LENS SUBLUXATION, RETINAL DETACHMENT

If Schlemm's canal is incorrectly identified and the trabeculotome is inserted into the suprachoroidal space, rotation into the anterior chamber can result in cyclodialysis, choroidal detachment and/or hemorrhage, lens subluxation, or retinal detachment. Correct placement in the canal with a too posterior rotation can similarly cause these problems. Fortunately, most of these serious complications are easily avoidable by correct identification of a "false passage" into the suprachoroidal space, usually just posterior to the canal. The most obvious indication of incorrect placement is resistance to the passage of the trabeculotomes, suture, or catheter. When correctly placed within the canal, there is usually very little (if any) resistance, and the instruments easily slide into place within the canal up to the connection between the 2 arms of the trabeculotome. Any significant resistance should raise suspicion and an immediate review and exploration of the anatomic landmarks.

Often it is easy to confuse the very anterior edge of the unroofed choroid with a somewhat opaque trabecular meshwork. Signs that the canal has been correctly identified include 1) absence of a small amount of blood backflowing from the cut ends of the canal; 2) the usually transparent and glistening nature of the anterior side of the trabecular meshwork; and 3) visualization. If the dissection has not proceeded anteriorly enough to unroof the canal, these 3 signs will be absent. Additionally, the scleral fibers will lack the radial orientation seen as the scleral spur is dissected posterior to the unroofed canal. If a small area of anterior choroid is exposed during dissection, it usually does not cause any problems if it is recognized and not cannulated. A small area of exposed anterior choroid in these cases does not cause a problem once the canal is correctly identified.

CONCLUSION

Most of the serious complications associated with the different techniques of adult trabeculotomy, except for hyphema, are directly related to problems with surgical technique. Careful attention to detail, anatomic landmarks, and correct positioning of instrumentation during the critical parts of the procedure usually result in a lack of serious problems. As noted in the literature, these techniques in general have associated fewer complications than trabeculectomy. This review of complications of the classic angle surgery forms a background for discussion of newer techniques discussed in subsequent chapters.

COMMENTARY

ROBERT M. FELDMAN

This chapter by Dr. Reynolds and Dr. Fellman is an excellent exploration of potential complications of a surgery rarely performed in adults. The reason this is important is the recent development of new surgeries that utilize trabeculotomy-like techniques. The advantages of accessing Schlemm's canal directly rely on obviating the need for a filtering bleb.

Trabeculotomy is uncommonly performed in adults but has been used in young adults and some uveitics with low levels of inflammation. The complications have never been explored separately but would be expected to be similar to those in children, the most common of which is hyphema. Hyphema is expected during surgery and can be limited by the use of ophthalmic viscoelastic devices prior to opening the trabecular meshwork. Postoperatively, it is not uncommon for synechiae to develop between the iris and Schlemm's canal. These tend to be peaked at areas of collector channel ostia and generally do not result in surgical failure. The early postoperative use of miotics may prevent this. Of course, the most common complication in adults is surgical failure, which is why this procedure has not become common in adults.

One complication Dr. Reynolds did not include is the development of a filtering bleb. These are common especially when creating a wide scleral flap with extensive unroofing of the canal by the techniques developed for some of the newer surgeries (e.g., viscocanalostomy and canaloplasty). Careful closure may prevent this, but full-thickness scleral flap sutures should be avoided as they lead to a passage for aqueous to reach the subconjunctival space. Smaller external access via a slit through sclera under a thin scleral flap is easier to close water-tight and may reduce the likelihood of bleb formation.

To call a bleb a complication may be overzealous on my part; this could be the mechanism by which these procedures lower IOP in adults. Blebs that form may be very low and diffuse making them difficult to identify, but the presence of microcysts in the conjunctiva around the area of scleral entry is a giveaway to transconjunctival filtration.

This chapter should serve as a cautious reminder that the new techniques developed to avoid complications of blebs have their own added difficulties, which can often be predicted from the results of previous generations of surgical techniques.

Dr. Feldman was supported by a Challenge Grant from Research to Prevent Blindness to The University of Texas Medical School at Houston and the Hermann Eye Fund.

REFERENCES

1. Godfrey DG, Fellman RL, Neelakantan A. Canal surgery in adult glaucomas. *Curr Opin Ophthalmol.* Mar 2009;20(2):116–121.
2. Spiegel D, Kobuch K. Trabecular meshwork bypass tube shunt: initial case series. *Br J Ophthalmol.* Nov 2002;86(11):1228–1231.
3. Babighian S, Rapizzi E, Galan A. Efficacy and safety of ab interno excimer laser trabeculotomy in primary open-angle glaucoma: two years of follow-up. *Ophthalmologica.* 2006;220(5):285–290.
4. Wilmsmeyer S, Philippin H, Funk J. Excimer laser trabeculotomy: a new, minimally invasive

procedure for patients with glaucoma. *Graefes Arch Clin Exp Ophthalmol.* Jun 2006; 244(6):670–676.

5. Chihara E, Nishida A, Kodo M, et al. Trabeculotomy ab externo: an alternative treatment in adult patients with primary open-angle glaucoma. *Ophthalmic Surg.* Nov 1993;24(11):735–739.

6. Mizoguchi T, Kuroda S, Terauchi H, Nagata M. Trabeculotomy combined with phacoemulsification and implantation of intraocular lens for primary open-angle glaucoma. *Semin Ophthalmol.* Sept 2001;16(3):162–167.

7. Park M, Hayashi K, Takahashi H, Tanito M, Chihara E. Phaco-viscocanalostomy versus phaco-trabeculotomy: a middle-term study. *J Glaucoma.* Oct 2006;15(5):456–461.

8. Tanihara H, Honjo M, Inatani M, et al. Trabeculotomy combined with phacoemulsification and implantation of an intraocular lens for the treatment of primary open-angle glaucoma and coexisting cataract. *Ophthalmic Surg Lasers.* Oct 1997;28(10):810–817.

9. Tanihara H, Negi A, Akimoto M, et al. Surgical effects of trabeculotomy ab externo on adult eyes with primary open angle glaucoma and pseudoexfoliation syndrome. *Arch Ophthalmol.* Dec 1993;111(12):1653–1661.

10. Gimbel HV, Meyer D. Small incision trabeculotomy combined with phacoemulsification and intraocular lens implantation. *J Cataract Refract Surg.* Jan 1993;19(1):92–96.

11. Gimbel HV, Meyer D, DeBroff BM, Roux CW, Ferensowicz M. Intraocular pressure response to combined phacoemulsification and trabeculotomy ab externo versus phacoemulsification alone in primary open-angle glaucoma. *J Cataract Refract Surg.* Nov 1995; 21(6):653–660.

12. Honjo M, Tanihara H, Negi A, et al. Trabeculotomy ab externo, cataract extraction, and intraocular lens implantation: preliminary report. *J Cataract Refract Surg.* Jun 1996; 22(5):601–606.

13. Tanihara H, Nakayama Y, Honda Y. Intraocular pressure elevation caused by massive and prolonged hemorrhage after trabeculotomy ab externo. *Acta Ophthalmol Scand.* Jun 1995;73(3):281–282.

14. Beck AD, Lynch MG. 360 degrees trabeculotomy for primary congenital glaucoma. *Arch Ophthalmol.* Sept 1995;113(9):1200–1202.

15. Verner-Cole EA, Ortiz S, Bell NP, Feldman RM. Subretinal suture misdirection during 360 degrees suture trabeculotomy. *Am J Ophthalmol.* Feb 2006;141(2):391–392.

16. Luke C, Dietlein TS, Luke M, Konen W, Krieglstein GK. A prospective trial of phaco-trabeculotomy combined with deep sclerectomy versus phaco-trabeculectomy. *Graefes Arch Clin Exp Ophthalmol.* Aug 2008;246(8):1163–1168.

17. Tanito M, Ohira A, Chihara E. Factors leading to reduced intraocular pressure after combined trabeculotomy and cataract surgery. *J Glaucoma.* Feb 2002;11(1):3–9.

18. Tanito M, Ohira A, Chihara E. Surgical outcome of combined trabeculotomy and cataract surgery. *J Glaucoma.* Aug 2001;10(4):302–308.

B. COMPLICATIONS SPECIFICALLY RELATED TO TRABECTOME® SURGERY

50

COMPLICATIONS SPECIFICALLY RELATED TO TRABECTOME® SURGERY (TRABECULOTOMY INTERNAL APPROACH)

BRIAN A. FRANCIS

COMPLICATIONS SPECIFICALLY RELATED TO TRABECTOME® SURGERY (TRABECULOTOMY INTERNAL APPROACH)

Current surgical therapy for open-angle glaucoma can be divided into procedures directed at decreasing aqueous inflow (such as cyclophotocoagulation) or increasing aqueous outflow. The latter group can be further subdivided into external filtering surgery (such as trabeculectomy and aqueous tube shunt implantation) and internal filtering surgery designed to enhance existing aqueous outflow pathways. Internal approaches provide an alternative to standard external filtering surgery and possibly reduce the complications, including hypotony, hypotony maculopathy, bleb leaks, blebitis, choroidal effusion and hemorrhage, bleb-related endophthalmitis, peripheral anterior synechiae (PAS) formation, posterior synechiae, cataract formation,[1-6] diplopia, tube obstruction, conjunctival erosion, tube migration, corneal decompensation, and plate encapsulation.[7-9] Anterior chamber angle surgery techniques include procedures performed by an internal approach (e.g., goniotomy, Trabectome® [NeoMedix Corporation, Tustin, California], trabecular stent [iStent®; Glaukos® Corp., Laguna Hills, California], excimer laser trabeculotomy) or by an external approach (e.g., canaloplasty [see Chapter 51] and viscocanalostomy). Trabeculotomy by internal approach with the Trabectome® is designed to create a direct pathway from the anterior chamber to Schlemm's canal (SC) and the aqueous collector channels by using electrocautery to selectively ablate a portion of trabecular meshwork (TM) tissue and the inner wall of SC in order to increase aqueous outflow.

TRABECTOME® DESIGN AND TECHNIQUE

The Trabectome® surgical device received FDA approval for clinical use in 2004. The system consists of 3 major components: a mobile stand with a gravity-fed bottle of balanced salt solution; a handpiece console with automated irrigation, aspiration, and microbipolar electrocautery; and a foot pedal to control these functions. The intraocular disposable handpiece (see Figure 50.1) tip contains a 19.5-gauge infusion sleeve and a 25-gauge irrigation and aspiration (I/A) port with a coupling for the ablation unit at the tip. The instrument incorporates a specially designed insulated triangular footplate that is bent at 90° at the end and is pointed in order to allow proper insertion through the TM into SC.[10] The insulation on the footplate is made of a multilayered polymer coating that allows the instrument to glide along within the canal and protects the outer wall of SC from thermal and electrical injury. This polymer film has good thermal stability (>500°C), mechanical strength, biocompatibility, and chemical resistance.[11]

The operative technique of Trabectome® surgery begins with the surgeon positioned temporal to the operative eye with the patient's head and microscope tilted to maximize a direct gonioscopic view of the angle. A 1.7-mm temporal clear corneal incision is made parallel to the iris with a keratome.[10,12,13] Preservative-free lidocaine, 1% and viscoelastic may be injected into the anterior chamber. Under direct visualization with a gonioscopy lens, the tip of the Trabectome® handpiece is advanced nasally across the anterior chamber, and the footplate is inserted through the TM into SC.[11] The cautery is activated, and the tip is maneuvered in an arcuate fashion along the angle in a counterclockwise direction to the farthest extent possible (usually 2 clock hours). The tip is then rotated 180 degrees, and the same procedure is repeated in the clockwise direction for a total ablation of approximately 3–4 clock hours. The instrument is then disengaged from the angle and removed from the eye. The viscoelastic material and any blood or cellular debris are aspirated, typically with an automated I/A device or Simcoe handpiece connected to the Trabectome® tubing (Figures 50.2 and 50.3).

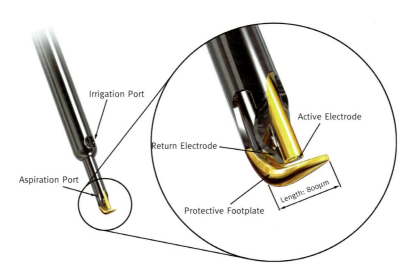

FIGURE 50.1 **Trabectome® handpiece**. The handpiece has irrigation and aspiration ports and active and return electrocautery electrodes. Additionally, there is a guiding footplate for placement of the tip in Schlemm's canal and to protect surrounding structures from thermal damage. Images courtesy of NeoMedix Corporation, Tustin, California. Adapted and reprinted with permission from Reference 14. © Expert Reviews Ltd.

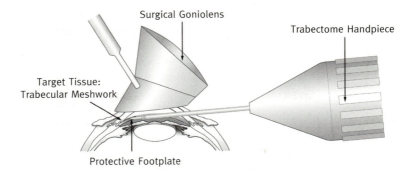

Surgical Goniolens

Trabectome Handpiece

Target Tissue:
Trabecular Meshwork

Protective Footplate

FIGURE 50.2 **Trabectome® procedure schematic**. The surgical goniolens is placed on the cornea, and the Trabectome® handpiece is guided into the anterior chamber via a temporal clear corneal incision. Using direct visualization through the goniolens, the tip is then advanced across the anterior chamber and inserted into Schlemm's canal through trabecular meshwork. Images courtesy of NeoMedix Corporation, Tustin, California. Adapted and reprinted with permission from Reference 14. © Expert Reviews Ltd.

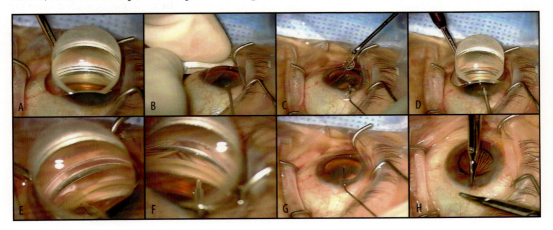

FIGURE 50.3 **Trabectome® procedure**. A) The surgical goniolens is placed on the cornea to confirm the angle view. B) A temporal clear corneal incision is made using the keratome blade. C) Lidocaine 1% preservative-free is flushed into the anterior chamber followed by viscoelastic. D) The handpiece tip is inserted into the anterior chamber, and the goniolens is returned back onto the cornea. E) The tip is inserted into Schlemm's canal through the trabecular meshwork. The electrocautery is activated and the tip rotated counterclockwise. Note the cleft formation to the right of the tip and reflux of blood from Schlemm's canal. F) The handpiece is rotated 180 degrees and ablation continued in a clockwise direction. G) The viscoelastic is removed by irrigation of balanced salt solution or by automated irrigation/aspiration. H) The corneal incision is sutured, and an air bubble is placed if necessary. Images courtesy of NeoMedix Corporation, Tustin, California. Adapted and reprinted with permission from Reference 14. © Expert Reviews Ltd.

INDICATIONS AND CONTRAINDICATIONS FOR TRABECTOME®

Trabeculotomy by internal approach is appropriate in patients with primary open-angle glaucoma, pseudoexfoliation, pigment dispersion, uveitic glaucoma, and possible steroid-induced glaucoma.[3,13] The procedure has also been performed in chronic angle closure glaucoma with lens extraction and goniosynechiolysis. Patients with advanced disease requiring a target intraocular pressure (IOP) in the low teens may not be appropriate candidates as the procedure typically results in an IOP of 15–16 mm Hg with IOP-lowering medications.[10,12–14] Trabectome®

requires a clear gonioscopic view of the angle throughout the procedure and is not possible if the view is blocked by corneal edema, opacities, or other obstructions, such as advanced pterygia. It is also contraindicated in neovascular glaucoma.

INCIDENCE OF TRABECTOME® COMPLICATIONS FROM CLINICAL STUDIES

The first clinical study of the Trabectome® procedure was reported by Minckler et al in 2005.[13] This prospective, interventional case series was a pilot study that evaluated 37 patients with uncontrolled open-angle glaucoma with or without prior ocular surgery or laser treatment. All patients underwent trabeculotomy by Trabectome® with or without viscoelastic, corneal suturing, and air instillation. Every patient experienced an intraoperative event with reflux of blood from SC, with persisting blood in the anterior chamber in 59% of patients (22 patients) on postoperative day one (the most common postoperative complication). On average, it took 6.4 days for the blood to clear. Visual acuity generally decreased in this period as well but recovered to within 2 lines of preoperative visual acuity by 3 weeks. Only one patient, who was not sutured at the time of surgery, had a hyphema at 3 weeks postoperatively after accidental blunt trauma. Other postoperative complications included peripheral anterior synechiae (24.3%; 9 patients), corneal epithelial or endothelial injury (16.2%; 6 patients), goniosynechiae (13.5%; 5 patients), and pressure spike (5.4%; 2 patients). There were no observations of many postoperative complications typically associated with filtration surgery by trabeculectomy, such as flat or shallow anterior chamber, iris injury, hypotony, infection, cataract progression, bleb formation, wound leaks, clinically significant pain, choroidal effusion, or choroidal hemorrhage.[13]

Minckler et al later expanded the pilot study and included 101 total eyes from both Mexico and the United States with extended follow-up of up to 30 months.[10] Postoperative complications included partial goniosynechiae (14%; 14 eyes) and epithelial defects (3%; 3 eyes).

There was one case of postoperative hypotony with IOP of 2 mmHg on postoperative day one. Sixteen eyes with complete IOP-lowering failure required additional surgery.[10]

A prospective, interventional case series of combined Trabectome® and cataract extraction by Francis et al in 2008 included 304 patients with open-angle glaucoma and clinically significant cataracts.[12] Intraoperative complications included blood reflux in approximately 78% (238 patients), iris injury in 4 patients, and lens capsule tear in 2 patients. An IOP spike was noted in 8.6% of patients (26 patients) on postoperative day one and in 2.0% at one week (6 patients).[12]

As of 2009,[14] 1688 eyes had undergone the Trabectome® procedure alone or with combined phacoemulsification cataract extraction. This number includes 1093 eyes with Trabectome® only, 576 eyes with Trabectome® combined with phacoemulsification, 7 eyes with Trabectome® combined with tube shunt (in order to lower IOP in the interim prior to ligature release), 5 eyes with Trabectome® combined with lysis of goniosynechiae, 3 eyes with bleb revision, and 2 eyes each with endoscopic cyclophotocoagulation and penetrating keratoplasty. Prior surgeries included selective laser trabeculoplasty (424 patients), argon laser trabeculoplasty (275 patients), trabeculectomy (133 patients), aqueous tube shunt (28 patients), Trabectome® (8 patients), and endoscopic cyclophotocoagulation (7 patients). The total number of secondary glaucoma procedures following failed Trabectome® was 162 (9.6%). Complications included 96 eyes (5.7%) with IOP elevation of greater than 10 mm Hg from baseline, 24 eyes (1.4%) with hypotony (IOP < 5 mm Hg) on postoperative day one, iris injury in 5 eyes (0.3%), corneal Descemet's membrane tear in 4 eyes (0.2%), aqueous misdirection (intraoperative, resolved) in one eye (0.06%), and choroidal hemorrhage in one eye (0.06%).[14]

COMPLICATIONS AND THEIR PREVENTION OR TREATMENT

Intraoperative complications

Anterior chamber bleeding. By far the most common intraoperative complication is anterior chamber bleeding,[10,12,13,15] estimated to occur in greater than 70% of all Trabectome® procedures. By removing the TM and opening SC, the collector channels are exposed to the anterior chamber, and reflux of blood from the aqueous veins is quite common. Vasoconstriction preoperatively with topical apraclonidine or brimonidine may reduce or prevent this complication. Additionally, preservative-free epinephrine can be flushed into the anterior chamber intraoperatively. Regardless whether blood is seen at the end of the ablation, a complete I/A should always be performed. For a standalone procedure, I/A should be performed with the Simcoe I/A attached to the Trabectome® tubing. During I/A, the goniolens can be used to check for further bleeding. If bleeding persists, the irrigation should be continued, and an air tamponade can be injected into the anterior chamber. Hypotony may lead to further blood reflux, so suturing the incision is generally recommended. See Chapter 5 for further information about management of intraoperative hyphema.

Surgical view. At times, the surgical view can be compromised, most commonly by corneal striae. The most common cause is compression with the goniolens or torque applied at the wound edges by the Trabectome® handpiece. To avoid the former, the goniolens should be resting on the cornea without any downward compression. A coupling solution, such as methylcellulose, may be useful for facilitating positioning of the goniolens. OcuCoat® viscoelastic (Bausch & Lomb, Inc., Rochester, New York; included in the surgical kit) also works well. The surgical technique should minimize torque at the wound entrance, with the incision used as a fulcrum to turn the instrument in an arc rather than move it side-to-side.

In a small minority of cases, there is iris obstructing the view when the pupil is widely dilated. This is more common with Trabectome® combined with phacoemulsification cataract extraction. Iris blocking the view is usually caused by fluid from the irrigation port of the handpiece diverting underneath the iris and billowing the handpiece anteriorly. In most cases, simply advancing the tip of the handpiece all the way to the angle will bring the irrigation port peripheral to the pupillary edge and cause the fluid to push the iris posteriorly. If this does not work, then the handpiece should be rotated so that the fluid is redirected anterior to the iris. Injection of cholinergic agonists to constrict the pupil or placement of viscoelastic in the peripheral angle can also treat this problem, but either of these requires removal of the handpiece.

Locating the TM. To aid in locating the TM, preoperative gonioscopy with attention to the nasal angle and identification of landmarks is critical. The angle view should again be verified with the surgical goniolens prior to the incision. Once an incision has been made, and even after the eye has been pressurized with viscoelastic, there is often visible blood reflux into SC, which makes targeting the TM in patients with little angle pigmentation easier (Figure 50.4). Pigmented TM is very easy to identify, but one must be careful to not mistake a pigmented Schwalbe's line for TM in patients with heavy angle pigmentation.

Narrow angle. If the angle is too narrow, the procedure is not possible. To deepen the angle, preoperative application of topical pilocarpine, 1% can sometimes help by pulling peripheral iris away from the angle. The use of viscoelastic is also helpful, but the irrigation from the console is usually sufficient to deepen the angle simply by raising the balanced salt solution bottle height. However, if

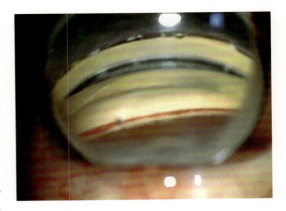

FIGURE 50.4 **Blood reflux into Schlemm's canal.** This may help in identifying the trabecular meshwork in patients with little pigmentation. Image courtesy of NeoMedix Corporation, Tustin, California.

the corneal incision is too large, the anterior chamber will not be stable and will shallow. In these instances, it is preferable to suture the incision and make a separate incision with the keratotomy blade.

Iris prolapse. The best treatment of iris prolapse is prevention with proper wound construction. This is most important in phakic patients with a shallow anterior chamber. For these patients, I recommend making a slightly beveled anterior incision rather than a single plane incision. If iris prolapse still occurs, then a small, self-sealing paracentesis is recommended with decompression of the anterior chamber and instillation of viscoelastic.

Corneal endothelial or Descemet's membrane damage. Corneal endothelial or Descemet's membrane damage[10,13] is rarely encountered if using the same precautions as would be taken with any intraoperative procedure. When entering the corneal incision, the Trabectome® tip should be angled to the side, parallel to the incision to prevent the edge of the tip from catching Descemet's membrane. While advancing the tip across the anterior chamber, the tip should be held close to the iris surface and away from the endothelium. When the handpiece tip is rotated in the middle of the procedure, the surgeon should bring the tip into the center of the eye or over the midperipheral iris. Once removal of the TM is complete, remnants of TM or other tissue on either side of the cleft often remain. The surgeon should avoid trying to remove these, as there is often a connection to the corneal endothelium anteriorly or the iris root posteriorly.

Corneal epithelial damage usually occurs due to the edge of the surgical goniolens rubbing the cornea near the temporal entrance site. Topical application of methylcellulose is helpful for prevention, as is avoiding indentation of the cornea with the lens. Even if damage occurs, it rarely compromises the procedure, but removal of sloughing epithelial tissue may become necessary.

Lens damage. Lens damage[12] is possible in phakic patients with a shallow anterior chamber. Pilocarpine, 1% or an intracameral miotic is recommended preoperatively or intraoperatively to reduce lens exposure. The highest risk for lens damage comes during the insertion of the Trabectome® tip into the anterior chamber. Thus, instillation of viscoelastic to deepen the anterior chamber (at least temporally at the incision site) is useful to prevent lens damage. Once the irrigation port is inside the anterior chamber, the iris and lens are pushed posteriorly and out of the way. If significant damage to the lens occurs, phacoemulsification can be performed after the Trabectome® procedure or concurrently if lens implant calculations are available.

Iris damage and cyclodialysis cleft. Iris damage[12] may occur during insertion of the handpiece or during tissue ablation. In the former case, the same precautions to prevent lens damage are used. During TM ablation, it is possible to cause iris damage, such as by an iris tear or iridodialysis. Damage usually occurs when the tip slips out of SC during the ablation process, and the sharp edge of the tip hits the iris. The Trabectome® tip is designed to stay within SC during the treatment and act as a guide, but may slip out, especially at the extreme extension of the arc. Thus, the surgeon should treat the tissue that is readily available and avoid extending too far laterally. If iris bleeding occurs, raising the bottle height or inserting viscoelastic can form a tamponade and wash out the anterior chamber. At the end of the procedure, irrigation and aspiration is carried out for a longer period than usual and air instilled if necessary. A small iridodialysis does not need treatment, but one greater than 2 clock hours should probably be repaired. Repair can be accomplished by suturing the iris with a double-armed 10–0 polypropylene on 2 straight needles passed across the anterior chamber (via the temporal wound), through the detached peripheral iris, into the iris insertion point behind the scleral spur, and out the sclera.[16–18] A preplaced scleral flap may assist burying the knot.[19] A radial iris defect can be repaired using a McCannel suture technique.[20,21]

Similarly, a cyclodialysis cleft due to trauma from the instrument is a possible, but quite rare, complication of Trabectome®. It is treated in the same manner as any other traumatic cyclodialysis. If the area is small, then conservative management with cycloplegia can be employed. Laser-assisted closure of the cleft at a later date can be performed if hypotony persists. Finally, a large cyclodialysis can be primarily closed with a suture reattachment of the ciliary body to the sclera[22–24] in a manner similar to that described above for an iridodialysis.

Overtreatment/undertreatment. Overtreatment during ablation can occur if the power level is set too high or the tip is advanced too slowly. Either way, charring of tissue can be seen in the TM remnants adjacent to the cleft. The resulting tissue damage may increase the risk of anterior synechiae formation and cleft closure but is thought not to cause damage to the outer wall of SC and collector channels due to the thermal protective properties of the coating on the handpiece tip.[11,14] Conversely, undertreatment results from moving the tip too quickly and/ or if the power setting is too low. A sign that not enough tissue is removed is if the resulting TM cleft is too narrow.

Aqueous misdirection. There has been one report of aqueous misdirection occurring intraoperatively[14] during Trabectome® with axial shallowing of the anterior chamber. The etiology is unknown and probably similar to its occurrence after other glaucoma surgeries. The one reported case resolved spontaneously during the procedure with continued irrigation and aspiration. Persistent aqueous misdirection would require aborting the surgery and returning to the operating room at a later date for a different procedure.

Postoperative complications

Hyphema. Due to the reflux of blood from the opened SC, a small hyphema is common during the immediate postoperative period and can take the form of a small amount of clotted blood at the nasal cleft site, a layered hyphema, or suspended red blood cells in the aqueous. The management is conservative, with topical steroids and IOP lowering as needed. A dense cloud of suspended red blood cells (not a layered hyphema) in the anterior chamber can decrease vision dramatically, but

hyphemas usually clear within one week without further sequelae.[13] A total hyphema has not yet been reported, but is theoretically possible and should be treated in the same manner as a traumatic hyphema. Treatment would include medical therapy and possibly surgery, such as anterior chamber washout or tissue plasminogen activator injection into the anterior chamber.[25–27] (See Chapter 23 for further information on postoperative hyphema.)

Late onset of blood in the anterior chamber. Rarely, late onset of blood may appear in the anterior chamber. This is thought to be related to an increase in episceral venous pressure (such as from Valsalva maneuver or bending) or from hypotony following the intraocular surgery. Because the trabecular meshwork has been removed as a barrier to aqueous flow to the collector channels, it is possible that blood from the aqueous veins can reflux into the eye. This is usually self-limited, and observational conservative management is usually all that is required. However, if the hyphema is recalcitrant, anterior chamber washout or even closure of the Trabectome® cleft may become indicated. To close the cleft, the posterior flap of the remaining TM along with some iris root can be treated with the argon laser to form peripheral anterior synechiae, much like the tepees that form after argon laser trabeculoplasty performed too posteriorly.

IOP spike. A significant IOP spike is possible after Trabectome® surgery[10,12] and should be divided into those occurring immediately after surgery (postoperative day one) versus short term (at one week). The former is probably related to retained viscoelastic, blood, or inflammatory cells in the anterior chamber and is usually self-limited and treatable medically. Rarely, this complication may require anterior chamber paracentesis, anterior chamber washout, or even trabeculectomy.

A later onset elevation in IOP (after a few weeks) is believed to be due to a *steroid response.*[14] The majority are relieved by using glaucoma medications and switching to a less potent corticosteroid, such as loteprednol, 0.5% or fluorometholone, 0.1%, along with lowering the frequency of administration and a rapid taper. While not common, a steroid-related rise in IOP is seen more frequently with Trabectome® than with external filtering surgery.

Hypotony. Hypotony[10,12] is rarely seen because IOP should not be able to decrease below episcleral venous pressure, and when it does occur, it is self-limited. Hypotony in the immediate postoperative period generally resolves within one week. A possible mechanism is a decrease of aqueous production due to inflammation of the ciliary body. Hypotony will resolve with continuation of topical steroids as per the usual postoperative protocol without requiring aggressive steroid use or cycloplegia. One must also check for a wound leak as a possible cause, and if present, the temporal incision should be resutured.

Anterior synechiae and cleft closure. The formation of anterior synechiae and closure of the cleft are possible complications leading to eventual failure of the procedure. Although pilocarpine use is helpful postoperatively to keep the cleft open,[13] longer term use may contribute to synechiae.[28] Once present, adhesions are difficult to treat except by repeat Trabectome® surgery with lysis of synechiae. The Nd:YAG laser can be used to open newly formed synechiae but may damage the collector channels and result in a less favorable outcome.

Loss of IOP control. Loss of IOP control can be due to several causes. The first is closure of the cleft with iris synechiae, as described above. The second is formation of a membrane occluding the TM cleft, which generally occurs weeks after the procedure. This membrane has not been histologically proven or studied, but there are anecdotal reports of its occurrence. Some surgeons have noted that failure of IOP lowering with an apparently open cleft can be retreated with the Trabectome®. During surgery, reflux of blood from SC and relaxation of the edges of the cleft have been noted just as if a membrane had been removed, reestablishing communication between the anterior chamber and SC. I have also noted the gonioscopic appearance of pigment *over* the cleft (not in the cleft) in patients with failed IOP control and hypothesize that this pigment has been deposited on the surface of such a membrane. Attempts to open the cleft with Nd:YAG laser have been unsuccessful in lowering IOP. Repeat Trabectome®, however, has had variable success in these cases. The final explanation for failure of the procedure is that the post-SC outflow pathway provides too much resistance. It is theorized that a chronic lack of aqueous outflow due to disease, previous TM obstruction, or IOP-lowering treatment with medications has resulted in collapse and closure of the post-SC outflow pathway. Unfortunately, there currently is no way to predict this preoperatively, but the presence of blood in SC on gonioscopy, especially with a Goldmann-3 mirror lens that compresses peripheral to the limbus, may indicate at least that there is still communication between SC and the aqueous veins.

CONCLUSION

Ab interno trabeculotomy with the Trabectome® is a surgical technique to remove a segment of the TM and inner layer of SC to increase aqueous outflow for the management of open-angle glaucoma. It provides a decrease in IOP adequate to reduce the need for glaucoma medications and may have fewer severe complications than trabeculectomy or aqueous tube shunt surgery. Those complications that do arise can usually be avoided or successfully treated with preoperative management, intraoperative technique, and diligent postoperative care.

Dr. Francis is a consultant for the NeoMedix Corporation, the maker of Trabectome®.

COMMENTARY

ROBERT N. WEINREB

Perhaps the most important goal of glaucoma surgery is to preserve or enhance vision by lowering IOP. However, one needs to be mindful of not making the patient worse by damaging their vision or causing other untoward effects such as hypotony maculopathy, suprachoroidal hemorrhage, and bleb-related complications. I view Trabectome® surgery as a procedure that offers an alternative to trabeculectomy and tube shunt surgery for optimizing the trade-offs among maximizing pressure lowering, minimizing risks (short- and long-term), and rapid rehabilitation. In my practice, it is most commonly employed with patients who have a target IOP of 16 mm Hg or more, the usual pressure outcome of the procedure. These patients typically have mild to moderate, but not severe, glaucoma and are administering 2 or more ocular hypotensive medications. It is particularly useful for patients undergoing combined cataract and glaucoma surgery. I routinely place patients on topical pilocarpine (1% for blue and 2% for brown irides) 4 times daily postoperatively and have found that this enhances the amount and duration of the pressure-lowering effect. Some patients tolerate the pilocarpine so well that they are maintained on it even after the immediate postoperative period.

The outcomes of Trabectome® surgery can likely be improved by better understanding TM biology. In my experience, Trabectome® surgery is successful in achieving target IOP only one-half of the time. Being able to predict success in an individual patient and achieving a successful outcome in a larger number of patients clearly are desirable. Moreover, it is not clear why postoperative pressure typically is higher than presumed episcleral venous pressure in most patients. Despite these unanswered questions, Trabectome® surgery unquestionably has a place in our repertoire of glaucoma surgical procedures.

Dr. Weinreb was supported by an Unrestricted Grant from Research to Prevent Blindness to the University of California at San Diego.

COMMENTARY

L. JAY KATZ

As with any new procedure, the Trabectome® may lead to new and unforeseen complications. With the removal of the tissue between SC and the reduction of the IOP below episcleral venous pressure, a "backflow" hyphema is commonly seen intraoperatively. It may also be seen with situations of elevated episcleral venous pressure postoperatively, such as bending over.

Although the procedure may reduce the risk of profound hypotony postoperatively, with all the attendant potential complications patients undergoing Trabectome® surgery are also at risk for IOP spikes with retained viscoelastic and steroid response. One should note that patients with a low starting IOP rarely benefit from this procedure and typically lower the IOP to a level around 16–18 mm Hg[29]; additionally, most of the preoperative glaucoma medications continue to be used after surgery.[30] If the patient needs a low target IOP or is nonadherent or intolerant of glaucoma medications, then Trabectome® *ab interno* trabeculotomy may not be a suitable operative choice.

Trabectome® use requires specific skills to properly perform the *ab interno* trabeculotomy. Intraoperative gonioscopy with a goniolens used with the operating microscope and clear knowledge of the angle anatomy are essential. Otherwise problems such as an inadvertent cyclodialysis cleft, iridodialysis, and corneal injury may occur.

REFERENCES

1. Bindlish R, Condon GP, Schlosser JD, D'Antonio J, Lauer KB, Lehrer R. Efficacy and safety of mitomycin-C in primary trabeculectomy: five-year follow-up. *Ophthalmology.* Jul 2002; 109(7):1336–1341; discussion 1341–1332.

2. DeBry PW, Perkins TW, Heatley G, Kaufman P, Brumback LC. Incidence of late-onset bleb-related complications following trabeculectomy with mitomycin. *Arch Ophthalmol.* Mar 2002; 120(3):297–300.

3. Filippopoulos T, Rhee DJ. Novel surgical procedures in glaucoma: advances in penetrating glaucoma surgery. *Curr Opin Ophthalmol.* Mar 2008;19(2):149–154.

4. Kobayashi H, Kobayashi K, Okinami S. A comparison of the intraocular pressure-lowering effect and safety of viscocanalostomy and trabeculectomy with mitomycin C in bilateral

open-angle glaucoma. *Graefes Arch Clin Exp Ophthalmol.* May 2003;241(5):359–366.

5. Soltau JB, Rothman RF, Budenz DL, et al. Risk factors for glaucoma filtering bleb infections. *Arch Ophthalmol.* Mar 2000;118(3):338–342.

6. Song A, Scott IU, Flynn HW Jr., Budenz DL. Delayed-onset bleb-associated endophthalmitis: clinical features and visual acuity outcomes. *Ophthalmology.* May 2002;109(5):985–991.

7. Gedde SJ, Herndon LW, Brandt JD, Budenz DL, Feuer WJ, Schiffman JC. Surgical complications in the Tube Versus Trabeculectomy Study during the first year of follow-up. *Am J Ophthalmol.* Jan 2007;143(1):23–31.

8. Guerrero AH, Latina MA. Complications of glaucoma drainage implant surgery. *Int Ophthalmol Clin.* Winter 2000;40(1):149–163.

9. Souza C, Tran DH, Loman J, Law SK, Coleman AL, Caprioli J. Long-term outcomes of Ahmed™ glaucoma valve implantation in refractory glaucomas. *Am J Ophthalmol.* Dec 2007;144(6):893–900.

10. Minckler D, Baerveldt G, Ramirez MA, et al. Clinical results with the Trabectome®, a novel surgical device for treatment of open-angle glaucoma. *Trans Am Ophthalmol Soc.* 2006;104:40–50.

11. Francis BA, See RF, Rao NA, Minckler DS, Baerveldt G. Ab interno trabeculectomy: development of a novel device (Trabectome®) and surgery for open-angle glaucoma. *J Glaucoma.* Feb 2006;15(1):68–73.

12. Francis BA, Minckler D, Dustin L, et al. Combined cataract extraction and trabeculotomy by the internal approach for coexisting cataract and open-angle glaucoma: initial results. *J Cataract Refract Surg.* Jul 2008;34(7):1096–1103.

13. Minckler DS, Baerveldt G, Alfaro MR, Francis BA. Clinical results with the Trabectome® for treatment of open-angle glaucoma. *Ophthalmology.* Jun 2005;112(6):962–967.

14. Liu J, Jung J, Francis BA. Ab interno trabeculectomy: Trabectome° surgical treatment for open-angle glaucoma. *Expert Review of Ophthalmology.* 2009;4(2):119–128.

15. Minckler D, Mosaed S, Dustin L, Ms BF. Trabectome® (trabeculectomy-internal approach): additional experience and extended follow-up. *Trans Am Ophthalmol Soc.* 2008;106:149–159; discussion 159–160.

16. Bardak Y, Ozerturk Y, Durmus M, Mensiz E, Aytuluner E. Closed chamber iridodialysis repair using a needle with a distal hole. *J Cataract Refract Surg.* Feb 2000;26(2):173–176.

17. Kaufman SC, Insler MS. Surgical repair of a traumatic iridodialysis. *Ophthalmic Surg Lasers.* Nov 1996;27(11):963–966.

18. Wachler BB, Krueger RR. Double-armed McCannell suture for repair of traumatic iridodialysis. *Am J Ophthalmol.* Jul 1996;122(1):109–110.

19. Kervick GN, Johnston SS. Repair of inferior iridodialysis using a partial-thickness scleral flap. *Ophthalmic Surg.* Jun 1991;22(6):354–355.

20. Shin DH. Repair of sector iris coloboma. Closed-chamber technique. *Arch Ophthalmol.* Mar 1982;100(3):460–461.

21. McCannel MA. A retrievable suture idea for anterior uveal problems. *Ophthalmic Surg.* Summer 1976;7(2):98–103.

22. Aminlari A. Inadvertent cyclodialysis cleft. *Ophthalmic Surg.* May 1993;24(5):331–335.

23. Aminlari A, Callahan CE. Medical, laser, and surgical management of inadvertent cyclodialysis cleft with hypotony. *Arch Ophthalmol.* Mar 2004;122(3):399–404.

24. Ioannidis AS, Barton K. Cyclodialysis cleft: causes and repair. *Curr Opin Ophthalmol.* Mar;21(2):150–154.

25. Kim MH, Koo TH, Sah WJ, Chung SM. Treatment of total hyphema with relatively low-dose tissue plasminogen activator. *Ophthalmic Surg Lasers.* Sept 1998;29(9):762–766.

26. Starck T, Hopp L, Held KS, Marouf LM, Yee RW. Low-dose intraocular tissue plasminogen activator treatment for traumatic total hyphema, postcataract, and penetrating keratoplasty fibrinous membranes. *J Cataract Refract Surg.* Mar 1995;21(2):219–224.

27. Williams DF, Han DP, Abrams GW. Rebleeding in experimental traumatic hyphema treated with intraocular tissue plasminogen activator. *Arch Ophthalmol.* Feb 1990;108(2):264–266.

28. Phillips CI, Clark CV, Levy AM. Posterior synechiae after glaucoma operations: aggravation by shallow anterior chamber and pilocarpine. *Br J Ophthalmol.* Jun 1987;71(6):428–432.

29. Vold, SD and the Trabectome® Study Group. Impact of Preoperative IOP on Trabectome Outcomes. *Clin Surg Ophthalmol.* 2010;28:11.

30. Mosaed S, Rhee DJ, Filippopoulos T, Tseng H, Deokule S, Weinreb RN. Trabectome® Outcomes in Adult Open Angle Patients—One Year Follow-up. *Clin Surg Ophthalmol.* 2010;28:8.

C. COMPLICATIONS SPECIFICALLY
RELATED TO CANALOPLASTY SURGERY

51

COMPLICATIONS SPECIFICALLY RELATED TO CANALOPLASTY SURGERY

RICHARD A. LEWIS

COMPLICATIONS SPECIFICALLY RELATED TO CANALOPLASTY SURGERY

Canaloplasty is a surgical approach for patients with open-angle glaucoma. The objective of the procedure is to enhance circumferential outflow of aqueous from Schlemm's canal to the collector system, improving outflow without creating a filtering bleb. In the procedure, a microcatheter is threaded into the canal using a standard nonpenetrating approach and then passed for 360 degrees. A polypropylene suture is attached to the catheter. The catheter is then retracted 360 degrees during which time viscodilation is performed. The suture remains in the canal, and the ends of the suture are tied together to place constant tension upon the trabecular meshwork (TM). Theoretically, the tension results in opening of the TM, improving outflow and lowering intraocular pressure (IOP). The procedure has

increased in popularity and may be a valuable option for patients with open-angle glaucoma who might be at high risk for filtering surgery complications, such as contact lens wearers, patients on blood thinners, and those patients who already failed filtering surgery in the other eye.

With the increased popularity of canaloplasty, knowing how to prevent and manage complications of this procedure are crucial skills for today's glaucoma surgeon.

CANALOPLASTY PROCEDURE

The notion of enhancing circumferential outflow arose from studies of an earlier nonpenetrating procedure, viscocanalostomy (see Chapter 52). In this procedure, a Descemet's membrane window is created under a scleral flap, and the outflow system is dilated with viscoelastic for 1–2 clock hours.[1] However, in canaloplasty, 360-degree viscodilation is performed, and a tensioning suture is left in Schlemm's canal to promote canal distension and aqueous outflow. Passing the microcatheter and completing a successful canaloplasty requires specific steps and careful attention to detail. The procedure may be performed under local, regional, or general anesthesia. Fixation of the globe is the first step, using either a corneal or rectus suture. Then, a half-thickness, 4 mm limbus-based scleral flap is created, followed by a deeper scleral flap, which unroofs the canal. The dissection is then taken forward onto Descemet's membrane to allow for creation of a Descemet's window, and the deep flap is excised. Schlemm's canal is next catheterized 360 degrees. As the illuminated microcatheter tip arises out the other end of Schlemm's canal, a 9–0 or 10–0 polypropylene suture is attached. The catheter is then gradually withdrawn back through the canal while viscoelastic is injected from the catheter into the canal. The polypropylene suture is left in the canal and tied to itself such that circumferential tension is placed on the TM. The superficial flap is tightly closed to avoid leakage, and the conjunctiva is sutured back to the limbus.[2]

INTRAOPERATIVE COMPLICATIONS

Creation of the scleral flaps is critical to the success of the surgery. If the dissection of the superficial flap is too thin, there is risk of causing a buttonhole. If the superficial flap is too thick, there is risk of perforation into the anterior or posterior chamber. Creating a deep flap in nonpenetrating surgery demands a clear understanding of the anterior segment anatomy. The deep flap's incision should start at the apex of the initial incision just over the ciliary body. The most common error is to dissect a deep flap that is too shallow, thereby passing directly over the canal without unroofing it. As you dissect forward toward the limbal gray zone and near the scleral spur, watch for the subtle change in the scleral texture. The "crossing scleral fibers" in this area are a useful dissection endpoint. Perforating into the anterior segment can be avoided by making a paracentesis to decompress the eye, thereby avoiding outward bulging of Descemet's

membrane. If a small perforation arises, you may be able to continue with the dissection. A large perforation will require converting to a standard trabeculectomy.

If the canal has been unroofed, threading the catheter is not difficult. On occasion, passage of the catheter through the canal can be blocked. This may be due to an incomplete Schlemm's canal, a scar in Schlemm's canal (as may happen from argon laser trabeculoplasty) or more likely the catheter hitting the opening of a collector channel. The first approach when this occurs is to inject viscoelastic through the catheter. The dilatory/lubricating effect usually facilitates passage. If dilation fails, gentle external pressure can be applied over the site of the stoppage (as indicated by the light beacon). Another option is to withdraw the catheter and pass it the opposite direction. It is important to avoid "forcing" the catheter as doing so may cause a tear in the trabecular meshwork through which the catheter may enter the anterior chamber.

The next step where complications may occur (although rarely) is during tying of the polypropylene suture (tensioning the trabecular meshwork). With ultrasound biomicroscopy (UBM), the amount of tension is noted as "distension."[2, 3] At this step, the suture may break while it is being tied, which is fixed by replacing the suture. Some surgeons place 2 sutures in the canal. The second serves as a "just-in-case" reserve and can be removed after the initial suture is appropriately tied.

Additionally, a detachment of Descemet's membrane may occur, which may be hemorrhagic.[3–6] With or without blood, Descemet's membrane detachments tend to occur 180 degrees away from the suture knot. Descemet's membrane detachments typically remain peripheral and are transient, self-limited complications that do not require intervention. (For more about Descemet's membrane detachment, see Chapter 8.)

Tight closure of the superficial scleral flap is necessary or a bleb will form. A thin superficial flap may also result in a bleb despite tight closure due to transscleral flow. The fornix-based conjunctival incision should be anchored back to the limbus in case there is aqueous flow out. The sutures from this closure tend to be a cause of postoperative irritation, but to my knowledge, endophthalmitis has not been reported after canaloplasty thus far.

POSTOPERATIVE COMPLICATIONS

One of the benefits of canaloplasty (and perhaps all nonpenetrating surgery) is the ease of care in the postoperative period. When compared to a trabeculectomy, canaloplasty appears to have fewer complications.[2,3,5] Other than occasional complaints of irritation from the incision and conjunctival closure, pain is uncommon. Anterior chamber reaction is generally limited.

However, early postoperative visual acuity may be reduced[2–5] if there is any closure-induced astigmatism or blood in the anterior chamber. Additionally, reflux bleeding in and around Schlemm's canal is not uncommon.[3,6] Gross hyphema occurs in less than 10% of cases[2,3,5,6] and usually resolves in 1–2 weeks. Persistent hyphema is rare but is a concern in patients on blood thinners. Hypotony has been reported in the early postoperative period but is uncommon.[2,4,5] If persistent hypotony is noted, it is important to examine for a wound leak or cyclodialysis cleft.

Elevated IOP may be noted in the first 1–2 weeks postoperatively, probably from retained viscoelastic,[2,3] but is usually transient and seldom requires anything more than medical treatment. If the IOP remains elevated, it is important to determine the cause. Gonioscopy is valuable for visualizing the location of the canal suture and morphology of the angle. UBM imaging is also helpful and should reveal a dilated scleral lake where the deep flap was excised near the site of the incision.[7] If the IOP remains elevated after surgery despite a well-placed suture and obvious scleral lake, hypotensive medications may be required. Other options for an uncontrolled IOP after canaloplasty include an Nd:YAG laser goniopuncture into the area of the scleral lake. If the IOP is uncontrolled despite these maneuvers, additional glaucoma surgery may be necessary.

There have been cases of late migration of the suture into the anterior chamber.[5] It can generally be left there without sequelae, but the long-term outcome remains unknown.

CONCLUSION

To date complications from canaloplasty have been few and can generally be managed without vision loss. However, long-term sequelae of canaloplasty are currently unknown. With its growing popularity, knowing how to prevent and manage complications from the procedure is important to prevent glaucoma progression and other unwanted outcomes.

COMMENTARY
STEVEN D. VOLD

In my clinical experience, postoperative hyphema is the most common complication following canaloplasty. Fortunately, hyphema is usually preventable and gradually resolves over a period of a few weeks without further surgical intervention. However, hyphema can slow visual recovery and potentially adversely impact postoperative outcomes due to increased scarring in the aqueous collector system. Prevention of hyphema is important. Although not necessarily mandatory, avoiding anticoagulants in the early perioperative period may be beneficial. Pressurizing the anterior chamber with balanced salt solution at the conclusion of surgery appears to be quite effective in preventing postoperative hyphema. If hyphema persists after 6 weeks or IOP control becomes problematic, anterior chamber washout should be considered.

High-quality scleral flap dissections are key to achieving good canaloplasty results. If the superficial scleral flap is amputated, moving to a different surgical location is recommended. If the deep scleral flap is too superficial, Schlemm's canal will not be unroofed. In this situation, deeper dissection to a scleral level just anterior to the choroid is required. Decompression of the anterior chamber assists in maintaining a soft eye that prevents perforation of the trabeculo-Descemet's window during this maneuver. Once the proper surgical plane is achieved and Schlemm's canal is unroofed, gentle dissection of the scleral flap is performed anteriorly. The scleral and corneal tissue typically separates easily from Descemet's membrane.

Early postoperative steroid-induced IOP elevation is more common following nonpenetrating glaucoma procedures than after filtration surgery. By using loteprednol (Lotemax, Bausch & Lomb, Rochester, New York) rather than prednisolone acetate postoperatively, surgeons can largely eliminate this potential complication. When postoperative IOP rises occur related to possible early canaloplasty failure, Nd:YAG laser treatment to the Descemet's window may effectively reduce IOP by essentially converting canaloplasty into a filtration-type procedure. When utilizing this approach, conscientious technique should be employed to avoid lysing the properly tensioned polypropylene suture in Schlemm's canal. Another potential method to manage a failing canaloplasty is to remove the polypropylene suture in Schlemm's canal from an *ab interno* approach in the operating room, essentially performing a 360-degree trabeculotomy. Trabeculectomy with an antifibrotic agent and tube shunt surgery are viable surgical alternatives in this setting as well.

COMMENTARY

ALAN S. CRANDALL

Many of the complications of canaloplasty are similar to the other nonpenetrating procedures; however, one can also see hyphema in multiple areas secondary to the viscodilation that is done 360 degrees. This does not normally require a surgical removal but can induce more inflammation postoperatively and can also cause a pressure spike that may need treatment. One unique area of concern with this procedure is related to the use of the polypropylene suture that is within Schlemm's canal. If the tension is too high, it can lead to tearing of the internal wall (goniotomy-like). The suture must be removed, and the procedure will likely fail, so one may need to convert this to a trabeculectomy.

Dr. Crandall was supported by an Unrestricted Grant from Research to Prevent Blindness to the University of Utah.

REFERENCES

1. Stegmann R, Pienaar A, Miller D. Viscocanalostomy for open-angle glaucoma in black African patients. *J Cataract Refract Surg.* Mar 1999;25(3):316–322.

2. Lewis RA, von Wolff K, Tetz M, et al. Canaloplasty: circumferential viscodilation and tensioning of Schlemm's canal using a flexible microcatheter for the treatment of open-angle glaucoma in adults: interim clinical study analysis. *J Cataract Refract Surg.* Jul 2007;33(7):1217–1226.

3. Shingleton B, Tetz M, Korber N. Circumferential viscodilation and tensioning of Schlemm canal (canaloplasty) with temporal clear corneal phacoemulsification cataract surgery for open-angle glaucoma and visually significant cataract: one-year results. *J Cataract Refract Surg.* Mar 2008;34(3):433–440.

4. Cameron B, Field M, Field M, Ball S, Kearney J. Circumferential viscodilation of Schlemm's canal with a flexible microcannula during non-penetrating glaucoma surgery. *Digit J Ophthalmol.* 2006;12(1). http://www.djo.harvard.edu/site.php?url=/physicians/oa/929. Accessed August 23, 2010.

5. Lewis RA, von Wolff K, Tetz M, et al. Canaloplasty: circumferential viscodilation and tensioning of Schlemm canal using a flexible microcatheter for the treatment of open-angle glaucoma in adults: two-year interim clinical study results. *J Cataract Refract Surg.* May 2009;35(5):814–824.

6. Grieshaber MC, Fraenkl S, Schoetzau A, Flammer J, Orgul S. Circumferential viscocanalostomy and suture canal distension (canaloplasty) for whites with open-angle glaucoma. *J Glaucoma.* Jun–Jul 2011;20(5):298–302.

7. Godfrey DG, Fellman RL, Neelakantan A. Canal surgery in adult glaucomas. *Curr Opin Ophthalmol.* Mar 2009;20(2):116–121.

PART SIX

NONPENETRATING SURGERY COMPLICATIONS

A. COMPLICATIONS COMMON TO NONPENETRATING SURGERIES

52

COMPLICATIONS COMMON TO NONPENETRATING SURGERIES

ANDREW C. CRICHTON

COMPLICATIONS COMMON TO NONPENETRATING SURGERIES

Nonpenetrating glaucoma surgery encompasses techniques that involve a deep dissection to the level of Descemet's membrane, allowing aqueous seepage. The major techniques covered by the term "nonpenetrating surgery" are deep sclerectomy with or without implant and viscocanalostomy. In large meta-analyses comparing nonpenetrating procedures to trabeculectomy, trabeculectomy resulted in lower intraocular pressures (IOP) but a higher risk of postoperative complications.[1,2] Although nonpenetrating surgery is successful in lowering IOP, the amount of IOP lowering is typically not as low as can be achieved with trabeculectomy. Consequently, patient selection with regard to the target IOP is important in the decision of whether or not to perform a nonpenetrating procedure.

The goal of nonpenetrating procedures is to lower IOP with fewer complications than are seen with trabeculectomy. The complications that can occur can be easily understood and predicted by an understanding of the techniques and modifications, as well as knowledge and mechanisms of the adjustments that can be used postoperatively to enhance success.

TECHNIQUE

After appropriate anesthetic, the techniques involve a deep dissection in the sclera to the limbus. In the case of deep sclerectomy, after the initial half-thickness flap is fashioned, a second deeper flap is created and excised. This dissection is taken to the level of Descemet's membrane, allowing controlled flow of aqueous. A fine forceps may be used to strip the outer wall of Schlemm's canal, further enhancing the flow. The space created by the excision can then be filled with an implant, such as collagen[3,4] (AquaFlow™ Collagen Glaucoma Drainage Device; STAAR® Surgical Company, Monrovia,

California) or hyaluronate (SK Gel®; Corneal Laboratories, Paris, France).[5,6] For viscocanalostomy, Schlemm's canal is identified and dilated by using viscoelastic.[7] With deep sclerectomy, intraoperative or postoperative antimetabolites may be used to try to increase success rates by limiting the inflammatory response.[8,9] Goniopuncture to the Descemet's window is often required postoperatively (in up to 67% of cases) to enhance flow and lower IOP.[10–13]

COMPLICATIONS

The available evidence on complications of nonpenetrating glaucoma surgery is relatively sparse and may be challenging to interpret. Comparative studies between trabeculectomy and nonpenetrating surgery would seem to show fewer complications in the nonpenetrating group. [14,15] However, these results were not supported in another study in which antimetabolites were used for many cases.[16] It is well accepted that nonpenetrating procedures are more difficult to perform, and training is marked by a significant learning curve.[17–20] Complication rates may therefore be expected to decrease as the surgeon becomes more skilled.[15,21] Supplementary procedures such as goniopuncture or needling are very individualized by surgeon experience and clinical situations, making success and complication rate comparisons difficult.

Complications follow logically from the sequence of steps. The major issues involve perforation of the Descemet's window, iris incarceration, hypotony, and inadequate IOP control. If antimetabolites (especially mitomycin-C) and goniopuncture are used to aim for low IOPs, all the bleb-related issues associated with trabeculectomy can occur.

Perforation

Intraoperative perforation of the Descemet's window has been reported to occur in up to 11.9% of cases,[6,18,21–24] with the occurrence higher during the learning curve phase.[17,21] Intraoperative perforation can occur at any time but is most likely to happen as the limbus is approached. If the perforation occurs posteriorly over the ciliary body, the procedure

can be continued as usual but with the flap directed more superficially. However, if the perforation occurs anteriorly with significant aqueous egress or if the hole is large with iris prolapse, the procedure should be converted to a trabeculectomy. Unfortunately, the trabeculectomy will now have a more posterior sclerostomy, possibly with a less than optimal result. In this case, tight closure of the superficial scleral flap should be performed to prevent iris incarceration or prolapse, or even vitreous prolapse. Although the procedure is no longer nonpenetrating and may have a higher rate of complications than a planned trabeculectomy, it can still be successful.[18,19] The perforation may also occur when the deeper flap is excised. Once the deep flap has been excised, it is difficult to achieve tight closure. Early overfiltration is likely, along with hypotony and hyphema.[18] As perforations are more frequent while the surgeon is becoming familiar with the techniques,[21] it is probably best to avoid mitomycin-C during the learning curve. Once the surgical techniques are mastered, and use of mitomycin-C is employed, the complication rates may be similar with or without antifibrotics but with better pressure lowering in the mitomycin-C group.[9]

Iris incarceration

Iris coming through a perforated Descemet's window during surgery is best handled by converting to a trabeculectomy with iridectomy; otherwise iris incarceration is likely. In the case of delayed incarceration, immediate intervention is required before scarring irreversibly attaches the iris to the sclerostomy. Delayed incarceration may occur spontaneously but more often is precipitated by goniopuncture.[24] Some authors suggest delaying goniopuncture until at least 3 weeks postoperatively to prevent hypotony or incarceration.[25,26] Aggressive goniopuncture with a high pressure[27] may predispose to incarceration. Even without goniopuncture, however, a delayed spontaneous incarceration (possible spontaneous perforation of Descemet's window) can occur, possibly due to trauma or eye rubbing.[28]

Pilocarpine and iridoplasty near the site of incarceration may pull the iris tissue centrally out of the perforation in Descemet's window. Additionally, an iridotomy should be performed adjacent to the perforation to reduce the likelihood of recurrence. If the incarceration cannot be released, surgical removal either through the initial surgical site or via a paracentesis is indicated. If revision is via the original surgical site, the procedure is essentially converted into a trabeculectomy.

Case 1. A 60-year-old female with thyroid ophthalmopathy underwent an uneventful implantation of an AquaFlow™ Collagen Glaucoma Drainage Device (also known as the collagen wick) with a resulting IOP of 8 mm Hg on the first postoperative day. Goniopuncture was performed 7 weeks postoperatively. Two weeks later, iris incarceration (Figure 52.1) was noted and subsequently relieved initially by laser iridotomy and laser to the synechiae. She was maintained on pilocarpine after recurrence of incarceration.

Case 2. A 65-year-old pseudophakic, previously highly myopic patient with glaucomatous visual field loss encroaching on fixation underwent nonpenetrating surgery with an AquaFlow™ Collagen Glaucoma Drainage Device. He had a microperforation at the time of surgery without iris prolapse. The day one postoperative pressure was 10 mm Hg. On the second day postoperatively, he sneezed and had iris incarceration (Figure 52.2). The iris remained incarcerated despite attempts at intervention, but IOP has been acceptable on medication.

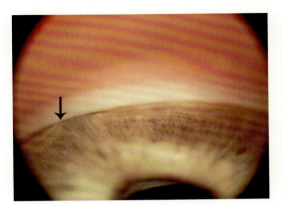

FIGURE 52.2 Iris incarceration (arrow) at site of microperforation of Descemet's window.

Hypotony

A study by Lim et al on cadaver eyes has shown that even without stripping the outer wall of Schlemm's canal, the IOP can be reduced to 5 mm Hg.[29] If the membrane is stripped, the IOP can be as low as 2 mm Hg. Therefore, even with a perfect surgery, all the usual hypotony-related complications, such as choroidal swelling and hemorrhage, can occur. (See Chapters 10, 21, 34, and 39 for more information about hypotony.) Of course, as mentioned previously, hypotony is even more likely to happen if perforation is encountered.

Hyphema

Hyphema may occur with or without visible perforation. The hyphema may occur from outside through a microperforation that was not noticed during surgery or from abnormal vessels inside the eye. Most are small or microscopic. The risk factors for hyphema without perforation are unknown but presumed to be abnormal vessels on the iris or angle, which bleed during decompression required for Descemet's window creation. See Chapter 23 for more information on hyphemas.

Descemet's membrane detachment

Another less frequent complication that may be seen with nonpenetrating surgery is Descemet's membrane detachment (Figure 52.3), with both

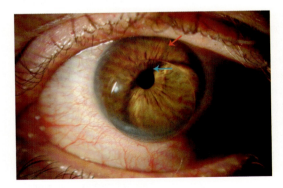

FIGURE 52.1 Iris incarceration 2 weeks after goniopuncture. Red arrow: slight tenting. Blue arrow: slight peaking of pupil.

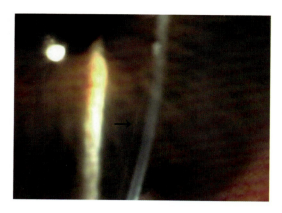

FIGURE 52.3 Focal Descemet's detachment after nonpenetrating surgery (arrow). Photo courtesy of Paul Harasymowycz, MD

intraocular tamponade by air is typically successful. For delayed detachment, as is more often seen in deep sclerectomy, IOP lowering and air tamponade should be helpful as well. Occasionally perfluoropropane (C_3F_8) or sulfur hexafluoride (SF_6) gas may be needed and, if unsuccessful in restoring normal corneal anatomy, fixation sutures may be required to reattach the membrane to the corneal stroma. See Chapter 8 for more information on Descemet's membrane detachment.

CONCLUSION

As with any surgical procedure, adverse events can and do occur. Although the literature may be conflicting, nonpenetrating surgery seems to be associated with fewer complications than trabeculectomy at the expense of less successful pressure lowering. However, with the use of antimetabolites and timely goniopuncture, pressure lowering comparable to trabeculectomy is possible. Avoiding mitomycin-C during the learning curve of the procedure and cautious approaches to goniopuncture (i.e., less power, smaller hole) may minimize many of the early learning curve related complications. Awareness of potential complications is the best way to avoid them.

deep sclerectomy and viscocanalostomy.[30-32] The detachments reported extended from the surgical site. With viscocanalostomy, the problem is usually detected early and may be caused by forceful injection of viscoelastic that regurgitates from the ostia of Schlemm's canal into the supra-Descemet's space.[30,31]

Treatment should be directed at the underlying cause and should be initiated promptly. In cases of immediate detachment, a Descemet's membrane incision with

COMMENTARY
E. RANDY CRAVEN

After Cairns first described a method for trabeculectomy,[33] he wanted to focus on aqueous getting into the normal outflow system, so he sought to avoid transscleral flow by describing a clear cornea trabeculectomy.[34] Since then, we have looked for the perfect way to get aqueous flowing. We peel off the outer wall of Schlemm's canal to get flow through the trabecular meshwork, ooze through Descemet's membrane by creating large "windows," create microperforation (or macroperforation) of these tissues to increase aqueous flow, create posterior windows or channels to get aqueous into the supraciliary space, and we put antimetabolites over the area to allow for a bleb (if we feel we need it) for pressure control. All in search of the best method to achieve a safe procedure with great IOP control.

Observations from the era when the clear-cornea trabeculectomy was described showed that the results were not as good as seen with scleral-incision trabeculectomy.[35] The IOP benefit from transscleral flow seemed to give us a clue over 25 years ago that we had better results when blebs were present. But we didn't want blebs. Success with using the conventional outflow system (Schlemm's canal and the collector channels) can happen, but not with the same IOP-lowering success as when you have transscleral flow or successful supraciliary and suprachoroidal flow. Now we have begun to modify many of the "nonpenetrating procedures" to allow for safety first with the procedure, then to increase the transscleral flow and allow for some bleb formation. With each modification of a deep sclerectomy, viscocanalostomy, nonpenetrating technique with sutures (canaloplasty), windows, and wicks, we will still have some need for the "escape" option for opening up the flow to "convert" the nonpenetrating procedure into a more full-thickness procedure. Perhaps the complications we see reported in this chapter, such as iris incarceration and overfiltration, will become less problematic as we learn how to plan ahead for conversions to avoid the problems.

COMMENTARY

ALAN S. CRANDALL

The chapter is well written and gives a logical approach to complications of nonpenetrating glaucoma surgery, both intraoperative and postoperative. However, another approach that one may need to use in the case of a large posterior penetration is to abandon the scleral incision, tightly close it, and find another spot.

Dr. Crandall was supported by an Unrestricted Grant from Research to Prevent Blindness to the University of Utah.

REFERENCES

1. Chai C, Loon SC. Meta-analysis of Viscocanalostomy Versus Trabeculectomy in Uncontrolled Glaucoma. *J Glaucoma*. Oct–Nov 2010;19(8):519–-527.

2. Cheng JW, Xi GL, Wei RL, Cai JP, Li Y. Efficacy and tolerability of nonpenetrating filtering surgery in the treatment of open-angle glaucoma: a meta-analysis. *Ophthalmologica*. 2010;224(3): 138–146.

3. Shaarawy T, Mermoud A. Deep sclerectomy in one eye vs deep sclerectomy with collagen implant in the contralateral eye of the same patient: long-term follow-up. *Eye (Lond)*. Mar 2005;19(3):298–302.

4. Shaarawy T, Nguyen C, Schnyder C, Mermoud A. Comparative study between deep sclerectomy with and without collagen implant: long term follow up. *Br J Ophthalmol*. Jan 2004;88(1):95–98.

5. Russo V, Scott IU, Stella A, et al. Nonpenetrating deep sclerectomy with reticulated hyaluronic acid implant versus punch trabeculectomy: a prospective clinical trial. *Eur J Ophthalmol*. Sept-Oct 2008;18(5):751–757.

6. Galassi F, Giambene B. Deep sclerectomy with SkGel® implant: 5-year results. *J Glaucoma*. Jan-Feb 2008;17(1):52–56.

7. Stegmann R, Pienaar A, Miller D. Viscocanalostomy for open-angle glaucoma in black African patients. *J Cataract Refract Surg*. Mar 1999;25(3):316–322.

8. Anand N, Atherley C. Deep sclerectomy augmented with mitomycin C. *Eye (Lond)*. Apr 2005;19(4):442–450.

9. Kozobolis VP, Christodoulakis EV, Tzanakis N, Zacharopoulos I, Pallikaris IG. Primary deep sclerectomy versus primary deep sclerectomy with the use of mitomycin C in primary open-angle glaucoma. *J Glaucoma*. Aug 2002;11(4):287–293.

10. Anand N, Pilling R. Nd:YAG laser goniopuncture after deep sclerectomy: outcomes. *Acta Ophthalmol*. Feb 2010;88(1):110–115.

11. Alp MN, Yarangumeli A, Koz OG, Kural G. Nd:YAG laser goniopuncture in viscocanalostomy: penetration in non-penetrating glaucoma surgery. *Int Ophthalmol*. Jun 2010;30(3): 245–252.

12. Bissig A, Rivier D, Zaninetti M, Shaarawy T, Mermoud A, Roy S. Ten years follow-up after deep sclerectomy with collagen implant. *J Glaucoma*. Dec 2008;17(8):680–686.

13. Wishart PK, Wishart MS, Choudhary A, Grierson I. Long-term results of viscocanalostomy in pseudoexfoliative and primary open angle glaucoma. *Clin Experiment Ophthalmol*. Mar 2008;36(2):148–155.

14. Chiselita D. Non-penetrating deep sclerectomy versus trabeculectomy in primary open-angle glaucoma surgery. *Eye (Lond)*. Apr 2001;15(Pt 2): 197–201.

15. Wang N, Wu H, Ye T, Chen X, Zeng M, Fan Z. [Analysis of intra-operative and early post-operative complications and safety in

non-penetrating trabecular surgery]. *Zhonghua Yan Ke Za Zhi.* Jun 2002;38(6):329–334.

16. Detry-Morel M, Pourjavan S, Detry MB. Comparative safety profile between "modern" trabeculectomy and non-penetrationg deep sclerectomy. *Bull Soc Belge Ophtalmol.* 2006(300):43–54.

17. Shaarawy T, Karlen M, Schnyder C, Achache F, Sanchez E, Mermoud A. Five-year results of deep sclerectomy with collagen implant. *J Cataract Refract Surg.* Nov 2001;27(11):1770–1778.

18. Sanchez E, Schnyder CC, Mermoud A. [Comparative results of deep sclerectomy transformed to trabeculectomy and classical trabeculectomy]. *Klin Monbl Augenheilkd.* May 1997;210(5):261–264.

19. Cabarga-Nozal C, Arnalich-Montiel F, Fernandez-Buenaga R, Hurtado-Cena FJ, Munoz-Negrete FJ. Comparison between phaco-deep sclerectomy and phaco-deep sclerectomy reconverted into phaco-trabeculectomy: series of fellow eyes. *Graefes Arch Clin Exp Ophthalmol.* May 2010;248(5):703–708.

20. Dahan E, Drusedau MU. Nonpenetrating filtration surgery for glaucoma: control by surgery only. *J Cataract Refract Surg.* May 2000; 26(5):695–701.

21. Carassa RG, Bettin P, Fiori M, Brancato R. Viscocanalostomy versus trabeculectomy in white adults affected by open-angle glaucoma: a 2-year randomized, controlled trial. *Ophthalmology.* May 2003;110(5):882–887.

22. Rebolleda G, Munoz-Negrete FJ. Phacoemulsification-deep sclerotomy converted to phacotrabeculectomy. *J Cataract Refract Surg.* Jul 2004;30(7):1597–1598.

23. Rebolleda G, Munoz-Negrete FJ. Comparison between phaco-deep sclerectomy converted into phaco-trabeculectomy and uneventful phaco-deep sclerectomy. *Eur J Ophthalmol.* May–Jun 2005;15(3):343–346.

24. Anand N, Kumar A, Gupta A. Primary phakic deep sclerectomy augmented with Mitomycin C: long-term outcomes. *J Glaucoma.* Jan 2011;20(1): 21–27.

25. Karlen ME, Sanchez E, Schnyder CC, Sickenberg M, Mermoud A. Deep sclerectomy with collagen implant: medium term results. *Br J Ophthalmol.* Jan 1999;83(1):6–11.

26. Mermoud A, Karlen ME, Schnyder CC, et al. Nd:Yag goniopuncture after deep sclerectomy with collagen implant. *Ophthalmic Surg Lasers.* Feb 1999;30(2):120–125.

27. Kim CY, Hong YJ, Seong GJ, Koh HJ, Kim SS. Iris synechia after laser goniopuncture in a patient having deep sclerectomy with a collagen implant. *J Cataract Refract Surg.* May 2002;28(5):900–902.

28. Li SN, Wang NL. Unusual ultrasound biomicroscopy appearance after non-penetrating trabecular surgery with SK Gel® implant. *Eye (Lond).* Dec 2006;20(12):1470–1471.

29. Lim KS, Sourdille P, Khaw PT. Intraocular pressure changes during experimental deep sclerectomy [ARVO abstract 437]. *Invest Ophthalmol Vis Sci.* 2000;41(4):S83.

30. Luke C, Dietlein T, Jacobi P, Konen W, Krieglstein GK. Intracorneal inclusion of high-molecular-weight sodium hyaluronate following detachment of Descemet's membrane during viscocanalostomy. *Cornea.* Jul 2000;19(4):556–557.

31. Ravinet E, Tritten JJ, Roy S, et al. Descemet membrane detachment after nonpenetrating filtering surgery. *J Glaucoma.* Jun 2002;11(3): 244–252.

32. Unlu K, Aksunger A. Descemet membrane detachment after viscocanalostomy. *Am J Ophthalmol.* Dec 2000;130(6):833–834.

33. Cairns JE. Trabeculectomy. Preliminary report of a new method. *Am J Ophthalmol.* Oct 1968; 66(4):673–679.

34. Cairns JE. Clear cornea trabeculectomy. *Trans Ophthalmol Soc UK.* 1975;104:142–145.

35. Keillor RB, Molteno AC. Twenty-two cases of clear cornea trabeculectomy. *Aus NZ J Ophthalmol.* Nov 1986;14(4):339–342.

INDEX

Antiinflammatories
  in preventing ptosis, 204
  and wound healing, 34
Antimetabolites
  adjusting amounts, 183
  caution during intraoperative use, 49
  and managing wound leaks, 86
  proper placement on sclera, 176
  and wound healing, 34
Antiplatelet therapy
  in elderly patients, 53
  reducing prior to surgery, 55
Antivascular endothelial growth factor, 35–37, 54
Aphakic patients
  and anticipating vitreous prolapse, 253
  and preventing hemorrhagic choroidal complications, 68–69
APT
  See Antiplatelet therapy
Aqueous hyposecretion, and hypotony, 172–173
Aqueous misdirection
  algorithm for surgical management, 95
  causal factors, 97
  diagnosis, 93–94
  encountered during Trabectome® surgery, 383
  risk factors, 93
  treatment, 94–97, 97, 98
Aqueous outflow
  after trabeculectomy, 5, 6
  after tube shunt surgery, 5, 6–7
  characteristics of normal outflow, 13–14
  mechanism of deep sclerectomy to restore, 22
  mechanism of trabeculotomy to restore, 16
  normal pathways, 14
  using Trabectome® surgery to improve, 19–20
Aqueous suppressants, 94
Argon laser
  for correcting underfiltration, 101–102
  to repair conjunctival buttonholes, 50–51
Astigmatic shift, 114
Astigmatism
  and corneal drying, 159
  following filtering surgery, 139, 140
  induced, 211
Atropine, preventing and managing hyptony, 86
Autoimmune disorders and scleral thinning, 78
Autologous blood injection
  and managing bleb leaks, 87
  to treat overfiltration, 173
Axial length changes, 315–319
  addressing with patients, 318
  after trabeculectomy and tube shunt implantation, 315–317, 316
  axial length shallowing, 93
  impact of, 317

B

Baerveldt, George, 19
Baik, Annie K., 100–106
Band keratopathy, 139
Banitt, Michael R., 74, 257, 267–275, 300, 339–340
Barkan, Otto, 14
Barnes, Catherine, xi
Bar-Sela, Shai, 156–161
Bell, Nicholas P., 85–91, 152, 236, 359–363, ix–x, viii
Bevacizumab
  and decreasing bleb vascularity, 102
  and other new wound healing modulators, 35–36
  reducing risk of early postoperative hyphema, 54

Biovascular, Inc., 33
Bleb failure
  late bleb failure, 123–127
    low, underfiltering bleb, 124
    preventing and managing, 123–124, 125
    risk factors for, 123
Bleb formation after trabeculotomy in adults, 371
Blebitis and bleb-related endophthalmitis, 162–164, 192–201
  blebitis, 196
  causative agents, 195
  clinical diagnosis, 194, 196, 198, 199
  organisms causing, 194
  outcomes, 198
  prevention and treatment, 196–198, 199
  risk factors for, 192–194
    antifibrotic usage, 193
    bleb leaks, 192–193
    bleb location, 194
    postoperative antibiotics, 194
    thin conjunctiva, 193–194
Bleb leaks
  and endophthalmitis, 192–193
  and hypotony, 172
  late bleb leaks, 128–135
    bleb leak revised by conjunctival advancement, 130
    characteristics favoring early intervention, 130
    etiology and risk factors, 128–129
    prevention, 129, 132–133, 133–134
    thin-walled avascular bleb, 129
    treatment, 129–131, 132–133, 133–134
  prevention and management, 86–87, 215–217
  Seidel-positive leak, 196
  treating, 199
Bleb morphology and managing hyptony, 86
Bleb needling and revision, 225–229
  advantages of, 228–229
  and antimetabolites, 226
  to correct postoperative fibrosis, 105
  expected complications, 226
  to revive a failing bleb, 124
  setting and anesthesia technique, 225–226
  surgical complications *not* unique to needle revision, 226–227
  surgical complications unique to needle revision, 227–228
Bleb-related infections, 217–218
Bleb-related vision loss, 156–161
  causes, 156, 158, 159, 160
  and low-lying blebs, 160
  management, 157–159
Blebs
  after nonpenetrating glaucoma surgery, 22–23
  aqueous outflow, 6
  bleb location, 194
  bubble formation over elevated bleb, 148
  characteristics of successful blebs, 123
  dysesthetic blebs, 143–155
    etiology of, 143–146
    images of, 144
    prevention of, 146–147
    proposed pathway of formation, 145
    risk factors for, 146
    treatment, 147–151, 152, 153
    types of, 148
  encapsulation *vs.* pathologic encysted bleb, 283
  encysted blebs, 283–288
    etiology, 283–284
    identifying, 284

Uveitic glaucoma and tube shunt implantation, 262
Uveitis, 162–170
    after tube shunt surgery, 346
    blebitis and bleb-related endophthalmitis, 162–164
    and early excessive iritis, 108
    noninfectious causes, 164–166
    treating, 167, 168
    varying severity of, 167

V

Vascular endothelial growth factor (VEGF), 102
Villarrubia, Hector J., 85–91
Viscocanalostomy
    histologic changes of Schlemm's canal, 24
    overview of, 20–23
    schematic of, 23
Viscoelastic
    caution during use to prevent Descemet's membrane detachment, 72
    injections to manage hypotony, 270
    and management of scleral flap complications, 80
    to prevent choroidal hemorrhage, 63, 64
    preventing intraoperative hyphema, 54
    preventing obstruction with, 104
    to repair conjunctival buttonholes, 49, 50
    treating Descemet's membrane detachment, 73, 74
    use in preventing vitreous prolapse, 69
    see also viscocanalostomy
Visual axis opacities after filtering surgery, 137–140
Visual loss
    after trabeculectomy, 113–120
    after tube shunt surgery, 309–314
        anterior segment complications, 310
        common causes of, 310

hypotony, 310–311
incidence of, 309–310
measures to prevent, 312–313
posterior segment complications, 310–312
Vitrectomy, 96, 197–198
Vitreous complications after tube shunt surgery, 350–354
Vitreous hemorrhage and retinal complications, 353
Vitreous prolapse, 67–69, 68–69, 253–257
    anticipating, 253–255
    managing, 255–257
Vitreo-zonuloido-vitrectomy
    schematic of, 96
Vold, Steven D., 293, 295–302, 391–392

W

Wand, Martin, 133–134
Wang, Nan, 336–341
Weinreb, Robert N., 384–385
Whitson, Jess T., 309–314
Wollan, Peter T., 187–191
Wound healing, 33–41
    and antiinflammatories, 34
    commonly used modulators, 34–35
    new modulators, 35–37
    three phases of, 33
Wound leaks
    fornix-based conjunctival flaps vs. limbus-based, 86
    vs. aqueous misdirection syndrome, 94
Wu, Huijuan, 13–30
Wudunn, Darrell, 5–9

Z

Zonulo-hyaloido-vitrectomy, 96